SALE

DATE: 12/03/01

Diagnosis and Management of Disorders of the Spinal Cord

Diagnosis and Management of Disorders of the Spinal Cord

Robert R. Young, M.D.
Professor and Vice Chairman
Department of Neurology
University of California, Irvine
College of Medicine
Irvine, California

Robert M. Woolsey, M.D.
Professor of Neurology
St. Louis University School of Medicine
Chief, Spinal Cord Injury Service
St. Louis Veterans Affairs Medical Center
St. Louis, Missouri

W.B. SAUNDERS COMPANY
A Division of Harcourt Brace & Company
Philadelphia London Toronto Montreal Sydney Tokyo

W.B. SAUNDERS COMPANY
A Division of
Harcourt Brace & Company

The Curtis Center
Independence Square West
Philadelphia, PA 19106

Library of Congress Cataloging-in-Publication Data

Diagnosis and management of disorders of the spinal cord / [edited by]
  Robert R. Young, Robert M. Woolsey.—1st ed.

      p.   cm.

    ISBN 0–7216–5447–9

    1. Spinal cord—Diseases.   I. Young, Robert R.
II. Woolsey, Robert M.
    [DNLM: 1. Spinal Cord Diseases—diagnosis.   2. Spinal Cord
Diseases—therapy.   3. Spinal Cord Injuries—diagnosis.   4. Spinal
Cord Injuries—therapy.   WL 400 D536 1995]

RC400.D49 1995   617.4′82—dc20

DNLM/DLC   94–30370

Diagnosis and Management of Disorders
of the Spinal Cord

ISBN 0–7216–5447–9

Some material in this work appeared in NEUROLOGIC CLINICS, Volume 9, Number 3, August
1991, copyright © 1991 by W.B. Saunders Company. All rights reserved.

Printed in the United States of America.

Last digit is the print number: 9   8   7   6   5   4   3   2   1

Preface

In 1991, we edited an issue of *Neurologic Clinics* on Disorders of the Spinal Cord. At that time, except for Sir Ludwig Guttman's monumental treatise on spinal cord injuries (and several smaller books on spinal trauma), no book on spinal cord disorders was available. We wanted our issue of *Neurologic Clinics* to be comprehensive and to emphasize management of the many problems associated with paraplegia and quadriplegia. Although we used the maximal number of pages allowed for an issue of *Neurologic Clinics* and used a reduced print size, we could only accommodate about half of the material that we thought should be included in a complete account of spinal cord medicine.

The aforementioned issue was well received by the readership and was reviewed favorably. A number of our colleagues in the spinal cord disorders field encouraged us to produce a monograph that would include the topics that space constraints had excluded from the *Neurologic Clinics* issue. Since publication of the issue, several excellent books on spinal cord disorders have appeared; however, they deal mainly with diagnosis and clinical features of the disorders and do not address management issues. It therefore seemed worthwhile to share our long experience, and that of many of our expert associates, in treating problems regularly associated with paraplegia and quadriplegia.

This book includes most of the material previously produced in the *Neurologic Clinics* issue on Disorders of the Spinal Cord. The authorship of several chapters has changed, and the authors of other original chapters have updated the contents where appropriate. In addition, ten new chapters have been added.

This book begins with reviews of spinal cord anatomy, physiology, and pathology to serve as a resource for authors of other chapters and to therefore avoid inclusion of this background information in their chapters, which would likely result in repetition, fragmentation, and incompleteness.

The clinical section of this book commences with three chapters that succinctly review the various disorders of the spinal cord in such a way that typical and important features are highlighted. Each chapter includes a selected bibliography to refer readers who require more detailed information to appropriate sources.

Following these six introductory chapters, the editors summarize what is known about the pathophysiology of spinal cord symptoms and physical findings and suggest a method of analysis that should facilitate a fairly simple and accurate diagnosis of the 30 or so clinical entities that affect the spinal cord.

Four chapters deal with imaging and electrophysiological techniques that, when appropriately used, can extend and validate clinical analysis.

The remaining 15 chapters deal with the management of problems regularly encountered in patients with spinal cord disorders, a few of which are rarely, if ever, encountered in patients with other neurological disorders.

Obviously, the value of a book of this type depends on the expertise and communication skills of the contributing authors. On perusing the table of contents, the reader will immediately recognize the eminence of the contributors, many of whom have themselves written books on the spinal cord. It is a privilege and pleasure to work with this outstanding group.

Though we have spent most of our careers managing patients with spinal cord disorders, and have tried to utilize this experience to produce a monograph that is succinct and useful, we are well aware that there is always room for improvement. We would be grateful for critiques and suggestions that might improve future editions of this book.

ROBERT R. YOUNG, M.D.
ROBERT M. WOOLSEY, M.D.

Contributors

Raymond D. Adams, M.D., D.Sc.
Chief (Emeritus), Neurology Service, Massachusetts General Hospital; Bullard Professor of Neuropathology, Harvard University Medical School; Director (Emeritus), E. K. Shriver Center, Boston, Massachusetts.
Chronic Nontraumatic Diseases of the Spinal Cord

Michael J. Aminoff, M.D., F.R.C.P.
Professor of Neurology, University of California School of Medicine; Director, Clinical Neurophysiology Laboratories, University of California Medical Center, San Francisco, California.
Segmentally Specific Somatosensory Evoked Potentials

Roy Ashford, M.D.
Rancho Los Amigos Medical Center, Downey, California.
Orthopedic Complications of Spinal Cord Disease

William E. Bradley, M.D.
Clinical Professor of Neurology and Urology, University of Washington Medical Center, Seattle, Washington.
The Urinary Bladder in Spinal Cord Disease

Thomas N. Byrne, M.D.
Clinical Professor of Neurology and Medicine, Yale University School of Medicine; Assistant Chief, Department of Neurology, Yale–New Haven Hospital, New Haven, Connecticut.
Spinal Cord Compression

Keith H. Chiappa, M.D.
Associate Professor, Department of Neurology, Harvard Medical School; Director, EEG/EP Laboratory, Massachusetts General Hospital, Boston, Massachusetts.
Motor and Somatosensory Evoked Potentials in Spinal Cord Disorders

George R. Cybulski, M.D.
Assistant Professor of Neurological Surgery, Department of Surgery, Northwestern University Medical School, Chicago, Illinois.
Spinal Cord Injury

Robert A. Davidoff, M.D.
Professor of Neurology, Molecular and Cellular Pharmacology, Physiology, and Biophysics, University of Miami School of Medicine; Chief, Neurology

Service, Director, Neurophysiology Laboratory, Veterans Affairs Medical
Center, Miami, Florida.
Some Observations on Spinal Cord Structure and Reflex Function

David M. Dawson, M.D.

Professor, Department of Neurology, Harvard Medical School, Boston;
Chief, Neurology Service, Brockton/West Roxbury Veterans Affairs Medical
Center, West Roxbury, Massachusetts.
Acute Nontraumatic Myelopathies

Donna Ferraro, M.D.

Physiatrist, Kessler Institute for Rehabilitation—West Orange Facility, West
Orange, New Jersey.
Rehabilitation in Patients with Spinal Cord Disorders

Manish Fozdar, M.D.

Clinical Fellow, Harvard Medical School; Fellow, Consultation-Liaison
Psychiatry, Brigham and Women's Hospital, West Roxbury Veterans Affairs
Medical Center, Boston, Massachusetts.
Psychiatric Aspects of Spinal Cord Injury

Jack O. Greenberg, M.D.

Professor of Neurology, Medical College of Pennsylvania; Medical Director,
Health Images of Philadelphia, Philadelphia, Pennsylvania.
Neuroimaging of the Spinal Cord

Michael H. Haak, M.D.

Fellow, Spine Injury Center, McGaw Medical Center, Northwestern University, Chicago, Illinois.
Spinal Cord Injury

John C. Hackman, Ph.D.

Associate Professor of Neurology and Molecular and Cellular Pharmacology, University of Miami School of Medicine; Research Physiologist and
Director, Spinal Cord Pharmacology Laboratory, Veterans Affairs Medical
Center, Miami, Florida.
Some Observations on Spinal Cord Structure and Reflex Function

Vincent R. Hentz, M.D.

Professor of Functional Restoration (Hand Surgery), Stanford University
School of Medicine, Stanford; Staff Surgeon, Palo Alto Veterans Affairs
Medical Center, Palo Alto, California.
Functional Restoration of the Upper Extremity in Tetraplegia

J. Trevor Hughes, M.D., F.R.C.Path., F.R.C.P.

Department of Neuropathology, Radcliffe Infirmary, Oxford, England.
Neuropathology of the Spinal Cord

Amie B. Jackson, M.D.

Assistant Professor, University of Alabama at Birmingham, Birmingham,
Alabama. Medical Director, Spain Rehabilitation Center, Interim Chairman,
Department of Rehabilitation Medicine, University of Alabama at Birmingham, Birmingham, Alabama.
Neurogenic Urinary Tract Infection

Lynette Kiers, M.B.B.S., F.R.A.C.P.

Clinical Instructor, University of Melbourne; Neurologist and Clinical Neurophysiologist, Clinical Neuroscience Centre, Royal Melbourne Hospital, Victoria, Australia.
Motor and Somatosensory Evoked Potentials in Spinal Cord Disorders

Amy L. Ladd, M.D.

Assistant Professor of Functional Restoration (Hand Surgery), Stanford University School of Medicine, Stanford; Staff Physician, Palo Alto Veterans Administration Medical Center, Palo Alto, California.
Functional Restoration of the Upper Extremity in Tetraplegia

L. Keith Lloyd, M.D.

Professor of Surgery (Urology), University of Alabama at Birmingham, Birmingham, Alabama.
Neurogenic Urinary Tract Infection

Walter E. Longo, M.D.

Assistant Professor, St. Louis University School of Medicine; Surgeon, Division of Colon and Rectal Surgery, St. Louis University Health Sciences Center, St. Louis, Missouri.
The Neurogenic Bowel

Michael E. Mayo, M.B.B.S., F.R.C.S.

Professor of Urology, University of Washington Medical Center; Director of Urology Residency Program, University of Washington Medical Center, Seattle, Washington.
The Urinary Bladder in Spinal Cord Disease

John D. McGarry, M.D.

Clinical Associate Professor of Neurology, St. Louis University School of Medicine; Assistant Chief, Spinal Cord Injury Service, St. Louis Veterans Affairs Medical Center, St. Louis, Missouri.
Cause, Prevention, and Treatment of Pressure Sores

Norma McKenzie, M.D.

Assistant Professor, Department of Psychiatry, Medical College of Virginia; Director, Emergency Psychiatry Service, Medical College of Virginia, Richmond, Virginia.
Medical Complications of Spinal Cord Disease

Paul R. Meyer, Jr., M.D.

Professor, Department of Orthopaedic Surgery, Northwestern University Medical School, Chicago, Illinois; Clinical Professor of Surgery, Uniformed Services University of Health Sciences, Bethesda, Maryland; Principal Investigator and Founder, Midwest Regional Spinal Cord Injury Care System, McGaw Medical Center; Director, Acute Spinal Cord Injury Trauma Unit/S.C.I. I.C.U., Northwestern Memorial Hospital, Chicago, Illinois.
Spinal Cord Injury

Meena Midha, M.D.

Associate Professor, Department of Physical Medicine and Rehabilitation, Medical College of Virginia/VCU; Chief, Spinal Cord Injury Service, Department of Veterans Affairs Medical Center, Richmond, Virginia.
Medical Complications of Spinal Cord Disease

Michael Mufson, M.D.
Instructor in Psychiatry, Harvard Medical School; Director of Psychiatry, West Roxbury Veteran's Affairs Hospital, Staff Psychiatrist, Brigham and Women's Hospital, Boston, Massachusetts.
Psychiatric Aspects of Spinal Cord Injury

John J. Mulcahy, M.D., Ph.D., F.A.C.S.
Professor of Urology, Indiana University School of Medicine; Chief of Urology, Wishard Memorial Hospital, Indianapolis, Indiana.
Disturbed Sexual Function in Patients with Spinal Cord Disease

P. Hunter Peckham, Ph.D.
Professor of Biomedical Engineering, Case Western Reserve University; Director, FES Center, Cleveland Veterans Affairs Medical Center, Metro Health Medical Center, Cleveland, Ohio.
Functional Electrical Stimulation and Its Application in the Management of Spinal Cord Injury

Frisso Potts, M.D.
Instructor, Department of Neurology, Harvard Medical School, Boston; Chief, Clinical Neurophysiology Laboratory, Brockton/West Roxbury Veterans Affairs Medical Center, West Roxbury, Massachusetts.
Acute Nontraumatic Myelopathies

Joseph J. Rusin, M.D.
Department of Orthopaedic Surgery, Medical College of Ohio, Toledo, Ohio.
Spinal Cord Injury

Maria Salam-Adams, M.D.[†]
Late Assistant Professor of Neurology, Harvard Medical School; Research Fellow in Neurology, Massachusetts General Hospital, Boston, Massachusetts.
Chronic Nontraumatic Diseases of the Spinal Cord

James Schmitt, M.D.
Assistant Professor, Department of Internal Medicine, Medical College of Virginia/VCU; Chief, Department of General Internal Medicine, Department of Veterans Affairs Medical Center, Richmond, Virginia.
Medical Complications of Spinal Cord Disease

Jean Schoenen, M.D., Ph.D.
Agrégé, Maître de Conférence, University of Liège, Liège, Belgium.
Clinical Anatomy of the Spinal Cord

Timothy R.D. Scott, Ph.D.
Research Associate, Case Western Reserve University, Cleveland, Ohio; Research Fellow, The Movement Disorder Foundation, New South Wales, Australia.
Functional Electrical Stimulation and Its Application in the Management of Spinal Cord Injury

---

[†] Deceased.

Jack L. Segal, M.D.

Associate Professor of Medicine, University of California, Irvine, College of Medicine; Staff Physician, Department of Veterans Affairs Medical Center, Long Beach, California.
Clinical Pharmacology of Spinal Cord Injury

Jeremy M. Shefner, M.D., Ph.D.

Assistant Professor, Department of Neurology, Harvard Medical School; Associate Physician, Brigham and Women's Hospital, Boston, Massachusetts.
Neurophysiology of Spinal Cord Injury

Marca L. Sipski, M.D.

Associate Professor of Clinical Physical Medicine and Rehabilitation, University of Medicine and Dentistry of New Jersey–New Jersey Medical School, Newark; Medical Director, Kessler Institute for Rehabilitation—West Orange Facility, West Orange, New Jersey.
Rehabilitation in Patients with Spinal Cord Disorders

Samuel L. Stover, M.D.

Professor Emeritus, Department of Rehabilitation Medicine, University of Alabama at Birmingham, Birmingham, Alabama.
Neurogenic Urinary Tract Infection

Ronald B. Tolchin, D.O., F.A.A.P.M.& R.

Assistant Professor and Chairman, Department of Physical Medicine and Rehabilitation, Nova Southeastern University, North Miami Beach; Staff, Hollywood Medical Center, THC Hospital of Hollywood, Hollywood, Florida.
Rehabilitation in Patients with Spinal Cord Disorders

Anthony M. Vernava III, M.D., F.A.C.S., F.A.S.C.R.S.

Associate Professor, St. Louis University School of Medicine; Chief, Division of Colon and Rectal Surgery, St. Louis University Health Sciences Center, St. Louis, Missouri.
The Neurogenic Bowel

Ken B. Waites, M.D.

Associate Professor, Departments of Pathology, Microbiology, and Rehabilitation Medicine, University of Alabama at Birmingham School of Medicine; Director of Clinical Microbiology, University of Alabama Hospital, Birmingham, Alabama.
Neurogenic Urinary Tract Infection

Stephen G. Waxman, M.D., Ph.D.

Professor and Chairman, Department of Neurology, Yale University School of Medicine; Neurologist-in-Chief, Yale–New Haven Hospital, New Haven, Connecticut.
Spinal Cord Compression

Robert M. Woolsey, M.D.

Professor of Neurology, St. Louis University School of Medicine; Chief, Spinal Cord Injury Service, St. Louis Veterans Affairs Medical Center, St. Louis, Missouri.
The Clinical Diagnosis of Disorders of the Spinal Cord; Cause, Prevention, and Treatment of Pressure Sores; Pain in Spinal Cord Disorders

Robert R. Young, M.D.

Professor and Vice Chairman, Department of Neurology, University of California, Irvine, College of Medicine, Irvine, California.
The Clinical Diagnosis of Disorders of the Spinal Cord; Spastic Paresis

Contents

Diagnosis
and
Management
of Disorders
of the
Spinal Cord

CHAPTER 1

Clinical Anatomy of the Spinal Cord

Jean Schoenen, M.D., Ph.D.

As is the case for diseases that affect other parts of the nervous system, knowledge of anatomic organization is a prerequisite for the correct diagnosis and management of spinal cord disease. This chapter discusses the external morphology and blood supply of the spinal cord, its internal neuronal organization, and some anatomic-functional correlations. For obvious reasons, attention is focused on the human spinal cord, and data from animal studies are mentioned only when appropriate information on humans is lacking.[8]

EXTERNAL MORPHOLOGY AND BLOOD SUPPLY

Gross External Anatomy

The spinal cord has a roughly cylindrical shape, tapering caudally to become the conus medullaris, which is attached by the filum terminale, a meningeal structure, to the fundus of the dural sac at the level of the second sacral vertebra. The length of the entire vertebral column is 70 cm, but the length of the spinal cord is approximately 45 cm in men and 41 to 43 cm in women. This discrepancy is explained by the fact that during development, the vertebral column grows at a faster rate than the spinal cord. In late adolescent years, the spinal cord attains its adult position, terminating at the level of the intervertebral disk between the first and second lumbar vertebrae (Fig. 1–1). Like the brain, the spinal cord is enveloped by three layers of meninges. Unlike the anatomy in the skull, at the spinal level the dura mater is separated from the periosteum of the vertebrae by an epidural space containing fatty and loose connective tissue and the epidural venous plexus. The dural sac and the subarachnoid space extend to the second sacral level. Consequently, at the lower lumbar area the dural sac contains only the spinal rootlets of the cauda equina bathed in cerebrospinal fluid, which can be removed by lumbar puncture (see Fig. 1–1).

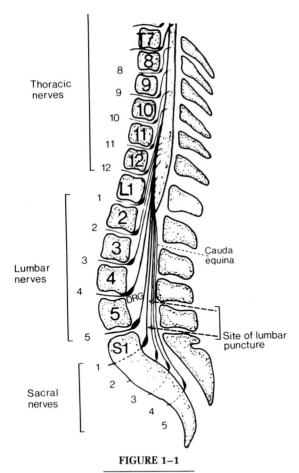

FIGURE 1–1

Schematic outline of the lower vertebral column, the lumbosacral spinal cord, and the cauda equina. The dorsal root ganglia (DRG) are located at the intervertebral foramina, where the spinal nerves emerge between the individual vertebrae. The spinal cord terminates at the level of the first lumbar vertebra, leaving at lower levels the epidural sac filled with cerebrospinal fluid and the cauda equina. Lumbar puncture can be performed at these levels.

A spinal cord segment is the portion of spinal cord and all of its rootlets that join to form the associated pair of spinal nerves. There are 31 spinal segments: 8 cervical, 12 thoracic, 5 lumbar, 5 sacral, and 1 coccygeal. The number of rootlets that form a spinal nerve varies between levels of the cord, as does the length of the cord segments. Cervical segments average 13 mm in length; midthoracic segments, 26 mm; lumbar segments, 15 mm; and sacral segments, 5 mm. Because of the difference in length between spinal cord and vertebral column, cervical and upper thoracic rootlets run at right angles to the cord, whereas lower thoracic, lumbar, and sacral rootlets are increasingly oblique. The diameter of the cord is increased at the level of the cervical (third cervical to second thoracic segments) and lumbar (first lumbar to third sacral segments or ninth to twelfth thoracic vertebrae) enlargements. The dorsal root ganglia (spinal ganglia) are located within the intervertebral foramina, explaining why the distance between the cord and the ganglia is much longer in lumbosacral than in cervicothoracic segments (see Fig. 1–1).

Blood Supply

The blood supply of the cervical spinal cord originates from collateral branches of the subclavian artery and that of the dorsal and lumbosacral cord from parietal branches of the thoracic and abdominal aorta. The major part of arterial blood supply is provided by the medullary (or radicular) arteries; the anterior spinal and the posterior spinal arteries contribute to the spinal cord blood supply to a lesser degree.[3]

RADICULAR (OR MEDULLARY) ARTERIES. The radicular arteries originate from the vertebromedullary arteries, the number of which is equal to that of spinal nerves. In a rostrocaudal direction, they successively derive from the extracranial portion of the vertebral artery, the ascending artery (a branch of the subclavian or other arterial branches of the neck), the superior intercostal artery (a branch of the subclavian artery), the aortic intercostal arteries, the lumbar arteries (branches of the abdominal aorta), the ilio-lumbar artery, and the sacral arteries. Each vertebromedullary artery divides into three branches (Fig. 1–2). Two of them, one anterior and one posterior, supply the meninges, ligaments, and bones of the vertebral canal. The third branch, the so-called neurospinal artery of Kadyi or lateral spinal artery, penetrates the dura together with the spinal nerve and divides into two terminal branches called anterior and posterior radicular arteries. These arteries follow the nerve root to the cord and then bifurcate into ascending and descending branches, forming numerous anastomoses with the posterior and anterior spinal arteries. From the end of the fourth month of embryonic life, only a few radicular arteries remain effective in carrying blood to the spinal cord (Fig. 1–3). The number of anterior radicular arteries varies between five and ten: one or two in the cervical region, usually at C6; one or two small arteries in the superior thoracic region; and one to three in the inferior thoracic and lumbosacral regions.

Frequently, one of the last group is larger and is referred to as the arteria radicularis anterior magna of Adamkiewicz or artery of the lumbar enlargement. Adamkiewicz's artery is found only on one side, more often on the left than on the right. The location is either high (T8–10 in 40% of individuals) or low (T11–L2 in 60%). If the location is high, the artery is the only blood supply for the lumbosacral cord, whereas if it is low, the artery is accompanied by a small radicular artery running with one of the roots of T7–8 or T9. The posterior radicular arteries are more numerous but smaller than the anterior ones. Their total number generally varies between 15 and 22. In the lumbosacral cord, the posterior radicular arteries are vestigial and of no physiologic significance.

ANTERIOR SPINAL ARTERY. Formed by two branches of the intracranial segments of the two vertebral arteries, the anterior spinal artery descends on the anterior surface of the medulla oblongata and upper cervical spinal cord and gives origin to the anterior anasto-

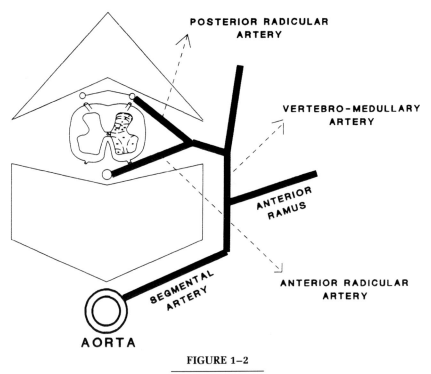

FIGURE 1–2

The segmental artery from the thoracic aorta gives rise to the vertebromedullary artery, which in turn provides the anterior and posterior spinal radicular arteries. The latter feed the anterior and the posterior anastomotic arterial tracts.

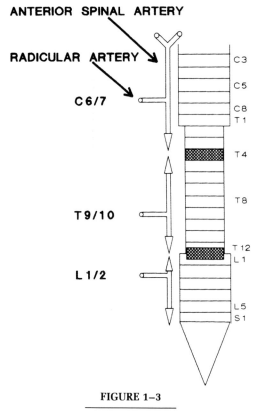

FIGURE 1–3

Diagram of supply of the anterior anastomotic arterial tract by three principal radicular arteries. Shaded areas represent "watershed zones" in which circulatory deficits may occur first. (Data from Zülch RJ. Rev Neurol 106:632, 1962).

motic arterial tract. Below the first cervical segments, this tract mainly receives blood via radicular (medullary) arteries. Its size changes considerably in different regions. It is largest just below the point of entry of Adamkiewicz's artery and smallest in the thoracic region, where radicular arteries are rare and slim. The anterior anastomotic arterial tract is responsible for the blood supply of much of the entire anterior two thirds of the spinal cord, including the anterior horn and most of the intermediate gray matter.

POSTERIOR SPINAL ARTERIES. The posterior spinal artery arises as a branch of the vertebral or the posterior inferior cerebellar artery (PICA) on the posterolateral surface of the medulla oblongata. Shortly after its origin, each artery splits into two anastomotic tracts, one larger and medial and the other smaller and lateral to the entering dorsal roots. These tracts, which are chiefly fed through numer-

ous anastomoses with the segmental medullary or radicular arteries, supply the posterior third of the cord.

VASOCORONA AND INTRASPINAL ARTERIES. The anterior and posterior anastomotic tracts vary considerably between individuals. They are interconnected by numerous anastomotic branches that run horizontally and vertically, giving origin to a network called the vasocorona, which encircles the cord. At each segment, the spinal parenchyma is penetrated by numerous small arteries that originate in the vasocorona. The network formed by the anterior median arteries, also called anterior sulcal arteries, is anatomically and functionally the most important.

SPINAL VEINS. No strict one-to-one relationship exists between spinal arteries and veins. The most striking difference is that the arterial network is denser on the anterior side of the cord and the venous network is denser on the posterior side. Blood from the intraspinal capillary network is drained through radial veins into the external veins, which include longitudinal venous channels analogous to the arterial tracts and lying deep to them. From the perispinal venous network, blood drains into the anterior and posterior radicular veins and then into a dense longitudinal vertebral plexus located posteriorly and anteriorly in the epidural space. Blood then reaches the external vertebral venous plexus through the intervertebral and sacral foramina.

INTERNAL NEURONAL ORGANIZATION

The white matter of the spinal cord consists of closely packed nerve fibers intermingled with blood vessels and glial cells. A few scattered neuronal cell bodies can normally be found in the white matter, but their exact significance is not known. The white matter, which contains more unmyelinated than myelinated axons, is continued at the base of the anterior median fissure via a slender lamina of nerve fibers called the anterior white commissure. Because the number of nerve fibers in the ascending and descending spinal tracts is greatest at cervical levels, the white matter is best developed in the cervical region and progressively decreases in size at successive caudal levels of the spinal cord. The white matter is subdivided into posterior, lateral, and anterior funiculi. The localization of the various fiber tracts in the spinal white matter is reviewed in the section on connections. Briefly, the white matter immediately surrounding the gray matter contains most of the propriospinal fibers of the cord, the so-called fasciculi proprii. Most of the posterior funiculi are occupied by the dorsal columns, which contain ascending fibers conveying sensory information to higher levels. Ascending as well as descending pathways are located in the lateral funiculi, whereas the ventral funiculi comprise chiefly descending pathways (Fig. 1–4).

The butterfly-shaped gray matter is divided into a dorsal (or posterior) horn, an intermediate zone, and a ventral (or anterior) horn that consists mainly of the motor neurons. The cytoarchitecture, dendroarchitecture, chemoarchitecture, and connections of the human spinal cord are described successively in the following text.

Cytoarchitecture

A laminar cytoarchitectonic scheme, such as the one initially described by Rexed[6] in thick histologic segments of cat spinal cord, can be recognized in mature and immature spinal cords of other mammals, including humans[7] (Figs. 1–4 to 1–6). Lamina I cuffs the tip of the dorsal horn and contains a small number of variable-sized fusiform or multi-

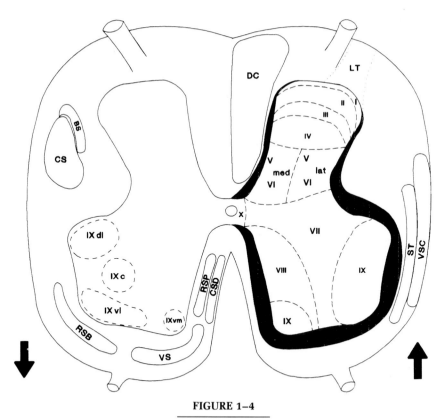

FIGURE 1–4

Diagram of a transverse section of the lumbar spinal cord illustrating Rexed's (1952) cytoarchitectonic lamination in the right hemicord and the various columns of motor neurons in the left ventral horn. IX dl, dorsolateral; IX c, central; IX vl, ventrolateral; Ix vm, ventromedial column. The shaded area represents the fasciculi proprii. The location of some descending (*left*) and ascending (*right*) white matter tracts is indicated. CS = Corticospinal tract; BS = bulbospinal serotoninergic tract; RSB = lateral or bulbar reticulospinal tract; VS = vestibulospinal tract; RSP = medial or pontine reticulospinal tract; CSD = ventral or direct corticospinal tract; ST = spinothalamic tract; VSC = ventral spinocerebellar tract; DC = dorsal column; LT = Lissauer's tract.

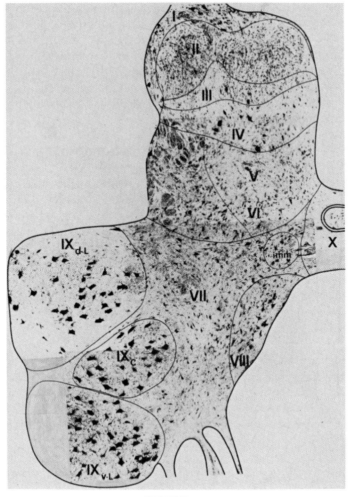

FIGURE 1–5

Montage of a 100 μm-thick, transverse, cresyl violet–stained section of the gray matter at the L5 level in the spinal cord of a normal 60-year-old man. Successive cytoarchitectonic laminae are marked by roman numerals. IXdl, IXc, IXvl: respectively, dorsolateral, central, and ventrolateral groups of motor neurons. imm = Intermediomedial nucleus. (Original magnification ×40.)

polar neurons. It corresponds to the marginal zone of Waldeyer found in classic anatomic descriptions. Lamina II, corresponding to the substantia gelatinosa of Rolando, is the portion of the spinal gray matter with the highest neuronal density. Its neurons are small and have their long axes oriented rostrocaudally. Lamina III is not well demarcated from adjacent laminae, has a lower cell density than lamina II, and contains larger neurons. Lamina IV is thicker than lamina III and contains neurons of varying size. In human spinal cords, laminae V and VI cannot be distinguished on a cytologic basis. They occupy the base of the dorsal horn. Their medial portion

contains numerous medium-sized dorsoventrally oriented neurons, corresponding at least in part to the nucleus proprius of Cajal. The lateral portion of laminae V–VI merges with the white matter of the lateral funiculus.

Lamina VII, which has fuzzy borders, occupies most of the intermediate gray matter containing medium-sized neurons of varying shapes. Lamina VIII consists of small, medium, and large neurons.

Lamina IX contains the various columns of motor neurons: the dorsolateral, ventrolateral, ventromedial, and central columns. The total number of motor neurons in segments L1 to S5 is between 52,000 and 62,000, with

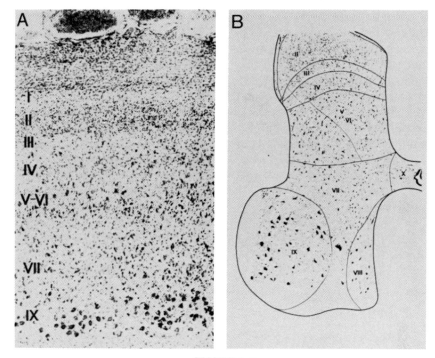

FIGURE 1–6

A, Thick sagittal Nissl-stained section through the lumbar spinal cord of a 26-week-old human fetus. Spinal laminae VIII and X are not within the plane of section. (Original magnification ×43.2). *B*, Montage of a 25 μm-thick transverse, cresyl violet–stained section of the gray matter at L5 in a 5-month-old child. (Original magnification ×18.)

segment L5 frequently containing the largest number of cells (±10,000) and segment S1 having the highest density of motor neurons per section.[4, 11] The number of motor neurons (as well as their size) decreases with age, approximately 200 neurons being lost per decade. Lamina X corresponds to the gray matter surrounding the central canal and comprises the posterior and anterior gray commissures. It is characterized histologically by the dense structure of its neuropil and the low density of small-sized neurons.

Over the length of the spinal cord, the laminar cytoarchitectonic organization undergoes important segmental variations. Certain laminae vary in size, orientation, or both according to the segmental level. In addition, some neuronal groups, such as the dorsal nucleus of Clarke, the intermediolateral nucleus, and the parasympathetic sacral nuclei, which are easily recognizable, are present only at certain segmental levels. In the human cord, three main region-dependent cytoarchitectural types can be recognized. The enlarge-

ment type (C4–8, L4–S2) is characterized by extensive dorsal and ventral horns, large laminae V–VI, a ventrally extended lamina VII, a medially confined lamina VIII, and an extensive lamina IX comprising several motoneuronal columns. The thoracic type (T2–12) has a much reduced gray matter, absence of large neurons in lamina IV, partial replacement of laminae V–VI by Clarke's column, an intermediolateral nucleus, spread of lamina VIII from the medial to the lateral border of the ventral horn, and the sole persistence of the ventromedial motoneuronal column. The transitional type is characterized by an intermediate cytoarchitectural organization, such as the one found in segments C1–3, L1–3, S3, and S4. From segments S1–2 to S4, a supplementary column of motor neurons appears in the ventral horn. This is Onuf's nucleus, which lies at the most ventral border of the ventral horn and is divided into a dorsomedial cell group innervating the bulbocavernosus and ischiocavernosus muscles and a ventrolateral group innervating external anal and urethral sphincters. The dorsomedial portion of Onuf's nucleus is sexually dimorphic, containing significantly more neurons in males than in females.

The laminar organization of the spinal gray matter appears during development as soon as neuroblasts migrate from the germinal plate laterally and differentiate. It is characteristic of mammals and is not found as such in lower, nonmammalian vertebrates.

Dendroarchitecture

Only the overall dendritic organization of spinal gray matter in humans is presented here. A detailed description of the dendroarchitecture of the various spinal laminae can be found elsewhere.[7, 9] Preferential dendritic orientation or dendritic spread, which can be quantified by morphometric analyses, clearly distinguishes neuronal populations. For this reason, cell types are represented by their dendritic domain or territory, that is, the main three-dimensional space of neuropil occupied by their dendritic trees (Fig. 1–7). Dendritic trees of lamina I neurons occupy a disklike domain tangentially oriented to the edge of the dorsal horn. In addition, these neurons have ventrally oriented dendrites penetrating deeply into underlying laminae II and even III and IV. These deep branches,

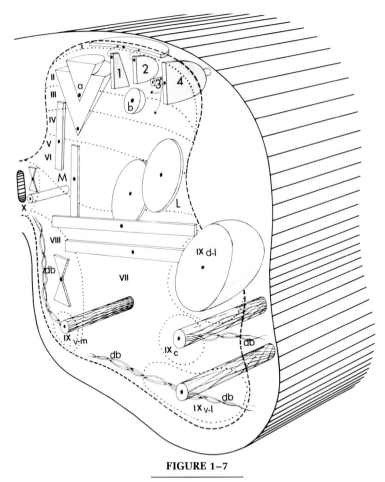

FIGURE 1–7

Dendroarchitectonic scheme of the human spinal cord at the lumbar level. Dendritic territories are three-dimensionally represented, cut in half by a transverse section through the center of the perikaryon (*large dot*). The four cell types of lamina II are represented, as is the direction of their main axonal projection (*dotted lines* and *arrows*): (1) filamentous cells; (2) curly cells; (3) islet cells; (4) stellate cells. The two cell types of lamina III are small antenna-like (*a*) and radiate (*b*) neurons. At the level of ventromedial (*IX v-m*), central (*IX c*), and ventrolateral (*IX v-l*) motoneuronal columns, the tightness of longitudinal dendritic bundling and transverse dendritic bundles (*db*) are schematized. M = Medial; L = lateral.

which are not represented in Figure 1–7, are of potential functional importance because they offer the possibility for lamina neurons to be contacted by axons running in the deeper laminae of the dorsal horn. Four cell types can be distinguished in lamina II: (1) filamentous cells, with a vertical trapezoid dendritic territory and an axon branching initially within the limits of the dendritic tree, then extending outside lamina II into lamina I or Lissauer's tract; (2) curly cells, with numerous spinous dendritic branches confined to a disklike sagittal domain and an axon directed toward lamina I or Lissauer's tract; (3) islet cells, with a narrow cylindrical longitudinal dendritic domain and an axonal network confined to the same territory; and (4) stellate cells, with the most extensive dendritic territory, similar to an ellipse with a sagittal long axis, overflowing dorsally into lamina I and ventrally into lamina III. Stellate cells are the only lamina II neurons of which the axon reaches deeper laminae III and IV. Lamina III contains radial cells with a small, spherical dendritic domain and small antennalike neurons. Lamina IV is characterized by large antennalike neurons of which the dendritic territory can be compared to a cone with a dorsal base lying in lamina II and a ventral apex at the cell body. In medial laminae V–VI, most neurons have their dendrites oriented dorsoventrally, giving a rectangular, dorsoventral dendritic domain. In contrast, neurons in the lateral portion of laminae V–VI are multipolar with an elliptic dendritic domain in the transverse plane. In lamina VII, dendritic domains also are rectangular in the transverse plane but they are mediolaterally oriented, slightly tilted ventromedially. In this lamina, subtle differences in dendritic orientation occur according to the medial, central, or lateral position of cells. Dendritic domains in lamina VIII can be compared to two dorsoventrally opposite triangles with a common summit at the perikaryon. In lamina IX, ventromedial, ventrolateral, and central motor neurons have in common cylindrical, longitudinal dendritic territories forming a plexus with dendritic microbundles that is very narrow and is meshed in the ventromedial column. These motoneuronal groups also differ by the orientation of transverse dendritic bundles, which

are dorsal in the ventromedial group, lateral in the central group, and both medial and lateral in the ventrolateral group (Fig. 1–8). In contrast, the dendritic domain of dorsolateral motor neurons is comparable to a sphere. Lamina X contains two neuronal types: one with a dorsoventral dendritic territory and the other with longitudinal orientation.

Chemoarchitecture

Since the increasing application of techniques such as immunocytochemistry, topobiochemistry, and receptor autoradiography, it is common to describe nervous system structures in terms of the localization of neuroactive compounds, including neurotransmitters, their metabolizing enzymes, and their receptors, a discipline called "chemical neuroanatomy." The data obtained with these techniques in the human spinal cord chiefly concern afferents to the gray matter, receptors, and, to a lesser extent, spinal neurons themselves. Tables 1–1 and 1–2 summarize some general chemoarchitectural features of the normal human spinal cord. A description of the regional chemoarchitecture and some functional applications demonstrated, in part, from the study of pathologic disorders in humans follows.

DORSAL HORN (LAMINAE I–IV) Each of the laminae and sublaminae of the dorsal horn has a distinctive chemoarchitecture. All neuropeptides are present in all or several laminae, and the highest concentrations of fibers containing substance P, enkephalin, calcitonin gene–related peptide (CGRP), and somatostatin are found in the dorsal horn. With the exception of CGRP-positive motor neurons, all peptide-containing cell bodies visualized in human autopsy material are localized in the superficial spinal laminae: enkephalin in lamina I neurons and lamina II stellate cells, somatostatin in lamina II islet cells, and substance P in lamina III radiate neurons.

The density of muscarinic cholinergic (mainly M_1 type), opiate, benzodiazepine, gamma-aminobutyric acid (GABA), CGRP, and thyrotropin-releasing hormone (TRH) receptors is also high in the dorsal horn. Because this portion of the spinal gray matter

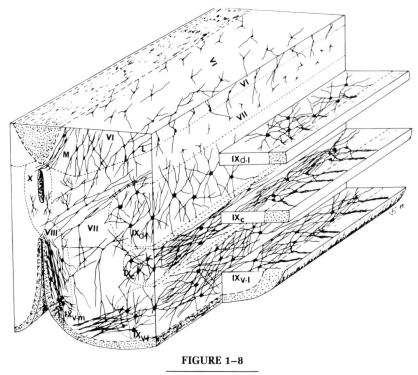

FIGURE 1–8

Synoptic three-dimensional view of dendroarchitectonics in the intermediate gray matter and ventral horns of the human spinal cord. (Abbreviations are as in previous figures.)

receives the termination of primary afferent fibers conveying nociceptive, mechanoreceptive, and thermoreceptive inputs to the central nervous system, the chemicals described are strategically placed to have major roles in processing sensory information.

The precise roles of these various neurotransmitters and receptors in sensory processing are still unknown. However, from the study of selected human disorders, such as limb amputations, interrupting afferent input from the periphery, or transections of thoracic spinal cord, disconnecting caudal segments from descending pathways, some insight has been gained into the origin of peptidergic fibers to the dorsal horn. Briefly, most substance P fibers to laminae I and II originate from spinal ganglion cells, whereas enkephalinergic fibers stem from intrinsic spinal neurons. Some of the somatostatin- and cholecystokinin-containing fibers have a peripheral origin, whereas the totality of oxytocin and vasopressin immunoreactivities is provided by descending afferent fibers. The observation of a marked reduction of lamina II substance P immunoreactivity in patients with familial dysautonomia and profound analgesia (Riley-Day syndrome) favors the hypothesis that substance P is important for the transmission of nociceptive input.

INTERMEDIATE GRAY MATTER (LAMINAE V–VIII, X, AND AUTONOMIC NUCLEI). The distribution of the various neuromediators and their receptors is rather nonselective. High concentrations of substance P, enkephalin, and cholecystokinin are found in the lateral portion of laminae V–VI, which has a role in processing muscular and visceral inputs and also receives a large contingent of descending afferent impulses. An interesting chemoarchitectural-functional correlation can be established from the finding of TRH innervation of medial lamina VII. In human volunteers, TRH in low intravenous doses modifies the excitability of motor neurons through an action on interneurons of the flexor reflex pathways. These interneurons are probably located in the medial portion of lamina VII, that is, in a region where TRH terminals can be identified. Lamina

TABLE 1–1

NEUROPEPTIDERGIC FIBERS IN HUMAN SPINAL CORD*

PEPTIDE	I	II$_o$	II$_i$	III	IV	V–VI MEDIAL	V–VI LATERAL	VII	VIII	IX	X	IML	PARA
SP	****	**	***	** + cells	*	**	**	*	*	*	**	***	***
M-ENK	** + cells	****	*** + cells	**	*	*	****	*	*	*	***	***	***
L-ENK	**	****	***	**	*	***	****	*	**	*	***	***	**
SYN	*	***	**	*	*	*	***	*	*	*	**	**	**
CCK	***	*	**	*	*	**	***	**	***	*	**	**	**
NPY	**	**	*	*	*	*	***	**	**	*	**	**	**

*Peptide-containing fibers (and cells when indicated) in the gray matter laminae of the human spinal cord. Symbols: * = sparse; ** = moderate; *** = dense; **** = very dense innervation; SP = substance P; M-ENK = methionine-enkephalin; L-ENK = leucine-enkephalin; SYN = synenkephalin; CCK = cholecystokinin; NPY = neuropeptide Y; IML = intermediolateral column; PARA = sacral parasympathetic nuclei.

TABLE 1–2

NEUROPEPTIDERGIC FIBERS IN HUMAN SPINAL CORD*

PEPTIDE	I	II$_o$	II$_i$	III	IV	LAMINA V–VI MEDIAL	V–VI LATERAL	VII	VIII	IX	X	IML	P
SOM	*	* + cells	**	*	O	O	O	O	O	*	*	*	*
OXY	*	O	O	*	*	*	O	O	O	*	O	O	O
VASO	O	*	*	*	*	*	O	O	O	O	O	O	O
TRH	O	**	**	O	O	O	O	*	O	*	*	O	O
CGRP	****	***	***	**	*	O	O	O	O	O + cells	O	O	*
VIP	**	*	O	O	O	O	O	O	O	O	*	*	**

*Peptide-containing fibers (and cells when indicated) in the gray matter laminae of the human spinal cord. Symbols: O = no fibers seen; * = sparse; ** = moderate; *** = dense; **** = very dense innervation; SOM = somatostatin; OXY = oxytocin; VASO = vasopressin; TRH = thyrotropin-releasing hormone; CGRP = calcitonin gene–related peptide; VIP = vasoactive intestinal polypeptide.

VIII is characterized by a dense network of cholecystokinin- and serotonin-containing fibers. Substance P and enkephalin levels in laminae V–VI appear unchanged after lesions of peripheral or descending afferents. In contrast, substance P in lamina VII is reduced below a spinal transection, whereas enkephalin immunoreactivity remains unchanged. In laminae V–VI, substance P and enkephalin are thus mainly of intrinsic origin, whereas in lamina VII, the origin of substance P is supraspinal and that of enkephalin is intrinsic.

The dorsal nucleus of Clarke is characterized by high levels of acetylcholinesterase and muscarinic cholinergic receptors. Fibers containing substance P and CGRP are found in close contact with neurons in the nucleus of Clarke, whereas other neuropeptides are virtually absent. This would suggest that Clarke's nucleus receives some small C or A delta peripheral afferent input in addition to the large input by thick myelinated fibers.

The autonomic nuclei in the intermediate gray matter have a specific chemoarchitecture. The intermediolateral, intermediomedial, and sacral parasympathetic nuclei and lamina X are characterized by high levels of muscarinic cholinergic receptor binding and high concentrations of several neuropeptides (substance P, enkephalin, cholecystokinin, neuropeptide Y, and vasoactive intestinal polypeptide). Acetylcholinesterase is also in high concentration in these structures, except in lamina X. GABA and glycine receptors are found in lamina X. A similar profuse peptidergic innervation of autonomic nuclei and lamina X has been shown in animals, and serotonin-containing lamina X neurons have been described in the monkey. The high concentrations of muscarinic receptors and acetylcholinesterase in both autonomic sensory (intermediomedial nucleus) and autonomic motor (intermediolateral) regions parallel their high concentrations in somatic sensory (lamina II) and somatic motor (lamina IX) regions.

Vasoactive intestinal polypeptide (VIP) has a distinct distribution in the spinal gray matter. Its concentration is very high in the lumbar region and even more so in the sacral regions of the spinal cord. VIP fibers are mainly distributed to lamina I, the intermediolateral nucleus, sacral parasympathetic preganglionic neurons, and lamina X. Evidence from animal experiments suggests that VIP is a transmitter in visceral afferents. Recently, lamina X neurons containing VIP have been found to contact the cerebrospinal fluid along the surface of the central canal of the cord in the cat and monkey.

MOTOR NUCLEI (LAMINA IX). Lamina IX contains high concentrations of acetylcholinesterase, choline acetyltransferase, and muscarinic cholinergic receptors of the M_1 and M_2 subtypes. Following degeneration of motor neurons in amyotrophic lateral sclerosis, there is a simultaneous reduction of cholinergic enzymes and receptors but also of glycinergic receptors. This reduction confirms theories that spinal motor neurons utilize acetylcholine as a transmitter and receive cholinergic innervation provided by recurrent collaterals of motor neurons or by supraspinal and propriospinal afferents, as well as innervation by fibers utilizing the inhibitory transmitter glycine, probably coming from Renshaw cells and Ia interneurons.

The presence of numerous serotoninergic fibers in lamina IX suggests that in the human spinal cord, serotonin has a role in motor function comparable to that demonstrated in animals. Serotoninergic fibers probably have a supraspinal origin because almost all of them disappear below a spinal transection. High levels of noradrenaline are also found in human ventral horn. The effect of this transmitter on motor functions is presumably mediated through an action on interneurons, because adrenergic receptors remain unchanged after degeneration of motor neurons with amyotrophic lateral sclerosis.

The density of peptide immunoreactive fibers in the ventral horn is relatively low in comparison with that in the dorsal horn. However, the fact that all peptides studied, except CGRP, vasopressin, and VIP, are found in terminals closely opposed to motor neurons and that peptide receptors are localized in this region suggests that various peptides may be involved in aspects of lower motor neuron control. Studies of human pathologic specimens indicate that the origin of oxytocin, TRH, and, in part, substance P and somatostatin fibers innervating lamina IX is supraspinal. Conversely, these studies suggest a predominantly local or dorsal root origin for enkephalin and cholecystokinin immunoreactive fibers. CGRP is the only peptide contained within the cell bodies of motor neurons (Fig. 1–9) and may exert a trophic action at the neuromuscular junction.

Connections

Thanks to modern tracing methods, which have complemented classical fiber degeneration techniques, our knowledge of connections in the mammalian spinal cord has greatly expanded. When studying material from humans, on which such techniques are not applicable, one must rely on data from anterograde degeneration or retrograde chromatolysis studies in selected pathologic conditions with circumscribed lesions.[10] Certain spinal connections differ markedly between different species (e.g., corticospinal connections), whereas others have roughly the same organization in all mammals (e.g., descending brain stem pathways). The following section is therefore based on data available from

studies in humans, but also, where appropriate, on experimental findings in subhuman mammalian cords.[1]

PROPRIOSPINAL PATHWAYS. Contrary to what has frequently been assumed to be the case, short-axoned neurons that distribute their fibers only through the gray matter to neighboring neurons are rare in the spinal cord. Such neurons probably exist only in the substantia gelatinosa (lamina II islet cells). Most spinal neurons, especially those located in laminae V to VIII, are propriospinal in nature; that is, they emit axons that penetrate into the white matter to make intrasegmental and intersegmental connections. On their way to the funiculi, they may establish connections with adjacent cells via collaterals of their main axonal trunk. Propriospinal neurons have a paramount role in spinal functions. Descending pathways, for example, are differentially distributed to subgroups of propriospinal neurons, which relay their action to motor neurons or other spinal cells.

Portions of the spinal white matter bordering the central gray matter, the so-called fasciculi proprii, contain most of the axons of propriospinal neurons (see Fig. 1–4). In humans,

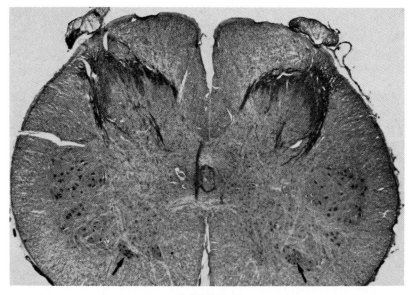

FIGURE 1–9

Calcitonin gene–related peptide (CGRP) immunoreactivity in a transverse section of human segment S1. Note a dense network of dark-appearing immunoreactive fibers in laminae I and II and dark immunoreactive product in most motor neurons including Onuf's nuclei (*arrows*). (Original magnification ×13.)

the fasciculi proprii are composed of the anterior, the lateral, and the posterior ground bundles. In addition, several white matter tracts, such as Lissauer's tract, contain propriospinal axons and dorsal root collaterals in a proportion that can vary between species. Propriospinal neurons can be subdivided schematically according to the length of their axons and their topography (Fig. 1–10).

Long propriospinal neurons distribute their axons throughout the length of the spinal cord mainly through the ventral funiculus. They are concentrated in lamina VIII and the dorsally adjacent part of lamina VII and terminate in the ventromedial part of the gray matter, i.e., lamina VIII, medial lamina VII, and the ventromedial motoneuronal column, which innervates axial and girdle muscles. Fibers from the long propriospinal neurons in the cervical cord descend bilaterally, but those from the corresponding neurons in the lumbosacral cord ascend mainly contralaterally.

Intermediate propriospinal neurons extend over shorter distances, chiefly in the ventral part of the ventrolateral funiculus. They are located in central and medial portions of lamina VII and distribute bilaterally with an ipsilateral preponderance to the homologous regions of the intermediate gray matter and the ventrolateral motor neurons, which innervate proximal extremity and girdle muscles.

Short propriospinal neurons, which are the main occupants of the lateral part of laminae V to VII, send their fibers primarily ipsilaterally through the lateral funiculus to terminate in the dorsal and lateral parts of the intermediate gray matter as well as in the dorsolateral column of motor neurons, which innervate intrinsic hand and foot muscles.

AFFERENT PATHWAYS

PRIMARY AFFERENTS. Primary afferent fibers reach the spinal cord via dorsal roots, which are segmentally arranged along the spinal cord. Peripherally, this segmental arrangement is reflected in the dermatomes, which can be used as clinically useful sensory landmarks. In humans, there are 31 pairs of roots (8 cervical, 12 thoracic, 5 lumbar, 5

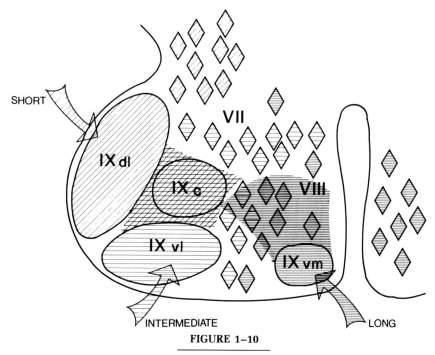

FIGURE 1–10

Schematic diagram of the three major propriospinal systems showing location of cells of origin in the intermediate gray matter and the area of fiber distribution in the ventral horn. Short propriospinal system: obliquely hatched area and neurons. Intermediate propriospinal system: horizontally hatched area. Long propriospinal system: horizontally narrow-hatched area (see text for comments).

sacral, and 1 coccygeal), the largest being those of the lumbar and cervical enlargements. Approximately 1,000,000 dorsal root fibers have been found on each side in the human adult. Caliber spectra in human roots show a bimodal distribution with a fine-caliber (diameters of 2–4 μm) and a thick-caliber (diameters of 8–9 μm) group. Most dorsal root fibers are unmyelinated (cutaneous C and muscular group IV afferents). The myelinated fibers (cutaneous A alpha, A beta, A delta, and muscular groups I, II, III) have their myelin produced by Schwann cells peripherally or by oligodendrocytes centrally to a transitional region called the dorsal root entry zone. Small-caliber axons are randomly distributed in the peripheral part of the dorsal rootlet (as they are in peripheral nerve). Centrally, however, the small-caliber axons take a ventrolateral course in the rootlet, whereas large-caliber axons are placed dorsolaterally, which permits selective destruction at this level of nociceptive afferents in certain chronic pain syndromes.

The neurons of the dorsal root ganglia (DRG) vary in diameter between 10 and 100 μm. Each cell is surrounded by satellite cells, which, like the neurons, are derived from the neural crest and seem to be modified Schwann cells. DRG neurons are unipolar, giving rise to a single process that bifurcates into a peripheral and a central branch. The proximal segment, which may be coiled, is referred to as the glomerular segment. DRG neurons are divided into three major classifications: (1) type I or large, light-colored cells; (2) type B or intermediate-sized, dark-colored cells; and (3) type C or small, dark-colored cells. Monoclonal antibodies have been produced that specifically label subsets of DRG neurons. Numerous neuromediators have been demonstrated, predominantly in type B and C DRG neurons. In addition to some classical transmitters, 50% of neurons contain neuropeptides, often with co-localization (CGRP, substance P, somatostatin, vasopressin, VIP, bombesin, galanin, and others).

The central processes of DRG neurons terminate in the spinal gray matter or ascend in the dorsal columns. The termination of primary afferent fibers in the gray matter is organized according to two principles. A mediolateral somatotopic organization exists (distal parts of the limb represented medially and proximal parts laterally) on which a ventrodorsal modality-related segregation principle (nociceptive fibers terminating in superficial parts, proprioceptive fibers in more deeper parts) is superimposed. Lamina II appears to receive afferent fibers almost exclusively from cutaneous receptors, whereas visceral as well as muscle afferents reach laminae I and V.

DESCENDING AFFERENTS. The *corticospinal (or pyramidal) system* has the highest level of development in higher primates, especially in humans. The cells of origin of the corticospinal tract are located in the precentral gyrus, mainly in its upper two thirds and in the paracentral lobule. Brodmann's areas 4 (primary motor cortex) and 6 (premotor cortex) contribute 80% of the pyramidal tract fibers. The number of axons in a pyramidal tract is roughly proportional to body and brain weight. In humans, approximately 1,000,000 axons are present in each tract. Thick fibers occur, especially in species that possess many direct corticomotoneuronal connections, such as humans. During postnatal development, myelination starts in the internal capsule and cerebral peduncles, where it is present in the 10- to 14-day-old neonate. Myelination is completed only in the second year. The trajectory of corticospinal fibers is well known. After crossing the midline in the caudal medulla, the bulk of corticospinal fibers continues in the dorsolateral fasciculus of the spinal cord as the lateral (crossed) corticospinal tract (see Fig. 1–4). Some fibers do not cross in the medulla but run in the ventral funiculus of the cord before crossing in the ventral white commissure. This is referred to as the ventral (uncrossed) corticospinal tract (see Fig. 1–4). The pyramidal tract is subject to much anatomic variation between individuals. For instance, in some subjects, the ventral tract may be absent or may not project into lumbosacral regions. The terminal distribution of corticospinal fibers, as determined in the human spinal gray matter by fiber degeneration methods, primarily involves contralaterally the lateral parts of laminae V–VI, VII, the dorsolateral motoneuronal column, and the lateral parts of the central and ventrolateral motor neurons. Terminals are also found contralaterally in the medial part of lamina VII and bilaterally in lamina VIII. A few cortical fibers are distributed to lateral lamina IV in the dorsal horn.

Unlike lower mammals, primates, especially humans, are characterized by a heavy projection of corticospinal fibers to the ventromedial gray matter containing long propriospinal neurons and to motoneuronal cell groups innervating distal and proximal extremity muscles. The corticospinal tract has a somatotopic arrangement. The few fibers from the postcentral gyrus are distributed mainly to dorsal gray matter (lamina IV and lateral part of laminae V–VI and VII), whereas those from the precentral cortex project in a topographically organized fashion to the intermediate gray matter and the motoneuronal cell groups. Moreover, at spinal levels, fibers innervating segments related to the lower limbs lie laterally, whereas those terminating in cervical segments are more medially placed.

As proposed by Kuypers,[5] *descending brain stem pathways to the spinal cord* can be subdivided into a *medial* and a *lateral* group on the basis of their terminal distribution and functional properties. The distribution area of the medial group overlaps with that of ventral corticospinal fibers, whereas that of the lateral group overlaps with that of the lateral corticospinal or pyramidal tract (Fig. 1–11).

Medial group A (medial reticulospinal, vestibulospinal, interstitiospinal, and tectospinal tracts) is characterized by location in the ventral and ventrolateral white matter and, frequently, bilateral termination in the ventromedial part of the gray matter (medial lamina VII, lamina VIII, ventromedial motor neurons), an area that contains long and intermediate propriospinal neurons (see Fig. 1–10). These fibers display a high degree of collateralization and have some direct connections with motor neurons of neck, back, and proximal extremity muscles. Functionally, this system is concerned with the control of posture, synergistic whole-limb movements, and orientation movements of the body and head.

Lateral group B (rubrospinal tract and lateral pontine reticulospinal tracts) comprises contralaterally descending fibers that are situated in the dorsolateral fasciculus and are characterized by their termination in the dorsal and lateral parts of the intermediate gray matter (lateral laminae V–VI, VII, and dorsolateral motor neurons), an area containing short propriospinal neurons. Group B pathways establish monosynaptic connections with motor neurons of distal extremity muscles in primates and cats. These pathways show a low degree of collateralization in contrast to group A. Group B brain stem pathways seem to supplement the control exerted by the group A pathways and provide the capacity for independent, flexion-biased movements of the extremities and the shoulder and particularly of the elbow and hand.

In addition, several other subcortical nuclei project to the spinal gray matter. Fibers from solitary and retroambiguous nuclei innervate phrenic motor neurons and thoracic motoneuronal cell groups, subserving respiratory activity. The hypothalamus sends fibers to spinal autonomic regions, such as the intermediolateral column and the sacral parasympathetic nuclei. Catecholaminergic innervation of the spinal gray matter is provided by two pathways: (1) the ceruleospinal noradrenergic projection originating in the locus ceruleus and subceruleus and distributing to all parts of the gray matter, and (2) the tegmentospinal noradrenergic system originating from lateral pontine groups A5 and A7 and projecting to the intermediolateral column and the dorsal horn. Serotoninergic fibers to the dorsal horn, considered to convey supraspinal control of nociception, come from the raphe magnus nucleus via the dorsolateral fasciculus and project to laminae I and V. Serotoninergic neurons located in the more caudal nuclei raphe obscurus and pallidus innervate the intermediate gray matter and ventral horn via the ventral and ventrolateral white matter.

EFFERENT PATHWAYS. Several groups of spinal neurons emit axons that reach structures lying outside the spinal cord, that is, supraspinal centers or the periphery. The spinal output from somatic motor neurons is well known. The pathways from autonomic preganglionic cells are now reviewed briefly, including data concerning ascending pathways to supraspinal structures.

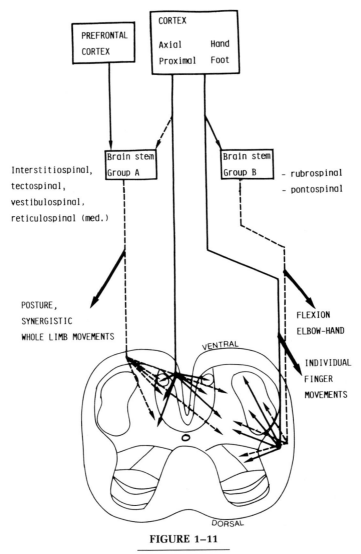

FIGURE 1–11

Descending systems to the spinal cord: origin, trajectory, spinal termination area, and major functions (see text for comments).

AUTONOMIC OUTFLOW. Preganglionic sympathetic and parasympathetic neurons of the spinal cord are located in the lateral aspect of the intermediate gray matter, that is, in the intermediolateral column and the parasympathetic sacral nuclei. Their myelinated axons exit the cord through ventral roots and then pass through the white ramus communicans. Preganglionic sympathetic neurons synapse either in the paravertebral sympathetic chain ganglia or in the prevertebral ganglia. The axons of the sympathetic ganglion cells are unmyelinated or thinly myelinated. Those that pass via the gray ramus communicans to spinal nerves supply the blood vessels, sweat glands, and hair follicles, and also form plexuses that supply the heart and bronchi. There are 3 cervical, 11 thoracic, and 4 to 6 lumbar paravertebral ganglia. The postganglionic fibers of the prevertebral ganglia (celiac and superior and inferior mesenteric ganglia) form the hypogastric, splanchnic, and mesenteric plexuses, which innervate the glands, smooth muscles, and blood vessels of the abdominal and pelvic viscera (Fig. 1–12). Preganglionic parasympathetic axons, conversely, travel all the way to the viscera being innervated and synapse

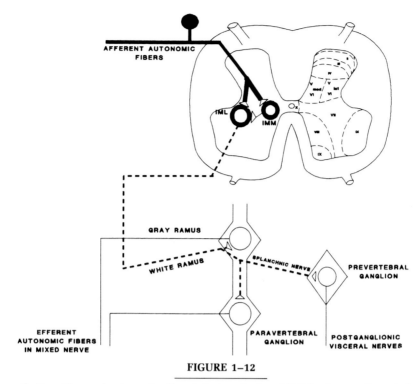

FIGURE 1–12

Sympathetic outflow and autonomic afferents in the spinal cord. IMM = Intermediomedial nucleus; IML = intermediolateral nucleus.

in either the myenteric plexus or the submucosal plexus.

ASCENDING PATHWAYS. Due to modern anatomic tracing methods and electrophysiologic experiments, data concerning the spinal ascending pathways are much more extensive and precise in animals than in humans. They are briefly summarized in the following text.

The *dorsal columns* comprise short, intermediate, and long systems of fibers. These fibers are not only from dorsal root afferents but also from second-order sensory neurons in the dorsal horn. The dorsal column pathway includes the fasciculus gracilis, containing ascending branches of afferents supplying the lower part of the body and hindlimbs, and the laterally located fasciculus cuneatus, which contains afferents from the upper part of the body and forelimbs. At the lower bulbar level, the gracile and cuneate fascicles synapse in the nuclei gracilis and cuneatus, respectively, also called the dorsal column nuclei (Fig. 1–13). Functionally, the dorsal column pathway is responsi-

ble for discriminative touch and limb proprioception.

Ventrolateral ascending pathways include portions of both the lateral and ventral funiculi. They contain spinothalamic and spinoreticular projections and convey pain, temperature, touch, and pressure information (see Fig. 1–13). The ventrolateral system is not compactly organized but is somewhat diffusely structured, intermingling with other ascending pathways. There is a general somatotopic tendency, such that axons arising from lower segments are located in a more dorsolateral position and those from higher levels in a more ventromedial position.

The *dorsal* and the *ventral spinocerebellar tracts* project sensation primarily from the lower extremities. The dorsal spinocerebellar tract is located at the periphery of the dorsolateral fasciculus and arises from the ipsilateral nucleus dorsalis of Clarke. It projects via the inferior cerebellar peduncle to the vermis and paravermal areas of the cerebellum in the hindlimb areas. Functionally, the dorsal spinocerebellar tract conveys in-

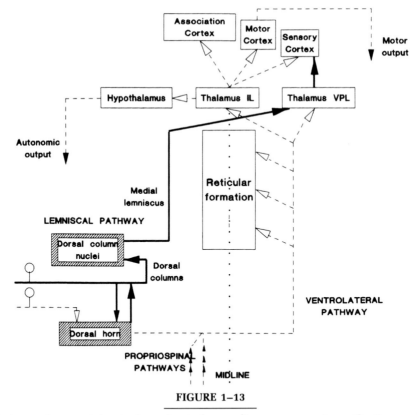

FIGURE 1–13

Trajectory, relays, and termination of spinal ascending sensory systems. Continuous lines: the lemniscal (dorsal column) pathway responsible for touch and proprioception. Dashed lines: the ventrolateral (spinothalamic) pain-conducting pathway. Arrowheads: propriospinal pain-conducting pathways. Thalamus IL = intralaminar thalamic nuclei; thalamus VPL = ventro-posterolateral thalamic nucleus (see text for comments).

formation from muscle spindles, Golgi tendon organs, joints, and touch and pressure receptors of the lower extremities. The ventral spinocerebellar tract is located at the periphery of the ventrolateral fasciculus (see Fig. 1–4). Its cells of origin are distributed in laminae V and VII of the lumbosacral segments. The tract enters the superior cerebellar peduncle to terminate in the vermal and paravermal regions of the anterior lobes of the cerebellum. As a result of its numerous polysynaptic inputs and larger receptive fields, the ventral spinocerebellar tract appears to relay information regarding the status of muscle groups and the entire extremity.

FUNCTIONAL ASPECTS AND CLINICAL IMPLICATIONS

Sensory Control at the Spinal Level

Somatic sensation is conveyed at the spinal level by two major ascending systems: the dorsal columns and the ventrolateral system (see Fig. 1–13). These systems relay afferent information to the brain for three purposes: perception, arousal, and motor control. They are parallel ascending pathways, and even though each subserves somewhat different functions, there is a degree of redundancy. Consequently, if one pathway is damaged, the other can provide residual perceptual capability.

TOUCH AND LIMB PROPRIOCEPTION: THE DORSAL COLUMN–MEDIAL LEMNISCUS SYSTEM. Afferents carrying tactile and proprioceptive information mostly ascend in the ipsilateral dorsal column; a small proportion of them terminate on dorsal horn neurons, the axons of which join the dorsal column. After a relay in the dorsal column nuclei, sensory information crosses through the medial lemniscus to the ventroposterolateral nucleus of the thalamus, from which it reaches the somatosensory cortex.

The dorsal columns are considered to be important for tactile discrimination as well as for vibratory and joint sensations. However, surgical lesions of the dorsal columns in humans produce only a minimal persistent sensory deficit. This is probably due to the fact that crude touch and pressure sensation can be mediated by the ventrolateral system. Recent findings suggest that the dorsal column pathways are involved in highly complex discriminative sensory tasks, such as two-point discrimination, judging the magnitude of cutaneous pressure, and the ability to detect the speed and direction of moving stimuli. Nevertheless, in clinical conditions in which the dorsal columns are affected, such as in subacute combined degeneration accompanying pernicious anemia or in neurosyphilis, there is loss of position and vibratory perception in the legs, causing unsteadiness of gait, i.e., sensory ataxia.

PAIN AND TEMPERATURE SENSE: THE VENTROLATERAL SYSTEM. Pain in humans is subserved by two distinct populations of peripheral afferent fibers. One consists of small, thinly myelinated A delta fibers, activated primarily by noxious heat and mechanical stimuli. The other consists of small, unmyelinated C fibers, the free nerve endings of which are activated by a variety of high-intensity mechanical, chemical, and thermal stimulation; they are therefore called polymodal nociceptors. Both types of fibers synapse on neurons in the superficial laminae of the dorsal horn (laminae I to III). Some A delta fibers terminate on lamina V cells. Several neuropeptides have been identified

within primary nociceptive afferent neurons. Among these, substance P is the best known. Evidence exists that neuropeptide-containing DRG neurons that convey afferent nociceptive information from peripheral tissues to the spinal cord are also involved in efferent regulation of the tissues they innervate. Efferent functions of these sensory neuropeptides include vasodilation, plasma extravasation, accumulation of leukocytes, mast cell degranulation, and regulation of the inflammatory, immune, and wound healing responses.

Second-order neurons, i.e., neurons postsynaptic to nociceptive afferents, give rise to the ascending ventrolateral system. Axons of most relay cells in lamina I project directly to the thalamus through the neospinothalamic tract. Cells located in deeper layers of the dorsal horn, especially lamina V, make up the phylogenetically older paleospinothalamic tract. In fact, this tract terminates primarily in the reticular formation of the brain stem and is therefore more appropriately called the spinoreticular tract. The ventrolateral system, especially the neospinothalamic component, is crossed in humans, but a small, albeit significant, ipsilateral component also exists. Crossing of axons occurs at the segmental level in the spinal cord through the ventral gray commissure (see Fig. 1–13).

Schematically, the spinothalamic tract mediates fast pain, whereas the spinoreticular tract is important in slow pain. The large contingent of fibers that goes to the reticular formation presumably explains the capability of noxious stimuli to produce behavioral activation and arousal. The periaqueductal gray matter of the midbrain, which also receives ventrolateral fibers, is probably a convergent area for limbic forebrain and sensory information; it may therefore be important in modulating pain input on the basis of emotional state.

During recent years, mainly from data obtained in animals, evidence has accumulated that processing of sensory information in the dorsal horn of the spinal cord is based on complex interactions between peripheral afferents, spinal neurons, and descending pathways. Two major classes of dorsal horn neurons have been recognized: nociceptive specific neurons located in lamina I and neurons responding to both non-noxious and noxious stimuli, called wide dynamic range or polymodal neurons, mainly confined to laminae IV and V. Sensory input is transferred to these neurons either directly by afferent terminals or indirectly via excitatory interneurons located in lamina II. Considering their axonal projections, lamina II curly and stellate cells could act as relays between peripheral afferents and spinothalamic neurons, respectively, in laminae I and IV of the human spinal cord. Several theories on the spinal modulation of pain inputs have been proposed, for example, the "gate control theory" or the model of "reciprocal sensory interaction." All of them postulate the presence of inhibitory interneurons in the superficial dorsal horn. In a strict anatomic sense, only lamina II islet cells are typical inhibitory interneurons. These neurons have an axonal network strictly confined to their dendritic territory. Nonetheless, they may influence laminae I and V projection neurons, which have dendrites crossing lamina II. Although definite experimental proof is still needed, the gate control theory has produced useful clinical predictions, for example, the suggestion that stimulation of the large-diameter peripheral and dorsal column fibers should close the gate and, thus, diminish pain. Indeed, direct or transcutaneous electrical stimulation of sensory nerves, particularly the dorsal columns, is used effectively for pain relief.

The anatomic organization of pain pathways in the spinal cord has important clinical implications. For instance, because axons of spinothalamic neurons cross segmentally in the ventral gray commissure, a lesion in the center of the spinal cord can abolish pain and temperature sensations, while touch as well as position and vibration sense, which are conveyed in the dorsal columns, can be spared. This type of dissociated sensory loss is found in syringomyelia. Alternatively, when a lesion such as a tumor arises in the innermost portion of the thoracic or cervical cord, it first compresses the most medial fibers from higher segments but may not affect the most lateral fibers originating in the sacral region. In such instances, all cutaneous sensation may be abolished below the level of the lesion, with the exception of the perineum, a phenomenon referred to as "sacral sparing." Neurosurgeons take advantage of the somatotopic organization of the spinothalamic tracts in anterolateral cordotomies performed for the control of intractable pain in the pelvis or legs. The spinothalamic tracts can be sectioned selectively under local anesthesia. When the scalpel enters the outer aspect of the spinal cord, it encounters the sacral fibers first. Unfortunately, recurrence of pain may follow the operation after variable delays, explained, in part, by the presence of uncrossed fibers in the ventrolateral system and by intraspinal polysynaptic, propriospinal pain-conducting pathways (see Fig. 1–13). The latter pathways also may be relevant concerning the efficacy of another procedure used to relieve intractable pain, commissural myelotomy.

Motor Control at the Spinal Level

The motor system is hierarchically organized and consists of separated neural circuits that are linked to each other: the spinal cord, the brain stem and reticular formation, the motor cortex, and the premotor cortical areas. The motor neurons of the spinal cord are the "final common pathway" of the motor systems. However, motor actions are chiefly coordinated at the interneuronal or proprioneuronal levels. The spinal cord is responsible for organizing the most automatic and stereotypical responses to stimuli. Even if disconnected from supraspinal input, the circuitry of the spinal cord is sufficient to generate a variety of automatic behaviors. In the intact nervous system, descending pathways onto interneurons or directly onto motor neurons control the final motor response. For example, automatic behaviors, such as segmental reflexes or locomotion that relies on networks of spinal interneurons called "step generators," are governed by inputs from higher centers. Some functional data on motor neurons, interneurons, and proprioneurons and their descending inputs are reviewed in the following text.

MOTOR NEURONS. The motor neurons are assembled in longitudinal columns located in lamina IX of the ventral horns. They can be subdivided into alpha and gamma motor neurons, the latter being of smaller size. Both types of neurons are intermingled in the motoneuronal columns. As described earlier, the motor neurons are somatotopically organized. Neurons that innervate proximal muscles are situated medially and those to distal muscles are situated laterally; in addition, motor neurons projecting to flexor muscles lie more dorsally than those innervating extensor muscles (Fig. 1–14). Alpha motor neurons innervate extrafusal muscle fibers. One motor axon contacts many muscle fibers, constituting the "motor unit." Gamma motor neurons project to the intrafusal fibers of the muscle spindles.

The dendritic organization found in the different motoneuronal columns can be related to their functional specialization. The longitudinal dendritic plexus with microbundles, observed in ventromedial motor neurons acting in the maintenance of posture, favors spatial summation along the longitudinal axis of a column and, consequently, synchronization and synergy, because motor neurons innervating a single muscle are grouped into a single longitudinal column and columns corresponding to synergistic muscles line up in the rostrocaudal axis of the cord. In contrast, the radial dendritic organization of the dorsolateral motor neurons, involved in fine, delicate movements of the extremities, permits only slight interactions between adjacent neurons and selective contacts with afferents. The transverse dendritic bundles found in ventromedial, central, and ventrolateral columns have a local, intrasegmental organization, because only adjacent motor neurons in the longitudinal axis participate in a given bundle. They could therefore act in phasic, focal modulation of the excitability of a motoneuronal pool. However, because of their close spatial relationship with the medial (group A) afferent system of the brain stem and the propriospinal system, they could also have at the lumbosacral level a function in centrally programmed activities such as walking. In accordance with the latter hypothesis, a parallelism between the ontogenic development of the transverse dendritic bundles of motor neurons and that of certain coordinated motor activities has been demonstrated in the cat and in humans.

Alpha motor neurons receive direct synaptic input from Ia afferents coming from the

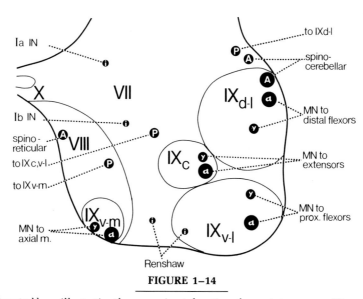

FIGURE 1–14

Diagram of ventral horn illustrating the approximate location of some interneurons (i), propriospinal neurons (P), ascending projection neurons (A), and the somatotopic organization of alpha (α) and gamma (γ) motor neurons.

spindles of the muscle they innervate. These afferents branch longitudinally within the motoneuronal columns. Such a parallel organization of terminals and motoneuronal dendrites permits multiple contacts with neurons projecting to the same muscle and to synergistic muscles. It has been estimated in the cat that a single Ia afferent may send synaptic terminals to several hundred motor neurons. The direct monosynaptic excitatory connection between alpha motor neurons and their corresponding Ia fibers is the anatomic basis of the stretch or myotatic reflex (Fig. 1–15). Stretch reflexes are most highly developed in physiologic extensors, the predominant action of which is to oppose gravity. Tapping a muscle tendon with a reflex hammer perturbs the corresponding muscle and produces an afferent volley that excites its motor neurons, leading to a brief contraction of the muscle. Tendon reflexes are clinically useful to assess at certain segmental levels the integrity of both afferent and motor connections as well as the general excitability of the spinal cord.

When activated, gamma motor neurons, which innervate intrafusal muscle fibers, can increase the sensitivity of the intrafusal muscle spindles, provoking increased Ia fiber firing from the muscle. The gamma loop may thus regulate the stretch reflex. It has been hypothesized that activation of the somatic muscle can also be brought about indirectly by activation of gamma motor neurons from higher centers. Some evidence suggests that coactivation of both alpha and gamma motor neurons occurs during movement. Although still controversial, the current view is that the gamma loop might function only to provide servo assistance in an auxiliary capacity; it is not responsible for the initiation of a movement, but it may still operate to assist in load or length compensation.

INTERNEURONS AND PROPRIONEURONS. Interneurons are cells that establish synapses with other neurons at the segmental level. All interneurons involved in motor control are localized in laminae V to VIII of the spinal gray matter. Axons of most of these neurons travel for a short distance in the white matter before reaching their targets. Interneurons are of paramount importance in spinal cord functions. They are interposed between peripheral or supraspinal afferents and the motor neurons but are also organized in networks capable of generating stereotypical

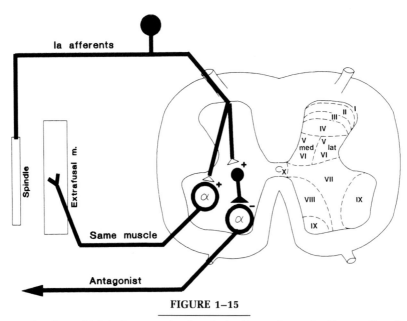

FIGURE 1–15

In the stretch reflex, which is the most simple spinal reflex pathway, Ia afferents directly excite alpha motor neurons to the same muscle. Concomitantly, they activate the inhibitory Ia interneuron, which inhibits alpha motor neurons to the antagonist muscle (reciprocal inhibition).

motor activities such as walking. One of the most fascinating recent advances in spinal cord physiology has been the ability to assess, in the living human subject, the activities of identified interneuronal classes.[2] This clinical neurophysiologic approach has led to a better understanding of the role of specific interneurons in the normal human cord and in several clinical syndromes. It has also provided insight into the neurotransmitters mediating spinal functions in humans and into the mechanisms of action of drugs used in neurologic therapy, such as antispastic agents. The following text is a summary of the physiology and function of some interneurons that can be assessed in humans.

The Ia inhibitory interneuron is intercalated between excitatory Ia fibers and alpha motor neurons controlling muscles that are antagonistic to those from which the Ia fibers originate (see Fig. 1–15). This permits Ia fibers to inhibit the antagonist motor neurons disynaptically, a phenomenon called reciprocal inhibition. Thus, as motor neurons to homonymous and synergist muscles are excited, motor neurons to antagonist muscles are inhibited. In addition to Ia afferents, the

Ia inhibitory interneuron receives input from many other sources (Fig. 1–16).

The Renshaw cell, another important inhibitory spinal interneuron, is directly excited from collateral branches of motor neurons. It inhibits many motor neurons, including the ones that give rise to its input. This process is called recurrent inhibition (Fig. 1–17). Its functional consequences are a tendency to curtail the motor output from a particular collection of motor neurons—a motor pool—and to highlight the output of motor neurons that are strongly activated. Moreover, because Renshaw cells also project directly to Ia inhibitory interneurons, they can limit the duration and magnitude of a Ia afferent-mediated reflex response by adding disinhibition of the antagonist motor neurons to inhibition of homonymous motor neurons. The inhibitory neurotransmitter used by Renshaw cells is probably glycine.

The Ib interneuron is excited by Ib afferents from Golgi tendon organs in the muscle. Ib inhibitory interneurons inhibit motor neurons to the muscle of origin and its synergists, whereas Ib excitatory interneurons excite the antagonists (Fig. 1–18). Central connections

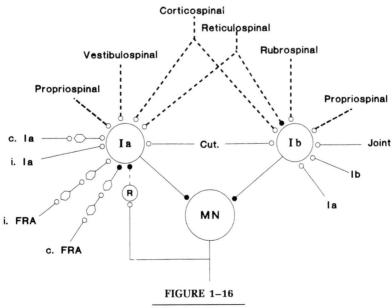

FIGURE 1–16

Diagram of peripheral, propriospinal, and descending afferents converging on Ia and Ib interneurons. Ia = Ia interneuron; MN = motor neuron; c. Ia = contralateral Ia afferents; i. Ia = ipsilateral afferents; i. FRA = ipsilateral flexor reflex afferents; c. FRA = contralateral flexor reflex afferents; Cut. = cutaneous afferents. Open circles: excitatory synapses; filled circles: inhibitory synapses.

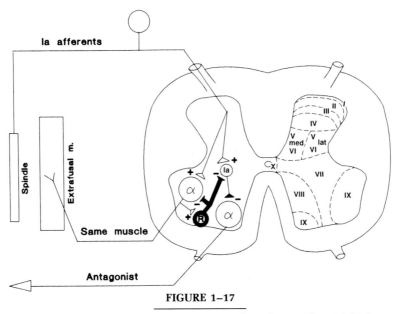

FIGURE 1–17

Renshaw cells (R), when stimulated by recurrent motor collaterals, are able to inhibit homonymous motor neurons as well as Ia inhibitory interneurons to antagonistic motor neurons. This recurrent inhibition limits the response induced by activation of a motor neuron pool.

of these afferents are more widespread than those of Ia afferents. The Golgi tendon system measures tension, whereas the spindle system measures length. It has therefore been proposed that the reflex action of Ib afferents functions as a tension feedback system, protecting the muscle from producing excessive tension. Some evidence suggests that Ib interneurons receive convergent short-latency excitation from low-threshold cutaneous afferents and from joint afferents, but also that they are modulated by descending inputs (see Fig. 1–16).

Interneurons of the flexor reflex pathway

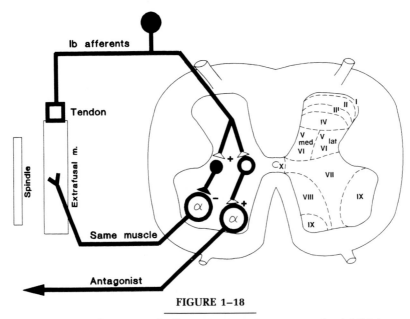

FIGURE 1–18

Afferents from Golgi tendon organs (Ib afferents) activate interneurons that inhibit homonymous motor neurons but excite antagonists. They may act as a tension feedback system.

are interposed between secondary afferent terminals from muscle spindles (group II), afferents from deep muscle receptors (group III), afferents from skin or joints, and interneurons or the motor neurons themselves. These afferents are collectively called flexor reflex afferents. Generally, these afferents produce a flexion response. Because most of them carry information about painful stimuli, the reflexes that they initiate serve as protective or escape responses. Flexor reflex afferents also project polysynaptically on Ia and Ib interneurons (see Fig. 1–16). They may give rise to ipsilateral flexion, usually accompanied by contralateral extension. However, the type of reflex action is strongly dependent on the quality and the location of the stimulus, as well as on the control from supraspinal afferents.

Proprioneurons (or propriospinal neurons) establish connections between distant spinal segments (see Fig. 1–10). Short proprioneurons send axons in the lateral funiculi that extend only a few segments. Long proprioneurons project mainly into the ventral funiculi and can extend the entire length of the spinal cord connecting the cervical with the lumbar enlargement. The latter are important for coordinating axial muscles during postural adjustments and limb girdle muscles during locomotion. Long priopriospinal neurons located in cervical regions can also be used for transfering supraspinal inputs to lower spinal segments. Short propriospinal neurons permit coordination of distal limb movements.

DESCENDING PATHWAYS. All spinal reflexes and interneuronal networks are under the control of descending efferents from the brain stem and the cerebral cortex. The descending pathways that act preferentially in motor control consist of the medial (or ventrolateral) group of fibers from the brain stem, the lateral (or dorsolateral) group of fibers from the brain stem (see the foregoing discussion), and the corticospinal (or pyramidal) tract.

The pyramidal tract establishes direct monosynaptic connections with motor neurons; the number of these connections progressively increases in the phylogeny of higher mammals from prosimians to apes and finally to humans. These connections are responsible for highly fractionated distal move-

ments, such as individual finger movements. Medial reticulospinal and lateral vestibulospinal fibers probably establish monosynaptic excitatory connections with motor neurons of neck and back muscles. The medial vestibulospinal tract has oligosynaptic inhibitory connections with many motor neurons of neck and back muscles. Rubrospinal fibers may, at least in the rhesus monkey, connect monosynaptically with motor neurons of the distal extremity muscles. As mentioned previously, the corticospinal pathway amplifies the motor control exerted by the descending brain stem pathway. Among the latter, the medial group is chiefly concerned with the control of posture, synergistic whole-limb movements, and orientation movements of the body and head. In contrast, the lateral group of brain stem pathways provides the capacity for independent flexion-biased movements of the extremities and the shoulder, and particularly of the elbow and hand (see Fig. 1–11).

In addition to the direct monosynaptic connections with motor neurons, the bulk of descending fibers establish contact with the various groups of spinal interneurons and proprioneurons described earlier (see Fig. 1–16). Interneurons can act as gates that enable or prevent peripheral input from affecting motor output. The way in which this gating is achieved is controlled by descending pathways that can engage spinal interneurons to enhance or suppress specific reflex actions. Gating also can be achieved directly by descending fibers through presynaptic actions on the terminals of afferent fibers due to axo-axonic contacts. Higher centers are thus capable of preselecting which of several possible responses will follow a certain stimulus at a given moment. This capability decreases the information processing required and eliminates the need for decisions in the interval between stimulus and response.

CONCLUSIONS

Recent structural and functional research on the spinal cord has produced an impressive body of information about this complexly organized nervous system structure. Particularly in human subjects and patients, the clinical neurophysiologic approach has provided invaluable data on spinal reflexes and interneuronal networks as well as on their selective modulation by higher centers. Morphologic studies of the human spinal cord have made major advances due to the application, to normal and pathologic human material, of morphometric studies and immunocytochemical or autoradiographic techniques permitting the identification of neurotransmitter systems and receptors.

Nonetheless, the gaps in our knowledge of the organization of the spinal cord in animals, and even more so in humans, remain varied and formidable. In coming years, the principal challenge in research on the human spinal cord will be to match physiologic and morphologic data. This will necessitate many more studies of normal subjects and selected pathologic disorders. Addressing specifically human material remains mandatory because of several organizational features that distinguish the human spinal cord from that of other mammals.

Acknowledgments

The work on which this chapter was based has been supported by research grants from the National Fund for Scientific Research (Brussels), the Queen Elisabeth Medical Foundation (Brussels), and the Research Fund of the University of Liège Faculty of Medicine (Liège), Belgium.

REFERENCES

1. Davidoff RA (ed): Handbook of the Spinal Cord, vols 2 and 3: Anatomy and Physiology, vol 1: Pharmacology. New York, Marcel Dekker, 1984.
2. Delwaide PJ: Electrophysiological testing of spastic patients: Its potential usefulness and limitations. In Delwaide PJ, Young RR (eds): Clinical Neurophysiology in Spasticity. Amsterdam, Elsevier Science Publishers, 1985, p 185.
3. Fazio C: Vascular pathology of the spinal cord. In Minckler J (ed): Pathology of the Nervous System, vol II. New York, McGraw-Hill, 1971, p 1548.
4. Irving D, Rebeiz JJ, Tomlinson BE: The numbers of limb motor neurones in the individual segments of the human lumbosacral spinal cord. J Neurol Sci 21:203, 1974.
5. Kuypers HG: Anatomy of the descending pathways. In Brooks VB (ed): Handbook of Physiology, sect 1, vol II, part I. Bethesda, American Physiological Society, 1981, p 597.
6. Rexed B: The cytoarchitectonic atlas of the spinal cord in the cat. J Comp Neurol 100:415, 1952.
7. Schoenen J: L'organisation neuronale de la moelle épinière de l'Homme. Liège, Belgium, Editions Sciences et Lettres, 1981.
8. Schoenen J: Spinal cord. In: Dulbecco R (ed): Encylopedia of Human Biology, vol 7. San Diego, Academic Press, 1991, pp 191–220.
9. Schoenen J, Faull RLM: Spinal cord: Cytoarchitectural, dendroarchitectural and myeloarchitectural organization and spinal cord: Chemoarchitectural organization. In Paxinos G (ed): The Human Nervous System. San Diego, Academic Press, 1990, p 19.
10. Schoenen J, Grant G: Spinal cord: Connections. In Paxinos G (ed): The Human Nervous System. San Diego, Academic Press, 1990, p 77.
11. Tomlinson BE, Irving D, Rebeiz JJ: Total numbers of limb motor neurones in the human lumbosacral cord and an analysis of the accuracy of various sampling procedures. J Neurol Sci 20:313, 1973.

CHAPTER 2

Some Observations on Spinal Cord Structure and Reflex Function

Robert A. Davidoff, M.D.
John C. Hackman, Ph.D.

For the most part, current interpretation of the neurologic examination and neurologic dysfunction in spinal disease is based on three assumptions: (1) that the spinal cord consists of simple circuits through which afferent inputs are converted into reflex responses; (2) that separate and isolated spinal reflex mechanisms use exclusive pathways to serve single muscles or small groups of synergistic muscles; and (3) that the spinal circuitry for reflex actions is separate and distinct from the circuitry governing automatic voluntary movement and the circuitry activated by descending pathways. These assumptions have resulted from attempts to view complicated questions of human motor and sensory function in terms of the conclusions drawn by Sherrington and colleagues from observing reflexes in simplified animal preparations. As a result, most analyses of reflexes and reflex pathways written for medical students, neurology residents, and clinical neurologists provide an oversimplified picture of the spinal cord, replete with primitive and misleading wiring diagrams of reflex connectivity.

This chapter presents and evaluates some important aspects of contemporary evidence about spinal reflex organization and function. The goal is to introduce research developments since the mid-1960s, which have disclosed a spinal cord apparatus composed of several kinds of neurons exquisitely fashioned to coordinate information from a variety of sources. These neuronal elements consist not only of fibers descending to the spinal segment from supraspinal sources, but also of all the neurons in the spinal segment, including the intraspinal portions of primary afferent fibers, interneurons whose axons do not exit from the neuraxis, and alpha and gamma motoneurons whose axons emerge from the cord in the ventral roots. Neurons in the spinal segment receive inputs from afferent, reflex, pattern-generating, and descending neuronal systems and act as nodal points onto which a variety of control mechanisms converge. Afferent impulses from the periphery and motor command signals descending from supraspinal centers combine with spinal reflex mechanisms and complex motor patterns for locomotion originating in spinal interneuronal generators. Such sensorimotor integration occurs largely at interneuronal levels where interneurons are shared by many descending, afferent, and segmental pattern-generating inputs[3] (Fig. 2–1). The spinal output funneled to muscle via alpha motoneurons is therefore not stereotyped but can be modified in ways determined by the moment-to-moment needs of the organism. Such flexible integration of information provides the substrate for rapid changes in reflex responses, for generation of

coordinated patterns for locomotion, and for error detection to improve the efficiency of motor responses.

CELLULAR ORGANIZATION OF THE SPINAL CORD

The spinal cord itself is organized in nine cell layers (laminae I–IX), together with a region around the central canal (lamina X) (Fig. 2–2). Seven of the laminae follow each other in a regular dorsoventral fashion; most of the ten extend the entire length of the cord.[74] This division into laminae is based on neuronal cell size, density, and staining characteristics determined by examination of thick Nissl-stained sections.

The ten laminae demonstrate a high degree of correlation with neuronal structure and function.[6] Thus, laminae I to V constitute the primary sensory receiving regions of the spinal gray matter and receive most of the cutaneous and visceral afferent inputs entering

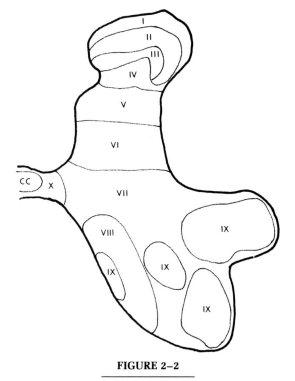

FIGURE 2–2

Cytoarchitectonic scheme for the human lumbar spinal cord; transverse section of segment L5. The laminae are designated by roman numerals. CC = central canal. (Adapted from Carpenter MB: Human Neuroanatomy. Baltimore, Williams & Wilkins, 1976.)

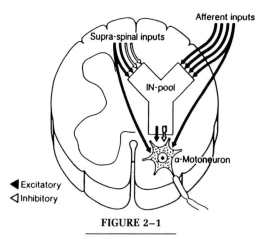

FIGURE 2–1

Schematic representation of a spinal cord segment showing how the majority of descending and afferent spinal inputs converge on interneurons (*IN-pool*). Only a small number of spinal inputs make monosynaptic connections with motoneurons. (Courtesy of Sandoz Pharmaceuticals Corporation.)

the cord via the dorsal roots. Interneurons involved in reflex transmission (e.g., Renshaw cells, Ia inhibitory interneurons, interneurons mediating group I nonreciprocal inhibition) are located in laminae V to VII. Lamina VIII contains many commissural neurons. Lamina IX contains alpha and gamma motoneurons. Lamina X consists of the area around the central canal and appears to process nociceptive information.

The intraspinal arborizations and terminations of primary afferent fiber axons are also organized according to the laminae of the cord.[6] For example, the small myelinated group III (A delta) and unmyelinated group IV (C) afferents originating in nociceptors and thermoceptors end mainly in laminae I and II, although group III fibers also send branches to lamina V. Coarse myelinated fibers go to deeper laminae. Mechanoceptive fibers of a wide range of axonal diameters project to laminae III, IV, and V and to the dorsal parts of VI. Group Ia, Ib, and II (A beta) muscle spindle and Golgi tendon organ afferents have terminals synapsing on interneurons in the intermediate region of the spinal cord (laminae V, VI, and VII). Group Ia and II afferents from muscle spindles also synapse on motoneurons in lamina IX (for a more detailed discussion, see Chapter 1).

THE MONOSYNAPTIC STRETCH REFLEX

The monosynaptic stretch reflex is usually depicted as the simplest or most basic of the reflexes. According to the traditional view, the group Ia afferents from primary endings on muscle spindles make excitatory synaptic contact with the alpha motoneurons that innervate the extrafusal muscle fibers of the same (homonymous) muscle. The resistance of muscle to stretch, however, involves a variety of interacting mechanisms that occur at peripheral, spinal, and supraspinal levels. These interacting mechanisms are different when the muscle is rapidly stretched (as when the tendon is tapped), when it is slowly stretched, or when the muscle that is being stretched is contracting (see following sections on The Tendon Jerk and Tone). In other

words, depending on the circumstances, the so-called simple stretch reflex may involve secondary group II afferents from the muscle spindle and group Ib afferents from the Golgi tendon organ, as well as several important classes of inhibitory interneurons (e.g., Renshaw cells, Ia inhibitory interneurons, interneurons mediating group I nonreciprocal inhibition). The reflex also involves presynaptic modulation (presynaptic inhibition), recruitment of various types of alpha motoneurons and their motor units, and interactions with other reflex mechanisms and descending fiber systems.

MUSCLE SPINDLES

The monosynaptic stretch reflex begins in the muscle spindle.[38, 46, 51, 63] The muscle spindle is a complex proprioceptive receptor that consists of specialized intrafusal muscle fibers, 4 to 20 of which are enclosed by a spindle-shaped connective tissue capsule. There are several major types of intrafusal muscle fibers: bag 1, bag 2, and chain fibers.[63] Intrafusal muscle fibers are striated except at the central portions where the sensory receptor endings are located (Fig. 2–3A). The striated portions of the intrafusal muscle fibers are innervated by fusimotor nerve fibers derived from gamma motoneurons.[67] The alpha motoneurons innervate the extrafusal muscle fibers. Because the tendinous ends of the intrafusal fibers project beyond the capsule to attach either to the tendon or to the perimysium of adjacent extrafusal muscle fibers, the intrafusal fibers are said to be arranged *in parallel* with ordinary extrafusal muscle fibers. Because the intrafusal fibers are organized *in parallel* with extrafusal muscle fibers, stretch of the extrafusal muscle containing the spindle stretches (*loads*) the central sensory region of the intrafusal muscle fibers and excites the afferent nerve endings.

Spindles contain two types of sensory receptor endings—primary endings located on all three types of intrafusal fibers of the spindle and secondary endings located principally on chain and bag 2 fibers. Both primary and secondary endings are stretch receptors, which respond to sustained, slower, steady-

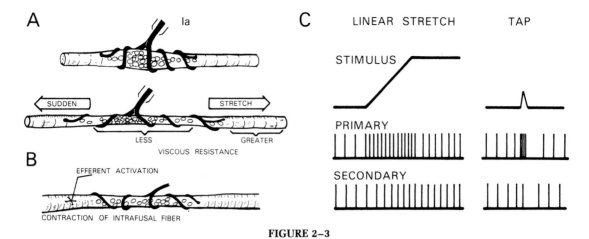

FIGURE 2–3

A, The primary spindle ending is distributed over the nucleated central region of the intrafusal muscle fibers and follows the length changes that are undergone by this central region. The noncontractile central portion has less viscous resistance to stretch than do the striated polar regions, and it would "give" under a stretch. *B*, Effect of fusimotor activation of intrafusal muscle fiber. Shortening of the striated contractile poles of the muscle fiber stretches the noncontractile nucleated central zone of the fiber. Sensory terminals wrapped around this zone are stretched and their discharge is increased. (*A* and *B* adapted from Eldred E: Peripheral receptors: their excitation and relation to reflex patterns. Am J Phys Med 46:69–87, 1967). *C*, Diagrammatic responses of 'typical' primary and secondary spindle endings to stretch and tendon tap. (Adapted from Matthews PBC: Muscle spindles and their motor control. Physiol Rev. 44:219–288, 1964).

state changes in the length of the nonstriated central region of the intrafusal muscle fibers (*static component*). In addition to signaling changes in length, primary endings are very sensitive to the rate of change and therefore have the capacity to signal the velocity at which the central region is being lengthened (*dynamic component*). Because of its sensitivity to the rate of change of length, the primary ending is the only proprioceptor capable of responding to rapid, small muscle stretches. In contrast, both primary and secondary endings respond to more sustained, slower stretches of muscle (Fig. 2–3*C*).

Two types of fusimotor nerve fibers—static and dynamic—innervate the striated contractile polar regions of intrafusal fibers. The dynamic fusimotor fibers dramatically increase the responsiveness of primary spindle sensory endings to transient length changes and lead to a relatively large afferent input for rapid, small extensions of muscle length. Such an effect is necessary not only to produce rapid corrections for the changes of muscle length seen during postural variations but also to provide regulation of alpha motoneuron firing and consequent muscle

contractions when small fluctuations in resistance are encountered.

Because spindles lie in parallel with the extrafusal muscle fibers, contraction of the latter unloads the spindles, and they stop firing unless the striated portion of the intrafusal fibers contracts and shortens enough to compensate for the effects of extrafusal muscle shortening. Firing of static fusimotor fibers rapidly shortens the intrafusal muscle fibers and maintains the sensitivity of spindles to changes in extrafusal fibers over a wide range of muscle lengths during reflex and voluntary contraction. Firing of dynamic fusimotor fibers cannot cause contraction of the intrafusal fibers rapidly enough to overcome the unloading effects of extrafusal muscle shortening. As seen in Figure 2–3*B*, the spindle receptors can also be stretched and excited to discharge by fusimotor firing in the absence of any change in extrafusal muscle length.

Gamma motoneurons, the source of fusimotor fibers, are small (10–30 μm) cells located in lamina IX of the ventral horn; they are scattered among the pool of alpha motoneurons that innervate the extrafusal muscle fibers of the same muscle. The two subgroups of gamma motoneurons—those that give rise to dynamic fusimotor fibers and those that give rise to static fusimotor fibers—can be differentially controlled by several different descending fiber systems.[63] Although some details are lacking, it is clear that many of the same descending neuronal pathways as well as segmental neuronal pathways synapse on both the alpha and gamma motoneurons supplying the extrafusal and intrafusal muscle fibers in a given muscle or a group of synergistic muscles. This means that activation of many descending and reflex systems evokes parallel effects in alpha and gamma motoneurons. A largely congruent synaptic input from descending and segmental fibers permits simultaneous activation (coactivation) of alpha and gamma motoneurons during motor and reflex acts.

The lack of monosynaptic Ia-mediated excitation of gamma motoneurons is a notable exception to the parallel ordering of synaptic inputs to alpha and gamma motoneurons, although excitation from Ia fibers may reach gamma motoneurons by means of polysynaptic pathways.[23] In addition to fusimotor fibers from gamma motoneurons, significant numbers of beta axons (skeletofusimotor fibers) innervate both extrafusal and intrafusal muscle fibers.[57] Skeletofusimotor fibers are collaterals of motor axons going from alpha motoneurons to extrafusal muscle fibers and receive a monosynaptic input from muscle spindles. Firing of skeletofusimotor fibers ensures a fixed coactivation of extrafusal and intrafusal muscle fibers and helps to preserve spindle sensitivity during muscle contraction.

ANATOMY OF GROUPS Ia AND II AFFERENT FIBERS

The primary endings on muscle spindles give rise to group Ia afferent fibers, the largest of the myelinated afferent fibers and the ones that conduct impulses the most rapidly. On entering the spinal cord, Ia fibers branch in such a way that rostral and caudal stem axons ascend and descend in the dorsal columns. From these stem axons about six to eight ma-

jor collateral branches arise. As illustrated in Figure 2–4A, the branches arborize in lamina VI to synapse on spinocerebellar tract cells, move laterally to branch in the area of Ia inhibitory interneurons (lamina VII), and terminate on alpha motoneurons in the motor nuclei of lamina IX.[7] Generally, a single Ia afferent fiber makes multiple synaptic contacts on the surface of each alpha motoneuron (Fig. 2–4C). Some branches of Ia fibers project monosynaptically to alpha motoneurons of the same muscle from which they arise (homonymous connections) and, in general, a single Ia afferent sends terminals to virtually all homonymous alpha motoneurons. In turn, each alpha motoneuron receives monosynaptic innervation from all of the Ia fibers originating in the homonymous muscle.[66] But, substantial monosynaptic connections of Ia fibers with alpha motoneurons of synergistic muscles are also made.[24, 25] Moreover, disynaptic and trisynaptic pathways activated by Ia afferents dispense excitation onto an extensive assortment of motoneuron species.

After entering the spinal cord via the dorsal root, group II afferent fibers from secondary muscle spindle sensory endings send collaterals to synapse on interneurons in the intermediate gray matter (laminae VII) before projecting to the motoneuron nuclei in lamina IX. The group II input to lamina IX is less extensive than that of Ia fibers.

ALPHA MOTONEURONS

The cell bodies of all alpha motoneurons lie within circumscribed motor cell columns (pools) in lamina IX within the ventral horn. The alpha motoneurons innervating a particular muscle are tightly packed in elongated, longitudinal nuclear columns that have a somatotopic arrangement.[75] Accordingly, motoneurons from related muscles are located near one another so that a dorsolateral group innervates distal musculature, while a ventromedial group innervates axial muscles.

Alpha motoneurons are large cells whose soma diameters range from approximately 30 to 70μm.[12, 14, 39] Cell size correlates with

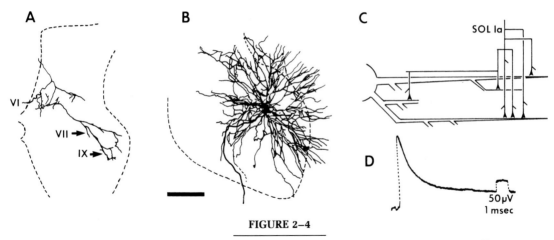

FIGURE 2–4

A, Reconstruction in the transverse plane of a collateral branch of a cat gastrocnemius Ia afferent fiber. The collateral gives off other branches that arborize in laminae VI, VII, and IX. (Adapted from Brown AG, Fyffe REW: Morphology of group Ia afferent fibre collaterals in the spinal cord of the cat. J Physiol (Lond) 274:111–127, 1978). B, Reconstruction of a horseradish peroxidase–injected cat lumbar alpha motoneuron. This is a composite of tracings made from serial cross sections. Scale = 0.5 mm. Note the extensive branching dendritic tree that provides an ample surface area for the very large number of synaptic connections. (From Ulfhake B, Kellerth J-O: Electrophysiological and morphological measurements in cat gastrocnemius and soleus α-motoneurons. Brain Res 307:167–179, 1984). C, Diagram of the location of the synapses of a single soleus Ia fiber on a cat soleus motoneuron. The synapses are on proximal dendrites. (From Burke RE, Walmsley B, Hodgson JA: HRP anatomy of group Ia afferent contacts on alpha motoneurons. Brain Res 160:347–352, 1979). D, Excitatory postsynaptic potential (EPSP) produced in a cat gastrocnemius motoneuron by an impulse in a single Ia afferent fiber. (From Munson JB, Sypert GW: Properties of single fibre excitatory post-synaptic potentials in triceps surae motoneurones. J Physiol (Lond) 296:329–342, 1979).

function, which is discussed in subsequent sections. Between 8 and 20 primary dendrites leave each cell body and branch many times (Fig. 2–4B). Each dendrite ranges in length from 1.0 to 1.5 mm and provides the surface membrane for the estimated 20,000 to 50,000 synaptic endings present on a given cell, the number of synapses being a function of alpha motoneuron size.

Electrophysiologic analysis and anatomic data indicate that most synapses made by Ia fibers on alpha motoneurons are located on the proximal half of the dendritic tree (Fig. 2–4C).[9] Such synapses make up approximately 5% of the synapses on an alpha motoneuron.[84] Each alpha motoneuron acquires monosynaptic innervation from the Ia fibers that originate from spindles in the homonymous muscle, and each Ia fiber establishes multiple excitatory synaptic contacts on the surface of a single homonymous alpha motoneuron. In addition, alpha motoneurons re-ceive significant synaptic connections from Ia afferents emanating from muscle spindles in heteronymous synergistic muscles acting at the same and even at distant joints.

Stimulation of the Ia fibers releases the neurotransmitter L-glutamic acid, which produces a depolarizing potential—the monosynaptic excitatory postsynaptic potential (EPSP)[73] (Fig. 2–4D). If the EPSPs produced by activation of Ia-fiber alpha motoneuron synapses and other excitatory synapses (from group II afferents, interneurons, and descending fibers) attain a critical threshold level, the alpha motoneuron discharges an impulse. Impulses are normally generated in the initial unmyelinated segment of the motoneuron axon because this is the most excitable region of the motoneuron.[13] The force developed by a muscle in response to firing of alpha motoneurons in the pool is established in large measure by the number of alpha motoneurons recruited by the excitatory synaptic input and by the rate of discharge of the recruited alpha motoneurons.

MOTOR UNITS

Sherrington defined the motor unit as an alpha motoneuron together with the bundle of muscle fibers innervated by that motoneuron. Under normal circumstances, when an alpha motoneuron fires, all of the muscle fibers innervated by that motoneuron contract. Although there is wide variation among motor units, the membrane properties and firing characteristics of alpha motoneurons are correlated with the speed of contraction, tension output, and histochemistry of the muscle fibers innervated by them.[11]

There appear to be two principal types of motor units in limb and trunk muscles of mammals. Chiefly on the basis of the mechanical properties of the innervated muscle fibers, the two types of motor units are designated as slow-twitch (S) and fast-twitch (F) types. Type S motor units consist of small numbers of small-diameter muscle fibers that contract slowly, develop small tetanic and twitch tensions, and are notably resistant to fatigue when stimulated repetitively. The muscle fibers of type S motor units are red, have a high rate of oxidative metabolism, and have a low glycogen content. The alpha motoneurons in type S motor units have both smaller cell bodies and smaller-diameter, slower-conducting axons than do type F alpha motoneurons. They typically discharge at a slow rate but can do so for a long time. Type S motor units are important for the maintenance of posture when muscle fibers have to contract for prolonged periods.

In contrast, F type motor units contain large numbers of large-diameter muscle fibers that contract rapidly and develop large tetanic and twitch tensions. Type F units are divided into relatively fatigable and fatigue-resistant subgroups. Relatively fatigable fibers fatigue rapidly when stimulated repetitively, but fatigue-resistant fibers are almost as resistant to fatigue as are S type muscle fibers. In general, relatively fatigable muscle fibers appear pale, are equipped with the appropriate enzymes for anaerobic metabolism, and contain a high glycogen content. In contrast, fatigue-resistant fibers tend to resemble slow units and are more dependent upon oxidative metabolism than fatigable fibers. Alpha motoneurons that innervate type F motor units are larger and have larger-diameter, faster-conducting axons than do type S alpha motoneurons. Relatively fatigable type F alpha motoneurons typically discharge in brief, high-frequency bursts. These motor units are used for all types of movements but are essential for the high velocities and forces of contraction needed for strenuous muscle activity.

SIZE PRINCIPLE

Most of the time when voluntary or reflex contractions occur, alpha motoneurons appear to fire in order of increasing size (size principle).[4, 39, 40] Accordingly, when excitation provided by afferent and descending synaptic inputs to motoneuron pools causes individual alpha motoneurons to fire, cell size (e.g., surface area of soma and dendrites), together with morphologic, electrophysiologic, and synaptic factors that correlate with motoneuron size, determines the order of firing (recruitment). Small motor units are recruited earliest by muscle stretch; the larger units are engaged later.

The pattern of recruitment is a reflection, in part, of an inverse relationship between the number of functional Ia boutons per unit of membrane surface area and the motor unit type. Thus, the smaller type S alpha motoneurons receive a greater number of functional Ia boutons per unit of membrane surface area than do type F alpha motoneurons and, as a result, Ia EPSPs are generally larger in cells of type S units than in cells of type F units. In addition, type S alpha motoneurons have electrical membrane properties that make them more excitable to synaptic inputs than type F alpha motoneurons.[70]

The size principle is of functional significance for it determines, in part, how the central nervous system uses the firing alpha motoneurons in a motoneuron pool to control the production of muscle force. Orderly recruitment of small motor units that produce low-twitch and tetanic forces before recruitment of large motor units that produce high-twitch and tetanic tensions permits increments of force to develop at any level of muscle contraction.

INTERNEURONS

In the past, alpha motoneurons were regarded as the principal nodal points for the integration of synaptic information derived from interneurons, afferents, and descending fibers. Interneurons were considered simple relay stations intercalated in some spinal reflexes. However, increasing data now indicate that most integrative functions in the spinal cord are in fact mediated by interneurons. Both descending command signals to the segmental motor system and spinal inputs from peripheral sensory receptors are largely directed to interneurons. Thus, the interneurons involved in every segmental reflex pathway are excited, inhibited, or both by several sets of peripheral afferent and descending fiber systems and can be shared by these systems.[59] Interneurons operate as common paths for impulses from different sources much in the same way that alpha motoneurons operate as final common paths for all signals that contribute to muscle activation.

It is an outdated assumption that afferent fibers of different types and various descending fiber systems exert their reflex actions completely independently of one another via separate and distinct groups of interneurons. In reality, transmission through a reflex pathway involving a particular set of interneurons is not simply determined by the excitatory input from a single set of primary afferents. The pathway is also opened or closed (gated) by virtue of the summation of excitatory and inhibitory inputs from other afferent systems, from other interneurons, and from descending fibers. It is no longer acceptable to assume that activation of peripheral receptors produces stereotyped responses. In other words, stimulation of a set of peripheral receptors can produce different motor responses at dif-

ferent times depending on the activity *at that time* of other sensory receptors and descending pathways.

RENSHAW CELLS

Renshaw cells are a type of interneuron located in lamina VII of the ventral horn medial to the motoneuronal cell columns.[3, 13, 71, 86] Renshaw cells are excited by collateral branches of alpha motoneuron axons, and in turn Renshaw cell axons make inhibitory synaptic contacts (which release the neurotransmitters glycine and gamma-aminobutyric acid [GABA]) with alpha motoneurons and produce hyperpolarizing inhibitory postsynaptic potentials (IPSPs) in alpha motoneurons. Thus, when an alpha motoneuron discharges, the collaterals of the motoneuron axon excite the Renshaw cells and, in turn, the Renshaw cells inhibit the alpha motoneuron (Fig. 2–5). Synaptic excitation of alpha motoneurons innervating a given muscle and activation of the Renshaw cell pathway produce recurrent IPSPs that are largest in alpha motoneurons of the same motor nucleus, but other alpha motoneurons innervating muscles with synergistic actions are also strongly inhibited. The alpha motoneuron–Renshaw cell–alpha motoneuron pathway forms a "negative feedback" circuit and serves to both stabilize and limit the discharge frequency of strongly activated alpha motoneurons.

Renshaw cells may, however, have functions more complex than that of simple negative feedback.[3, 71] For example, as can be seen in Figure 2–5, Renshaw cells inhibit not only alpha motoneurons but also gamma motoneurons and Ia inhibitory interneurons.[55] In addition, Renshaw cells are subject to direct excitatory and inhibitory influences via segmental afferents originating from both peripheral cutaneous and muscle receptors and also from descending fibers from supraspinal structures. The existence of an elaborate convergence from a number of reflex pathways and descending tracts indicates that, under certain conditions, the amount of Renshaw cell activity can determine the amount of mo-

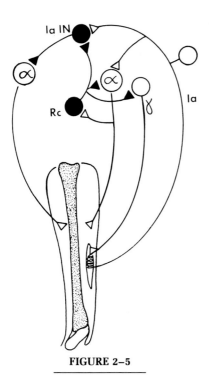

FIGURE 2–5

Schematic illustration of inhibitory connections made by a Renshaw cell (*Rc*) on an alpha motoneuron (α), a gamma motoneuron (γ), and an Ia inhibitory interneuron (*Ia IN*). The Ia afferent fiber (*Ia*) to the alpha motoneuron synapse is also shown. Inhibitory interneurons (Renshaw cells, Ia inhibitory interneurons) are shown in black. (From Pompeiano O: Recurrent inhibition. *In* Davidoff R (ed): Handbook of the Spinal Cord, vol 2 and 3. New York, Dekker, 1984, pp 461–557.)

toneuronal firing and the corresponding amount of muscle force.

INTERNEURONS THAT MEDIATE RECIPROCAL Ia INHIBITION

Stretch of a muscle that activates Ia afferent fibers not only produces monosynaptic excitation of homonymous alpha motoneurons, but also results in disynaptic inhibition of the alpha motoneurons that innervate antagonist muscles (reciprocal inhibition)[20,47] (Fig. 2–6). As illustrated in Figure 2–6C, the inhibition is mediated by Ia inhibitory interneurons interposed between the Ia afferent fibers and the alpha motoneurons. Like Renshaw cells, Ia inhibitory interneurons secrete the neurotransmitter glycine. Ia inhibitory interneurons are located within an area just

dorsal and dorsomedial to the motor nuclei in lamina VII (Fig. 2–6A).

The Ia inhibitory interneuron was formerly regarded as a convenient device that enabled a single spinal afferent input to produce both excitation of one set of alpha motoneurons and concomitant inhibition of another set. However, it is now solidly established that Ia inhibitory interneurons receive the same wide and diverse convergence of excitatory and inhibitory inputs from a variety of segmental and supraspinal sources as do alpha motoneurons (Fig. 2–6C).[48,49] Presumably, collateral branches of the same afferents and descending fibers innervate both sets of neurons. This ensures that spinal cord inputs from a variety of sources (e.g., primary afferents, corticospinal, rubrospinal, and vestibulospinal tracts) produce excitation of alpha motoneurons and contraction of synergistic muscles and excitation of Ia inhibitory interneurons with inhibition of alpha motoneurons to antagonist muscles during activation of the monosynaptic stretch reflex as well as during more complex activities, such as maintenance of postures and performance of volitional and locomotory movements.[29]

GROUP II AFFERENT FIBERS

The role of group II afferents in reflex activity has been the subject of dispute. According to most texts, volleys in group II afferents disynaptically excite flexor alpha motoneurons and inhibit extensor alpha motoneurons. In other words, excitation of secondary spindle endings elicits a flexion reflex. More recent evidence, however, indicates that group II afferents also contribute significantly to the stretch reflex. There are convincing data that discharges in group II fibers make monosynaptic excitatory connections with alpha motoneurons of homonymous muscles in parallel with the pathway from primary spindle endings involving Ia fibers.[83] The monosynaptic connection is relatively weak, however, and the main connections of group II afferents to alpha motoneurons are polysynaptic.

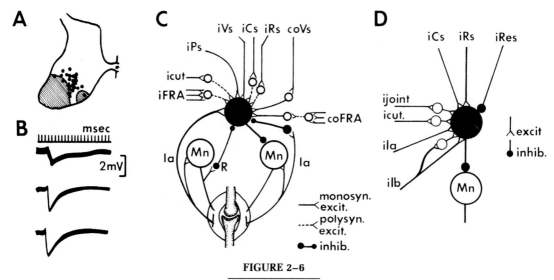

FIGURE 2–6

Ia inhibitory interneurons and interneurons mediating group I nonreciprocal inhibition. *A*, Diagram illustrating the location of Ia inhibitory interneurons dorsomedial to the motor nuclei (*shaded area of ventral horn*) in cat lumbar spinal cord. (From Hultborn H, Jankowska E, Lindström S: Recurrent inhibition of interneurones monosynaptically activated from group Ia afferents. J Physiol (Lond) 215:613–635, 1971). *B*, Inhibitory postsynaptic potentials (IPSPs) produced by increasing strengths of stimulation of group Ia afferents in nerve from quadriceps muscle and recorded in antagonistic hamstring alpha motoneuron. Records formed from superimposition of about 40 oscilloscope traces. (Adapted from Curtis DR, Eccles JC: The time courses of excitatory and inhibitory synaptic actions. J Physiol (Lond) 145:529–546, 1959.) *C*, Connections of Ia inhibitory interneuron (*large black central circle*) showing convergence of excitatory and inhibitory inputs from a variety of segmental and supraspinal sources. i = Ipsilateral; co = contralateral; Vs = vestibulospinal tract; Cs = corticospinal tract; Rs = Rubrospinal tract; Res = reticulospinal fibers; Ps = propriospinal tract; cut = cutaneous afferents; FRA = flexor reflex afferents; Mn = alpha motoneuron; R = Renshaw cell. *D*, Circuit diagram summarizing most of the neuronal connections to interneurons mediating group I nonreciprocal inhibition. Again, note extensive convergence of synaptic input. (Abbreviations as in *C*.) (*C* and *D* adapted from Baldisera F, Hultborn H, Illert M: Integration in spinal neuronal systems. *In* Brooks VB (ed): Handbook of Physiology, vol 2. Bethesda, Md, American Physiological Society, 1981, pp 509–595.)

GOLGI TENDON ORGANS, GROUP Ib AFFERENTS, AND INTERNEURONS MEDIATING GROUP I NONRECIPROCAL INHIBITION

Tendon organs are tension receptors. They consist largely of collagenous fascicles and sensory nerve endings encased in spindle-shaped connective tissue capsules that lie in the myotendinous or myoaponeurotic junction in series with the ends of extrafusal muscle fibers. Tendon organs respond selectively to *active* tension produced by contraction of any one of the 10 to 20 single extrafusal muscle fibers that insert on the tendinous fascicle associated with the receptor.[42] Tendon organs have a very high threshold for excitation by passive extension of the muscle.

Group Ib afferent fibers arising from tendon organs end on interneurons located in lamina VI.[8] These interneurons form widespread inhibitory synapses with alpha motoneurons to both homonymous and heteronymous muscles. The inhibitory circuit formed by Ib afferents, Ib inhibitory interneurons, and alpha motoneurons suggested to early investigators that Ib fibers from tendon organs provided the afferent limb of an inhibitory safety mechanism that reflexly reduced muscle contraction whenever tension became dangerously high. This concept must be discarded because (1) tension produced by *passive* extension of the muscle does not excite tendon organs, and (2) group Ib afferents from many muscles acting at the same and at different joints converge onto single interneurons and, in turn, each interneuron forms widespread inhibitory synapses with both homonymous and heteronymous alpha motoneurons.[30, 37, 52, 60]

The inhibitory interneurons activated by Ib afferent fibers were originally designated as Ib inhibitory interneurons, but most not only are excited by Ib afferents, but also are controlled by group Ia muscle spindle afferents.[30] Thus, these interneurons are excited in a parallel manner by *both* Ia and Ib afferents, and, as a result, they have been designated as interneurons mediating group I nonreciprocal inhibition.[35–37, 52, 53] In addition, similar to Renshaw cells and Ia inhibitory interneurons, interneurons mediating group I nonreciprocal inhibition receive a wealth of convergent inputs. Interneurons mediating group I nonreciprocal inhibition are shared by many segmental and supraspinal systems and, as a result, their activity may only partially convey information about the activity of Ib afferents (Fig. 2–6D). Because the afferent information furnished by Ib afferents is integrated with the information from these other sources, the effects of tendon organs should be viewed as part of a complex system that regulates muscle tension during maintenance of posture and during movement.

PRESYNAPTIC INHIBITION

Not only do volleys of impulses in appropriate sets of afferent fibers entering the spinal cord evoke reflex responses, but the same volleys can also cause long-lasting (100–150 msec) decrements in the amplitude of EPSPs produced in alpha motoneurons by afferent activity from muscle, tendon, joint, and cutaneous receptors.[22, 81] Because neither detectable changes in alpha motoneuron membrane potential and excitability nor the production of IPSPs accompanies this inhibition of EPSPs, it is thought to result from a decrease in the presynaptic release of excitatory transmitter from primary afferent terminals, i.e., the inhibition is presynaptic.[22, 76] Presynaptic inhibition is hypothesized to result from the release of the neurotransmitter GABA from axo-axonic synapses formed by the terminals of specific interneurons and the terminals of primary afferent axon terminals (Fig. 2–7).[21, 31]

The afferent volleys that cause presynaptic inhibition generate a slow depolarization of the terminals of primary afferent fibers—a process called primary afferent depolarization (PAD). It has been hypothesized that either the PAD itself or the processes responsible for the generation of PAD—namely, an increase in chloride conductance—are the causal factors in the inhibition responsible for the EPSP reduction.[22]

Several relatively complex input-output patterns have been described for primary afferent depolarization and presynaptic inhibition (Fig. 2–8). These input-output patterns depend on which type of afferent fiber is stimulated and which type of afferent fiber receives primary afferent depolarization.[81] In

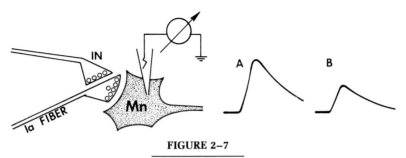

FIGURE 2–7

Presynaptic inhibition of group Ia-induced excitation of an alpha motoneuron. Schematic diagram illustrates axoaxonic synapse made by the terminal of an interneuron (*IN*) on the presynaptic terminal of a Ia afferent (*Ia fiber*). *A*, An impulse in the Ia afferent produces EPSPs recorded with a microelectrode placed in an alpha motoneuron (*Mn*). *B*, An EPSP of reduced amplitude is produced by stimulation of same Ia fiber when the stimulation is preceded by a discharge of the interneuron. The membrane potential of the motoneuron is unchanged during the inhibitory process. (Adapted from Schmidt RF: Fundamentals of Neurophysiology. New York, Springer-Verlag, 1975.)

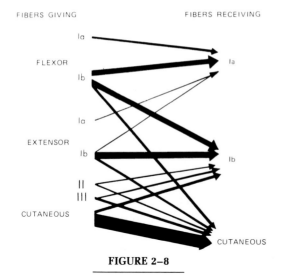

FIBERS GIVING   FIBERS RECEIVING

FIGURE 2–8

Diagram of afferent fibers producing depolarization of group I and large cutaneous fibers. The widths of the arrows are approximately proportional to the amounts of primary afferent depolarization (PAD) that are produced in each case. (Adapted from Eccles JC, Schmidt RF, Willis WD: Depolarization of central terminals of group Ib afferent fibers from muscle. J Neurophysiol 26:1–27, 1963.)

general, activity in muscle afferents inhibits other muscle afferents. For example, release of transmitter by Ia afferents is reduced mainly by volleys in Ia and Ib afferents from ipsilateral muscles. Presynaptic inhibition can also be generated by activation of pathways descending from the sensorimotor cortex, red nucleus, reticular formation, and vestibular nuclei.[79]

A polysynaptic pathway that includes at least two interneurons is involved.[54] Some of the interneurons, however, synapse both on afferent fibers and on alpha motoneurons.[78, 82] Thus, they can diminish reflexes by causing presynaptic inhibition of transmitter release from afferent fiber terminals and by producing IPSPs in alpha motoneurons.[78]

Because both descending and afferent volleys can presynaptically influence the efficacy of afferent proprioceptive and cutaneous inputs to the spinal cord, it appears that the transmitter release from activated afferent fibers involved in reflex activity is not an inflexible process. Thus, the ability of afferent proprioceptive spinal inputs varies over time depending on what other afferent and descending spinal inputs are firing. Moreover,

the balance between Ia and Ib inputs converging on interneurons and motoneurons can be manipulated by spinal presynaptic inhibitory mechanisms.[77] The presynaptic inhibitory circuits can be optimized to favor either muscle spindle–determined position feedback or Golgi tendon organ–determined tension feedback. Moreover, the system has the ability to selectively suppress particular sensory signals while leaving interneurons and motoneurons free to receive information from other uninhibited afferent and descending systems.

FLEXOR REFLEX AFFERENTS

In general, when high-threshold myelinated muscle, cutaneous, and joint afferents are stimulated electrically, a flexion reflex occurs, i.e., EPSPs are produced in flexor motoneurons and IPSPs are produced in extensor motoneurons.[26] As a result of observation of these phenomena, high-threshold myelinated afferents have long been thought to constitute a system of flexor reflex afferents with a more or less uniform reflex function. This unitary and simplistic formulation, however, is not adequate.[3] In fact, the term *flexor reflex afferents* is itself misleading because it connotes a stereotyped withdrawal response to stimulation of high-threshold afferents, even though it has been realized for many years that responses to flexor reflex afferents are highly dependent on supraspinal structures that have the ability to gate and switch pathways activated by flexor reflex afferents by affecting the excitability of interneurons intercalated in the spinal pathways. Furthermore, interneurons intercalated in the reflex pathways activated by discharges in the flexor reflex afferents are excited by different supraspinal structures and therefore may be used by the central nervous sytem to mediate descending commands for movement.[59] It is now hypothesized that flexor reflex afferents from joints and skin excited during movements of a limb set the excitability of a variety of interneurons and thereby facilitate or inhibit transmission of information through reflexes activated by excitation of muscle and tendon receptors.[47, 59, 61]

DESCENDING PATHWAYS

Descending fiber systems make extensive monosynaptic contacts with different types of alpha motoneurons and interneurons.[13, 56, 68] These fiber systems can be classified into two major categories. One category consists of the pontine reticulospinal and the lateral vestibulospinal tracts. Both tracts descend in the ventral funiculus of the spinal cord and terminate on ventromedially situated alpha motoneurons, which innervate proximal musculature mainly concerned with postural activities including extension of lower limbs and flexion of upper limbs. The pontine reticulospinal and the lateral vestibulospinal tracts also terminate on interneurons that synapse on these motoneurons. The second set of descending fibers consists of the corticospinal, the rubrospinal, and the medullary reticulospinal tracts. These tracts descend in the lateral funiculus and terminate in areas of the cord spatially related to the dorsolaterally localized alpha motoneurons, which innervate the distal extremity musculature engaged in phasic and manipulatory movements. In addition, all of the fibers descending from supraspinal structures have extensive terminations on gamma motoneurons. They can also influence the monosynaptic stretch reflex by acting on Renshaw cells and interneurons intercalated in reflex arcs and by exciting interneurons responsible for presynaptic inhibition.

LONG-LATENCY RESPONSES

During volitional motor acts, during maintenance of a posture, or during passive stretch of a muscle, long-latency responses, which occur at about twice the latency of the monosynaptic reflex, act to supplement the short-latency segmental components of the stretch reflex.[15, 58, 62, 65] The long- and short-latency reflex responses are thought to act together to compensate for perturbations of a limb produced by changes in load or resistance to movement. Thus, when a subject initiates a movement or maintains an intended limb posture and the limb is disturbed, the stretched muscles react first with spinal stretch reflexes of short latency. The initial spinal reflex is followed by longer-latency reflex responses and finally, if necessary, by a voluntary movement (Fig. 2–9). Typically the long-latency responses are substantially more effective than the monosynaptic response. Long-latency responses appear to play a more important role for distal muscles engaged in manipulative movements than for more proximal limb muscles engaged largely in posture and locomotion.

Because they have longer latencies than the early reflexes, it was believed that long-latency responses are relayed through a "long-loop" transcortical neural pathway involving muscle spindles, dorsal columns, sensorimotor cortex, and the corticospinal tract. But long-latency responses can be elicited by stimulation of cutaneous afferents, and it has been suggested that skin (and possibly joint) afferents may play a role. Long-latency responses are, however, under some voluntary control because their amplitude is affected by both preceding instructions to the individual concerning the stimulus and the

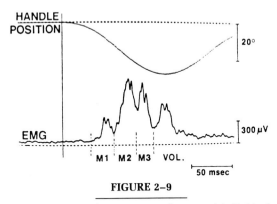

FIGURE 2–9

Sequential muscular responses of a normal individual resisting a sudden displacement from an intended posture. Average of 20 rectified electromyographic (EMG) responses recorded from wrist extensors following sudden flexor displacement of the wrist. Downward deflection of upper trace represents flexion at the wrist by handle position, which starts at the vertical line. The first response (M1) begins at a latency (32 msec) consistent with an origin in the Ia monosynaptic pathway. The other two peaks (M2, M3) occasionally combine into a single response and are considered to be long-latency responses. The last response (VOL.) is attributed to the onset of a voluntary contraction. (Adapted from Lee R, Tatton WG: Long loop reflexes in man: Clinical applications. In Desmedt JE (ed): Progress in Clinical Neurophysiology, vol 4. Basel, S. Karger, 1978, pp 320–333.)

individual's contemplated reaction to displacement of a limb.

FAST AND SLOW SPINAL SYNAPSES

For the most part, the reflex and descending pathways described previously use simple synaptic mechanisms whereby binding of conventional transmitters (e.g., amino acids such as L-glutamate, glycine, and GABA) to postsynaptic neuronal receptors rapidly and briefly opens ionic channels in postsynapic membranes within a millisecond time frame. The increase in permeability produced by the opening of membrane channels permits the passive flow of ions down their electrochemical gradients and results in changes in membrane potential known as postsynaptic potentials (PSPs). Such synapses act as the switches (fast "on" and "off" devices) in the "hard-wiring" of the spinal cord's circuitry. By means of such fast synapses, individual impulses can be transmitted rapidly across the synaptic cleft.

However, a complete extra tier of chemical control mechanisms is superimposed on this fast-switching circuitry. These chemical mechanisms modify the input-output functions of reflex pathways that use conventional transmitters. Accordingly, monoamines, such as serotonin, norepinephrine, and dopamine, released by descending bulbospinal fibers affect the excitability of spinal neurons and reflex pathways by means that do not fit the ordinary concepts of excitation or inhibition. The monoaminergic pathways employ slow (occurring within seconds to minutes) synaptic processes and intracellular second messengers both to activate and to inactivate specific voltage-sensitive ionic channels. Such influence of monoamines on reflex transmission can be pronounced at times. Thus, descending monoaminergic pathways have been reported to regulate the excitability of primary afferent terminals, interneurons, and motoneurons to control segmental reflex transmission and to modulate locomotion.[16, 27, 28, 33, 41, 87]

Under certain conditions, activation of Ia afferents can lead to a long-lasting increase of up to several minutes in the excitability of alpha motoneurons of homonymous and synergistic muscles.[50] The increase in excitability is brought about by changes in the intrinsic membrane properties of the alpha motoneurons such that the brief depolarization evoked by conventional excitatory transmitters changes into a prolonged depolarization (plateau potential) accompanied by repetitive motoneuron discharges. The plateau potential results from activation of a particular calcium conductance that appears after the conventional depolarization when either serotonin or norepinephrine is released from the terminals of descending bulbospinal fibers.[17, 44, 45] This change in the properties of alpha motoneuron membranes in the presence of particular monoamines means that a large amplification of synaptic excitation can occur. The phenomenon may be a major factor in regulating the motoneuron output of the spinal cord, but its significance is still unclear.

CONTROL OF MUSCLE LENGTH AND TENSION

How does the spinal cord integrate afferent information from peripheral proprioceptors and descending inputs to regulate muscle length and tension?[43, 80] In this regard, the motor servo diagram in Figure 2–10 can be considered a basic functional spinal motor unit. The motor servo consists of muscle fibers and the length and tension reflex (feedback) pathways from spindles and tendon organs that regulate muscle contraction. The motor servo seems to function as an automatic feedback system activated by signals from peripheral proprioceptors, which give it the power to restore the position of a limb following a perturbation or a displacement.

However, both muscle length and muscle force cannot be well maintained when external loads are altered because the effects of the reflex circuits activated by alterations in length and by changes in force oppose each other. As a result, it has been suggested that neither length nor tension constitutes an independent property that is regulated separately.[43] Thus, the muscle servo may not pri-

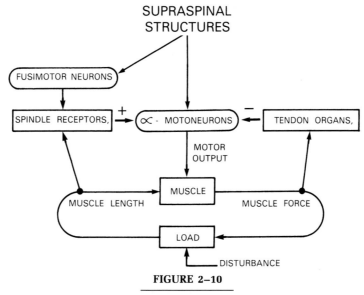

FIGURE 2–10

Basic organization of the motor servo involved in the stretch reflex. Arrows indicate central control signals to alpha and gamma motoneurons. (Adapted from Houk JC, Rymer WZ: Neural control of muscle length and tension. *In* Brooks VB (ed): Handbook of Physiology, vol 2. Bethesda, Md, American Physiological Society, 1981, pp 257–323.)

marily adjust muscle *length* but rather, regulate muscle *stiffness*. Stiffness is a measure of the springlike qualities of muscle and is defined as the ratio of the muscle tension to the muscle length. Stiffness depends in large part on nonreflex, mechanical mechanisms—mainly the mechanical, or viscoelastic, properties of muscle.[69, 72] Muscle tension increases with increasing muscle length, but the relationship depends in large measure on the amount of muscle contraction, which, in turn, is a function of alpha motoneuron activity. In this formulation, neither muscle length nor muscle tension can be thought of as a controlled quantity; rather it is their ratio, or stiffness, that is kept constant by the Ia, II, and Ib systems acting concurrently to compensate for unwanted irregularities in the mechanical properties of muscle.[43] In other words, the stiffness of muscle is the factor that resists displacement.

THE TENDON JERK

The tendon jerk (deep tendon reflex [DTR], phasic stretch reflex) activates the primary muscle spindle endings and the monosynaptic stretch reflex.[64] The primary spindle end-

ings are the only proprioceptors with adequate dynamic sensitivity to react to the rapid increases of muscle length caused by tendon percussion. In addition, as indicated in previous sections, the degree of alpha motoneuron firing activated by impulses in Ia afferents is affected by the excitability of afferent presynaptic terminals, discharges in Ia inhibitory interneurons, Renshaw cells, and interneurons mediating group I nonreciprocal inhibition; by the level of activity in other reflex pathways; and by descending systems.[22, 59, 76, 81]

TONE

The term "tone" as defined by clinical neurologists is the resistance offered by muscles to slowly applied stretch when the patient is in a state of voluntary relaxation.[19] It is tested at the bedside by passive flexion or extension of a muscle. Activation of the monosynaptic stretch reflex by muscle stretch has been *assumed* by most neurologists to be responsible for the resistance to stretch observed during such testing. In normal, relaxed human muscles, however, inertial and mechanical properties of muscle are much more potent in resisting slow stretches than the force generated as a result of reflex activity.[1, 2, 5] The stretch reflex is activated only at rapid rates of stretch in most normal relaxed humans. The stretch reflex may, however, be activated by either voluntary contraction of the muscles being tested or previous instruction regarding the stimulus and the expected response. Voluntary contraction of muscles to assist the examiner's (presumably) passive movement of a limb occurs in many alert individuals. Such voluntary contractions may account for a large part of the resistance to movement that is felt when testing tone.[85] Moreover, voluntary contraction of muscles increases fusimotor drive to the appropriate spindles, and stretch reflexes, as well as tendon jerks, are augmented.[10] Long-latency responses are used when appropriate guidelines are supplied to an individual to resist the movement. Prior instruction also seems to have a modest effect on the magnitude of short-latency monosynaptic reflexes.[18, 32]

LOCOMOTION

Substantial data now support the hypothesis that the alternating pattern of muscle contraction needed for locomotion is generated by an intraspinal interneuronal network that sequentially activates the alpha motoneurons that supply the different limb muscles.[34] In other words, the neuronal substrate for coordinated locomotion is thought to exist within the lumbar spinal cord and to constitute a central pattern generator for locomotion. The neuronal mechanisms within the central pattern generator are not known, but most models propose that groups of interneurons mutually excite and inhibit one another. Some data suggest that the centrally generated rhythm produced by the central pattern generator includes interneurons that are also intercalated in reflex pathways. For example, Ia inhibitory interneurons are driven by the central pattern generator in the absence of any excitation from Ia afferents. Peripheral feedback from muscle, joint, and cutaneous receptors and spinal reflex circuits provides potent control of the central pattern generator. This control regulates the duration and amplitude of the

different phases of the step cycle. In addition, activity in the central pattern generator is initiated and controlled from several regions in the brain stem.

SUMMARY

Current textbooks still feature overly simplistic approaches to spinal cord function. Medical training still emphasizes the notion of stereotyped spinal reflex responses fixed by rigid neuronal connections. These assumptions must be replaced by recognition that (1) descending and sensory information converges on the same sets of interneurons and motoneurons; (2) the effects of different classes of afferents from muscle, joints, and skin act together in different combinations as a result of convergence; (3) synaptic actions initiated by activity in proprioceptive afferents are exerted not only on homonymous alpha motoneurons, but also on motoneurons of synergic (heteronymous) muscles; (4) transmission along the premotoneuronal reflex path can be altered by presynaptic inhibition, which in turn is affected by activity in other afferent and descending fibers; (5) the flexibility of reflex responses is determined in large measure by the excitability of interneurons; (6) conventional and monoamine transmitters act and interact to adjust neuronal excitablity and transmission in reflex pathways; and (7) rhythmic movements are largely determined by intraspinal circuitry.

Acknowledgments

Preparation of this chapter was supported in part by Veterans Administration Medical Center Funds (MRIS 1769 and 3369) and a U.S. Public Health Service grant (NS 17577).

REFERENCES

1. Allum JHJ: Responses to load disturbances in human shoulder muscles: The hypothesis that one component is a pulse test information signal. Exp Brain Res 22:307–326, 1975.
2. Allum JHJ, Büdingen HJ: Coupled stretch reflexes in ankle muscles: An evaluation of the contributions of active muscle mechanisms in human posture stability. Prog Brain Res 50:185–195, 1979.
3. Baldissera, F., Hultborn, H, Illert M: Integration in spinal neuronal systems. In Brooks VB (ed): Hand-

book of Physiology, vol II. Bethesda, Md, American Physiological Society, 1981, pp 509–595.

4. Bawa P, Binder MD, Ruenzel P, et al: Recruitment order of motoneurons in stretch reflexes is highly correlated with their axonal conduction velocity. J Neurophysiol 52:410–420, 1984.

5. Bizzi, E, Dev P, Moraso P, et al: Effect of load disturbances during centrally initiated movements. J Neurophysiol 41:542–556, 1978.

6. Brown AG: Organization in the Spinal Cord. Berlin, Springer-Verlag, 1981.

7. Brown AG, Fyffe REW: Morphology of group Ia afferent fibre collaterals in the spinal cord of the cat. J Physiol (Lond) 274:111–127, 1978.

8. Brown AG, Fyffe REW: The morphology of group Ib afferent fibre collaterals in the spinal cord of the cat. J Physiol (Lond) 296:215–228, 1979.

9. Brown AG, Fyffe REW: Direct observations on the contacts made between Ia afferent fibres and alpha motoneurons in the cat's lumbosacral spinal cord. J Physiol (Lond) 313:121–140, 1981.

10. Burke D: The activity of human muscle spindle endings in normal motor behavior. Int Rev Physiol 25:91–126, 1981.

11. Burke RE: Motor units: Anatomy, physiology, and functional organization. In Brooks VB (ed): Handbook of Physiology, vol II. Bethesda, Md, American Physiological Society, 1981, pp 345–422.

12. Burke RE: Spinal cord: Ventral horn. In Shepard GM (ed): The Synaptic Organization of the Brain. New York, Oxford University Press, 1990, pp 88–132.

13. Burke RE, Rudomin P: Spinal neurons and synapses. In Kandel E (ed): Handbook of Physiology vol 1. Bethesda, Md, American Physiological Society, 1977, pp 877–944.

14. Carlen PL, McCrea DA, Durand D: Dendrites and motoneuronal integration. In Davidoff RA (ed): Handbook of the Spinal Cord, vols 2 and 3. New York, Dekker, 1984, pp 243–267.

15. Chan CWY: Segmental versus suprasegmental contributions to long-latency stretch responses in man. In Desmedt JE (ed): Motor Control Mechanisms in Health and Disease. New York, Raven, 1983, pp 467–487.

16. Commissiong JW, Sedgwick EM: Modulation of the tonic stretch reflex by monoamines. Eur J Pharmacol 57:83–92, 1979.

17. Conway BA, Hultborn H, Kiehn O, et al: Plateau potentials in α-motoneurones induced by intravenous injection of l-DOPA and clonidine in the spinal cat. J Physiol (Lond) 405:369–384, 1988.

18. Crago PE, Houck JC, Hasan A: Regulatory actions of human stretch reflex. J Neurophysiol 39:925–935, 1976.

19. Davidoff RA: Skeletal muscle tone and the misunderstood stretch reflex. Neurology 42:951–963, 1992.

20. Davidoff RA, Hackman JC: Spinal inhibition. In Davidoff RA (ed): Handbook of the Spinal Cord, vols 2 and 3. New York, Dekker, 1984, pp 385–459.

21. Davidoff RA, Hackman JC: GABA: Presynaptic actions. In Rogawski MA, Barker JL (eds): Neurotransmitter Actions in the Vertebrate Nervous System. New York, Plenum, 1985, pp 3–32.

22. Eccles JC: Presynaptic inhibition in the spinal cord. Prog Brain Res 12:65–89, 1964.

23. Eccles JC, Eccles RM, Iggo A, et al: Electrophysiological studies on gamma motoneurons. Acta Physiol Scand 50:32–40, 1960.

24. Eccles JC, Eccles RM, Lundberg A: The convergence of monosynaptic excitatory afferents onto many species of alpha-motoneurones. J Physiol (Lond) 137:22–50, 1957.

25. Eccles JC, Lundberg A: Integrative pattern of Ia synaptic actions on motoneurones of hip and knee muscles. J Physiol (Lond) 144:271–298, 1958.

26. Eccles RM, Lundberg A: Synaptic actions in motoneurons by afferents which may evoke the flexion reflex. Arch Ital Biol 97:199–221, 1959.

27. Ellaway PH, Trott JR: The mode of action of 5-hydroxytryptophan in facilitating a stretch reflex in the spinal cat. Exp Brain Res 22:145–162, 1975.

28. Engberg I, Ryall RW: The inhibitory action of noradrenaline and other monoamines on spinal neurons. J Physiol (Lond) 185:298–322, 1966.

29. Feldman AG, Orlovsky GN: Activity of interneurons mediating reciprocal Ia inhibition during locomotion. Brain Res 84:181–194, 1975.

30. Fetz EE, Jankowska E, Johannisson T, et al: Autogenetic inhibition of motoneurones by impulses in group Ia muscle spindle afferents. J Physiol (Lond) 293:173–195, 1979.

31. Fyffe REW, Light AR: The ultrastructure of group Ia afferent fiber synapses in the lumbosacral spinal cord of the cat. Brain Res 300:201–209, 1984.

32. Gottlieb GL, Agrawal GC: Response to sudden torques about ankle in man: Myotatic reflex. J Neurophysiol 42:91–106, 1979.

33. Grillner S: Locomotion in vertebrates: Central mechanisms and reflex interaction. Physiol Rev 55:247–304, 1975.

34. Grillner S: Control of locomotion in bipeds, tetrapods, and fish. In Brooks VB (ed): Handbook of Physiology, vol II. Bethesda, Md, American Physiological Society, 1981, pp 1179–1236.

35. Harrison PJ, Jankowska E: Sources of input to interneurones mediating group I non-reciprocal inhibition of motoneurones in the cat. J Physiol (Lond) 361:379–401, 1985.

36. Harrison PJ, Jankowska E: Organization of input to interneurones mediating group I non-reciprocal inhibition of motoneurones in the cat. J Physiol (Lond) 361:403–418, 1985.

37. Harrison PJ, Jankowska E, Johannisson T: Shared reflex pathways of group I afferents of different cat hindlimb muscles. J Physiol (Lond) 338:113–127, 1983.

38. Hasan Z, Stuart DG: Mammalian muscle receptors. In Davidoff R (ed): Handbook of the Spinal Cord, vols 2 and 3. New York, Dekker, 1984, pp 559–607.

39. Henneman E, Mendell LM: Functional organization of motoneuron pool and its inputs. In Brooks VB (ed): Handbook of Physiology, vol II. Bethesda, Md, American Physiological Society, 1981, pp 423–507.

40. Henneman E, Somjen G, Carpenter DO: Functional significance of cell size in spinal motoneurons. J Neurophysiol 28:560–580, 1965.

41. Holohean AM, Hackman JC, Davidoff RA: Changes in membrane potential of frog motoneurons induced by activation of serotonin receptor subtypes. Neuroscience 34:555–564, 1990.

42. Houk J, Henneman E: Responses of Golgi tendon organs to active contractions of the soleus muscle of the cat. J Neurophysiol 30:1482–1493, 1967.

43. Houk JC, Rymer WZ: Neural control of muscle length and tension. In Brooks VB (ed): Handbook of Physiology, vol. II. Bethesda, Md, American Physiological Society, 1981, pp 257–323.

44. Hounsgaard J, Kiehn O: Ca^{++} dependent bistability induced by serotonin in spinal motoneurons. Exp Brain Res 57:422–425, 1985.

45. Hounsgaard J, Kiehn O: Serotonin-induced bistability of turtle motoneurones caused by a nifedipine-sensitive calcium plateau potential. J Physiol (Lond) 414:265–282, 1989.

46. Hulliger M: The mammalian muscle spindle and its central control. Physiol Biochem Pharmacol 101:1–110, 1984.

47. Hultborn H: Transmission in the pathway of reciprocal Ia inhibition to motoneurones and its control during the tonic stretch reflex. Prog Brain Res 44:235–255, 1976.

48. Hultborn H, Illert M, Santini M: Convergence on interneurons mediating the reciprocal Ia inhibition of motoneurones: II. Effects from segmental flexor reflex pathways. Acta Physiol Scand 96:351–367, 1976.

49. Hultborn H, Illert M, Santini M: Convergence on interneurones mediating the reciprocal Ia inhibition of motoneurones: III. Effects from supraspinal pathways. Acta Physiol Scand 96:368–391, 1976.

50. Hultborn, H, Wigström H, Wangberg B: Prolonged activation of soleus motoneurones following a conditioning train in soleus Ia afferents—A case for a reverberating loop. Neurosci Lett 1:147–152, 1975.

51. Hunt CC: Mammalian muscle spindle: Peripheral mechanisms. Physiol Rev 70:643–661, 1990.

52. Jankowska E, Johannisson T, Lipski J: Common interneurones in reflex pathways from group Ia and Ib afferents of ankle extensors in the cat. J Physiol (Lond) 310:381–402, 1981.

53. Jankowska E, McCrea D: Shared reflex pathways from Ib tendon organ afferents and muscle spindle afferents in the cat. J Physiol (Lond) 338:99–111, 1983.

54. Jankowska E, McCrea D, Rudomin P, et al: Observations on neuronal pathways subserving primary afferent depolarization. J Neurophysiol 46:506–516, 1981.

55. Jankowska E, Roberts WJ: Synaptic actions of single interneurons mediating reciprocal Ia inhibition of motoneurons. J Physiol (Lond) 222:623–642, 1972.

56. Kuypers HGJM: Anatomy of the descending pathways. In Brooks VB (ed): Handbook of Physiology, vol II. Bethesda, Md, American Physiological Society, 1981, pp 597–666.

57. Laporte Y, Emont-Dénand F, Jami L: The skeletofusimotor innervation of mammalian muscle spindles. Trends Neurosci 4:97–99, 1981.

58. Lee R, Tatton WG: Long loop reflexes in man: Clinical applications. In Desmedt JE (ed): Progress in Clinical Neurophysiology, vol 4. Basel, Karger, 1978, pp 320–333.

59. Lundberg A: Multisensory control of spinal reflex pathways. Prog Brain Res 50:11–28, 1979.

60. Lundberg A, Malmgren K, Schomburg ED: Convergence from Ib, cutaneous and joint afferents in reflex pathways to motoneurones. Brain Res 87:81–84, 1975.

61. Lundberg A, Malmgren K, Schomburg ED: Reflex pathways from group II muscle afferents: 3. Secondary spindle afferents and the FRA: A new hypothesis. Exp Brain Res 65:294–306, 1987.

62. Marsden CD, Rothwell JC, Day BL: Long-latency automatic responses to muscle stretch in man: Origin and function. Adv Neurol 39:509–539, 1983.

63. Matthews PBC: Muscle spindles: Their messages and their fusimotor supply. In Brooks VB (ed): Handbook of Physiology, vol II. Bethesda, Md, American Physiologcal Society, 1981, pp 189–228.

64. Matthews PBC: The knee jerk: Still an enigma. Can J Physiol Pharmacol 68:347–354, 1990.

65. Matthews PBC: The human stretch reflex and the motor cortex. Trends Neurosci 14:87–91, 1991.

66. Mendell LM, Henneman E: Terminals of Ia fibers: Location, density and distribution within a pool of 300 homonymous motoneurons. J Neurophysiol 34:171–187, 1971.

67. Murthy KSK: Vertebrate fusimotoneurones and their influences on motor behavior. Prog Neurobiol 11:249–307, 1978.

68. Nyberg-Hansen R: Functional organization of descending supraspinal fibre systems to the spinal cord: Anatomical observations and physiological observations. Ergebn Anat 39:1–48, 1966.

69. Partridge LD, Benton LA: Muscle, the motor. In Brooks VB (ed): Handbook of Physiology, vol II. Bethesda, Md, American Physiological Society, 1981, pp 43–106.

70. Pinter MJ: The role of motoneuron membrane properties in the determination of recruitment order. In Binder MD, Mendell LM (eds): The Segmental Motor System. New York, Oxford University Press, 1990, pp 165–181.

71. Pompeiano O: Recurrent inhibition. In Davidoff RA (ed): Handbook of the Spinal Cord, vols 2 and 3. New York, Dekker, 1984, pp 461–557.

72. Rack PMH: Limitations of somatosensory feedback in control of posture and movement. In Brooks VB (ed): Handbook of Physiology, vol II. Bethesda, Md, American Physiological Society, 1981, pp 229–256.

73. Redman S: Junctional mechanisms at group Ia synapses. Prog Neurobiol 12:33–83, 1979.

74. Rexed B: Some aspects of the cytoarchitectonics and synaptology of the spinal cord. Prog Brain Res 11:58–90, 1964.

75. Romanes GJ: The motor cell columns of the lumbosacral spinal cord of the cat. J Comp Physiol 94:313–363, 1951.

76. Rudomin P: Presynaptic control of synaptic effectiveness of muscle spindle and tendon organ afferents in the mammalian spinal cord. In Binder MD, Mendell LM (eds): The Segmental Motor System. New York, Oxford University Press, 1990, pp 349–380.

77. Rudomin P, Jiménez I, Solodkin M, et al: Site of action of segmental and descending control of transmission on pathways mediating PAD of Ia- and Ib-afferent fibers in cat spinal cord. J Neurophysiol 50:743–769, 1983.

78. Rudomin P, Solodkin M, Jiménez I: Synaptic potentials of primary afferent fibers and motoneurons evoked by single intermediate nucleus interneurons in the cat spinal cord. J Neurophysiol 57:1288–1313, 1987.

79. Rudomin P, Solodkin M, Jiménez I: PAD and PAH response patterns of group Ia and Ib fibers to cutaneous and descending inputs in the cat spinal cord. J Neurophysiol 56:987–1006, 1986.

80. Rymer WZ: Spinal mechanisms for control of muscle length and tension. In Davidoff RA (ed): Handbook of the Spinal Cord, vol 2. New York, Dekker, 1984, pp 609–646.

81. Schmidt RF: Presynaptic inhibition in the vertebrate central nervous sytem. Ergeb Physiol 63:20–101, 1971.

82. Solodkin M, Jiménez I, Rudomin P: Identification of common interneurons mediating pre- and post-synaptic inhibition in the spinal cord. Science 224:1453–1456, 1984.

83. Stauffer EK, Watt DGD, Taylor A, et al: Analysis of muscle receptor connections by spike-triggered averaging: II. Spindle group II afferents. J Neurophysiol 39:1393–1402, 1976.

84. Sypert GW, Munson JB: Excitatory synapses. In Davidoff RA (ed): Handbook of the Spinal Cord, vols 2 and 3. New York, Dekker, 1984, pp 315–384.

85. Van Der Meché FGA, Van Gijn J: Hypotonia: An erroneous clinical concept? Brain 109:1169–1178, 1986.

86. Windhurst U: Activation of Renshaw cells. Prog Neurobiol 35:135–179, 1990.

87. Wohlberg CJ, Hackman JC, Ryan GP, et al: Epinephrine and norepinephrine-evoked potential changes of frog primary afferent terminals: Pharmacological characterization of α and β components. Brain Res 327:289–301, 1985.

CHAPTER 3

Neuropathology of the Spinal Cord

J. Trevor Hughes, M.D., F.R.C.P., F.R.C.Path.

The spinal cord is affected by a large number of pathologic processes, but in many of these, the main damage occurs to the brain or some other part of the body. These conditions are mentioned briefly in this chapter which focuses on those few diseases and special traumas involving the spinal cord. This discussion is arranged under the following headings: congenital and developmental disorders, vascular disorders, inflammatory disorders, trauma, and diseases of the spine affecting the spinal cord.

CONGENITAL AND DEVELOPMENTAL DISORDERS

Myelodysplasia, myeloschisis, and spinal dysraphism are disorders in which the neural groove fails to develop normally into a spinal cord or other posterior midline structures. The conditions to be mentioned here are spina bifida occulta and spina bifida cystica, the latter being subdivided into meningocele, meningomyelocele, and meningomyelocystocele. There are other nomenclatures for this complex subject, which is the topic of many specialized monographs, to which reference should be made not only for pathologic details but also for theories of etiology and possibilities of prevention. The names given above are arranged in a progressive order of maldevelopment. In meningomyelocele and meningocystocele, profound errors of structural anatomy occur not only of the spinal cord but also of the brain. In spina bifida occulta and spinal meningocele, the maldevelopment affects mainly, but not exclusively, the spinal cord. These two conditions are described in this chapter, as is hydromyelia, a common accompaniment of all these maldevelopments. Syringomyelia is described separately because there are important differences between it and hydromyelia. The conditions of diplomyelia, diastematomyelia, iniencephalus, and the Klippel-Feil syndrome are also briefly described.

Spina Bifida

Spina bifida is the incomplete closure of the vertebral canal commonly seen as posterior spina bifida, in which the defect occurs in the posterior lamina of the spinal canal, most frequently in the lumbosacral region. It may be covert (occulta) or overt, associated with a bulging cystic sac in communication with a spinal cord that is opened posteriorly. There are gradations of this defect, and the degree of structural malformation varies along the whole neuraxis. This realization is important to the surgeon operating on a localized deformity that may be associated with a generalized defect on the spine, the spinal cord, and, possibly, the brain. Anterior spina bifida is a condition in which the vertebral bodies are malformed and an anterior deficiency exists. There may be fistulous connections between the spinal canal and either the mediastinum or the intestine. Entodermal cysts within the spinal canal are associated with this anterior malformation of the spine.

Hydromyelia

Hydromyelia is a common condition in which the central canal of the spinal cord is enlarged into a central midline cavity lined with ependyma. A minor degree of hydromyelia, particularly in the upper cervical region, can occasionally be found at necropsy in otherwise normal spinal cords from persons living a normal life span without evidence of neurologic disease. These instances are probably examples of minimal maldevelopment

of the neuraxis too slight to cause an obvious clinical neurologic deficit. When any maldevelopment of the neuraxis is examined pathologically, hydromyelia is found. It is seen in association with spina bifida occulta, spina bifida cystica, Arnold-Chiari deformity, and diastematomyelia.

Diastematomyelia, Klippel-Feil Syndrome, and Iniencephalus

Diastematomyelia (Fig. 3–1), Klippel-Feil syndrome, and iniencephalus represent a spectrum of deformity and are discussed here in a progression of severity of the structural changes. Diastematomyelia (also called diplomyelia) is a disorder in which some part of the spinal cord is divided longitudinally into two similar structures. Spina bifida is usually present. The spinal canal is abnormal, ranging from being unusually wide to being duplicated. When there are two canals, they are separated by an anteroposterior septum made of fibrous tissue, cartilage, or bone. The meninges may be duplicated, the pia-arachnoid is always duplicated, and the dura is duplicated in approximately half of patients. The duplication of the spinal cord can affect some 10 spinal cord segments usually below the mid-thoracic region. In one of the patients examined by the author, hydromyelia was present in the upper thoracic region. As the cord was examined caudally, a point was reached at which the dilated and elliptical central canal divided into two; more caudally, there were two almost complete spinal cords joined posteriorly, each being rotated through 90 degrees. Here the medial parts of the anterior horns and anterior roots of each cord were underdeveloped. Many of these patients present in childhood with varying degrees of neurologic deficit. Some attain adulthood and, as in the case just described, no apparent disability may be noted throughout life. Iniencephalus is the most extreme form of the disorder described by Klippel and Feil. The term *iniencephalus* derives from the deformity of the neck (*inion*), but in this gross malformation there is also profound abnormality of the brain, spinal cord, viscera, and other soft tissue structures. The

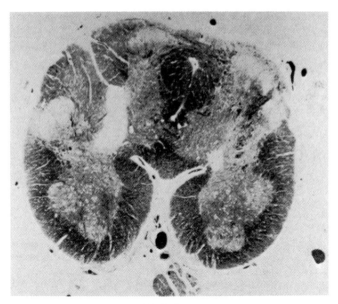

FIGURE 3–1

Diastematomyelia. Transverse section, stained for myelin, of the spinal cord in a case of diastemato-myelia. The lumbosacral enlargement has two halves of a partially divided cord united by the incomplete medial portions. (From Hughes JT: Pathology of the Spinal Cord, ed 2. London, WB Saunders, 1978; with permission of Hodder & Stoughton Ltd, London.)

neck is short and, due to the marked retro-flexion, the face looks upward. The spinal canal is grossly malformed and, due to absence or fusion, fewer vertebrae are present. The spinal cord is always maldeveloped and may be rudimentary or absent. In the Klippel-Feil syndrome, shortness and webbing of the neck are present due to maldevelopment of the cervical vertebrae. The bodies of these vertebrae may be fused, and posterior spina bifida is present. The spinal cord is always abnormal, the most consistent finding being hydromyelia.

Syringomyelia

Syringomyelia can be congenital or ac-quired (secondary), the latter condition being caused by tumors, vascular infarctions, and, notably, trauma.[1] Primary syringomyelia (Fig. 3–2) is a condition rarely seen by the neuropathologist; I have examined fewer than 10 cases. By contrast, I have examined many hundreds of spinal cords with hydro-myelia for the reasons explained previously. Syringomyelia is a primary spinal cord disor-der, the pathologic basis of which is a pro-gressive longitudinal spinal cord cavitation in the form of a syrinx. It becomes clinically manifest in the second or third decade, but a feature such as scoliosis may be noted much earlier. Macroscopically a distended cord is present that collapses on cutting. A perfect central cavity is rare, the more common find-ing being a slit passing transversely across the cord, the location of which is often asym-metrical. An extension into the medulla (sy-ringobulbia) can occur, and occasionally two or more separate cavities are present in the spinal cord and brain stem. The extent and nature of the cavity can be seen on histologic examination, but many sections are required to determine its extent and the presence of any communication with the subarachnoid space. The gray commissure is regularly de-stroyed, but in the asymmetrical extensions one or both of the posterior horns may be involved. The wall of the cavity consists of a glial layer of variable thickness often con-taining connective tissue. Ependyma as an inner lining is present only where the syrinx approaches the central canal, distinguishing the condition of syringomyelia from hydro-

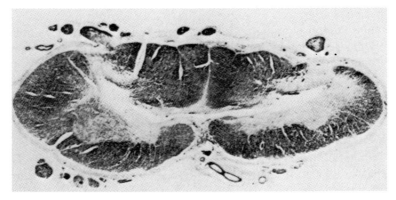

FIGURE 3–2

Transverse section through the cervical spinal cord in a case of syringomyelia. The syrinx is symmetrical and involves both of the posterior horns and the anterior commissure. (From Hughes JT: Pathology of the Spinal Cord, ed 2. London, WB Saunders, 1978; with permission of Hodder & Stoughton Ltd, London.)

myelia. A characteristic feature of the wall of the syringomyelic cavity is the frequent presence of small peripheral-type nerve fibers clothed in Schwann cells, ramifying in the connective tissue and derived from the nearby posterior nerve roots.

VASCULAR DISORDERS

The spinal cord is much less susceptible than the brain to ischemia and infarction; this relative sparing is due to anatomic and physiologic features of its complex blood supply. Simple arterial obstruction is not the only syndrome seen, and other categories of vascular disturbance are described under the headings of aortic obstruction; vertebral, intercostal, and radicular artery obstruction; anterior spinal artery syndrome; posterior spinal artery syndrome; spinal venous obstruction; and hypoxia/ischemia. Arteriovenous vascular malformation must also be mentioned because this strange angioma is seen more frequently than any other vascular condition of the spinal cord.

Aortic Conditions

Aortic causes of spinal cord ischemia may be more common than is realized because severe aortic atheroma, often combined with

aortic thrombosis, leads to a confusing neurologic state that may be diagnosed as motor neuron disease or even multiple sclerosis. In dissecting aneurysm of the aorta, the clinical syndrome is more easily recognized, and involvement of the spinal cord by ischemia is readily understood. Dissection of the tunica media by a hematoma compresses the origin of the intercostal or lumbar arteries. If a major arterial tributary to the anterior spinal artery is obstructed, the syndrome of the occlusion of that artery is seen.[3, 8, 20] Rarely, trauma to the aorta can cause exactly the same result; in one case that I observed, a traumatic tear of the aorta caused a mural hematoma that compressed the second through fifth intercostal arteries at their origin and infarcted the spinal cord from T3 to T7 segments.[12]

Vertebral, Intercostal, and Radicular Artery Obstruction

Vertebral artery obstruction is probably underdiagnosed, because in neck injuries, which are frequently combined with head injuries, damage may occur to one or more vertebral arteries in their course through the foramina of the transverse processes of the upper six cervical vertebrae.[16] The intercostal and lumbar arteries are the most frequently injured or ligated in surgical procedures.[19] Thoracoplasty, pneumonectomy, and sympathectomy have all caused arterial obstruction. The mechanism of such obstruction is the occlusion, often by ligation, of an artery that feeds directly into an important tributary to the anterior spinal artery. The radicular tributary arteries are occluded by pathologic processes nearer the spinal cord, the most common being the infiltration of the intervertebral foramina by a mass of malignant tumor. Psoas abscess due to tuberculous osteitis can operate in this anatomic location by causing an inflammatory arteritis; I have seen similar pathologic findings in herpes zoster.

Occlusion of the Anterior Spinal Artery

Although any part of the anterior spinal artery can be occluded, the instances described tend to involve the major part of either the upper or the lower parts of the artery. This division has an anatomic explanation in that the upper part of the spinal cord to about T2 is supplied from the subclavian arteries via the vertebral arteries, whereas the lower part from T3 to the conus derives its blood supply from arterial branches arising directly from the aorta. Arterial thrombosis (Fig. 3–3) is the common pathologic entity and nearly always has a primary cause in some arterial disease or in an effect on the artery of some other process. Formerly, syphilis accounted for many of these instances, but now this cause is rare. Minor localized trauma is often a feature, and in one patient, the pressure on the anterior spinal artery by a central protuberance of cervical spondylosis was directly related anatomically to the site of spinal cord infarction.[18]

Necropsy shows antemortem thrombus in the anterior spinal artery in the form of the widespread occurrence of small occlusive portions of thrombus. Many sections are required to demonstrate the full extent of the arterial obstruction, which a single section

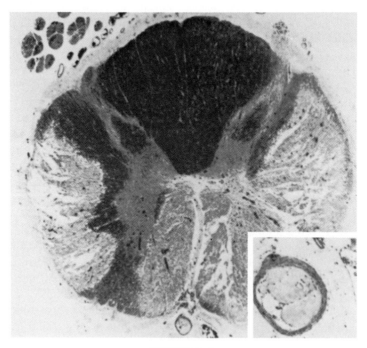

FIGURE 3–3

Anterior spinal artery thrombosis. The large image shows the spinal cord at T12 segmental level. An acute infarction of the anterior parts of the spinal cord is present, with asymmetry due to the anatomy of the sulcal arteries. The inset shows an enlarged view of the thrombus in the anterior spinal artery. (From Hughes JT: Pathology of the Spinal Cord, ed 2. London, WB Saunders, 1978; with permission of Hodder & Stoughton Ltd, London.)

may not confirm. There also may be portions of thrombus in some sulcal arteries. The pattern of spinal cord infarction is characteristic, being anterior and central due to the centrifugal flow of the blood from this artery. The other remarkable feature is the asymmetry of the infarction due to the sulcal arteries turning either left or right in their supply.

Occlusion of the Posterior Spinal Artery

Instances of obstruction of the posterior spinal arteries are much rarer than those just reviewed. When describing a case with necropsy confirmation of the diagnosis, I could find only seven previous case reports.[14] Clinically the onset begins with pain or dysesthesia, but paresis or paralysis of the lower limbs and trunk rapidly supervenes. The bladder and bowel are also paralyzed. This description refers to the period immediately following the onset of the neurologic syndrome when, because of swelling and edema, there is a temporary disability of the spinal cord amounting to a cord transection. If the patient survives this acute phase, considerable neurologic improvement can occur, and recovery can be almost complete. The predisposing cause of the occlusion of the posterior spinal artery is usually apparent in the case history, and in a case of my own, the thrombosis was caused by an intrathecal phenol injection. Thrombosis is generally present, and in the earlier reports, this occurred in the setting of syphilitic arteritis. Cases have been reported following minor indirect trauma, and in others the posterior spinal arteries were obstructed by embolic atheromatous material.[21]

Venous Obstruction

Acute venous obstruction is rare; my review revealed only seven reports.[15] The primary causes have included tumor and extensive generalized septicemia; in a case of my own, a thrombotic diathesis was present associated with an adenocarcinoma of the pancreas. In the reviewed cases, the poor prognosis was due to the gravity of the associated illness that caused the venous infarction of the spinal cord. The actual prognosis of the condition can be less grave, because, usually, only cases verified by necropsy have been diagnosed. A milder form of the condition may exist but is not recognized clinically. At necropsy the spinal veins are always greatly distended and are usually extensively thrombosed. The venous obstruction can, however, be sited in the plexus of veins in the spinal canal or in the veins in the pelvis and abdomen. The spinal cord itself is disrupted by severe hemorrhagic necrosis in which small hematomas are conspicuous. The parts of the spinal cord affected most greatly are the central areas, and the infarction is much more hemorrhagic than after arterial occlusion. The extent of the infarction both longitudinally and in cross-sectional area is even greater than that caused by an extensive thrombosis of the anterior spinal artery.

The previous description refers to an acute infarction caused by an acute thrombophlebitis. Instances of a subacute or chronic spinal cord syndrome also occur that are produced by either a more caudal venous thrombotic occlusion or a recurrence of episodes of spinal cord damage due to recurrent thrombosis. These instances should be differentiated from spinal vascular malformations, in which venous thrombosis can be found.

Hypoxia/Ischemia

In addition to spinal cord damage due to the occlusion of some part of the spinal vascular system, the spinal cord can be damaged by hypoxia/ischemia, most evident in the perinatal period, and associated with cerebral damage from the hypoxia, the ischemia, or a combination of the two causes.[5]

Arteriovenous Malformation of the Spinal Cord

Arteriovenous malformation of the spinal cord, formerly a curiosity of neuropathologists, is now discussed in a voluminous literature including reports on the new techniques in neuroradiology[4, 6, 7] for demonstrating the anatomy of the condition and on the experience of neurosurgeons who have devised new surgical measures of treatment. In this chapter only the pathology of the condition is described (Fig. 3–4 A and B). The anterior spinal artery is normal or slightly enlarged. The posterior spinal arteries are normal. The spinal venous system is normal in its fundamental anatomy but abnormal in the hypertrophy and distension of most of the spinal veins. The anterior spinal vein, for example, is always normally situated. A constant finding is a very abnormal large, thick-walled, tortuous vessel pursuing an irregular course longitudinally on the posterior surface of the spinal cord. At necropsy this tortuous, convoluted vessel can be dissected away from the spinal cord as a single continuous vascular channel greatly exceeding in length that of the whole spinal cord. This abnormal vessel is now known from angiographic studies in living humans to be part of an abnormal vascular communication between the arterial and venous systems of the spinal cord. It is difficult at necropsy, but easy during life with the angiographic techniques mentioned, to determine the artery or arteries feeding into this large complex vessel and the veins that drain it.

The microscopic findings are so unusual that, in many of the published reports, attention has been directed away from the more informative macroscopic appearances. Furthermore, the anatomy of the malformation described earlier becomes difficult to elucidate after the spinal cord is cut transversely and tissue blocks are taken. The histologic changes are more advanced in the caudal part of the spinal cord, being very evident in the lumbosacral enlargement. There are many capillaries and other small thick-walled channels, the size and position of which suggest that they are altered capillaries and veins. The vessels have thick hyaline walls that are sometimes calcified. Recent thrombosis can be seen within these intramedullary vessels, and others show changes indicative of the organization of earlier thrombus. Thrombosis also can be seen in the large extramedullary vessels. Examination by elastin stains of the tunica media of the large abnormal vessels reveals the structure of arterialized veins.

The substance of the spinal cord is affected by an unusual form of incomplete necrosis that involves gray and white matter but particularly the central parts of the cord. Most of the neuronal cell bodies are lost, but some, although apparently dead, are encrusted with material that stains for iron and calcium. Lipid phagocytes are common, but acute inflammatory cells are usually absent. The upper parts of the spinal cord show wallerian degeneration of the upward-directed long tracts.

INFLAMMATORY DISORDERS

Many inflammatory diseases can affect the spinal cord. Due to space constraints, mention is made only of those that are most important. However, certain rare conditions that may be encountered by the specialized readers of this text are also discussed. Most of the conditions referred to have a known microbial cause that is viral, bacterial, fungal, or parasitic.

Viruses

The viral diseases affecting the spinal cord are caused by infection with neurotropic viruses, e.g., rabies, acute anterior poliomyelitis (Figs. 3–5 A–C), herpes zoster, and herpes B encephalomyelitis. Details of these important infections cannot be given here, and the reader is referred to the references cited earlier. The slowly infecting viruses of kuru and Creutzfeldt-Jakob diseases also involve the spinal cord.

Bacteria

The bacterial infections of the various types of leptomeningitis affect the subarachnoid space around the brain and spinal cord, and special mention is not needed here. Bacterial infections in the other spaces around the spinal cord produce more localized

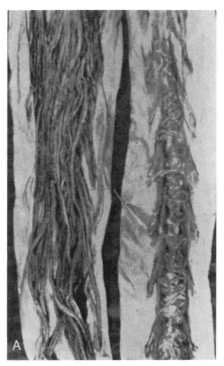

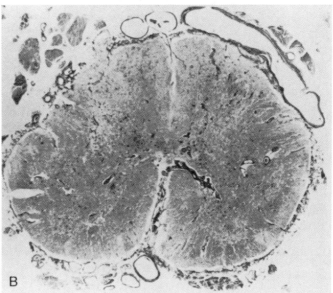

FIGURE 3–4

Arteriovenous angiomatous malformation of the spinal cord. A, Posterior aspect of the spinal cord. B, Transverse section through the sacral level of the spinal cord of the case shown in A. Many abnormal vessels are present inside the spinal cord. With one exception, the anterior and posterior spinal arteries and spinal veins are normal. The exception is the single large abnormal anastomotic vessel on the posterolateral aspect of the cord. (From Hughes JT: Pathology of the Spinal Cord, ed 2. London, WB Saunders, 1978; with permission of Hodder & Stoughton Ltd, London.)

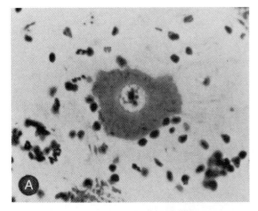

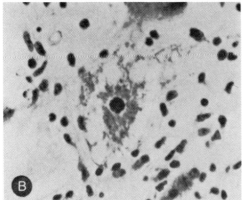

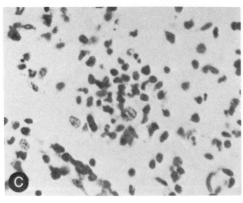

FIGURE 3–5

Cellular damage caused by the virus of anterior poliomy-elitis. A–C, three images show the progressive stages of infection of a neurone. (From Hughes JT: Pathology of the Spinal Cord, ed 2. London, WB Saunders, 1978; with permission of Hodder & Stoughton Ltd, London.)

pathologic findings. Extradural (epidural) abscess is seen from a neighboring source of infection, such as osteomyelitis of the spine, from the infection introduced by a penetrating wound or from metastatic spread from an abscess. The common organisms found in extradural abscess are *Staphylococcus aureus, Diplococcus pneumoniae,* and *Pseudomonas pyocyanea.* Pachymeningitis (infection of the dura) and subdural abscess are more rare and are due to the spread of infection from outside (extradural abscess) or inside (leptomeningitis) the spinal cord. Penetrating wounds and, occasionally, lumbar punctures are rare causes.[25] Intramedullary abscess, although less common than its counterpart in the brain, is a rare remedial cause of cord expansion and is usually seen as a metastatic abscess. Pyogenic infections in and around the spinal cord are now being seen in drug addicts, particularly those using heroin intravenously. Tuberculosis is briefly described in the next section, but syphilis in the spinal cord is now so rare that the reader must review the many previous reports in the historical literature.

Tuberculosis and Pott's Paraplegia

Tuberculosis affects the spinal cord in several ways. As part of a generalized leptomeningitis, the spinal cord is extensively involved by the chronic granulomatous infection, and in partially treated patients, localized pockets of infection are frequently located around the spinal cord (Fig. 3–6A). The effect on the cord is for the most part due to the ischemia of the inflammatory arteritis (Fig. 3–6B and C). Tuberculous osteitis of the spine, often accompanied by a psoas abscess, can affect the spinal cord by direct extension of the inflammatory process, and a sudden paraplegia can be caused by the occlusion of a large tributary artery directed into the major spinal cord arteries.

Pott's paraplegia is the most well known effect of tuberculosis on the spinal cord. The pathologic lesion is caused by pressure due to kyphosis caused by the collapse of the spine by a localized destruction of tuberculous osteitis. The angled spine (kyphosis) compresses the spinal cord due to the gibbus of the kyphos pressing backward into the spinal canal and crushing the cord against the spinal laminae behind.

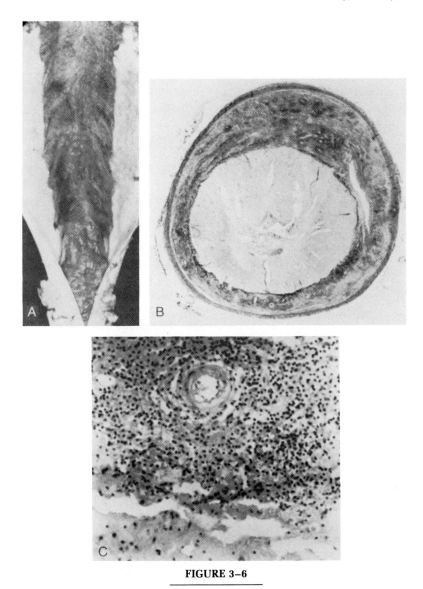

FIGURE 3–6

Tuberculous leptomeningitis. *A*, Posterior aspect of upper cervical cord. *B*, Appearances in a transverse section at T7, which at higher magnification (*C*) shows arteritis in a small artery buried in the tuberculous exudate. (From Hughes JT: Pathology of the Spinal Cord, ed 2. London, WB Saunders, 1978; with permission of Hodder & Stoughton Ltd, London.)

Fungal Infections

Cryptococcosis (torulosis), histoplasmosis, coccidioidomycosis, blastomycosis, and aspergillosis can all involve the spinal cord.[24] *Cryptococcus hominis* is a spherical or oval yeastlike organism, widespread throughout the world. The common form of cryptococcal leptomeningitis affects the brain and spinal cord, but, occasionally, this organism causes a large necrotic mass involving the caudal part of the cord and the cauda equina. *Histoplasma capsulatum*, which enters the body by inhalation and causes pulmonary lesions and hilar lymphadenopathy, particularly attacks the reticuloendothelial system. Rarely, the spinal cord is involved. *Coccidioides immitis*, a filamentous fungus that thrives in the arid soils of hot countries, causes a granulomatous leptomeningitis affecting brain and spinal cord. It can also cause spinal extradural granulomata spreading from an osteitis.

The last fungus to be mentioned is *Aspergillus fumigatus*, which is today a pathogen because of diminished immunologic tolerance from various treatments. The spinal cord is involved by a granulomatous leptomeningitis and, occasionally, from an inflammatory mass of the spine compressing the spinal cord.

Parasitic Infestations

The main parasitic conditions that give rise to a localized involvement of the spinal cord are cysticercosis, hydatid disease, and schistosomiasis. Some spinal cord involvement has been reported in paragonimiasis and gnathostomiasis.

Cysticercosis arises from the ingestion of the ova of the pork tapeworm *Taenia solium*. A few reports exist of the parasitic cysts in the spinal cord; most likely, more would be discovered by a more thorough search at necropsy or by modern imaging techniques. Hydatid disease is caused by the larval form of the parasite *Taenia echinococcus*, the life cycle of which is manifested in the sheep and the dog. The spinal cord may harbor a primary cyst from an initial infection or may receive secondary (metastatic) cysts. More commonly, hydatid disease causes an inflammatory mass in the spine, which extends into the spinal canal, and causes pressure on the spinal cord. Schistosomiasis is caused by infestations of any of three members of a group of trematode parasites. Man is the primary host; the secondary host is a water snail whose species differs for each trematode. The three parasites that give rise to disease in humans are *Schistosoma haematobium*, found mainly in Africa, *Schistosoma mansoni*, found mainly in Africa but also in South America, and *Schistosoma japonicum*, found in the Far East. Involvement of the central nervous system is uncommon, but there are interesting differences between the three parasites. *S. haematobium* predominantly affects the spinal cord. *S. mansoni* causes lesions equally in the brain and spinal cord, and *S. japonicum*, with two reported exceptions, affects only the brain. The parasites affect the lower thoracic and lumbosacral re-

gions of the spinal cord and, less frequently, the cauda equina, causing a myelopathy and sometimes a radiculopathy. Paragonimiasis, caused by a lung fluke, the most commonly identified organism being *Paragonimus westermani*, has involved the spinal cord, although the infection predominantly affects the lungs. Most cases have been reported from China, Korea, and Japan. Reports of gnathostomiasis involving the spinal cord have come from Thailand. The disease is caused by the adult form of the nematode worm *Gnathostoma spinigerum*, which burrows into the spinal cord (and brain) and paraspinal structures. Clinical and pathologic changes caused by the presence of this nematode in the spinal cord are dramatic.

TRAUMA TO THE SPINAL CORD

Traumatic lesions of the spinal cord can be either direct (from a stab wound or the penetration of a high-velocity missile) or indirect (from fractures, fracture dislocations, or subluxations of the spine) (Fig. 3–7A and B). Both mechanisms are often combined in the gross trauma of warfare or in civilian injuries, such as road accidents. The gross structural details of these injuries have been discussed elsewhere. The histologic findings in the spinal cord differ according to the interval after the trauma and can be divided into three stages.

The immediate consequences of a spinal cord contusion or laceration are damage or total severance of nerve fibers, traumatic effects on neuronal cell bodies, and exudative phenomena. Both the axon and its myelin sheath become swollen and may disintegrate. When mildly damaged, the axons show beading in silver stains; in a more severe state, a line of silver droplets of axonal material is seen in the former position of the axon, whereas in grossly contused specimens, appropriate methods demonstrate only a silver-impregnated dust of scattered displaced axonal fragments. The cell bodies of the neurons are either disrupted or show the phenomenon of axonal reaction, also called central chromatolysis.

The early exudative changes are edema, red

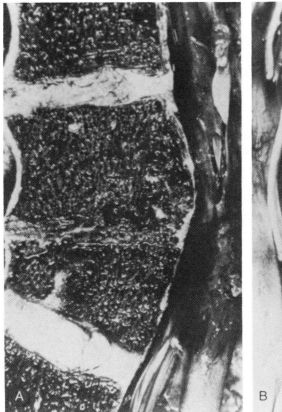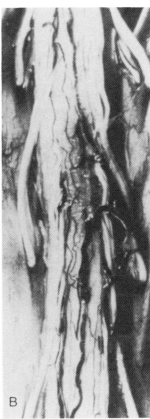

FIGURE 3–7

Traumatic paraplegia: findings several years after trauma. *A,* T11 to L2 of a sagittally sawn spine, with angulation at T12. *B,* Posterior aspect of the spinal cord with the dura reflected. Note localized discoloration and atrophy. The posterior spinal veins and a major radicular vein are distended. (From Hughes JT. *In* Adams JH, Duchen LW (eds): Greenfield's Neuropathology, ed 5. London, Edward Arnold, 1992, chap 17; with permission of Oxford University Press, New York.)

cell diapedesis, and an inflammatory cellular reaction of polymorphs and lymphocytes, these changes being accompanied by edema. All of these changes cause swelling of the spinal cord, which becomes rounded and tense within the leptomeninges and dura, with obliteration of the subarachnoid and subdural spaces. In addition to the swelling, purple discoloration arises from the initial hemorrhage, which is added to later by venous stasis. The final form usually assumes the shape of a spindle. This comprises a fusiform region of softening, which affects one or more segments and tapers to end above and below a small round area of necrosis usually situated in the posterior columns. Measures in the immediate post-traumatic period to combat this cord swelling have frequently

been advocated, but the majority opinion favors conservative treatment. Recently, the richness of neuropeptides in the spinal cord has been documented.[9] Some are destroyed, but the production of others is stimulated by trauma. The action of neuropeptides and other active compounds in the early stage of spinal cord injury merits study.

The acute changes just described subside and are gradually replaced after 2 to 3 weeks by a reparative phase that can continue for up to 2 or more years.[11] The edema has by this time subsided, and the smaller hemorrhages have been absorbed. The polymorphs of the acute reaction are replaced by lymphocytes and large macrophages. The most striking cell is the lipid phagocyte. These phagocytes are present wherever necrosis has destroyed neurons, nerve fibers, and other elements with the liberation of breakdown products. The presence and location of a reactive astrocytic gliosis in any particular part of the traumatic lesion depends on the degree of damage and occurs when this is moderate. In severely damaged areas, the glia are destroyed along with the neuron cell bodies and their processes, and, here, organization is carried out by young fibroblasts to form the beginnings of a connective tissue scar. Changes in any surviving neurons consist of central chromatolysis. These neurons, with their swollen cytoplasm and eccentric nuclei, can persist for as many as 3 years.

Gradually the pathologic presentation changes. When the survival period is 5 to 10 years or more, a traumatic scar forms, with acellular collagenous connective tissue uniting meninges to the spinal canal and to the spinal cord (Fig. 3–8A and B). The grossly damaged regions of the cord are replaced by connective tissue occupying the position of the former blood clot and the severe parenchymal necrosis. The less damaged regions of the cord and always a zone above and below the main damage show an intense astrocytic fibrous gliosis. A glial network with occasional astrocyte cell bodies replaces the damaged nerve fibers and the destroyed

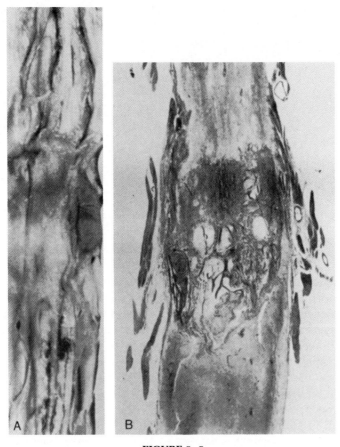

FIGURE 3–8

Trauma. *A*, Anterior aspect of the spinal cord showing late appearance of a traumatic lesion. Above and below, the spinal cord is discernible, but in the region of injury, a connective tissue scar replaces the damaged cord and blends with the thickened dura mater. *B*, Longitudinal section through the traumatic scar of a patient with long survival. The injured spinal cord segments are telescoped and three segments occupy the normal space of one. The center of the scar is filled with regenerating nerve fibers and clothed with Schwann cells. The nerve fibers are invading the scar from the posterior nerve roots. (From Hughes JT: Pathology of the Spinal Cord, ed 2. London, WB Saunders, 1978; with permission of Hodder & Stoughton Ltd, London.)

cell bodies. An interesting regenerative phenomenon is frequently seen in these traumatic scars. The cell bodies of the posterior root ganglia regenerate their central processes into the region of the connective tissue scar. These fibers, which are myelinated by Schwann cells, ramify in the connective tissue in the manner of an amputation neuroma of peripheral nerve. They do not enter the glial scar and do not penetrate intact nervous tissue.[10, 11, 17]

Post-traumatic Syringomyelia

In a few patients, long after the initial injury and at a time when the neurologic state has been stable for several months, signs of an upward extension of the spinal cord lesion become evident.[22] This development can progress rapidly and can reach the level of the medulla. The central part of the spinal cord is the most affected, with neurologic signs and myelographic appearances similar to those seen in idiopathic syringomyelia. Although in most instances the syringomyelia is an upward cavitation from the original trauma, downward cavitation can also occur but is clinically silent because of the existing cord lesion above. A combination of upward and downward syringomyelia extending from the trauma may be found. The anatomic extent of these post-traumatic syringes can be demonstrated postmortem provided that many sections are examined. A communication or several communications between the syrinx and the subarachnoid space is nearly always demonstrable, the usual location being near the posterior root entry zone.

DISEASES OF THE SPINE AFFECTING THE SPINAL CORD

The bony, cartilaginous, and fibrous components of the vertebral column normally protect the spinal cord, but some diseases or malformations of the spine can cause local or widespread pressure either on the spinal cord or on the blood vessels that supply it.[23] The effects of this type of pressure resemble those of slowly growing tumors. In some in-

stances the pressure is widespread, in others it is sharply localized, and in most patients the onset is insidious and progressive. Primary spinal diseases are discussed in this section, but tumors, primary and secondary, of the spine are also a common cause of spinal cord compression, and a similar effect can be produced by inflammatory disease, notably kyphosis due to tuberculous osteitis (Figs. 3–9 through 3–14).

Osteitis Deformans (Paget's Disease of Bone)

The skull and vertebral column are common sites of osteitis deformans, which can produce lesions in the brain, spinal cord, or spinal nerve roots.[26] The rarefaction of the body trabeculae, which constitutes the early stage of the disease, makes the bone less able

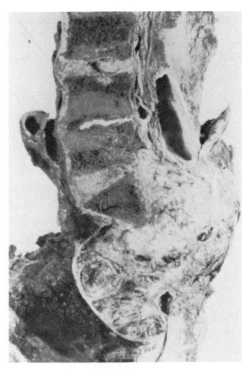

FIGURE 3–9

Chordoma involving the spinal cord. The lumbosacral spine has been sawn sagittally to show the destruction and replacement of the sacrum by tumor. (From Hughes JT: Pathology of the Spinal Cord, ed 2. London, WB Saunders, 1978; with permission of Hodder & Stoughton Ltd, London.)

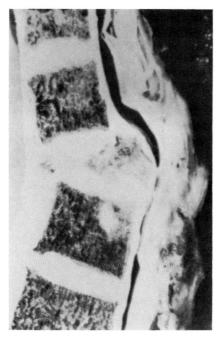

FIGURE 3–10

Malignant paraplegia from carcinoma of the bronchus. There is angulation at the T2 body that has collapsed owing to infiltration by metastatic tumor. Another tumor is seen in the T3 body. (From Hughes JT: Pathology of the Spinal Cord, ed 2. London, WB Saunders, 1978; with permission of Hodder & Stoughton Ltd, London.)

to resist the effects of gravity despite its increased thickness, so that as it thickens it becomes moulded into new shapes. Osteoporosis from other causes can result in a similar deformity. In osteitis deformans of the spine, some degree of kyphosis is usually present, and in some patients a sharp curvature may be manifest. However, the paraplegia that occasionally results is more often due to a general reduction in the size of the lumen of the canal or to local pressure by bony prominences, which can form on the dorsal surfaces of the vertebral bodies.

Ossification of the Posterior Longitudinal Ligament

Several recent reports have described compression of the spinal cord due to spinal stenosis in the cervical or thoracic region, caused by ossification of the posterior longitudinal ligament.

Bony Abnormalities in the Region of the Foramen Magnum

Abnormalities in the floor of the posterior fossa or in the articulation of the skull with the atlas or of the atlas with the axis can cause serious neurologic symptoms. Three common abnormalities have been described: occipitalization or assimilation of the atlas, in which there is partial or complex bony fusion of the atlas with the ring of the foramen magnum; basilar invagination or impression; and anomalies either of the odontoid process itself or of its relation to the atlas.

Intervertebral Disk Protrusion

The central part of the intervertebral disk consists of soft cellular fibrocartilage, with very fine collagenous fibers, forming the nucleus pulposus, which is the structure that protrudes, usually posteriorly, to injure the spinal nerve roots or occasionally the spinal cord. Protrusions upward or downward into the adjacent vertebral body cause Schmorl's node.

Spondylosis Deformans

Degeneration of the intervertebral disks is common after the age 50 years owing to gradual desiccation of the nucleus pulposus. This causes bony outgrowths from the margins of the upper and lower surfaces of the vertebral bodies, forming the lipping that is commonly seen after middle age.[2] Anterior lipping causes no neurologic symptoms, and many patients in whom minor degrees of posterior lipping are present are also asymptomatic. In a few patients, however, bony transverse ridges on the dorsal surface of the cervical vertebrae associated with protrusions of disk substance are the cause of paraparesis or tetraparesis (see Figs. 3–13A and B).

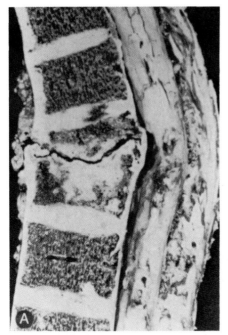

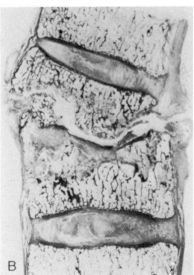

FIGURE 3–11

Pott's paraplegia. *A*, Right half of a sagittally sawn thoracic spine. T7 and T8 vertebral bodies have collapsed owing to tuberculous osteitis. The anterior aspect of the spinal cord is compressed by kyphosis. *B*, Decalcified section of left half of the spine seen in *A*. The histologic appearances are a mirror image of those seen in *A*. (From Hughes JT: Pathology of the Spinal Cord, ed 2. London, WB Saunders, 1978; with permission of Hodder & Stoughton Ltd, London.)

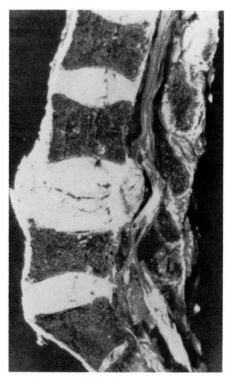

FIGURE 3–12

Spinal osteoporosis. Sagittally sawn lumbosacral spine shows collapse of L4 body and pressure on the cauda equina. (From Hughes JT: Pathology of the Spinal Cord, ed 2. London, WB Saunders, 1978; with permission of Hodder & Stoughton Ltd, London.)

Rheumatoid Arthritis Involving the Spinal Cord

Rhematoid arthritis is an arthropathy in which destruction is present not only in the articular joint surfaces and joint capsules but also in the ancillary ligaments that support the joints. Characteristically, relatively little reactive bone formation is seen, and in the intervals when the disease is inactive, little bony repair takes place. When rheumatoid arthritis affects the spine, the arthritis does not itself create the osteophytes characteristic of spondylosis deformans, although this disorder can coexist. Rheumatoid arthritis involving the spine produces a myelopathy by cervical dislocations, which may occur between C1 and 2 (atlantoaxial) or below C2 (subaxial) (see Figs. 3–14*A* and *B*). Subaxial dislocations are less common, and in neither

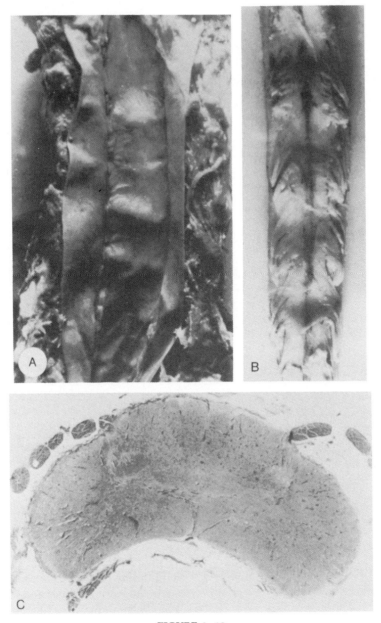

FIGURE 3–13

Cervical spondylosis. A, Spinal canal opened from behind with removal of the spinal cord. B, Anterior view of the spinal cord. C, Histologic section of the spinal cord at C6. (From Hughes JT: Pathology of the Spinal Cord, ed 2. London, WB Saunders, 1978; with permission of Hodder & Stoughton Ltd, London.)

dislocation has the pathologic abnormality of the spinal cord been studied in more than a few patients. My report described two patients with severe longstanding rheumatoid arthritis involving the cervical spine.[13] A progressive spinal cord syndrome developed in which spastic paraparesis was combined with a lower motor neuron paresis affecting the upper limb. In both instances, necropsy showed the cause to be subluxation between the C4 and 5 vertebral bodies and backward encroachment into the spinal canal of the upper and posterior part of the C5 vertebral body. A feature of the spinal cord abnormal-

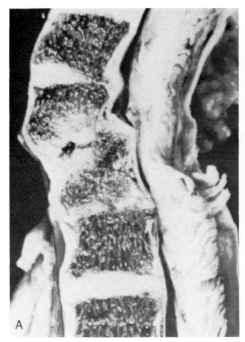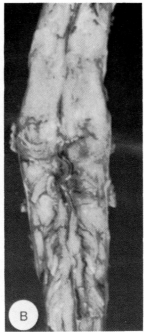

FIGURE 3–14

Rheumatoid arthritis with myelopathy. *A*, Sagittally sawn cervical spine for C3 to C7. Forward subluxation of the spine has occurred down to C4 with respect to the part from C5 downward. Note the deformity of the spinal cord. *B*, Anterior aspect of the spinal cord showing compression of the C4 segment. (From Hughes JT: Pathology of the Spinal Cord, ed 2. London, WB Saunders, 1978; with permission of Hodder & Stoughton Ltd, London.)

ity was central infarction, apparently caused by an effect on a patent anterior spinal artery and manifested not only at the site of spinal cord compression but also for several spinal cord segments caudal to this level.

SUMMARY

The neuropathology of the spinal cord is described and illustrated from the viewpoint of a neuropathologist observing at necropsy the many traumas and pathologic diseases affecting the spinal cord. The clinician is provided with an insight into the disease processes and anatomic derangements underlying the neurologic deficits in paraplegia and quadriplegia.

The clinical examination of patients with spinal cord trauma or spinal cord disease is greatly assisted by many ancillary investigations, notably, radiology and the new imaging techniques now applied so successfully to

the spinal cord. Comparison of the patient's neuropathology with the classical neuropathology of the spinal cord provided in this chapter remains important for the clinician.

REFERENCES

1. Barnett HJM, Foster JB, Hudgson P: Syringomyelia. WB Saunders, London, 1973.
2. Brain WR, Northfield D, Wilkinson M: The neurological manifestations of cervical spondylosis. Brain 75:187–225, 1952.
3. Braunstein H: Pathogenesis of dissecting aneurysm. Circulation 28:1071–1080, 1963.
4. Chiro G, Wener L: Angiography of the spinal cord. J Neurosurg 39:1–29, 1973.
5. Clancy RR, Sladky JT, Rorke LB: Hypoxia-ischemic spinal cord injury following perinatal asphyxia. Ann Neurol 25:185–189, 1989.
6. Djindjian R: Angiography of the Spinal Cord. Baltimore, University Park Press, 1970.
7. Hassler W, Thon A, Grate EH: Hemodynamics of spinal dural arteriovenous fistulas. J Neurosurg 70:360–370, 1989.
8. Hills S, Vasquez JM: Massive infarction of spinal cord and vertebral bodies as a complication of dissecting aneurysm of the aorta. Circulation 25:997–1000, 1962.

9. Hughes JT: The new neuroanatomy of the spinal cord. Paraplegia 27:90–98, 1989.

10. Hughes JT: Pathology of spinal cord damage in spinal injuries. In Feiring EH (ed): Brock's Injuries of the Brain and Spinal Cord, ed 5. New York, Springer, 1974, pp 668–687.

11. Hughes JT: Regeneration in the human spinal cord: A review of the response to injury of the various constituents of the human spinal cord. Paraplegia 22:131–137, 1984.

12. Hughes JT: Spinal-cord infarction due to aortic trauma. Br Med J 2:356, 1964.

13. Hughes JT: Spinal cord involvement by C4–C5 vertebral subluxation in rheumatoid arthritis. A description of two cases examined at necropsy. Ann Neurol 1:575–582, 1977.

14. Hughes JT: Thrombosis of the posterior, spinal arteries. A complication of an intrathecal injection of phenol. Neurology 20:659–664, 1970.

15. Hughes JT: Venous infarction of the spinal cord. Neurology 21:794–800, 1971.

16. Hughes JT: Vertebral artery insufficiency in acute cervical spine trauma. Int J Paraplegia 2:207–213, 1964.

17. Hughes JT, Brownell B: Aberrant nerve fibres within the spinal cord. J Neurol Neurosurg Psychiatry 26:528–534, 1963.

18. Hughes JT, Brownell B: Cervical spondylosis complicated by anterior spinal artery thrombosis. Neurology 14:1073–1077, 1964.

19. Hughes, JT, MacIntyre AG: Spinal cord infarction occurring during thoraco-lumbar sympathectomy. J Neurol Psychiatry 26:418–421, 1963.

20. Lindsay J, Hurst JW: Clinical features and prognosis in dissecting aneurysm of the aorta. Circulation 35:880–888, 1967.

21. Perier O, Demanet JC, Henneaux J, et al: Existe-t-il un syndrome des arteres spinales posterieures? Rev Neurol 113:396–409, 1960.

22. Rossier AB, Foo D, Shillito, et al: Posttraumatic cervical syringomyelia. Brain 108:439–461, 1985.

23. Schmorl G, Junghans H: The Human Spine in Health and Disease, 1st Am. ed. (Trans and ed, Wilk SP). New York, Grune and Stratton, 1959.

24. Wolstenholme GEW, Porter R: Systemic Mycoses. (Ciba Foundation Symposium held in Ibadan, 1987.) London, Churchill, 1968.

25. Wright RL: Intramedullary spinal cord abscess: Report of a case secondary to stab wound with good recovery following operation. J Neurosurg 23:208–210, 1965.

26. Wyllie WG: The occurrence in osteitis deformans of lesions of the central nervous system with a report of four cases. Brain 46:336–351, 1923.

CHAPTER 4

Acute Nontraumatic Myelopathies

David M. Dawson, M.D.
Frisso Potts, M.D.

Acute myelopathies include two major groups consisting of inflammatory and vascular disorders. The clinical presentations conform to the patterns described elsewhere (see Chapter 7). With modern imaging techniques, particularly magnetic resonance imaging (MRI), exclusion of compressive lesions is relatively easy, but differentiation between an inflammatory/demyelinative lesion and a vascular/ischemic lesion can be difficult. This is best illustrated by the myelopathies seen in lupus erythematosus which are described later. This chapter describes the clinical features of both types of acute myelopathy.

We do not discuss multiple sclerosis as a separate entity. One of the most common causes of myelopathy in American and European clinics, this condition is naturally included in the differential diagnosis of any spinal cord lesion, especially if it is recurrent or progressive. Nothing is clinically distinctive about acute lesions of multiple sclerosis in the spinal cord, with the possible exception of the marked prominence of Lhermitte's sign in some patients. The diagnosis of disseminated disease therefore depends on the discovery of lesions in the cerebrum by MRI or in the optic pathways by visual evoked responses (VER) or by some other paraclinical observation.

ACUTE TRANSVERSE MYELITIS (AUTOIMMUNE TYPE)

Acute inflammatory lesions of the spinal cord have been seen for many decades. The fact that some of these lesions occur within a week or two of a viral illness or an immunization indicates that an immune response to an antigenic stimulus may be involved. It is clinically important to distinguish patients who have an autoimmune cause of a lesion from those with vascular insufficiency, vascular malformations, multiple sclerosis, or compressive lesions of the cord. Thus, several investigators have gathered series of patients with acute transverse myelitis and attempted to discern specific clinical features that would be diagnostically useful.[1, 11, 129]

The general features are as follows:

1. The time course typically encompasses several days to several weeks.

2. An antecedent viral illness is recorded in approximately a third of patients.

3. Initial symptoms can include ascending paresthesis, back pain, weakness, or urinary retention. The patients with the most acute onset and with pain have the poorest prognoses.[129]

4. The thoracic cord is affected in most patients and the cervical cord in only 10%; T8 and T12 upper levels of dysfunction are the most common.

5. Pathologic study (available in only a few instances) shows a primary demyelinating process with significant inflammation. Despite the name of the disorder, which implies a localized transverse lesion, the process often extends through many segments of the cord.

6. The illness is rare. From 1955 to 1975 in Israel, the incidence was 0.13 patient per 100,000 population.[11]

7. The relationship to multiple sclerosis remains controversial. In an American series, later development of multiple sclerosis after initial presentation with acute transverse myelitis occurred in 5% to 10% of patients. In Israel (where multiple sclerosis is less common), later development of this condition is very rare.[11] Both illnesses are demyelinating and inflammatory, but significant differences exist in the pathologic findings, e.g., acute transverse myelitis causes much more necrosis. Acute perivenous encephalomyelitis, which may present with acute myelopathy along with optic neuropathy, encephalopathy, and other disorders, is also distinguishable from acute transverse myelitis.

8. Lymphocytes from patients with acute transverse myelitis show immune reactivity to myelin basic protein or to P2 protein.[1] Similar immune responses also occur in acute perivenous encephalomyelitis, and the latter illness (but not necessarily acute transverse myelitis) closely resembles experimental encephalomyelitis in which myelin basic protein is the standard antigen. The antigen in acute transverse myelitis is undefined.

9. MRI scans in those few patients who have undergone study show high signal intensity on long TR sequences, often over six or more segments.[10]

MYELOPATHY IN LUPUS ERYTHEMATOSUS

A variety of neurologic syndromes have been observed in patients with systemic lupus erythematosus. In patients with clinically apparent systemic lupus erythematosus, seizures, confusion, and delirium are the most common presentations.[81] Peripheral neuropathy and optic neuropathy also occur.

Myelopathy is an infrequent neurologic manifestation of systemic lupus erythematosus. Most of the available information on spinal cord syndromes in systemic lupus erythematosus is derived from case reports or reviews of the literature summarizing anecdotal experience. After reviewing this literature, we believe these cases can usefully be classified into two groups.

Group 1: Acute Transverse Myelitis

The case reported by Propper and Bucknall[125] is illustrative. They describe a 16-year-old girl with a history of arthralgia and vasculitis in the fingers, positive antinuclear antibodies, and reduced complement levels in whom an acute paraplegia developed over the course of 4 hours. The patient had midscapular pain and a dense sensory level to T7, with sparing of dorsal column function. Study of cerebrospinal fluid (CSF) showed a protein level of 1100 mg/mL with pleocytosis and reduced glucose content. She was treated intensively and had a partial recovery after many months.

In their review, Propper and Buchnall found 44 reported cases of acute myelopathy, although only half of these were described in detail. There have been many representative case reports.[8, 16, 61, 85] The clinical features of these cases resemble those of acute transverse myelitis of the autoimmune type:

1. Acute onset over a few hours or days.

2. Back pain at the level of the sensory loss.

3. Severe paralysis, often with flaccidity.

4. Easily demonstrated sensory level.

5. CSF showing elevated total protein, pleocytosis, and reduction of glucose (in 50% of patients).

6. Myelography showing local swelling of the cord.

7. MRI[16] showing enlargement and edema of the cord.

The pathologic substrate of this clinical presentation appears to be incomplete spinal cord infarction. In a review published in 1978, reports of 12 autopsies were summarized.[87] Most of the patients had had myelomalacia, vasculitis, and occluded vessels. Recovery in most instances was either poor or long-delayed, although favorable responses to intensive immunosuppression occurred, typically with high-dose steroids, intravenous cyclophosphamide, or short-term plasma exchanges.

Group 2: Subacute Myelopathy

By contrast, patients with systemic lupus erythematosus in whom subacute myelopathy develops do not have acute transverse lesions. This myelopathy is less intense, can recur, or can progress over some time. For example, in a 10-year-old girl, Lhermitte's phenomenon developed, and several months later a subacute spinal syndrome was manifest.[98] Examination showed a right hemiparesis, weakness of the left leg, and no sensory level. Over the course of a year, she experienced three mild relapses. Although she had hematologic test results compatible with systemic lupus erythematosus (positive antinuclear antibody, decreased complement, and histone antibodies) and a skin biopsy suggested immune abnormalities, she did not have signs or symptoms of involvement of other organs.

From the clinical standpoint the disorder in these patients more closely resembles multiple sclerosis. The rather unfortunate term *lupoid sclerosis* was used in several reports,[46, 62] indicating the resemblance to multiple sclerosis. The common features in cases reported thus far include (1) subacute onset, progression over weeks or months, or recurrence; (2) asymmetrical weakness; (3) sensory level poorly defined or partial;[97] and (4) presence of other neurologic signs, such as optic neuropathy,[85] tonic spasms,[76] or dystonia.[98]

The pathologic substrate of this illness is poorly understood because of the lack of autopsy data. In one of the cases reported by Johnson and Richardson,[81] a subacute degenerative process without occluded vessels was present; this may be a pathologic correlate. Another autopsy report describes widespread demyelination in the cord, although one area of necrosis was noted in the midthoracic region.[90]

The role of anticardiolipin antibodies in the production of myelopathy is unknown.[94] Both group 1 and group 2 patients can have these serum antibodies in high titer, whereas in other instances they are absent.

The more widespread use of MRI assists in evaluation but will not clear up the ambiguities about the pathogenesis of group 2 disorders. Both multiple sclerosis and systemic lupus erythematosus can cause lesions with similar MRI appearances in cerebrum or spinal cord. Multiple sclerosis appears to be a primary autoimmune illness with a component of myelin as the target, possibly a sequence of myelin basic protein.[121] Few patients with multiple sclerosis have any anti-

DNA or antiphospholipid antibodies. The true nature of the illness in disputed cases may be best evaluated by serologic means.

MYELOPATHY CAUSED BY HERPES VIRUS

The herpesviruses, which are enveloped DNA viruses, include herpes simplex virus (HSV), types 1 and 2, varicella-zoster virus (VZV), cytomegalovirus (CMV), Epstein-Barr virus (EBV), and herpes simiae (monkey B virus). Of these viruses, the only one known to cause myelopathy as a frequent clinical outcome of infection is herpes simiae in laboratory workers exposed to this agent.[165]

Myelopathy has been reported in association with VZV and with both types of HSV. The number of cases is small with respect to all three viruses, and the status of acute myelopathy in herpetic infection is far from clear. The known proclivity of each of these viruses to produce another syndrome must also be taken into consideration: VSV, an acute local sensory ganglionitis with rash; HSV-1, an acute limbic encephalitis; and HSV-2, an acute lumbosacral radiculopathy with urinary retention. The appearance of acquired immunodeficiency syndrome (AIDS)–related myelopathy syndromes has caused further confusion. In particular, CMV, another DNA virus of the herpes group, can cause myelopathy in patients with AIDS, sometimes associated with severe radiculopathy. A definitive diagnosis may therefore require isolation of virus from autopsy tissue or demonstration of viral protein or nucleic acids within tissue by immunohistochemical techniques. Demonstration of herpesvirus infection in other organs (e.g., CMV retinopathy) or isolation of virus from CSF (common in HSV-2 meningoencephalitis), although indicating an association, would not constitute proof of cause.

Wiley and others[165] described a 57-year-old diabetic man who died of a rapidly ascending necrotizing myelopathy that extended from C4 to the conus, with additional lesions in the mid-brain, cerebellum, nerves, and dorsal root ganglia. HSV antigen was demonstrable by the immunoperoxidase technique, and HSV-2 was grown by culture from the cord. Hogan and Krigman[69] described a 59-year-old woman with severe myelopathy at T8–11 segments, serpentine extensions above and below this point, and isolation of VZV at autopsy. Less well-documented cases of possible VZV myelopathy (with or without rash) also have been recorded.[63, 108] A patient with myelopathy at T2, with good subsequent recovery, had HSV-2 isolated from CSF.[5]

In a patient with AIDS, both CMV and HSV-2 were found in the spinal cord following a progressive ascending myelitis that began with arreflexia and urinary retention.[159] In retrospect, we wonder whether CMV infection, as in the case of Mahieux and colleagues,[101] caused the radiculopathy.

No clear pattern emerges from the reported cases of herpesvirus myelopathy. All occurrences seem rare. The spread of AIDS will obviously increase their number. Severe ascending necrosis of the cord seems to be a typical version of infection in the few well-studied cases.

MYELOPATHY WITH TOXOPLASMOSIS

Toxoplasma gondii, a protozoan parasite, is a common cause of infectious focal encephalitis in the AIDS population. We are aware of two reports of invasion of the cord by this organism, producing in both instances a well-localized expansion of the cord.[66, 110] One patient with myelopathy had a laminectomy at T1–5 to reduce pressure, with a poor outcome.

SCHISTOSOMIASIS

Spinal involvement in schistosomiasis is due to either Schistosoma mansoni or S. haematobium. Its true incidence is unknown because it is rarely reported, but as many as 200 million persons in the world may be infected (World Health Organization data). Granulomata form around the lumbar roots and the conus, and most instances involve only the lumbar cord. Immunologic tests are often positive; rectal biopsy may be needed to establish the diagnosis. Eosinophilia is frequently absent.

Early treatment with praziquantel can be curative. Delay in treatment can lead to irreversible paraplegia.[154]

BORRELIOSIS—LYME DISEASE

A spectrum of peripheral and central nervous system disorders can occur after infection with *Borrelia burgdorferi* (Lyme disease). Frequently, the clinical presentation is dominated by painful radiculopathy with mental confusion.[99] In one patient, a spastic quadriparesis developed as part of Lyme disease, and cervical MRI showed a small intramedullary cavity or syrinx.[92] Another patient had painful cramps, stiffness, and spasms of one leg, interpreted as gray matter infection.[106] This patient had spontaneous and reflex myoclonus.

TOXIC MYELOPATHY

Several chemotherapeutic agents can cause acute myelopathy when injected intrathecally; methotrexate and cytosine arabinoside seem to be the most common offenders.[34]

Chemonucleolysis with chymopapain has been associated rarely with transverse myelopathy.[41]

Injection of penicillin into the buttock in infants can cause infarction of the cord in the thoracolumbar region, probably due to inadvertent intra-arterial injection.[153]

ISCHEMIC MYELOPATHY

Spinal cord strokes are a rare, although devastating, cause of myelopathy. The overall incidence of spinal cord ischemia is not known and is difficult to determine from the literature because published reports often fail to describe the patient population in which the cases were encountered or how many cases were reviewed in a given series. It is clear, however, that spinal cord ischemia is much less frequent than cerebral ischemia.[138] In a recent study in which admissions to a general hospital over a 52-month period were reviewed, eight cases of ischemic myelopathy were found, representing 1.2% of all admissions for stroke.[137] In a retrospective study of 2500 patients seen at a spinal cord injury center, Eltorai and Juler[40] found 92 nontraumatic occurrences of myelopathy (excluding those due to malignancy). Of these, 25 instances (37.5%) were attributable to ischemia. In a later series from the same center, in which 1535 patients admitted between 1975 and 1986 were reviewed, only 25 occurrences of ischemic myelopathy were found.[89] Other studies describe an even lower incidence of this condition. Blackwood[12] found 7 instances of nontraumatic ischemic or hemorrhagic myelopathy among 3737 postmortem examinations carried out over a 50-year period at National Hospital, Queen Square. Van Wieringen[162] reviewed a 30-year experience at a general neurology clinic and found only 9 cases of this condition but did not report the total number of case records reviewed.

Mechanisms of Spinal Cord Ischemia

Much information is available on the anatomy and physiology of the spinal circulation (see Chapter 1). However, no obvious explanation is available regarding why spinal strokes occur less frequently than do cerebral strokes.

One explanation that has been advanced has to do with the presence of rich anastomotic channels connecting various levels of the cord through coronal vessels.[40] However, well-designed experiments have demonstrated that these anastomotic channels are probably inadequate to perform the task of redistributing blood flow further than one or two adjacent segments and that, at best, they may protect only the peripheral or superficial white matter.[78, 95] Much the same is true of the medullary vessels. Although their capillary bed appears more extensive than that found in the cerebral circulation, they act as end arteries and provide little or no flow between anterior and posterior circulation in the cord.

Extraspinal anastomoses do exist and may

provide functionally adequate redistribution of flow in instances of occlusion of spinal or segmental vessels. These are most evident in the cervical region[157] and less well-defined caudally, a possible explanation for the relatively greater incidence of caudal ischemia. These extraspinal anastomotic channels may also account for the observation that the closer vascular occlusion occurs to the aorta or vertebral arteries, the less likely the cord is to suffer ischemia.[64]

In addition to the adequacy of the blood supply, another important factor in determining ischemic damage is the tissue's vulnerability to ischemia. In this respect, the spinal cord may have an advantage over the brain. The greater metabolic requirements of the brain are suggested by the brain's greater blood flow (both brain and spinal cord autoregulate blood flow). The total blood flow in the brain is 50 mL/minute/100 g. The blood flow in the cord varies according to the spinal level and the species studied, but a rate of 19.7 ± 1.2 mL/minute/100 g of tissue probably represents maximal flow in the resting cord.[116]

Indeed, experiments designed to study the spinal cord's resistance to ischemia suggest that no permanent ischemic damage occurs in the cord with as much as 30 minutes of interruption in blood supply by aortic clamping.[122] This experiment, carried out in dogs, is one of many suggesting that the cord can survive relatively long periods of ischemia.[86, 135] Clinical data also suggest that aortic clamping times of less than 30 minutes are attended by a lower incidence of permanent spinal ischemia.[18]

It is also clear that when ischemia occurs, the most vulnerable region of the spinal cord is the gray matter[104] because its metabolic rate may be three to five times that of white matter. This would account for the many cases reported in the literature of severe paraparesis with little or no sensory involvement and for instances of progressive lower motor neuron syndrome on an ischemic basis.

Aortic Dissection

Spinal cord infarction is a well-recognized complication of spontaneous aortic dissection,[109, 150] which may be the most common cause of vascular cord injury.[45] DeBakey and co-workers[137] reported an incidence of just under 2% in a series of 527 patients with spontaneous aortic dissection and noted that this complication is not as common as cerebral ischemia or peripheral nerve ischemia. The differentiation between peripheral nerve ischemia and spinal ischemia can be difficult clinically in some patients.[164] It is an important distinction, because peripheral nerve ischemia can be reversible with reestablishment of the blood flow and has a better prognosis. At times, however, peripheral nerve ischemia and spinal ischemia can coexist as a complication of aortic aneurysm dissection or rupture. The location and extent of the dissection are important factors in determining the degree of cord ischemia.

Aortic dissections are classified as type I when they involve the ascending as well as descending aorta, type II when they are proximal to the take-off of the left subclavian artery, and type III when distal to it. The last type is further subdivided into type IIIa when only the thoracic descending aorta is involved and type IIIb when the dissection extends below the diaphragm. Ischemic myelopathy is equally common in types I and III, with a vanishingly small incidence in type II.[37, 141, 169]

The clinical presentation is variable. Descriptions range from syndromes resembling those of complete spinal cord transection[139] to anterior spinal artery syndrome.[169] Most patients, however, typically present with sudden onset of paraplegia accompanied by chest or abdominal pain. The pain is described as very sharp or tearing and may radiate into the lower extremities.[150] Sensory loss below the lower thoracic dermatomes is the rule.[67, 89] Some reports have stressed that the aneurysmal dissection can occur without pain;[49] however, it appears that none of the patients with painless dissection could be unequivocally determined to have myelopathy and may have had peripheral nerve ischemia instead.[49, 67] The motor deficits in all pathologically proved cases of ischemic myelopathy are bilateral.[139] Occasionally, the deficit starts as a monoparesis but soon becomes bilateral. In some patients, the symptoms may be intermittent before the onset of a more permanent deficit.[39, 139] Although paraparesis is the most common presentation, tetraparesis or triparesis has been described as a result of more proximal dissections.[139]

This mechanism of cord ischemia appears to be occlusion of the mouth of segmental spinal arteries by the dissection. The greatest incidence of ischemia is encountered in dissections involving the descending thoracic aorta and upper abdominal aorta, which give rise to thoracic spinal arteries and the artery of Adamkiewicz. For this reason, lesions below the level of the renal arteries tend to cause little or no spinal ischemia.[3, 37, 164]

Atherosclerosis and Other Occlusive Diseases of the Aorta and Its Branches

Atherosclerosis commonly affects the aorta and causes narrowing of the ostia of segmental arteries but may account for only 1% of all instances of ischemic myelopathy.[79] The process of atheroma formation can be slow enough to permit adequate collateralization,[45] which can spare the cord. This may be one of the situations in which, by virtue of the slowness of the occlusion and the cord's circulation autoregulatory abilities, the coronal vessels can actually become important channels for redistribution of flow between widely separated segments.

Unlike the aorta, the segmental and spinal vessels are rarely involved by atheroma or by hypertensive vasculopathy.[72] In the rare documented case of acute ischemic myelopathy secondary to atherosclerosis, a progressive ischemic myelopathy is described.[143] It tends to occur in the elderly, presenting as a combination of upper and lower motor neuron signs with preferential cervical cord involvement.[103] The pathologic findings in the reported cases support an ischemic etiology.[74, 79] Although progression over weeks to years is emphasized, acute exacerbations can occur due to superimposed hypotensive episodes.[74]

Atherosclerosis also has been blamed for the syndrome of spinal cord claudication,[64] a syndrome distinct from cauda equina claudication. These patients experience intermittent exercise-induced painless lower extremity weakness, sometimes accompanied by sphincter disturbances. A similar syndrome has been produced experimentally in dogs by radicular artery ligation[126] but no pathologic or radiologic evidence has been found to confirm atherosclerosis as the cause of this syndrome in humans.

Other causes of aortic occlusion can also result in spinal ischemia. Sumpio and Gusberg[155] have reviewed instances of blunt abdominal trauma resulting in aortic occlusion, noting the rarity of this complication. They emphasize that both cord and peripheral nerve ischemia can occur under these circumstances and that the latter has a better prognosis.

Spinal Cord Ischemia Due to Embolic Etiologies

Thromboemboli as a cause of spinal cord infarction have rarely been documented.[51, 60] A review of several published studies of subacute and acute bacterial endocarditis, comprising more than 1300 reported cases, failed to reveal any definite instances of ischemic myelopathy.[24, 38, 43, 53, 58, 71, 82, 120] Although some of the patients reported by Jones and others[82] may have had myelopathy, no clearcut clinical or pathologic evidence of this exists.

Atheromatous emboli also have been implicated in spinal cord infarctions. Again, documented cases are few.[119, 123] In a retrospective study of 1000 autopsies, Slavin and co-workers[149] found 28 cases of histologically documented atheromatous emboli to abdominal viscera. Despite careful and exhaustive examination of the spinal cord in this group, only one patient had had symptoms of ischemic myelopathy and demonstrated atheromatous embolization of the anterior spinal artery. Eleven patients had had evidence of atheromatous emboli to the spinal vessels, two with evidence of focal cord ischemia but without obvious clinical myelopathy.

Fibrocartilaginous embolization was described as a cause of ischemic cord lesion in 1961.[114] Since then, a total of 25 cases have been reported in the American literature.[14] The origin of the emboli appears to be the intervertebral disk. Infarction can occur at any cord level, and it is not clear how disk fragments get into the circulation to cause the infarction. Although some form of trauma is thought to be necessary to cause extrusion of disk material into the spinal circulation, in most reported cases no history of major trauma is present to explain the event. The patients tend to have had a painful onset, with pain at or close to the spinal level of the lesion. Severe, bilateral motor deficit develops very quickly. Little or no recovery has been described.

Decompression sickness (caisson disease) has been implicated in air embolization of the spinal cord. Kim and colleagues[89] reported acute myelopathy in three divers who ascended quickly from a depth of more than 100 feet. Two of the patients had partial motor/sensory deficits at the low thoracic level and one at the mid-cervical level, and partial recovery of function was noted. Previous reports describe a similar clinical presentation.[64] The pathophysiology of the lesion appears to be occlusion of epidural venous sinuses by nitrogen gas bubbles that come out of solution during rapid decompression. This impairs venous return from the cord and results in patchy hemorrhagic myelopathy.[58]

A patient with atrial myxoma with presumed embolization to the cord was reported by Wolman and Bradshaw.[168] At postmortem examination, intramedullary vessels in the infarcted region showed fibrinous material with evidence of organization. No myxomatous emboli were found, but it was assumed that the fibrin adherent to the myxoma had embolized the cord. Malarial infestation[64] has also been implicated in embolic cord pathology. Despite the worldwide abundance of malaria, only one or two case reports of cord ischemia can be found. A slightly more common cause of spinal cord vessel embolization is schistosomiasis. The usual presentation is a slowly progressive radiculopathy or myelopathy, most likely due to inflammatory reaction to the parasitic ova,[154] but occasionally a strokelike onset of the deficit is seen. The most common route for the parasites to reach the cord appears to be by embolization of the venous plexus; however, embolization of the arteria radicularis magna can be equally

common and might account for why the majority of patients demonstrate lumbosacral involvement.[144]

Embolization, of whatever origin, is clearly a rare etiology of spinal strokes.

Spinal Cord Ischemia as a Complication of Vascular Surgery

Spinal cord ischemia has been a recognized attendant of cardiovascular surgery since the early practice of this discipline.[3] The incidence of this complication varies with the procedure performed, being highest in surgery involving the thoracic aorta[35, 147] and lowest in procedures involving the coronary arteries[40, 41] or the abdominal aorta below the level of the renal arteries.[36] In one of the largest series describing complications of thoracoabdominal aneurysm repair, Crawford and others[30] noted that the highest incidence of paraplegia (presumably cord ischemia) occurred in patients in whom aneurysm replacement involved the descending thoracic as well as the abdominal aorta. The incidence of paraplegia was 28% in this group as compared with 2% in patients in whom the aneurysm involved only the abdominal aorta. The incidence of spinal ischemia was much higher (as much as 42% for thoracoabdominal aorta replacement) in patients in whom the aneurysm had ruptured or had dissected before operation. It is not clear, however, how much neurologic deficit was present before operation in these patients. The study by Debakey and co-workers[36] on surgical intervention in the abdominal aorta does not report a single instance of spinal cord ischemia among 1719 patients whose lesions were below the level of the renal arteries. Nevertheless, later studies have shown that this complication can occur with infrarenal procedures.[124]

Repair of coarctation of the aorta also has been associated with spinal cord ischemia. Brewer and colleagues[18] reported an incidence of 0.41% in a series of 12,532 patients. Costello and Fischer[29] reported an incidence of 2.8% in a series of 84 patients; none of the 14 neonates included in their report had ischemic complications. Although the incidence of spinal strokes is clearly lower than that with aneurysmectomy, untreated coarctation of the aorta rarely leads to myelopathy.[18]

The vertical extent of cord damage varies depending on the individual patient's vascular pattern. Postoperative spinal cord syndromes tend to be catastrophic, with complete flaccid paraplegia, severe sensory loss, and loss of autonomic functions. However, reports have been made of remarkable improvements in neurologic function.[52]

Factors that are clearly related to the development of spinal ischemia are the extent of the aneurysm, rupture or dissection, and reattachment of intercostal vessels. Clamp time and development of hypotension in the segment distal to the occlusion do not appear by themselves to be correlated highly with cord pathology.[30]

Given the fact that repair of aortic aneurysms prolongs life expectancy, several procedures have been used to prevent spinal injury. The most popular operations have been shunt procedures designed to bypass the operative site and maintain distal perfusion. Left-atrium to femoral artery pump bypass,[35] artery to artery external shunting,[83] and femoral artery to vein shunt with oxygen perfusion[115] were among the leading techniques. Although the initial results were promising, these methods have not gained universal acceptance because they do not appear to consistently improve survival rates or to prevent ischemic myelopathy.[30] Some surgeons still find them useful, however, in selected patients.[93, 107] The relationship between CSF pressure and spinal cord perfusion also has been investigated because experimental data suggest that very low CSF pressure may protect against paraplegia.[70] Intraoperative recording of somatosensory evoked potentials has not proved reliable as a predictor of poor outcome.[33] Other methods that remain controversial are treatment with high doses of corticosteroids,[57] use of free-radical scavengers, and thiopental and papaverine therapy.[93] In an attempt to decrease metabolic demands of the spinal cord during operation, hypothermia is widely used and is believed to be effective in decreasing ischemic complications.

Although much effort has gone into preventing cord ischemia, there may be an irreducible minimum incidence of this complication that will prove refractory to anyone's best efforts.[30, 31]

Other Iatrogenic Causes

In addition to direct manipulation of the aorta, other surgical procedures have been implicated in cord ischemia. When sympathectomy was a commonly performed surgical procedure, cord strokes were reported, presumably as a consequence of unwitting ligation of segmental arteries.[75, 112] Radicular artery ligation also has been implicated in the cord syndromes following thoracoplasty,[132] pneumonectomy,[64] and correction of scoliosis.[108] Review of the recent literature suggests a decreasing incidence of ischemic myelopathy due to these procedures.

Intra-aortic balloon counterpulsation is a useful and relatively safe support measure in a variety of hypotensive syndromes.[27] Paraplegia has been reported following intra-aortic balloon counterpulsation. Criado and co-workers[31] reported a case of anterior spinal artery syndrome with a midthoracic motor and sensory level and referred to a previous description of this complication. Orr and colleagues[119] reported a case of myelopathy following intra-aortic balloon counterpulsation and reviewed six additional cases. Paraplegia was the most common clinical syndrome. In one patient a lower extremity monoparesis developed and was attributed to spinal cord infarction, but autopsy failed to show spinal ischemia.

Of patients with definite ischemic myelopathy, one had cholesterol emboli to the spinal vessels and another had a dissecting aortic wall hematoma that had apparently occluded segmental vessels supplying the spinal cord. Little or no recovery is reported in the patients who survived.

Spinal infarctions also have been reported as a result of continuous epidural or spinal anesthesia.[2, 84] The patients in whom paraplegia developed (with or without sensory deficit) as a complication have shown no significant recovery. Although hypotension as a result of the anesthetic may have a role, it appears that the main culprit is vasoconstriction of spinal vessels by the epinephrine or phenylephrine used in the anesthetic solution.[59] These vasoconstrictive agents greatly prolong the duration and analgesic effect of local anesthetics. This is an unusual complication but tends to occur in patients who may not be otherwise predisposed to spinal ischemia and has raised questions about the methodology of spinal anesthesia.[2, 59]

Catheterization of thoracic or abdominal vessels can also cause ischemic myelopathy. A case has been reported of spinal cord infarction following therapeutic renal artery embolization with absorbable gel sponge.[47] In this instance the material embolized spinal vessels. Ischemic complications of spinal and aortic angiography are few. A review of several large series[40, 44, 89] encompassing a total of 110 patients with ischemic myelopathy revealed only two separate instances of this complication. Szilagyi and others[156] reported an incidence of 0.01% in more than 17,000 patients examined, and Riche and coworkers[127] found no complications in 38 pediatric patients.

Occlusion of the Spinal Arteries and Microvasculature of the Cord

As may be gathered from the previous discussion on atherosclerosis, occlusion of spinal vessels themselves is not a major cause of ischemic myelopathy. Even in patients who present with the classic findings of anterior spinal artery syndrome, occlusion of the anterior spinal artery can rarely be documented, the ischemia being most likely due to occlusion of a more proximal vessel.[44]

In the past, a major, if not the major, cause of spinal vessel occlusion was syphilitic arteritis. In 1909, Spiller[152] reported a patient with acute myelopathy associated with meningovascular syphilis and anterior spinal artery thrombosis; he also mentioned another patient with acute myelopathy associated with syphilis. In this series and in a later one,[151] he suggested a vascular etiology for some of the cases of syphilitic myelitis. Adams and Merritt,[4] however, dubbed syphilitic ischemic myelopathy "a rarity." In a study of 2231 syphilitic patients at the Boston City Hospital, they found only 31 instances of spinal cord involvement; of these patients, 10 had evidence of cord ischemia on the basis of occlusion of meningeal or spinal vessels. In their review of vascular myelopathy, Winkelman and Eckel[166] could find no cases of syphilis and cited Spiller's[152] description of this entity. Foo and Rossier[44] reported only two cases of syphilitic etiology in a review of 60 patients with anterior spinal artery syndromes. With the advent of antibiotic therapy, the role of syphilis in central nervous system pathology has waned. Nevertheless, meningovascular infiltration from other causes can result in spinal strokes.

In a clinicopathologic study of 58 patients with ischemic myelopathy, Gruner and Lapresle[55] stressed the importance of meningeal infiltration by neoplastic or infectious disease as a mechanism for occlusion of spinal vessels. They found no patients with syphilitic involvement but described 13 patients with epidural metastases and 7 instances of meningeal tuberculosis resulting in cord infarctions. Van Wieringen[162] reported on two patients with anterior spinal artery syndrome associated with vertebral metastasis from malignant melanoma and prostatic carcinoma. In a series of eight patients, Sandson and Friedman[37] reported three instances of non-Hodgkin's lymphoma and one instance of prostatic carcinoma associated with acute ischemic myelopathy. In the last two series, however, only one autopsy is reported, and no definite evidence of vascular or meningeal involvement by the malignancy is shown. Other factors, such as radiation myelopathy or paraneoplastic myelopathy, may have been responsible for the clinical presentation.

With the increasing longevity of cancer victims, these two entities have become more apparent. Neither in postradiation myelopathy nor in paraneoplastic myelopathy does vascular occlusion appear to have a prominent role.[117] Only an occasional instance of vascular occlusion is reported in radiation myelopathy.[80]

Hypercoagulable states are well-known causes of central nervous system infarctions.[105] Arterial infarctions of the cord rarely occur during these circumstances. Thrombocytosis may have been a causative factor in a patient with giant cell arteritis leading to myelopathy.[50]

The relatively rare entity of venous infarctions appears to be more clearly related to hypercoagulable states,[26, 73] either hemorrhagic or nonhemorrhagic. The former are of relatively sudden onset and tend to be painful; the latter have a more subacute course, and pain is less frequent.[88]

Vascular Malformations of the Cord and Meninges

Vascular malformations of the cord and meninges can be divided into true spinal cord arteriovenous malformations and spinal dural arteriovenous fistulas. The former have been further subdivided into intramedullary malformations, which occupy the substance of the cord, and intrathecal perimedullary malformations, which surround the cord.[25, 56]

Clinically, there are differences in the presentation of these malformations. Dural fistulas tend to present relatively late in adult life, with a progressive myelopathy sometimes exacerbated by exercise.[118] Dural fistulas drain into the venous system of the spinal cord; the pathogenesis of the symptoms appears to involve chronic venous hypertension causing cord ischemia, rather than a steal phenomenon, as has been proposed for the cerebral arteriovenous malformations. Hemorrhage is a rare, if not unheard of, complication of this type of arteriovenous malformation. By contrast, spinal cord arteriovenous malformations can present with subarachnoid hemorrhage or acute myelopathy; this appears to be more common with intramedullary malformations, particularly when the arteriovenous malformation is complicated by aneurysm.[23, 130] Intradural arteriovenous malformations affect a younger age group, and the patients more commonly present with stepwise progression of symptoms.[56]

Once selective angiography delineates the extent of the lesion and the primary feeding and draining vessels, endovascular embolization, surgical excision, or a combination of both is undertaken. The best results are obtained with dural arteriovenous malformations; spinal cord malformations carry a higher incidence of permanent neurologic deficit from the therapy.[163]

Trauma and Degenerative Disease of the Spine

Several case reports describe ischemic myelopathy as a result of trauma to the cervical spine.[7, 54] The consequences of spinal trauma are discussed elsewhere in this book (see Chapter 6). A vascular etiology also has been proposed for the myelopathy associated with cervical spondylosis,[15] and some of these patients are reported to have an acute presentation.[42]

Systemic Hypotension

Spinal cord necrosis is known to occur as a result of severe systemic hypotension after cardiac arrest or hemorrhage. In most reported cases, the pathologic abnormalities are distributed primarily in the gray matter of the lumbosacral segments of the cord.[13, 148] Infarction in the arterial border zones of the spinal cord is less frequent. Wolf and others[167] reported on such a patient with pathologically proved necrosis in longitudinal (junction of thoracic and lumbosacral supply) as well as transverse (junction of anterior and posterior circulation) border zones. They suggest that this type of infarction is the result of hypotension superimposed on a previously compromised spinal circulation.

Approach to the Patient with Presumed Spinal Cord Ischemia

CLINICAL CONSIDERATIONS. A vascular etiology must be suspected in any acute, nontraumatic spinal cord lesion. This is particularly true if the patient also presents with abdominal or chest pain. A vascular etiology is virtually certain if the onset of symptoms is accompanied by limb ischemia or loss of peripheral pulses.

Ischemic etiologies also should be suspected in patients who give a history of prior brief neurologic deficits of spinal cord origin. Similar to that of the brain, the spinal circulation can be affected by transient ischemic attacks. The tempo of these attacks appears to be different in both organs. In the few documented cases of spinal infarction preceded by transient ischemia, the interval between the initial symptoms and final event has been as short as a few hours in some cases and as long as a year in others.[20] Although no data exist on how often spinal infarcts are preceded by transient ischemia, the clinician must have a high index of suspicion when transient spinal neurologic deficits are encountered in a patient because they may be the harbinger of correctable vascular pathologic abnormalities.[68]

Because multiple pathologic processes can result in spinal ischemia, once the lesion has been established clinically, further investigations should be undertaken to discover the cause.

LABORATORY INVESTIGATIONS. The role of laboratory investigations is to define the site and nature of the vascular occlusion, to determine the reason for the occlusion, and to exclude etiologies such as cord compression and demyelinating, inflammatory, or infectious disease.

MRI is fast becoming the examination of choice in spinal cord injury (see Chapter 11). It can provide a very fast, noninvasive assessment of the presence or absence of spinal cord compression. Additionally, because of its ability to display the cord itself, it can demonstrate intramedullary pathology, such as vascular malformations, tumors, syringes, infarctions, hemorrhages, or demyelinating disease. It can also suggest the presence of meningeal arteriovenous malformations, malignancy, and inflammatory or infectious processes involving the spinal canal. If MRI is not available, CT, preferably with myelography, should be carried out. Although this procedure is probably as accurate as MRI for determining the presence or absence of cord compression and some types of extramedullary pathology, it has the disadvantage of giving a poor image of the cord itself.

Plain films of the spine are useful in demonstrating bone and joint abnormalities, but they do not provide enough information about the contents of the spinal canal to be universally useful. They can be used as adjuncts, but not as substitutes, for spinal CT or MRI. Similarly, plain films of the chest and abdomen can hint at pathology involving the aorta, but the presence of aneurysm or dissection is usually best established by CT or MRI.

Angiography has a limited role. It is indicated when there is a suspicion of aortic occlusion or of spinal vascular malformation. These conditions are amenable to surgical repair, and timely intervention can prevent further morbidity or death. Selective angiography is required to demonstrate spinal vascular malformations. This procedure is usually not indicated in patients with suspected occlusion of segmental vessels or of the spinal arteries themselves because it carries potential dangers as a result of the amount of contrast material required and the need for prolonged instrumentation of vessels. Furthermore, no surgical technique is currently available for repair of stenosed or occluded spinal vessels or for revascularization of the cord.

Cerebrospinal fluid examination can be extremely useful in patients with ischemic myelopathy and should be carried out once spinal canal block has been ruled out by the appropriate studies. The presence of blood or xanthochromia suggests hemorrhagic infarction or bleeding vascular malformation. Although spinal cord infarction is rarely the presenting symptom of meningovascular inflammatory or infectious processes, CSF examination can indicate such involvement. High protein and low glucose levels can be an indication of neoplastic infiltration of the meninges, and microscopic examination of the sediment can corroborate the presence of malignancy. Blood or CSF serologic tests for parasites are usually not indicated unless the patient lives in or has visited an endemic region.

Additionally, a search for embolic sources (although rare) should include echocardiography and, if sepsis is a consideration, blood cultures.

Treatment of Spinal Ischemia

If investigation yields a reversible cause for the spinal ischemia, appropriate treatment can be undertaken to prevent progression or recurrence of morbidity. This is particularly true in patients demonstrating intermittent or stepwise ischemia. Unfortunately, most patients who sustain spinal strokes present with a completed deficit that would be unaffected by treatment directed at etiologic factors.

Preventive measures in patients facing surgery of the great vessels have been discussed earlier. These measures and the removal of risk factors are the most helpful in reducing the incidence, as well as mortality and morbidity, of cord infarctions. Specific treatment measures that have been advocated are anticoagulation in suspected thromboembolic disease,[22] use of high-dose steroids,[57] sympathectomy,[77] revascularization of the cord,[146] use of opiate antagonists,[128] and combined use of magnesium and hypothermia.[161] Of all these treatments, only the use of naloxone and steroids[17] has been studied in controlled therapeutic trials, and the latter has shown promise.

REFERENCES

1. Abramsky O, Teitelbaum D: The autoimmune features of acute transverse myelopathy. Ann Neurol 2:36, 1977.
2. Ackerman WE, Juneja MM, Knapp RK: Maternal paraparesis after epidural anesthesia and cesarean section. South Med J 83:695, 1990.
3. Adams HD, VanGeertruyden HH: Neurologic complications of aortic surgery. Ann Surg 144:574, 1956.
4. Adams RD, Merritt HH: Meningeal and vascular syphilis of the spinal cord. Medicine 23:181, 1944.
5. Ahmed I: Survival after herpes simplex type II myelitis. Neurology 38:1500, 1988.
6. Albin MS, White RJ: Epidemiology, physiopathology and experimental therapeutics of acute spinal cord injury. Crit Care Clin 3:441, 1987.
7. Allen JP: Birth injuries to vertebral arteries. In Vinken PJ, Bruyn GM (eds): Handbook of Clinical Neurology, vol 26: Injuries to the Spine and Spinal Cord. Amsterdam, Elsevier–North Holland, 1976, pp 51–56.
8. Andrianakos AA, Duffy J, Suzuki M, et al: Transverse myelopathy in systemic lupus erythematosis: Report of three cases and review of the literature. Ann Intern Med 83:616, 1975.
9. Babikian VL, Stefannson K, Dieperink K, et al: Paraneoplastic myelopathy: Antibodies against protein in normal spinal cord and underlying neoplasm. Lancet 2:49, 1985.
10. Barakos JA, Mark AS, Dielon WP, et al: MR imaging of acute transverse myelitis and AIDS myelopathy. J Comp Assist Tomogr 14:45, 1990.
11. Berman M, Feldman S, Alter A, et al: Acute transverse myelitis: Incidence and etiologic considerations. Neurology 31:966, 1981.
12. Blackwood W: Discussion on vascular disease of the spinal cord. Proc R Soc Med 51:543, 1958.
13. Blumbergs PC, Byrne E: Hypotensive central infarction of the spinal cord. J Neurol 43:751, 1980.
14. Bockeneck WL, Bach JR, Alba AS, et al: Fibrocartilaginous emboli to the spinal cord: A case report. Arch Phys Med Rehabil 71:754, 1990.
15. Bohlman HH, Emery SE: The pathophysiology of cervical spondylosis and myelopathy. Spine 13:843, 1988.
16. Boumpas DT, Patronas NJ, Dalakas MC, et al: Acute transverse myelitis in systemic lupus erythematosus: magnetic resonance imaging and review of the literature. J Rheumatol 17:89, 1990.
17. Bracken MB, Shepard MJ, Collins WF, et al: A randomized controlled trial of methylprednisolone or naloxone in the treatment of acute spinal cord injury: Results of the second national acute spinal cord injury study. N Engl J Med 322:1405, 1990.
18. Brewer LA, Fosburg RG, Mulder GA, et al: Spinal cord complications following surgery for coarctation of the aorta. J Thorac Cardiovasc Surg 64:368, 1972.
19. Britton CB, Mesa-Tejeda R, Fenoglio CM, et al: A new complication of AIDS: Thoracic myelitis caused by herpes simplex virus. Neurology 35:1071, 1985.
20. Brusa A, Firpo MP, Gambini G, et al: Recurrent vascular myelopathy: Report of a case with autopsy. Eur Neurol 28:194, 1988.
21. Brusa A, Stoehr R, Brusa G, et al: Some little-known aspects of spinal cord softening. Ital J Neurol Sci 8:487, 1987.
22. Buchan AM, Barnett HJM: Infarction of the spinal cord. In Barnett HJM, Stein BM, Mohr JP, et al (eds): Stroke, Pathophysiology, Diagnosis and Management. New York, Churchill Livingstone, 1986, p 716.
23. Caroscio JT, Brennan T, Budabin M, et al: Subarachnoid hemorrhage secondary to spinal arteriovenous malformation and aneurysm: Report of a case and review of the literature. Arch Neurol 37:101, 1980.
24. Cates JE, Christie RV: Subacute bacterial endocarditis: A review of 442 patients treated in 14 centers of the Penicillin Trials Committee of the MRC. Q J Med NS 20:93, 1951.
25. Choi IS, Berenstein A: Surgical neuroangiography of the spine and spinal cord. Radiol Clin North Am 26:1131, 1988.
26. Clarke CE, Cuming WJ: Subacute myelopathy caused by spinal venous infarction. Postgrad Med J 63:669, 1987.

27. Cleveland JE, Lefemine AA, Mardoff I: The role of intrathoracic balloon counterpulsation in patients undergoing cardiac operation. Ann Thorac Surg 20:652, 1975.

28. Coleman JB: Dissecting aneurysm. Lancet 2:317, 1898.

29. Costello TG, Fisher A: Neurological complications following aortic surgery. Anaesthesia 38:230, 1983.

30. Crawford ES, Crawford JL, Safi JJ, et al: Thoracoabdominal aortic aneurysms: Preoperative and intraoperative factors determining intermediate and long term results in 605 patients. J Vasc Surg 3:389, 1986.

31. Criado A, Agosti J, Horno R, et al: Paraplegia following balloon assistance after cardiac surgery. Scand J Thorac Cardiovasc Surg 15:103, 1981.

32. Criscuolo GR, Oldfield EH, Doppman JL: Reversible acute and subacute myelopathy in patients with dural arteriovenous fistulas. J Neurosurg 70:354, 1989.

33. Cunningham JN, Laschinger JC, Spencer FC: Monitoring of somatosensory evoked potentials during surgical procedures on the thoracoabdominal aorta. J Thorac Cardiovasc Surg 94:275, 1987.

34. Dawson DM: Antineoplastic drugs. In Asbury AK, McKhann GM, McDonald WI (eds): Diseases of the Nervous System. ed 2. Philadelphia, WB Saunders, 1990.

35. DeBakey ME, Cooley DA, Crawford ES, et al: Aneurysms of the thoracic aorta: Analysis of 170 patients treated by resection. J Thorac Surg 36:393, 1958.

36. DeBakey MC, Crawford ES, Cooley DA: Aneurysm of the abdominal aorta: Analysis of results of graft replacement therapy one to eleven years after the operation. Ann Surg 160:622, 1964.

37. DeBakey ME, McCollum CH, Crawford ES: Dissection and dissecting aneurysm of the aorta: Twenty-one year follow-up of 527 patients treated surgically. Surgery 92:1118, 1982.

38. DeJong RV: Central nervous system complications in subacute bacterial endocarditis. J Nerv Ment Dis 85:397, 1937.

39. East T: Dissecting aneurysm of the aorta. Lancet 2:317, 1898.

40. Eltorai I, Juler G: Ischemic myelopathy. Angiology 30:81, 1979.

41. Equro H: Transverse myelitis following chemonucleolysis. J Bone Joint Surg Am 65:1328, 1983.

42. Ferguson RJ, Caplan LR: Cervical spondylotic myelopathy. Neurol Clin 3:373, 1985.

43. Fetterman JL, Ashe WF: Cerebral debut of certain cases of cardiac disease. Ohio State Med J 34:1354, 1938.

44. Foo D, Rossier AB: Anterior spinal artery syndrome and its natural history. Paraplegia 21:1, 1983.

45. Fosburg R, Brewer LA III: Arterial vascular injury to the spinal cord. In Vinken PJ, Bruyn GM (eds): Handbook of Clinical Neurology, vol 26: Injuries to the Spine and Spinal Cord. Amsterdam, Elsevier–North Holland, 1976, pp 63–79.

46. Fulford KWM, Catteral RD, Delhanty JJ, et al: A collagen disorder of the nervous system presenting as multiple sclerosis. Brain 95:373, 1972.

47. Gang DL, Dole KB, Adelman LS: Spinal cord infarction following therapeutic renal artery embolization. JAMA 237:2841, 1977.

48. Garland H, Greenberg J, Harriman GF: Infarction of the spinal cord. Brain 89:649, 1966.

49. Gerber O, Heyer EJ, Vieux U: Painless dissection of the aorta presenting as acute neurological syndrome. Stroke 17:644, 1986.

50. Gibb WRG, Ury PA, Less AJ: Giant cell arteritis with spinal cord infarction and basilar artery thrombosis. J Neurol Neurosurg Psychiatry 48:945, 1985.

51. Gowers WR, Taylor J: Manual of Diseases of the Nervous System, ed 3. London, Blakiston & Son, 1898.

52. Grace RR, Mattox KL: Anterior spinal artery syndrome following abdominal aortic aneurysmectomy: Case reports and review of the literature. Arch Surg 112:813, 1977.

53. Greenlee JE, Mandell GL: Neurological manifestations of infective endocarditis. A review. Stroke 4:958, 1973.

54. Grinker RR, Guy CC: Sprain of cervical spine causing thrombosis of anterior spinal artery. JAMA 88:1140, 1927.

55. Gruner J, Lapresle J: Etude anatomo-pathologique des medullopathies d'origine vasculaire. Rev Neurol 106:592, 1962.

56. Guegen B, Merland JJ, Riche MC, et al: Vascular malformations of the spinal cord: Intrathecal and perimedullary arteriovenous fistulas fed by medullary arteries. Neurology 37:964, 1987.

57. Hall ED, Braughler JM: Glucocorticoid mechanisms in spinal cord injury: A review and therapeutic rationale. Surg Neurol 18:320, 1982.

58. Hallenbeck JM, Bove AA, Elliott DH: Mechanisms underlying spinal cord damage in decompression sickness. Neurology 25:308, 1975.

59. Hammond DL: Intrathecal administration: Methodological considerations. Prog Brain Res 77:313, 1988.

60. Harrington AW: Embolism of the spinal cord. Glasgow Med J 103:28, 1925.

61. Hardie RJ, Isenberg DA: Tetraplegia as a presenting feature of systemic lupus erythematosus complicated by pulmonary hypertension. Ann Rheum Dis 44:491, 1985.

62. Harris EN, Gharavi AE, Mackworth-Young CG, et al: Lupoid sclerosis: A possible role for antiphospholipid antibodies. Ann Rheum Dis 44:281, 1985.

63. Heller HM, Carnevale NT, Steigbigel RT: Varicella-zoster virus transverse myelitis without cutaneous rash. Am J Med 88:550, 1990.

64. Henson RA, Parsons M: Ischemic lesions to the spinal cord: An illustrated review. Q J Med 36:205, 1967.

65. Herregods P, Chappel R, Mortier G: Benzene poisoning as a possible cause of transverse myelitis. Paraplegia 22:305, 1984.

66. Herskovitz S, Siegel SE, Schneider AT, et al: Spinal cord toxoplasmosis in AIDS. Neurology 39:1552, 1989.

67. Hirst AE, Johns JJ, Kime SW: Dissecting aneurysms of the aorta: A review of 505 cases. Medicine 37:217, 1958.

68. Hoffman TG, Harati Y, Witaker SH: Transient paraplegia caused by aortic occlusion. Arch Neurol 38:668, 1981.

69. Hogan EL, Krigman MR: Herpes zoster myelitis: Evidence for viral invasion of spinal cord. Arch Neurol 29:300, 1973.

70. Hollier LH: Protecting the brain and spinal cord. J Vasc Surg 5:524, 1987.

71. Horder TJ: Infectious endocarditis with an analysis

of 150 cases and with special reference to the chronic form of the disease. Q J Med 2:289, 1909.

72. Hughes JT: Vascular disorders of the spinal cord. *In* Vinken PJ, Bruyn GW, Klawans HL, et al (eds): Handbook of Clinical Neurology, vol 55 (revised series). Amsterdam, Elsevier Science Publishers, 1989, p 101.

73. Hughes JT: Venous infarction of the spinal cord. Neurology 21:575, 1971.

74. Hughes JT, Brownell B: Spinal cord ischemia due to arteriosclerosis. Arch Neurol 15:189, 1966.

75. Hughes JT, McIntyre AG: Spinal cord infarction occurring during thoracolumbar sympathectomy. J Neurol Neurosurg Psychiatry 15:189, 1963.

76. Hutchinson M, Bresnahan B: Neurological lupus erythematosus with tonic seizures simulating multiple sclerosis. J Neurol Neurosurg Psychiatry 46:583, 1983.

77. Ikeda M, Mohri K, Tsunekawa K: Surgical treatment of vascular lesions of the spinal cord. Vasc Surg 10:257, 1976.

78. Jellinger K: Circulation disorders of the spinal cord. Acta Neurochir (Wien) 26:327, 1972.

79. Jellinger K: Spinal cord arteriosclerosis and progressive vascular myelopathy. J Neurol Neurosurg Psychiatry 30:195, 1967.

80. Jellinger K, Sturm KW: Delayed radiation myelopathy in man: Report of 12 necropsy cases. J Neurol Sci 14:389, 1971.

81. Johnson RT, Richardson EP: The neurological manifestations of systemic lupus erythematosus: A clinical-pathological study of 24 cases and review of the literature. Medicine 47:337, 1968.

82. Jones HR, Siekert RG, Geraci JE: Neurological manifestations of bacterial endocarditis. Ann Intern Med 71:21, 1969.

83. Kahn DR, Vathayanon S, Sloan H: Resection of descending thoracic aneurysms without left heart bypass. Arch Surg 97:336, 1968.

84. Kane RE: Neurologic deficits following epidural or spinal anesthesia. Anesth Analg 60:150, 1981.

85. Kenik JG, Krohn K, Kelly RB: Transverse myelopathy and optic neuritis in systemic lupus erythematosus: A case report with magnetic resonance imaging findings. Arthritis Rheum 30:947, 1987.

86. Kennedy C, DesRosiers MH, Jehle J, et al: Mapping of functional neural pathways by autoradiographic survey of local metabolic rate with ^{14}C deoxyglucose. Science 187:850, 1975.

87. Kewelramani LS, Saleem S, Bertrand MT: Myelopathy associated with systemic lupus erythematosus. Paraplegia 16:282, 1978.

88. Kim R, Smith HR, Henbest ML, et al: Nonhemorrhagic venous infarction of the spinal cord. Ann Neurol 15:379, 1984.

89. Kim SW, Kim RC, Choi BH, et al: Non-traumatic ischemic myelopathy: A review of 25 cases. Paraplegia 26:262, 1988.

90. Kinney EL, Berdoff RL, Rao NS, et al: Devic's syndrome and systemic lupus erythematosus. Arch Neurol 36:643, 1979.

91. Klastersky J, Cappel R, Snoock JM, et al: Ascending myelitis in association with herpes simplex virus. N Engl J Med 287:182, 1972.

92. Kohler J: Lyme borreliosis: A case of transverse myelitis with syrinx cavity. Neurology 39:1553, 1989.

93. Laschinger JC, Izumoto H, Kouchoukos NT: Evolving concepts in prevention of spinal cord injury during operations on the descending thoracic and thoracoabdominal aorta. Ann Thorac Surg 44:667, 1987.

94. Lavalle C, Pizarro S, Drinkard C, et al: Transverse myelitis: A manifestation of systemic lupus erythematosus strongly associated with antiphospholipid antibodies. J Rheumatol 17:34, 1990.

95. Lazorthes G: Blood supply and vascular pathology of the spinal cord. *In* Pia HW, Djindjian R (eds): Spinal Angiomas. Berlin, Springer-Verlag, 1978, p 10.

96. Lazorthes G: Pathology, classification and clinical aspects of vascular diseases of the spinal cord. *In* Vinken PJ, Bruyn GW (eds): Handbook of Clinical Neurology, vol 12. Vascular Diseases of the Nervous System, part II. Amsterdam, Elsevier North-Holland, 1972, pp 492–506.

97. Liu GT, Greene JM, Charness ME: Brown-Séquard syndrome in a patient with systemic lupus erythematosus. Neurology 40:1474–1475, 1990.

98. Liussen WHJP, Fiselier TJW, Gabreels FJM, et al: Acute transverse myelitis as the initial manifestation of probable systemic lupus erythematosus in a child. Neurol Pediatr 19:212, 1988.

99. Logigian EL, Kaplan RF, Steere AC: Chronic neurologic manifestations of Lyme disease. N Engl J Med 323:1438, 1990.

100. MacEwen GD, Bunnell WP, Siram K: Acute neurological complications in the treatment of scoliosis. J Bone Joint Surg 57:404, 1975.

101. Mahieux F, Gray F, Fenelon G, et al: Acute myeloradiculitis due to cytomegalovirus as the initial manifestation of AIDS. J Neurol Neurosurg Psychiatry 52:270, 1989.

102. Mancall EL, Rosales RK: Necrotizing myelopathy associated with visceral carcinoma. Brain 87:639, 1964.

103. Mannen T: Vascular lesions in the spinal cord in the aged. Geriatrics 4:151, 1966.

104. Marcus ML, Heistad DD, Ehrhardt JC, et al: Regulation of the total regional spinal cord blood flow. Circ Res 41:128, 1977.

105. Martin EA, Lavin PJ, Thompson AJ: Painful extremities and neurological disorder in essential thrombocytemia. J R Soc Med 77:372, 1984.

106. Martin R, Meinck HM, Schulte-Mattler W, et al: *Borrelia burgdorferi* myelitis presenting as a partial stiff-man syndrome. J Neurol 237:51, 1990.

107. Marvosti MA, Meyer JA, Ford BE, et al: Spinal cord ischemia following operation for traumatic aortic transection. Ann Thorac Surg 42:425, 1986.

108. Mayo DR, Booss J: Varicella-zoster associated neurologic disease without skin lesions. Arch Neurol 46:313, 1989.

109. McCloy RM, Spittel JA, McGoon DC: The prognosis of aortic dissection. Circulation 31:665, 1965.

110. Mehren M, Burns PJ, Mamani F, et al: Toxoplasmic myelitis mimicking intramedullary spinal cord tumor. Neurology 38:1648, 1988.

111. Miller RG, Storey JR, Greco CM: Ganciclovir in the treatment of progressive AIDS-related polyradiculopathy. Neurology 40:569, 1990.

112. Mosberg WH, Voris H, Duff J: Paraplegia as a complication of sympathectomy for hypertension. Ann Surg 139:330, 1954.

113. Muder RR, Lumish RM, Corsello GR: Myelopathy after herpes zoster. Arch Neurol 40:445, 1983.

114. Naiman JL, Donhue WL, Prichard JS: Fatal nucleus

pulposus embolism of spinal cord after trauma. Neurology 11:83, 1961.

115. Neville WE, Cox WD, Leininger RB, et al: Resection of the descending thoracic aorta with femoral vein to femoral artery oxygenation perfusion. J Thorac Cardiovasc Surg 56:39, 1968.

116. Nystrom B, Stjernschantz J, Smedegard G: Regional spinal cord blood flow in the rabbit, cat, and monkey. Acta Neurol Scand 70:307, 1984.

117. Ojeda VJ, Walters M: Spinal cord disorders in patients with cancer. Pathol Annu 19:63, 1984.

118. Oldfield EH, Doppman JL: Spinal arteriovenous malformations. Clin Neurosurg 34:161, 1988.

119. Orr E, McKittrick J, DiAgostino R, et al: Paraplegia following intra-aortic balloon support: Report of a case. J Cardiovasc Surg 30:1013, 1989.

120. Osler W: Gulstonian lectures. Lancet 1:415–418, 459–464, 505–508, 1885.

121. Ota K, Mattui M, Milford EL, et al: T-cell recognition of an immunodominant myelin basic protein epitope in multiple sclerosis. Nature 364:183, 1990.

122. Otomo E, VanBuskirk C, Workman JB: Circulation of the spinal cord studied by autoradiography. Neurology 10:112, 1960.

123. Perier O, Demanet JC, Henneux J, et al: Existe-t-il un syndrome des arteries spinales posterieures? Rev Neurol 103:396, 1960.

124. Picone AL, Green RM, Ricotta JR, et al: Spinal cord ischemia following operations of the abdominal aorta. J Vasc Surg 3:94, 1986.

125. Propper DJ, Bucknall RC: Acute transverse myelopathy complicating systemic lupus erythematosus. Ann Rheum Dis 48:512, 1989.

126. Reichert FL, Rytand DA, Bruck EL: Arteriosclerosis of the lumbar segmental arteries producing ischemia of the spinal cord and consequent claudication of the thighs. Am J Med Sci 187:794, 1934.

127. Riche ML, Modenosi-Freites J, Djindjian M, et al: Arteriovenous malformation of the spinal cord in children: Review of 38 cases. Neuroradiology 22:171, 1982.

128. Robertson CS, Foltz R, Grossman RG, et al: Protection against experimental ischemic spinal cord injury. J Neurosurg 64:6333, 1986.

129. Ropper AH, Poskanzer DC: The prognosis of acute and subacute transverse myelopathy based on early signs and symptoms. Ann Neurol 4:51, 1978.

130. Rosenblum B, Oldfield EH, Doppman JL, et al: Spinal arteriovenous malformations: A comparison of dural arteriovenous fistulas and intradural AVM's in 81 patients. J Neurosurg 67:795, 1987.

131. Ross RT: Spinal cord infarctions in disease and surgery of the aorta. Can J Neurol Sci 12:289, 1985.

132. Rouges L, Passelcq A: Syndrome de Brown-Séquard apres la thoracoplastie. Rev Neurol 97:146, 1957.

133. Rousseau JJ, Lust C, Zangerle PF: Acute transverse myelitis as presenting neurological feature of Lyme disease. Lancet 2:1222, 1986.

134. Rutan G, Martinez AZ, Fieschko JT, et al: Primary biliary cirrhosis, Sjogren's syndrome and transverse myelitis. Gastroenterology 90:206, 1986.

135. Sandler AN, Tator CH: Review of the measurement of normal spinal cord blood flow. Brain Res 118:181, 1976.

136. Sands ML, Ryczal M, Brown RB: Recurrent aseptic meningitis followed by transverse myelitis as a presentation of lupus erythematosus. J Rheumatol 15:862, 1988.

137. Sandson TA, Friedman JH: Spinal cord infarction. Report of 8 cases and review of the literature. Medicine 68:282, 1989.

138. Satran R: Spinal cord infarction. Stroke 19:529, 1988.

139. Scott RW, Sanatta SM: Dissecting aneurysm of the aorta with hemorrhagic infarction of the spinal cord and complete paraparesis. Am Heart J 38:747, 1949.

140. Shaw PG: Neurological complications of cardiovascular surgery: II. Procedures involving the heart and thoracic aorta. Int Anaesthesiol Clin 24:159, 1986.

141. Shaw PJ, Bates D, Cartlidge NEF, et al: Early neurological complications of coronary bypass surgery. Br Med J 291:1384, 1985.

142. Shepard DI, Downie AW, Best PV: Systemic lupus erythematosus and multiple sclerosis (abstract). Arch Neurol 30:423, 1974.

143. Shinhoj E: Arteriosclerosis of the spinal cord. Acta Psychiatr Scand 29:139, 1954.

144. Siddorn JA: Schistosomiasis and anterior spinal artery occlusion. Am J Trop Med Hyg 27:532, 1978.

145. Silver JR, Buxton PH: Spinal stroke. Brain 97:539, 1974.

146. Sindou M, Chignier E, Mazoyer J-F: Revascularization of the spinal cord by microanastomoses in dogs. Surg Neurol 12:492, 1979.

147. Skillman JJ: Neurological complications of cardiovascular surgery: Part I. Procedures involving the carotid arteries and abdominal aorta. Int Anaesthesiol Clin 24:135, 1986.

148. Sladky JT, Rorke JB: Perinatal hypoxic/ischemic spinal cord injury. Pediatr Pathol 6:87, 1986.

149. Slavin RE, Gonzalez-Vitale JC, Marin OSM: Atheromatous emboli to the lumbosacral spinal cord. Stroke 6:411, 1975.

150. Slater EE, DeSantis RW: The clinical recognition of dissecting aortic aneurysm. Am J Med 600:625, 1976.

151. Spiller W: Syphilis as a possible cause of systemic degeneration of the motor tract. J Nerv Ment Dis 39:584, 1912.

152. Spiller W: Thrombosis of the cervical median anterior spinal artery: Syphilitic acute anterior poliomyelitis. J Nerv Ment Dis 36:601, 1909.

153. Stafford WW, Mena H, Piskun WS, et al: Transverse myelitis from intra-arterial penicillin. Neurosurgery 15:552, 1984.

154. Suchet I, Klein C, Horwitz T, et al: Spinal cord schistosomiasis: A case report and review of the literature. Paraplegia 25:491, 1987.

155. Sumpio BE, Gusberg RJ: Aortic thrombosis with paraplegia: An unusual consequence of blunt abdominal trauma. J Vasc Surg 6:412, 1987.

156. Szilagyi DE, Hageman JH, Smith RF, et al: Spinal cord damage in surgery of the abdominal aorta. Surgery 83:38, 1978.

157. Thron AK: Vascular Anatomy of the Spinal Cord. New York, Springer-Verlag, 1988, p 106.

158. Toone E: Cerebral manifestations of bacterial endocarditis. Ann Intern Med 14:1551, 1941.

159. Tucker T, Dix RD, Katzen C: Cytomegalovirus and herpes simplex virus ascending myelitis in a patient with acquired immune deficiency syndrome. Ann Neurol 18:74, 1985.

160. Tyler KL, Gross RA, Cascino GD: Unusual viral causes of transverse myelitis: Hepatitis A virus and cytomegalovirus. Neurology 36:855, 1986.

161. Vacanti FX, Ames A III: Mild hypothermia and Mg^{++} protect against irreversible damage during cerebral CNS ischemia. Stroke 15:695, 1984.

162. Van Wieringen A: An unusual case of occlusion of the anterior spinal artery. Eur Neurol 1:363, 1968.

163. Vinuela F, Dion J, Lylyk P, et al: Update on interventional neuroradiology. AJR 153:23, 1989.

164. Weisman AD, Adams RD: The neurological complications of dissecting aortic aneurysm. Brain 67:67, 1944.

165. Wiley CA, VanPatten PD, Carpenter PM, et al: Acute ascending necrotizing myelopathy caused by herpes simplex virus type III. Neurology 37:1791, 1987.

166. Winkelman NW, Eckel JL: Focal lesions of the spinal cord due to vascular disease. JAMA 99:1919, 1932.

167. Wolf HK, Anthony DC, Fuller GN: Arterial border zone necrosis of the spinal cord. Clin Neuropathol 9:60, 1990.

168. Wolman L, Bradshaw P: Spinal cord embolism. J Neurol Neurosurg Psychiatry 330:446, 1967.

169. Zull DN, Cydulka R: Acute paraplegia: A presenting manifestation of aortic dissection. Am J Med 84:765, 1988.

CHAPTER 5

Chronic Nontraumatic Diseases of the Spinal Cord

Raymond D. Adams, M.D.
Maria Salam-Adams, M.D.†

Peculiarities of anatomy and biochemistry undoubtedly explain the localization of certain diseases in the spinal cord. Its elongate, slender structure enclosed within tight, confining meningeal sheaths, its position in relation to the bony structures forming the spinal canal, the extensive aposition of myelinated tracts to the pia, and the special arrangement of its blood supply from extravertebral vessels all contribute to the pathogenesis of spinal diseases.[1] However, a number of pathologic states exist that defy our concepts of anatomic localization and remain as matters of speculation. Why, for example, do spinal neurons wither gradually and die at a certain period of life, sometimes as a manifestation of a genetic disease; why is the cervical cord so disposed to cavitation; why do the myelin sheaths in the central parts of posterior and lateral funiculi degenerate from lack of cobalamin (vitamin B_{12})?

THE MOST COMMON CHRONIC DISEASES OF THE SPINAL CORD SEEN AT THE MASSACHUSETTS GENERAL HOSPITAL

A late stage of spinal multiple sclerosis, cervical spondylosis, and amyotrophic lateral sclerosis are the three most common chronic progressive myelopathies seen on the Neurological Service at the Massachusetts General Hospital. Secondary epidural and meningeal tumors and syringomyelia, although less common, occur with some regularity. Subacute combined degeneration from B_{12} deficiency, other nutritional myelopathies, Friedreich's ataxia, and vascular malformations are rare, being observed only a few times in a year. Acquired immunodeficiency syndrome (AIDS) myelopathy, although not one of the frequent manifestations of this disease, has largely replaced spinal syphilis, but, like subacute or chronic necrotizing myelitis, is still unusual and remarkable when it does occur.

SPINAL MULTIPLE SCLEROSIS

It always is somewhat of a surprise that multiple sclerosis, the natural form of which is a widespread disease of the central nervous system usually affecting adolescents and young adults, should present as a chronic progressive spinal cord disease late in life. However, this happens not infrequently, both in patients known to have had this disease in earlier years and in some who have had no earlier symptoms. There is no doubt that the spinal cord and optic nerves are sites favored by the disease process and that either may be the first and only part to be involved symptomatically. If the early symptoms are slight and overlooked or forgotten, only the late and more often progressive stage of the disease comes to medical attention.[2]

Definition

The usual presentation of chronic spinal multiple sclerosis is that of a slowly progressive, asymmetrical spastic paraparesis with variable sensory ataxia. Although the patient tends to complain of only one leg being weak or stiff, examination often discloses increased tendon reflexes in both legs and bilateral Babinski's signs. The Romberg sign can be elicited in many instances, and vibratory and position senses in the legs are reduced or absent. Micturition may have a precipitant quality because of spastic weakness of the bladder. Usually the patient has difficulty in recalling whether the neurologic disorder has progressed step-wise or slowly and steadily,

but it is not unusual for little change to be detected over periods of months or years. Unfortunately, the patient's estimate of the degree of disability is influenced by his or her prevailing mood and outlook.

Detailed clinical examination is helpful by giving hints of more widespread disease: an inequality of tendon reflexes in the arms in a predominantly paraplegic patient or a slight ataxia of one arm, a numbness and clumsiness of one hand, Lhermitte's sign (tingling in shoulders and arms on neck flexion), a numbness of one side of the trunk, or a slight ocular weakness or nystagmus or pallor of an optic disk, all of which incriminate other parts of the central nervous system. A rapid worsening of symptoms on exposure to high environmental temperatures is of some value. Inexplicable fatigue is common, yet fever and signs of systemic infection are not parts of the demyelinative process.

Variants of this spinal syndrome include an acute worsening of the paralysis or sensory deficit superimposed on a background of chronic myelopathy, circumscribed lesions of the lower parts of the spinal cord resulting in an areflexic paralysis without much atrophy of muscles, and sacral sensory disorder and hypotonic weakness of the bladder. A unilateral lesion of the cervical or thoracic cord may present as a partial Brown-Séquard syndrome. A mainly posterior column lesion of the cervical cord is expressed as an ataxia and numbness of the hands.

Pathogenesis and Pathology

The study of the pathology of chronic spinal multiple sclerosis leaves much to be desired from the clinician's standpoint. Data are for the most part lacking in large series of cases coming to postmortem examination; the frequency of a purely spinal form of multiple sclerosis, devoid of lesions in the brain stem, optic nerves, and cerebrum is rare. Incompleteness of the examination of the spinal cord deprives the clinician of data concerning the localization of the lesions in all segments of the spinal cord and the age of the lesions. Not fully explained also is the way in which a multifocal disease, known to occur in acute episodes, can cause a functional loss that is gradual and progressive. Is it from a fortuitous combination, in additive form, of many small subclinical lesions? Or are old lesions reactivated in their margins by fresh demyelination, which gradually increases the deficit? The answers to such questions may eventually be clarified by studies combining functional deficits with MRI.[15]

Differential Diagnosis

From the clinical analysis alone, the physician can eliminate a number of suspected diseases of the spinal cord. An early onset of asymmetrical spastic weakness before posterior column signs become manifest nearly always excludes subacute combined degeneration due to pernicious anemia. The finding of slight signs at a higher level (upper spinal cord or brain stem) tends to rule out a solitary spinal cord tumor. Cervical spondylosis can be more difficult to exclude because laterally directed x-rays will frequently show a few cervical osteophytes, and a cervical myelogram viewed by computed tomographic (CT) scan may demonstrate a slight inconsequential indentation of the spinal dural sheath. It is necessary to search for signs and symptoms that point toward lesions at other levels of the neuraxis than the site of the spondylosis. On more than one occasion, a cervical laminectomy has been performed because of such findings in patients with spinal multiple sclerosis. Symmetry of clinical presentation, early age at onset, extreme chronicity, and slow progressivity differentiate some of the familial degenerative diseases to be discussed later.

Laboratory Aids

Helpful diagnostic aids in patients with spinal multiple sclerosis are visual, auditory, and somatosensory evoked potentials and magnetic resonance imaging (MRI) of the brain and spinal cord. These tests are used in a search for asymptomatic lesions remote from those in the spinal cord. If the diagnosis is still in doubt, a lumbar puncture also should be done for pleocytosis (seen in some cases of multiple sclerosis) and measurement of oligoclonal bands (increased gamma globulin or IgG index) in the cerebrospinal fluid. The MRI scan, although the most effective means of imaging any cerebral lesion, must be interpreted with some caution because it often reveals foci of indeterminate type (increased signal in T2-weighted images) near the lateral ventricles in normal individuals.

Treatment

The treatment of multiple sclerosis at a late progressive stage has been for the most part unsatisfactory. A 2- to 3-month trial of corticotropin or prednisone may halt the progress in only a few patients. Many patients insist on receiving low-dose steroids even though there is little evidence that they are beneficial. Immuran is of questionable value. Beta interferon, given parenterally every other day, is said to reduce the number of acute attacks. Intense immunosuppression by use of combined cyclophosphamide (Cytoxan) and corticotropin is being tried in certain centers, but the results have been difficult to assess. Supportive medical measures designed to keep the patient active and in a good frame of mind in the presence of ongoing disability are certainly worthwhile objectives. Neurorehabilitative measures, including therapy for spasticity, are recommended.

CERVICAL SPONDYLOSIS

The development of bony spurs and ridges that stud the surfaces of the vertebral bodies and protrude backward into the spinal canal is part of the aging process of the skeleton. These changes are often associated with bulges of intervertebral disks or frank rupture of disk tissue from weakened ligaments. Together, they narrow the spinal canal and intervertebral foramina. They are most evident and most likely to become sources of neurologic symptoms in the most mobile parts of the spine, i.e., the mid to lower cervical and lumbar segments. Either the cervical roots or the spinal cord or both may be compressed.

Injury, even trivial, of the structurally altered spine can precipitate either acute or chronically recurrent neurologic syndromes.

Definition

In briefest outline, cervical spondylosis presents clinically as a triad of painful stiff neck, pain and numbness in the arms and hands, and spastic weakness with variable ataxia of the legs. The onset is gradual and progression takes place over months or years, often punctuated by acute exacerbations. The most frequently affected spine segments are C4–5, C5–6, and C6–7.

Clinical Syndromes

The first component of this triad is usually pain. As an isolated symptom, it varies in degree. In some patients it is not prominent even at an advanced state of spinal cord compression. When pain occurs alone, it is always difficult to interpret, because some degree of creaking, stiffness and discomfort on turning, and tipping or flexing and extending of the neck are so common in older adults (older than 50 years) that they hardly attract medical attention and alone do not deserve investigation. Acute onset of neck, shoulder, and arm pain is more demanding of explanation. Trauma may be a factor in the aggravation of a chronic disorder but not infrequently, the exacerbation has no apparent cause. Immobilization of the neck affords relief in a few days or weeks.

When present as a second component, brachialgia varies in location with the site of radicular involvement. With C5 root involvement (C4–5 spine segments), pain is present in the deltoid region; with C6 root involvement (C5–6 spine segments), pain is present in the thumb and index finger along with sensory impairment there and in the radial part of the forearm along with diminished biceps reflex; with C8 root involvement C7–T1 spine segments), pain is present on the ulnar side of the hand and sensory loss in the fourth and fifth fingers and medially on the forearm. In any given patient, only one or two of these findings may be present to provide a clue as to the level of disease in a compressive cord syndrome. Also, the pain may have been recorded only in the past history. An acute sense of a purely radicular syndrome should raise the suspicion of a ruptured disk.

The spinal cord component of the syndrome is usually an asymmetrical paraparesis with increased tendon reflexes (Achilles' reflexes may not contribute to this hyperreflexia in the elderly) and Babinski's signs. Spasticity tends to be more prominent than weakness. Sensory disturbances are reported as numbness and tingling and prickling in the hands and soles of the feet around the ankles. Vibratory and position senses are impaired in the feet and legs. Sharp flexion of the neck may cause discomfort or induce a typical Lhermitte sign. Infrequently, the sensory impairment includes the pain and thermal senses. As the condition progresses, the legs weaken and stiffen so as to interfere with locomotion, and precipitancy and incontinence of urine become troublesome.[1, 5]

Pathogenesis and Pathology

The obvious mechanism in the pathogenesis of radicular and spinal cord lesions would appear to be the osteophytic ingrowth and occasional subluxation of one vertebra on another, compressing these structures. Buckling of the ligamentum flavum posterolaterally also contributes to the narrowing. The tethering of the spinal cord to the dura by the laterally placed denticulate ligaments places it at risk by limiting its mobility. On measurement, the anteroposterior dimension of the canal (normally 17–18 mm in lateral radiographs) is reduced to 9 to 10 mm. These compressive effects can be observed when the head is moved passively during a laminectomy, presumably reproducing the usual compression mechanism. Laterally placed osteophytes or ruptured disk tissue also compresses spinal roots in or near the intervertebral canals. However, unexplained by this simple compressive mechanism is the fact that the degree of cord damage has not correlated well with the degree of spinal canal stenosis, and that some of the damage to the spinal cord is distributed in foci some distance from its surface. This suggests to some pathologists an additional ischemic factor. All of these changes can now have more disastrous effects if the spinal canal is congenitally narrow, as is known to be the situation in some stocky individuals and particularly in those with achondroplasia.

The physician should remember the threat of acute cervical cord injury in individuals with a stenotic canal. A fall that occurs with the neck extended may result in a permanent quadriplegia.[2, 5]

Distinct from lumbar disk ruptures, which are not the subject of this chapter, the entire cauda equina also may be compressed by this same so-called spondylosis deformans.[4] The lumbar spinal canal becomes stenotic, most commonly at L2–3, L3–4 or higher, and, gradually, a sensory-motor-reflex deficit is evinced. The fluctuant nature of this clinical state is notable. Standing and walking for prolonged periods induces or aggravates the symptoms; sitting and lying with the hips flexed assuages or relieves them. This postural influence is explained by the fact that the natural lumbar lordosis increases in the standing position, narrowing the lumbar spinal canal even further and increasing the radicular pressure. The clinical state, incorrectly thought to be increased by locomotion, was traditionally believed to be a spinal circulatory claudication similar to the circulatory claudication of the legs described earlier by Charcot.

Laboratory Aids

Lateral radiographs, CT, MRI, myelography, and electromyography (EMG) are the most helpful tests in cervical spondylosis.

Differential Diagnosis

Important from the clinical standpoint is the demonstration that the spinal cord is significantly compromised by the vertebral abnormalities and that the neurologic findings (radicular and spinal cord symptoms and signs) correspond to that abnormality. The physician must also prove that the patient does not exhibit evidence of another more diffuse abnormality of the spinal cord, such as amyotrophic lateral sclerosis. Usually the aforementioned cervical myelogram and CT scan or MRI are essential. Spinal multiple sclerosis can be ruled out by this lack of correspondence of symptoms to stenosis and by other tests mentioned earlier. Motor system disease and amyotrophic lateral sclerosis reveal themselves by evidence of denervation atrophy at other levels of the neuraxis. In our experience, there are nearly always sensory findings in cervical spondylosis affecting the spinal cord and roots that are not observed in amyotrophic lateral sclerosis.

Treatment

Treatment of cervical and lumbar stenoses is controversial.[5] The slow intermittently progressive course with long periods of relatively unchanging symptomatology in elderly, often infirm individuals makes generalization difficult. Assuming the aforementioned mechanisms of cord injury to be correct, the obvious treatment is laminectomy with decompression. The spinal cord disturbance has priority, mandating either relief or the institution of measures to prevent progression. Brachialgia is in itself seldom severe enough to warrant surgical therapy. If the patient is old and relatively immobile for other reasons and spinal cord symptoms are not prominent, a soft collar to prevent anteroposterior motion of the neck can be prescribed. If the cord lesion disables an otherwise healthy, active individual, laminectomy, either an anterior or posterior surgical decompression of the spinal cord, is indicated. Roughly two thirds of such patients improve to some extent and in most of the others progression is halted. Many patients still retain some symptoms and may be dissatisfied with the outcome. The most frequent cause of failure of therapy is an inadequate decompression or the error of falsely attributing symptoms of some other spinal cord disease to the changes in the cervical spine.

MOTOR SYSTEM DISEASES INCLUDING AMYOTROPHIC LATERAL SCLEROSIS

Subsumed under the classification of "motor system diseases" are a heterogeneous assortment of clinical states bound together only loosely by the common clinical feature of progressive paralysis without sensory changes. Most reports on motor system diseases include progressive muscular atrophy (Aran-Duchenne disease and Werdnig-Hoffman disease), progressive bulbar palsy (Duchenne's disease), amyotrophic lateral sclerosis (Charcot's disease), and primary lateral sclerosis (Erb and Strumpell disease), each of which have been named after the neurologist who proffered the first published account. We believe the wide differences in age at onset, rate of progression, genetic background, and the presence or absence of either amyotrophy or spastic weakness favor the idea that these are separate motor disorders.

Clinical Manifestations

The most frequently seen and dreaded member of this group is amyotrophic lateral sclerosis in which lower motor neuron degeneration (with atrophic paralysis) is combined with corticospinal and corticobulbar tract degeneration.[2] The amyotrophy may begin in one arm or hand but within months extend to the other muscles of the limb and eventually to the other side of the body. Alternatively, it may first affect bulbar muscles (those of face, tongue, pharynx, and larynx) or those of the foot and leg. Over a period of a few years, the affection becomes more diffuse, and variable degrees of corticospinal paralysis with hyperactive tendon reflexes, spasticity, and Babinski's signs are added. Again, the latter symptoms may appear early and, for a time, dominate the clinical picture. The sparing of ocular musculature and all sensory functions are notable identifying and differentiating characteristics. Sphincteric control tends to be preserved until late in the course of the disease. Complete conservation of intellect permits the patient to appreciate fully the inexorable course of the "creeping paralysis." Loss of articulate speech, inability to swallow food, and the need for respiratory aid pose vexatious problems, i.e., whether to resort to a feeding gastrostomy and a respirator in view of the hopeless prognosis. Life usually ends in 4 to 7 years.

Diagnostic Aids

Electromyography reveals widespread denervation, even at an early stage when the clinical findings are localized. Biopsy of muscle discloses "group atrophy" without muscle fiber degeneration. Nerve conduction velocity measurements demonstrate only slight slowing of motor impulses in keeping with the axonal pathology. Deceptive at times are a slight elevation of the creatine kinase level, for which there is no explanation, and a slight elevation of cerebrospinal fluid protein.

Pathogenesis and Pathology

There are no convincing leads as to the causative factors in motor system diseases. Most of our patients present in late adulthood, but we have seen instances of the disease in early adult years; most occurrences are sporadic, but familial coincidence over two or more generations is recorded in approximately 5% of patients. Familial incidence is higher in the purely lower motor neuron amyotrophics (progressive muscular atrophy) and the course of the disease tends to be more protracted (see Hereditary Spinal Muscular Atrophies). There is no evidence suggestive of an earlier infection with one of the poliomyelitis viruses. In Guam, where the disease has been noted in 10% of individuals in some villages (sometimes in association with dementia and Parkinson's disease symptoms), the ingestion of flour from the cycad nut has been incriminated, but this still remains an unproven cause.

Gradual shrinkage (atrophy) and degeneration of motor nerve cells of the spinal cord and brain stem with a mild astroglial reaction are the principal findings. The degeneration of the corticospinal and corticobulbar tracts in the spinal cord and brain stem is easily traced to the motor cortices by the trail of fat-filled macrophages left by the disintegrating myelin and axons. All other parts of the nervous system are preserved.

Differential Diagnosis

Recently, two interesting findings have permitted the separation of two potential subgroups of motor system disorders, which are probably newly recognized diseases. One is the finding of a deficit in hexosaminidase A, the same enzyme lacking in infantile Tay-Sachs disease. This deficit leads to a chronic intraneuronal accumulation of GM_2 ganglioside, presumably in motor nerve cells. This variant presents in adult years, mainly as a pure amyotrophy. The second finding is a group of patients in whom there are elevated levels of antimyelin-associated glycoprotein (antiMAG) antibodies, extremely slow and multifocal motor nerve conduction velocities, and a response to immunosuppressive drugs (corticosteroids, cyclophosphamide).

Treatment

Unfortunately, supportive measures are all that can be offered at this time.

SPINAL CORD COMPRESSION BY TUMOR

Definition

A useful clinical rule states that spinal epidural tumors are metastatic (carcinoma or lymphoma), intradural-extramedullary tumors are neurofibromas or meningiomas, and intramedullary tumors are gliomas. Notable exceptions are instances of neurofibromas that extend outside the spinal canal, forming a dumbbell-shaped mass, leptomeningeal seedings of carcinomas and gliomas; and intramedullary metastatic deposits. The extramedullary tumors induce neurologic symptoms by a combination of compression and venous ischemia, and the intramedullary tumors by direct invasion of the spinal cord tissue.

EXTRADURAL TUMORS. Unfortunately, epidural tumors are the highest in frequency, and the ultimate prognosis is most grave, even when the localized lesion is successfully diagnosed and treated. Usually the growth is heralded by localized pain in some region of the back, which may be associated with radicular segmental pain, the latter being intensified by movement and strain. In the first several weeks, the diagnosis may remain in doubt but should be suspected in a patient known to harbor a malignancy or an obvious destructive vertebral lesion (as seen on a radiograph or bone scan). Evolving over a period of days or weeks, a paraparesis and sensory changes below the level of the lesion appear, followed by loss of sphincter control. Occasionally, the neurologic symptoms advance rapidly over a few days, and once they are well established, even decompressive laminectomy may fail to restore function. Lung and breast cancer are the most frequent causes of extradural tumors, followed by lymphomas (lymphocytoma, lymphoblastoma, multiple myeloma). The latter group is responsive to radiotherapy directed to the lesions localized by the neurologic symptoms, myelography and MRI scan, and to steroid therapy.

When malignant tumors invade the subarachnoid space and spread along the spinal canal, they may affect roots and the spinal cord at numerous levels and even higher nervous structures, such as cranial nerves and brain (carcinomatosis of the meninges). Such lesions may be demonstrable by MRI scans and myelography, and tumor cells can be found in ultrafiltrates of the cerebrospinal fluid in one third to one half of patients. The cerebrospinal fluid also offers a route for therapy. Antineoplastic agents can be injected into the lumbar subarachnoid space as a supplement to systemic therapy. Some of the lymphomas and carcinomas respond rapidly to steroids and radiotherapy.[11]

It is important to differentiate epidural spinal tumors from the myelopathy that is associated with malignancy (see discussion on paraneoplasic myelopathy). Rare instances of spinal cord compression with paraparesis have been traced to pronounced epidural hematopoiesis or to proliferation of lipocytes after prolonged treatment with steroids.

INTRADURAL EXTRAMEDULLARY TUMORS. As would be expected, spinal cord syndromes associated with neurofibromatosis and meningioma develop more chronically over months and years. In the type of neurofibromatosis that involves cranial and spinal nerves (type II), cutaneous lesions may be absent, and the diagnosis is made exclusively from biopsy results and clinical, genetic, and radiologic data. Radicular pain is more prominent in the syndromes due to neurofibroma than in those due to meningioma. Usually, the spinal cord manifestations develop asymmetrically. The neurofibromas may be multiple and in some instances can be associated with one or more spinal or cranial meningiomas. The onset tends to be in early adulthood in both sexes; the meningioma-associated syndrome is more frequent in middle-aged women.

Diagnosis of epidural and subdural extramedullary growths is confirmed by MRI or CT scan with myelography. Surgical excision should restore function, even after weeks of compression.

INTRAMEDULLARY TUMORS. The intrinsic tumors of the spinal cord are predominantly ependymomas and less commonly astrocytomas[19] (benign or malignant). They progressively invade the tracts of the spinal cord over a period of months or years. Vascular malformations, hemangioblastomas, and other[13] tumors such as oligodendrocytomas are observed less frequently. Schistosomiasis is a known cause in South America and Africa. Apart from vascular abnormalities in the other intramedullary lesions, the clinical presentation is one of progressively failing spinal cord function. Motor and sensory tracts are successively involved and, later, sphincteric function fails. Regional spinal and radicular pain are usually absent or not at all prominent. The segmental level is sometimes indicated by localized sensory and motor functional disorders. However, the first symptomatic manifestation of tract involvement by an intrinsic cord tumor (or a compressive tumor) may be far below the level of the lesion and gradually rise, or, rarely,

the level may descend from the site of the lesion as the tumor enlarges. This is explained by the lamination of sensory and motor fibers in the tract itself, the largest and longest fibers being affected first. Although this can be misleading in the clinical analysis, the error can be rectified by radiologic procedures. The treatment is surgical decompression and radiation. Some ependymomas can be shelled out of the spinal cord and long-standing remission of symptoms can be obtained.

Other causes of cord compression include unusual neoplasms, cysts, or bone diseases (chondrosarcomas, angioendotheliomas, dermoid cysts, Paget's disease, etc.). Space limitations do not permit further discussion of these conditions.

HEREDITARY SPINAL MUSCULAR ATROPHIES

Definition

Progressive spinal muscular atrophies follow Duchenne muscular dystrophy in frequency of occurrence as causes of paralysis in children. The variable age of the patient at presentation from birth to middle age, the genetic origin, the extremely slow progression of the atrophic areflexic paralysis, either predominantly proximal or distal pattern of muscle involvement, and the exclusive degeneration of the motor neurons of the spinal cord and brain stem are identifying features.

Clinical Description

The most common forms of progressive spinal muscular atrophies (Werdnig-Hoffmann type) present as a generalized weakness of autosomal recessive geneologic pattern in the first months or years of life. The weakness is diffuse and some movement is retained. Fasciculations of the tongue may be seen but not of limb muscles. The tendon reflexes are absent. The patient is otherwise normal. Admittedly, diagnosis can be difficult at this early age because sensory testing is impossible. In the past, the differentiation from limb-girdle dystrophies, chronic poly-neuropathies, and congenital myopathies was often inaccurate.

Laboratory Aids

The clinical recognition and distinctive boundaries of these entitites were not established until the wider application of electrophysiologic studies (EMG and nerve conduction) and muscle biopsy. In addition to three types of Werdnig-Hoffmann disease (varying only in age at onset, severity, and rate of progression), a proximal juvenile form (Kugelberg-Welander disease), an adolescent or adult form of scapulofemoral atrophy, a distal atrophic form, and a predominantly bulbar form (Fazio-Londe disease) have been identified.[2] Autosomal recessive, autosomal dominant (frequently variable in penetrance), and sex-linked patterns of inheritance are known to occur, but some of the cases appear to be sporadic mutations.

Pathology

In the simplest terms, the lesion in progressive spinal muscular atrophies consists of a degeneration of motor neurons and a reactive gliosis, not unlike that observed in amyotrophic lateral sclerosis. Shrinkage and pyknosis (atrophy) of neurons precedes their disappearance. Some of the nerve cells exhibit cytoplasmic swelling and chromatolysis, indicative of axonal injury as an early event.

Treatment

Thus far, therapeutic measures have proved to be valueless. In the more chronic situations of later onset, it is advantageous to encourage the patient to remain physically active as long as possible, i.e., to attend school or work. Genetic counseling to families is advised.

FAMILIAL SPASTIC PARAPLEGIA

Definition

In essence, familial spastic paraplegia consists of a progressive weakness and spasticity of the legs, beginning in childhood or adult life and afflicting more than one member of a family. Both sexes are affected, and the disease may be confined to members of a sibship or occur in a succession of generations in both sexes. In some families, it may be associated with dementia, cerebellar ataxia, or a hypertrophic form of polyneuropathy, but in most instances, it assumes a relatively pure form.

Clinical Manifestations

The gradual stiffening and weakening of the legs renders locomotion laborious and is associated with a tendency to scuff the toes of the shoes. Walking for a distance is increasingly hampered, and running becomes impossible. The tendon reflexes are hyperactive and Babinski's signs are present. Sphincteric control tends to be preserved until late in the disease. Sensation is spared. The arms are little affected, if at all, as is true of the bulbar musculature. No evidence of muscular atrophy can be found.

Laboratory Aids

All laboratory tests except transcranial magnetic stimulation of the motor cortices are uninformative. A slowing or loss of corticospinal conduction is demonstrable by the latter method.

Pathogenesis and Pathology

The pathologic changes in familial spastic paraplegia are simple: a loss of the largest motor neurons of the motor cortex and the depletion of the medullated fibers in the corticospinal systems. This is most obvious in the lower parts of the spinal cord. Unexplained, in view of the absence of sensory findings, is a slight pallor in myelin stains of the central part of the columns of Goll.

Treatment

Attempts to inhibit spasticity by the use of baclofen and threonine have been disappointing because as the stiffness is alleviated, leg weakness is exposed to a greater degree. Presently, there are no means of preventing the disease or halting its progress.

SYRINGOMYELIA

Definition

The term *syringomyelia*, long in use in medical parlance, refers to a cavitation of the central parts of the spinal cord, usually of uncertain origin. It is characterized by a peculiar disposition of spinal cord lesions of destructive type leading to longitudinal cavitation. Cerebrospinal fluid can enter such lesions from the subarachnoid space or from the central canal and extend vertically in the central gray matter over many segments. The most typical example is idiopathic cervical syringomyelia, which occurs during adult years and presents with a segmental sensory dissociation in the cervical region on one or both sides (loss of pain and temperature sensitivity with retention of other tactile modalities) and amyotrophy.

Clinical Manifestations

Syringomyelia may become manifest accidentally when the patient discovers that superficial injuries or burns of the arm and hand have caused no pain. Infrequently, there is unexplained neck and arm pain or muscle atrophy and weakness and areflexia of hand or forearm muscles. Examination then discloses loss of pain and temperature sensation not only in the hand and forearm but also in the shoulders and neck in a capelike distribution. Touch, pressure, sense of position, movement, and vibration are unaffected. Below the cervical and upper thoracic seg-

ments, pain and temperature sensitivity are retained. This segmental distribution is characteristic of a lesion of the pain and temperature fibers (which decussate within one or two segments after leaving the posterior horn of gray matter), extending over several adjacent segments of the cervical spinal cord. The principal site of the intramedullary lesion is the anterior commissure, but it usually also extends into the anterior and posterior horns of gray matter on one or both sides. When the anterior horn is involved, the aforementioned segmental amyotrophy occurs; with posterior horn lesions, segmental pain and other modalities of sensation may be lost. The lesion varies in size and symmetry from one spinal cord segment to another. Involvement of thoracic segments often results in kyphoscoliosis. Pain is prominent in approximately a third of patients. Occipital or generalized headache on exertion or cough is a feature of some cases, mainly those with a Chiari malformation. Some of the cavities extend upward into the lateral tegmentum of the medulla or even to higher parts of the brain stem, causing analgesia and thermoanesthesia of one or both sides of the face and other disorders of lower cranial nerves (syringobulbia). As the lesion advances, the long sensory and motor tracts of the upper part of the cervical cord become implicated, resulting in the expected functional disturbances of the legs and sphincters.[3, 14]

Approximately half of all instances of idiopathic cervical syringomyelia are associated with type I Chiari malformations and in some patients with the latter, the neck may be shortened due to congenital abnormalities of the cervical spine and base of skull. Presumably this is associated with cervical cord injury that progresses to cavitation. Other types of syringomyelia occur as well, such as obstruction to the foramen magnum by localized arachnoiditis, cysts, and tumors; however, they are infrequent. Frank fracture-dislocation injuries of the cervical spinal cord are infrequently accompanied at a later time by the extension of cavitation, manifested by neurologic symptoms and signs in segments above the level (cephalad) of the original lesion. Radiologically or on postmortem examination a syrinx is found. Tumors such as hemangioblastoma and glioma are other causes. In patients with glial tumors, the so-called cysts usually contain a high-protein yellow coagulum indicating disintegration of tumor tissue instead of the usual limpid low-protein cerebrospinal fluid of a true syrinx. In a few cases of syringomyelia there is evidence of a cervical arachnoiditis.

Laboratory Aids

An MRI scan of the spinal cord and brain stem taken in the sagittal plane provides a reliable corroboration in nearly every patient suspected of having syringomyelia. A coexistent Chiari malformation also can be seen. Myelography with water-soluble media usually shows that the cavity is filling from the subarachnoid space without passage via the fourth ventricle.[3]

Pathogenesis and Pathology

The affected segments of the spinal cord can be expanded by the syrinx and, at times, even the spinal canal is widened by the pressure it exerts. In other cases, the affected segments retain their normal size and contour. In microscopic sections, the walls of the syrinx are composed only of fibrous glia and a few vessels. At one or more points, the ependyma lined central canal is expanded and ruptured, permitting ready communication between the canal and syrinx. One or more direct connections between the subarachnoid space and the syrinx must also exist but are usually not obvious under the microscope. The ease with which myelographic media enter the cyst from the subarachnoid space indicates their presence. The postulation by Gardner[10] of a direct communication between the fourth ventricle and syrinx via a dilated central canal (a true hydromyelia) has not been found in several of our patients. With coexistence of a Chiari malformation, the typical protrusion of cerebellar tissue, its indentation of the posterior surface of the spinal cord, and downward displacement of the medulla and arachnoidal fibrosis are added. Hydrocephalus may or may not be present.

Differential Diagnosis

The most important condition to be excluded in the differential diagnosis of syringomyelia is an intramedullary tumor, particularly a hemangioblastoma. The latter is nearly always part of the von Hippel-Lindau syndrome of retinal lesion and cerebellar cyst, but only rarely is the spinal cord alone involved. In the patient with an intramedullary glioma or metastatic carcinoma, the tissue around a cavity often enhances with gadolinium in MRI scans.

Treatment

Decompression of the cervical cord at the foramen magnum relieves some of the symptoms of the syringomyelia presenting with a Chiari malformation. Attempts to shunt the syrinx by a tube containing a one-way valve that empties into the subarachnoid space or peritoneal cavity have achieved indifferent results. Usually, the shunt does not remain open and needs to be revised. By these measures the advance of sensory and motor deficits may be halted and occipital pain relieved. Arm pain seldom responds.

SPINOCEREBELLAR DEGENERATIONS

Definition

The classic example of a spinocerebellar degeneration is Friedreich's ataxia. This is a relatively rare, autosomal recessive disease that is characterized by progressive ataxia, skeletal deformities, and myocardiopathy. The onset is in childhood, less often in adolescence; the progression is slow, occurring over 2 to 3 decades, and death is usually the result of cardiac dysrhythmia and failure.

Clinical Manifestations

Spinocerebellar degeneration is not usually thought of in connection with spinal cord syndromes because ataxia, both sensory and cerebellar, is the predominant clinical finding. However, as in some of the other hereditary cerebellar ataxias of adolescence and adult life, there are always manifest signs of spinal cord and peripheral disease. Almost invariably the tendon reflexes are lost along with impairment of touch, vibratory, and position senses, because of degeneration of dorsal root ganglion cells and sensory tracts in the spinal cord. Speech becomes dysarthric, swallowing difficult, ocular movements jerky (nystagmus is often present), and arm movement clumsy. Within a few years, walking is impossible. Strangely, denervation atrophy of muscles does not occur in most patients. The spinocerebellar tracts also degenerate, but their contribution to the clinical syndrome remains unclear. The kyphoscoliosis and pes cavus are probably secondary to the spinal neurologic disorder.

Laboratory Diagnosis

The finding of electrocardiographic (ECG) abnormalities in a young person with progressive ataxia aids diagnosis, as does the autosomal recessive inheritance. Diabetes mellitus is frequently present.

Differential Diagnosis

Other forms of familial spinocerebellar atrophy begin in the same age period but present with retained tendon reflexes. Its relationship to Friedreich's ataxia is uncertain. Multiple sclerosis also must be distinguished, using the criteria described previously.

Pathology

The myelin-stained section of the spinal cord displaying the obvious pallor of the corticospinal and spinocerebellar tracts and posterior columns cannot be mistaken for any other disease. The spinal cord is reduced in size. More difficult to demonstrate, except by resorting to quantitative methods, is the loss of neurons in the dorsal root ganglia, poste-

rior horn of the spinal cord, motor cortices, and parts of the cerebellum.

Treatment

No therapy is known.

SUBACUTE COMBINED DEGENERATION OF SPINAL CORD

Subacute combined degeneration of the spinal cord has long been recognized as one of the classic types of pure spinal cord disease and is typified by its unique association with macrocytic anemia (pernicious because of its formerly fatal outcome). This disease has become relatively rare. Nevertheless, steps should always be taken to rule it out, because it is preventable or curable by administration of vitamin B_{12}.

Definition

In simplest form, this condition consists of a subacute degeneration of the posterior columns followed later by that of lateral columns of the spinal cord (i.e., combined sensory and motor systems). The clinical manifestations include paresthesias and sensory ataxia followed by spastic paraparesis. The peripheral nervous system is affected to some extent in most patients.

Clinical Manifestations

Generally, the first symptoms are tingling and numbness of the hands and arms spreading to the thorax and later to lower parts of the body. Once the legs are involved, unsteadiness of gait and a Romberg sign appear. Both legs are involved at about the same time in keeping with the bilateral symmetry of the posterior column lesions. As the disease advances over several weeks, the legs become weak and stiff, with either an increase or decrease in tendon reflexes and Babinski's signs. The syndrome is then one of an ataxic paraparesis. In the more advanced stages of the disease after the spinal cord disorder is well developed, new lesions may appear in the white matter of the brain stem, optic nerves, and cerebrum. In almost all patients who present with earlier spinal lesions, the symptoms of peripheral nerve disorder tend to be obscured by those referrable to the spinal cord. The macrocytic anemia with megaloblasts in bone marrow and leukopenia and polysegmentation of neutrophilic leukocytes accompanies or precedes the neurologic manifestations, but in approximately 20% of patients it may develop several months or a year or more later. Loss of lingual papillae and gastric achlorhydria are other findings. A claim has been made of cerebral disorder, treatable by vitamin B_{12}, that occurs without evidence of spinal cord abnormality.

Pathogenesis and Pathology

The disease is caused by a chronic inability to absorb cobalamin from the stomach because of lack of a protein (the Castle intrinsic factor). The parietal cells of the stomach, which are atrophied due to a possible autoimmune abnormality, fail to liberate both hydrochloric acid and the cobalamin-binding glycoprotein. The failure of production of the latter and its absorption in the ileum over a long period has two effects: (1) the blocking of DNA synthesis, leading to a megaloblastic anemia and (2) a failure of incorporation of fatty acids in myelinated fibers of central and peripheral nervous system. The latter is reflected in a rise of methylmalonic acid and total homocysteine in the serum and urine.[2]

A distinctive spongy appearance is caused by degeneration of the myelin sheaths and, to a lesser degree, of axons in the central parts of the posterior columns and lateral columns of the cervical and thoracic spinal cord. Groups of myelinated fibers near veins degenerate, liberating cholesterol esters that are phagocytized by histiocytes. Astrocytes, which are not numerous in the spinal cord, react but do not form a tight isomorphic scar for a long time, hence, the spongy appearance in untreated patients. No infiltration of inflammatory cells is present. As the disease

advances, all of the tracts in the spinal cord are involved. Later, the same small perivascular lesions appear in the white matter of the medulla, cerebellum, optic tracts, and cerebrum.

Differential Diagnosis

Multiple sclerosis, syphilitic meningomyelitis, cervical spondylosis, tropical paraparesis, subacute AIDS myelopathy, necrotizing and demyelinative myelitis, and chronic arachnoiditis also can present as a spastic, ataxic paraparesis. Gastric and bowel resection and a dietary deficiency are rare causes of this syndrome.

Treatment

As little as 100 mg/mL of cobalamin (B_{12}) per week is sufficient to cure the disease. Reticulocytes appear in the circulating blood within 4 to 5 days, and the anemia is gradually corrected. The spinal cord lesions regress more slowly but always improve. If there is a long delay in starting treatment, there may be residual ataxia, posterior column signs, and slight spastic weakness. The failure to respond should raise suspicion of some other metabolic diseases underlying the cobalamin and methylmalonic acid disorder. Folate deficiency can also cause a macrocytic anemia but probably not the neurologic abnormality, although the latter may worsen if folate alone is given for the pernicious anemia.

TROPICAL SPASTIC PARAPARESIS (HTLV-1–ASSOCIATED MYELOPATHY)

Definition

Tropical spastic paraparesis has only recently been recognized in Northern and Southern temperate zones and is rare. It consists of a slowly advancing spastic weakness of the legs with a variable degree of sensory and sphincteric disorder. Most patients have been middle-aged adults living in tropical regions of the West Indies and Northern Africa. Human T-cell lymphotropic virus (HTLV-1) is the established cause.

Clinical Manifestations

The symptom that causes the patient to come to the physician is a weakening and a stiffening of both legs. There also may be a complaint of backache in some instances. Unsteadiness of gait can add to the difficulty in locomotion. Only later do precipitancy of micturition or loss of sphincter control occur. On examination the tendon reflexes in the legs are increased and the plantar reflexes extensor. Vibratory and position senses are reduced and in a few patients, pain, temperature, and touch senses are also reduced. The arms usually remain normal. The progression of disease gradually advances over years but can progress more rapidly.

Laboratory Aids

Cerebrospinal fluid may contain an increased number of mononuclear cells and increased levels of protein and gamma globulin. Myelography is negative.

Pathogenesis and Pathology

The finding of HTLV-1 antibodies in the serum and cerebrospinal fluid and the isolation of the virus from white blood cells have established the viral etiology. Virus particles have been seen in the central nervous system by electron microscopy. In endemic areas, antibodies are found in 5% to 20% of the population, and asymptomatic individuals are more common than symptomatic persons. The disease can be transmitted by transfusion. An associated T-cell lymphoblastic leukemia can occur but has been rare.

The basic disease process is a chronic meningomyelitis as would be expected from the pleocytosis and increased protein in the cerebrospinal fluid. Destruction of myelinated fibers in the superficial parts of the spinal tracts with meningeal and perivascular infiltrates of lymphocytic and mononuclear cells with variable gliosis constitute the histologic reaction.

Differential Diagnosis

Heretofore, most of the patients with this syndrome were diagnosed as having chronic multiple sclerosis, syphilitic meningomyelitis, or adhesive arachnoiditis. In India, ingestion of the fava bean is known to induce a spastic paraplegia.

Treatment

Steroids have benefited some patients. Antiviral agents have not been given an adequate trial.

THE MYELOPATHY OF AIDS

Since the discovery of acquired immunodeficiency syndrome (AIDS) in 1981 and the isolation of the retrovirus called the human immunodeficiency virus (HIV), both acute and subacute associated myelopathies have been reported. Evidently, the AIDS virus can alter the function of the spinal cord in several ways. It may cause compression by a Kaposi sarcoma or lymphoma or a direct infection by another so-called opportunistic microorganism such as herpes simplex or zoster virus, or may attack the spinal cord directly. The last process takes the form of a subacute, noninflammatory vacuolar degeneration of myelinated tracts in the posterior and lateral columns of the cervical and thoracic cord. In many respects, the lesions resemble those of subacute combined degeneration due to cobalamin deficiency.[17] The lack of inflammation and failure to isolate the AIDS virus or another microorganism frequently observed in patients with AIDS tend to exclude an infective cause. Although patients are often subject to chronic diarrhea and inanition, a deficiency of cobalamin has not been found. This vacuolar myelopathy has been observed in 10% to 30% of patients with AIDS at postmortem examination, and frequently, it is combined with the well-known encephalitis, peripheral neuritis, or myositis common to this disease. The condition is less frequent in AIDS-infected children.

Clinical Manifestations

The symptoms of AIDS-associated myelopathy vary but include some combination of sensory loss, ataxia, spastic weakness, and sphincteric incontinence. Burning pain, prominent in some patients, probably is an indication of a coexistent peripheral neuritis. Proprioceptive sensory impairment is regularly described, as are the reflex changes associated with corticospinal tract involvement. The cerebrospinal fluid has been normal in some patients but contains inflammatory cells (lymphocytes and mononuclear cells) and increased protein in others.

Treatment

An effective therapy for the vacuolar myelopathy has not been developed.

MYELITIS

In ancient times, the term *myelitis* was used to designate almost any disease of the spinal cord. It has gradually been restricted to diseases of inflammatory type, either infective or noninfective. Of the former, the most familiar are those caused by viruses, such as poliomyelitis and herpes zoster, but the usual practice is to call these diseases by their proper names and not by the term *myelitis*. The second group of noninfective inflammations, meaning no infectious agent has been isolated, includes postinfectious and postvaccinial demyelinations, acute multiple sclerosis, and subacute necrotizing myelitis. The demyelinative disorders are thought to be inflammations due to autoimmune mechanisms. There is also a third group, the meningomyelitides, which may be caused by either an infective agent, such as the spirochetes of syphilis or Lyme disease, or a toxin, such as spinal anesthesia and my-

elographic dyes. In this instance, the noxious agent resides in the spinal subarachnoid space and damages the spinal cord by causing inflammation of the pia-arachnoid. The pial lesion may implicate the vasculature, or by progressive fibrosis, constrict the spinal cord. The latter process is termed *arachnoiditis*.

Demyelinative Forms of Myelitis

DEFINITION. Three forms of demyelinative myelitis are recognized: (1) acute myelitis after an exanthem or vaccination and, occasionally, a nonexanthematous viral infection, such as viral influenza; (2) acute multiple sclerosis; and (3) acute hemorrhagic leukomyelitis. All of these manifest an acute "transverse" myelitis with sensory, motor, reflex, and sphincteric syndromes indicative of demyelination of tracts of the spinal cord. In some patients, particularly those with acute multiple sclerosis and hemorrhagic leukomyelitis, a considerable degree of necrosis may occur, which accounts for the permanence of neurologic deficits.[2]

Because these syndromes are acute, they are not discussed further here. Occasionally, acute myelitis, instead of being an acute monophasic postinfectious myelitis, will prove by later recurrence of attacks to have been an initial episode of multiple sclerosis. The factors described previously under the section on chronic multiple sclerosis then become applicable to this form of myelitis. In other cases, the disease never recurs and follows the expected course of postinfectious myelitis, of which it is probably a subtype.

Progressive Necrotic Myelitis (Foix-Alajouanine Disease)

DEFINITION. Progressive myelitis has proved to be a condition that is very controversial. In 1925, Foix and Alajouanine[8] described this disease in two patients who died at the Salpetrière as a "myélite nécrotique subaigue." They emphasized the progressive nature of the necrosis (lesions of different ages and symptoms of an ascending amyotrophy) and a pathologically curious hypertrophy of blood vessels. It is the latter type of change, sometimes referred to as an *endomesovasculitis*, that has led to several different interpretations. Foix thought it was part of an inflammatory process, Wyburn-Mason[20] judged it to be a vascular malformation, and others have decided that in some instances the basic process is a spinal thrombophlebitis. It is generally agreed that the spinal cord necrosis is of ischemic origin from narrowing or occlusion of arteries or veins.

After a review of 80 cases, Folliss and Netzky[9] concluded that some of the cases are caused by vascular malformations (a group that they call *angiodysgenetic*) and others are idiopathic. One reason for the confusion has been the indiscriminate mixing of instances of acute infarction (myelomalacia) due to several types of extravertebral and intravertebral vascular occlusion with those due to progressive necrotic myelopathy. This neglects the characteristic clinical course and the peculiar vascular lesions described by Foix and Alajouanine.

CLINICAL MANIFESTATIONS. Progressive necrotic myelitis occurs in adult years in both sexes and has been preceded by a wide assortment of infections, both viral and bacterial. Nevertheless, in some instances, it has struck down a person in perfect health without warning. Nausea, malaise, and weakness of the legs, sometimes with limb pain, have initiated the clinical syndrome. Tingling, prickling numbness indicates sensory involvement. Loss of sphincteric control also occurs. All of this transpires in hours or days. Severe paralysis of "pyramidal" type is attended by spinal cord shock, which eventually gives way to spastic paralysis. In some instances, the limbs remain flaccid. As the disease progresses over months or a year or two, the sensory and motor level of the cord lesions rises, and spasticity may be replaced by amyotrophic areflexic paralysis indicative of destruction of the gray matter (anterior horn cells) of the spinal cord. Breathing may eventually be compromised, and in many instances, death is the consequence of intercurrent infection.

LABORATORY AIDS. The protein level in cerebrospinal fluid is elevated in some patients, and in a few, pleocytosis occurs, but the level of glucose remains normal, and all bacteriologic studies have been negative. EMG reveals motor unit denervation. The spinal cord is atrophied on CT and MRI.

DIFFERENTIAL DIAGNOSIS. Acute demyelinative forms of myelitis, myelopathy from epidural tumors and meningeal carcinomatosis, paraneoplastic myelopathy, the vacuolar myelopathy associated with AIDS, and spinal vascular malformations should be considered in the differential diagnosis.

PATHOLOGY. Varying degrees of necrosis and glial mononuclear–microglial reactions of differing ages along with marked thickening and increased cellularity of intramedullary arteries and veins characterize the lesions. Vascular occlusion is seldom found, either of meningeal or intramedullary vessels. The adventitial sheaths contain mononuclear cells and an occasional lymphocyte, but infiltrates of hematogenous inflammatory cells are seldom conspicuous.

TREATMENT. Steroids are usually given a trial, with rather indifferent results.

MYELOPATHY WITH SYSTEMIC CARCINOMA

Distinct from spinal cord compression and invasion caused by carcinomatous implants, a rapidly developing noninflammatory myelopathy appears in patients harboring a variety of malignant tumors.[16] The clinical syndrome includes symptoms and signs of a painless impairment of motor and sensory function below the level of the lesion. Postmortem examination has disclosed a necrosis of the tracts of the spinal cord without sign of neoplasm. In one patient, serum antibodies to the tumor cells have been found to cross-react with spinal cord tissue. This is postulated as the pathogenetic mechanism of the cord lesion. A similar disorder has been observed in patients who have no tumor. Perhaps in some instances, the necrosis is caused by fibrocartilaginous emboli (from an invertebral disk) to the spinal cord. The condition is rare, and there have been no systematic attempts at therapy. The subacute spinocerebellar degeneration associated with ovarian and lung carcinomas is a different illness.

The recently recognized fibrocartilaginous embolization of the spinal cord may have been overlooked in some patients.

RADIATION MYELOPATHY

Radiation myelopathy, which follows incidental exposure of the spinal cord during radiation treatment of visceral tumors, is a dreaded complication. A gradual symmetrical or asymmetrical sensory and motor tract lesion evolves over a period of weeks, and once fully installed, becomes permanent. The dose of ionizing radiation has ranged from 2500 to 6500 rads, but frequently the amount of ionizing radiation received by the spinal cord has not been measured accurately. The spacing of the exposures in a series of treatments is critical. A single dose of as little as 1500 to 2000 rads can destroy the exposed parts of the nervous system; a dose of 3000 to 4000 rads spaced over a month will not. There are, however, examples of a transient myelopathy in 3% of a series of patients receiving doses of less than 3500 rads given in 17 days. With doses of more than 3500 rads, the incidence was 23%, and the effects were irreversible.[12] Others have placed the tolerance dose at a slightly lower level but emphasize that the size of the radiated field also makes a difference. The interval between the time of irradiation and the first spinal cord symptom has ranged from 6 to 48 months. The radiation lesion is typically vascular, with fibrosis and occlusion of vessels and coagulative necrosis of spinal tissue.[6] Occasionally, steroids in large doses have caused some regression of symptoms.

SPINAL ARACHNOIDITIS

Definition

The term spinal arachnoiditis continues to appear in the medical literature despite its ambiguity. Actually, it refers to one aspect of a variety of pathologic entities that result in fibrosis of the arachnoid membrane of the spinal cord. However, because the arachnoid is inseparable from the pia and is always involved, it incompletely designates the pathologic change. Also omitted is reference to the neurologic disorder in which the spinal roots and spinal cord are involved. A more precise and inclusive term would be *chronic meningomyelopathy* and *meningoradiculopathy*, depending on whether the spinal cord or roots of the cauda equina are affected. The causes range from chronic spinal meningitis due to many types of infection to various toxins that are introduced into the spinal subarachnoid space for diagnostic or therapeutic purposes.

Generally, it would seem probable that any infective agent or toxin, if it remained long enough in the spinal subarachnoid space, would be capable of irritating sensitive tissues and exciting an inflammatory response in the pia-arachnoid.[7, 18] This ultimately leads to fibroblastic proliferation and scarring of the leptomeninges.

Clinical Manifestations

One of the most instructive examples of spinal arachnoiditis was occasioned by accidental introduction of chemically contaminated spinal anesthesia into the cerebrospinal fluid. The cause was found to be inadvertent leakage of a detergent into vials of procaine. The condition has been prevented by preparing the anesthesia at the time it is used.

The immediate effect of this chemical contaminant was severe back pain followed within 1 or 2 days by a rapidly advancing sensory and motor paralysis of the lower extremities. The nerve roots were the site of the disorder. The parts of the body innervated by the cauda equina rapidly lost innervation. The cerebrospinal fluid protein level rose precipitously and a mild pleocytosis was noted. If the toxic agent extended up over the spinal cord, this also could have been affected, with loss of function of sensory and motor tracts. After many months or a year or more, the radicular paralysis receded and nerves regenerated, even though by that time the spinal subarachnoid space had been obliterated by scar tissue. Then, in several patients after months to several years, the fibrosis that was progressive led gradually to a constrictive myelopathy or radiculopathy. Also, some patients later became blind or experienced obstructive hydrocephalus from a basilar intracranial arachnoiditis.

Pathogenesis and Pathology

Several pathogenetic mechanisms can be discerned in this sequence of events. First, immediate paralytic effects are evident of the injected agent acting on the spinal roots and spinal cord. Later, the constrictive effects of a progressive fibrosis became evident in the spinal cord and roots. The two mechanisms can be separated by an interval of time or merge. If the initial event is not severe, it can be asymptomatic, in which case only the later meningeal fibrosis eventually emerges.

This sequence of events can occur in patients sustaining a low-grade bacterial, viral, or syphilitic meningitis. In some instances, multiple factors may be operative, such as a series of pantopaque myelograms, one or more laminectomies, subarachnoid blood, and postoperative infections. In a few patients, no clue as to the original meningeal infection can be obtained. Such instances are classed as idiopathic chronic adhesive arachnoiditis.[7]

The clinical presentation, as would be expected, varies widely. The most frequent syndrome involves some of the roots of the cauda equina after rupture of one or more lumbar disks and multiple diagnostic myelograms and operations. In addition to the residual root damage from the disk rupture, intractable pain develops in the lower back, thighs, and legs, with rather few additional neurologic deficits. Attempts at myelography reveal pocketing of the dye between adhesions. Operation exposes dense adhesions around the roots and between pia and arachnoid and arachnoid and dura. Attempts to extricate the roots from the fibrous tissue are futile in most instances, and the patient is left with chronic pain that often defies all therapeutic measures.

Another syndrome is a chronic meningomyelopathy with a gradually evolving spastic-ataxic paraparesis. Again, myelography demonstrates an extensive blockage of the subarachnoid space, which is incomplete in places. Laminectomy exposes widespread adhesive arachnoiditis with scattered loculi of yellow cerebrospinal fluid. Dissection of the adhesions from the encased spinal cord can improve function, but the benefit is usually not lasting.

Differential Diagnosis

In the differential diagnosis, all forms of compressive myelopathy, radiculopathy, and tumor should be considered. Knowledge of the initiating events aids in establishing the correct diagnosis, as does a myelogram. The most difficult and frequent problem is distinguishing the lumbosacral arachnoiditis from disk rupture and from a variety of pathologic states in the spine itself.

REFERENCES

1. Adams CBT, Logue V: Studies in cervical spondylotic myelopathy. Brain 94:569, 1971.
2. Adams RD, Victor M: Principles of Neurology, ed. 5. New York, McGraw Hill, 1993.
3. Barnet HJM, Foster JB, Hudgson P: Syringomyelia. Philadelphia, WB Saunders, 1973.
4. Bartleson JO, Cohen MD, Harrington TM: Cauda equina syndrome secondary to longstanding ankylosing spondylitis. Ann Neurol 14:662, 1983.
5. Brain WR, Northfield D, Wilkinson M: The neurological manifestations of cervical spondylosis. Brain 75:187, 1952.
6. Burns RJ, Jones AN, Robertson JS: Pathology of radiation myelopathy. J Neurol Neurosurg Psychiatry 35:888, 1972.
7. Elkington JS: Arachnoiditis. In Feiling A (ed): Modern Trends in Neurology. New York, Hoeber-Harper, 1951.
8. Foix C, Alajouanine T: La myélite nécrotique subaigue. Rev Neurol 2:1, 1926.
9. Folliss AGH, Netzky MG: Progressive necrotic myelopathy. In Vinken PJ, Bruyn W (eds): Handbook of Clinical Neurology, ch 10, vol 9. Amsterdam, Elsevier, 1970.
10. Gardner WJ: Hydrodynamic mechanism of syringomyelia: Its relation to myelocele. J Neurol Neurosurg Psychiatry 28:247, 1965.
11. Gilbert RW, Kim JH, Posner JB: Epidural spinal cord compression from metastatic tumor: Diagnosis and treatment. Ann Neurol 3:46, 1978.
12. Jones A: Transient radiation myelitis. Br J Radiol 37:727, 1914.
13. Logue V: Angiomas of the spinal cord. Review of the pathogenesis, clinical features and results of surgery. J Neurol Neurosurg Psychiatry 42:1, 1979.
14. Logue V, Edwards MR: Syringomyelia and its surgical treatment—an analysis of 75 cases. J Neurol Neurosurg Psychiatry 44:273, 1981.

15. McDonald WL: Multiple sclerosis: Pathological and clinical dynamics. J Neurol Neurosurg Psychiatry 53:338, 1994.
16. Mancall EL, Rosales RK: Necrotizing myelopathy associated with visceral carcinoma. Brain 87:639, 1964.
17. Petito CK, Navia BA, Cho ES, et al: Vacuolar myelopathy pathologically resembling subacute combined degeneration in patients with AIDS. N Engl J Med 312:374, 1985.
18. Shaw MDM, Russell JA, Grossant KW: The changing pattern of arachnoiditis. J Neurol Neurosurg Psychiatry 41:97, 1978.
19. Sloof JH, Kernohan JW, MacCarty CS: Primary Intramedullary Tumors of the Spinal Cord and Filum Terminale. Philadelphia, WB Saunders, 1964.
20. Wyburn-Mason R: Vascular Abnormalities and Tumours of the Spinal Cord and Its Membranes. St. Louis, Mosby, 1944.

CHAPTER 6

Spinal Cord Injury

Paul R. Meyer, Jr., M.D.
George R. Cybulski, M.D.
Joseph J. Rusin, M.D.
Michael H. Haak, M.D.

Reports estimating the annual incidence of spinal cord injuries in the United States vary greatly, but the range of 8000 to 10,000 new cases is most commonly cited. The prevalence of traumatic spinal cord injury is estimated to be 906 per million population. Accidents involving motor vehicles are the principal cause of traumatic injury to the spinal cord. Other etiologies of traumatic spinal cord injury in descending order of frequency include falls, recreational activities (especially diving accidents), and penetrating injuries of the spinal column secondary to gunshot or knife wounds (Table 6–1). The cervical region and the thoracolumbar junction are the most commonly affected areas in traumatic spinal cord injury followed by the thoracic and lumbar segments of the spine (Fig. 6–1). Diagnostic and therapeutic consideration of spinal injury involves both a detailed analysis of the skeletal as well as the neurologic components of the spine. Skeletal evaluation includes more than the identification of obvious bony fractures because the range of potential injury can include ligamentous and intervertebral disk disruption as well as dislocation of the affected vertebral segments. Neurologic injury can therefore occur on the basis of spinal cord compression from bony fracture fragments, stretching of the spinal cord due to spinal instability as a consequence of disk/ligamentous injury, or additional mechanisms of vascular injury or direct injury from missiles.

TABLE 6–1

ETIOLOGY OF SPINE INJURY SEEN
AT THE NORTHWESTERN UNIVERSITY
ACUTE SPINE INJURY CENTER
FROM 1972–1990

ETIOLOGY	INJURIES	
	NO.	%
Automobile	1112	31.79
Fall	919	26.27
Gunshot	310	8.86
Diving	278	7.95
Other traumatic	254	7.26
Motorcycle	149	4.26
Other sports	142	4.06
Other medical	131	3.74
Pedestrian	94	2.69
Other	60	1.72
Unknown	49	1.40
Total	3498	100.00

CERVICAL SPINE INJURY

By virtue of its unique construction surrounding a centrally located spinal cord, its exposure, and its flexibility, the cervical spine is subject to forces and patterns of injury distinct from that affecting other areas of the spinal vertebral column. For example, in the upper cervical spine, the atlas or first cervical vertebra (C1) is a bony ring with its vertebral body having been joined during development to that of the second vertebral body (axis, C2) to form a structure known as the odontoid process. The ringlike atlas is thus perfectly suited for providing rotation around the odontoid process of the axis, accounting for as much as 50 degrees of rotation of the head and cervical spine. The ringlike atlas can undergo indirect injury when forces applied to the top of the head are transmitted by way of the occipital condyles to the lateral masses of the atlas. The ring of the atlas can burst under this axial compression load. This type of injury (Jefferson fracture) has occurred in 30 of the 3377 patients with cervical spine injuries treated at the Midwest Regional Spinal Cord Injury Center (Table 6–2).

Generally, it is not associated with neurologic deficit.

Trauma to the upper cervical spine involving rotational forces can produce a rotatory subluxation type injury at the C1–2 junction. This type of injury often occurs after an episode of horseplay or tumbling in which the head undergoes a low-velocity twisting or rotational movement. Disruption of the transverse ligament of the atlas and the alar ligaments, which prevent excessive shift of the atlas on the axis, leads to a shift of the atlas on the axis, producing posterosuperior cervical and occiput pain due to compression of the sensory root of C2 as it exits between C1 and C2, an abnormal tilting and rotation of the head (torticollis or wryneck, the so-called "cock robin" position after the posture of a listening robin), and loss of cervical spine rotary mobility.

The transverse ligamentous complex holding the odontoid process in alignment with the posterior portion of the anterior ring of C1 can rupture, leading to subluxation upon flexion (Fig. 6–2). This typically occurs in an elderly patient with a history of a fall involving a blow to the occiput.[3, 15] An identifiable bony fracture is not usually present, but the diagnosis is established by a lateral flexion-extension cervical spine film with measurement of the space or interval between the back of the anterior ring of C1 and the front of the odontoid process. A measurement of greater than 3 mm in the adult indicates damage of the transverse ligament. If displacement is more than 5 mm, the transverse ligament has probably ruptured.

The odontoid process itself can fracture in three different pattern types (I, II, III) (Fig. 6–3). Fortunately, in injuries of the upper cervical spine, the neural canal at the C1–2 level is the most capacious of the entire cervical spine, with a low incidence of neurologic injury. At the C1 level the canal is equally shared by the odontoid process, spinal cord, and free space—the so-called "rule of thirds."[40] This free space provides a margin of safety for the spinal cord when C1–2 subluxation or odontoid fractures occur. Type II fractures of the odontoid were associated with complete neurologic injury in 6.7% of

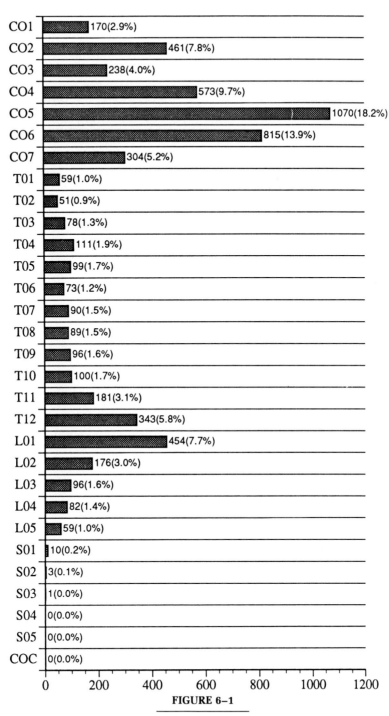

FIGURE 6–1

Incidence of spine injury by highest level (Northwestern University Acute Spine Injury Center: 1972–June 1990).

patients, incomplete injury in 19.1% of patients, and no neurologic injury in 73% of patients with intact cord in our series of 89 patients. Below C2, the spinal canal rapidly narrows, reaching its most narrow point between C4 and C6 (Fig. 6–4). Thus, the luxury of additional space for the spinal cord is lost. However, greater than 50% canal compromise may be necessary before neurologic injury occurs.[5]

TABLE 6–2

FRACTURE TYPE BY EXTENT (CERVICAL* FRACTURES), NORTHWESTERN UNIVERSITY ACUTE SPINE INJURY CENTER, 1972–1990

FRACTURE TYPE	TOTAL	COMPLETE		INCOMPLETE		INTACT		MISSING	
		NO.	%	NO.	%	NO.	%	NO.	%
Body-anticompression-wedge	488	192	39.3	196	40.2	96	19.7	4	0.8
Subluxation—unilateral	412	82	19.9	214	51.9	110	26.7	6	1.5
Lamina fracture—unilateral	348	135	38.8	150	43.1	61	17.5	2	0.6
Dislocation	325	144	44.3	140	43.1	38	11.7	3	0.9
Facet fracture—unilateral	265	82	30.9	118	44.5	62	23.4	3	1.1
Body-axial compression-burst	247	93	37.7	106	42.9	46	18.6	2	0.8
Spinous process fracture	166	62	37.4	59	35.5	45	27.1	0	0.0
Pedicle fracture—unilateral	153	45	29.4	74	48.4	34	22.2	0	0.0
Body-cervical compression—teardrop	127	41	32.3	59	46.5	25	19.7	2	1.6
Facet lock—unilateral	125	42	33.6	57	45.6	23	18.4	3	2.4
Lamina fracture—bilateral	107	39	36.5	55	51.4	11	10.3	2	1.9
Type II odontoid	89	6	6.7	17	19.1	65	73.0	1	1.1
Facet lock—bilateral	77	42	54.6	31	40.3	4	5.2	0	0.0
Hangman's	71	2	2.8	10	14.1	59	83.1	0	0.0
Subluxation—bilateral	67	15	22.4	22	32.8	30	44.8	0	0.0
Post longitudinal, ligament disruption	48	13	27.1	22	45.8	13	27.1	0	0.0
Type III odontoid	36	2	5.6	8	22.2	26	72.2	0	0.0
Jefferson	30	5	16.7	5	16.7	20	66.7	0	0.0
Transverse process fracture—unilateral	26	5	19.2	10	38.5	11	42.3	0	0.0
Spondylolisthesis	25	3	12.0	17	68.0	5	20.0	0	0.0
Posterior arch	24	6	25.0	8	33.3	10	41.7	0	0.0
Cord contusion	16	1	6.3	13	81.3	2	12.5	0	0.0
Lateral mass	13	2	15.4	6	46.2	5	38.5	0	0.0
Body-compression–split fracture	12	5	41.7	5	41.7	2	16.7	0	0.0
Facet fracture—bilateral	12	6	50.0	5	41.7	1	8.3	0	0.0
Anterior longitudinal ligament disruption	11	4	36.4	4	36.4	3	27.3	0	0.0
Disrupted/herniated disk	11	1	9.1	9	81.8	1	9.1	0	0.0
Type I odontoid	10	1	10.0	2	20.0	7	70.0	0	0.0
Slice/plate fracture	9	1	11.1	3	33.3	5	55.6	0	0.0
Interspinous ligament disruption	9	0	0.0	7	77.8	2	22.2	0	0.0
Pedicle fracture—bilateral	7	5	71.4	2	28.6	0	0.0	0	0.0
Atlantoaxial subluxation	3	1	33.3	0	0.0	1	33.3	1	33.3
Transverse process fracture—bilateral	3	1	33.3	1	33.3	1	33.3	0	0.0
Anterior arch	2	0	0.0	1	50.0	1	50.0	0	0.0
Body-compression-rotation shear	1	0	0.0	0	0.0	1	100.0	0	0.0
Chance fracture	1	1	100.0	0	0.0	0	0.0	0	0.0
Cord sever/cut	1	1	100.0	0	0.0	0	0.0	0	0.0
Totals[†]	3377	1086	32.2	1436	42.5	826	24.5	29	0.9

* C1–7 fractures.
[†] Totals represent actual number of injuries. Patients may have multiple injuries.

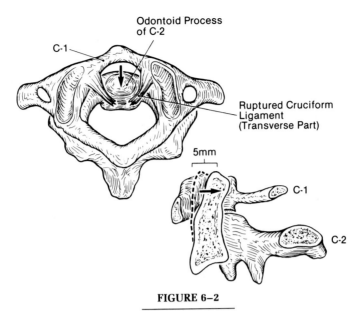

FIGURE 6–2

Rupture of C1 cruciform ligament (transverse part). (From Meyer PR: Surgery of Spine Trauma. New York, Churchill Livingstone, 1989 (Fig. 14–1); with permission.)

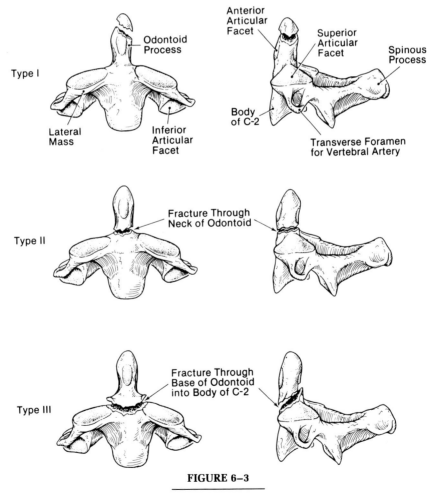

FIGURE 6–3

Variations in odontoid fractures (types I–III). (From Meyer PR: Surgery of Spine Trauma. New York, Churchill Livingstone, 1989 (Fig. 15–31); with permission.)

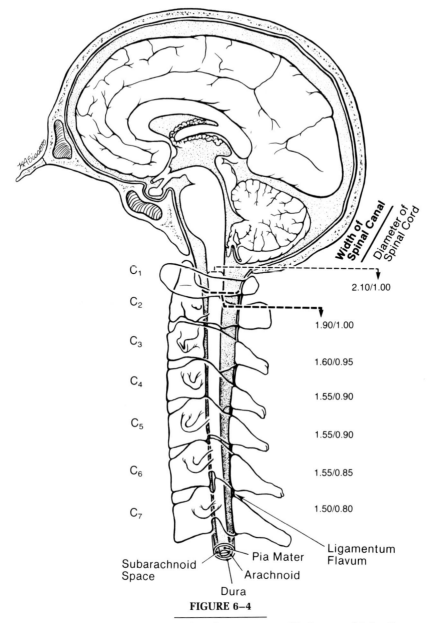

FIGURE 6–4

Measurement ratio of spinal canal to spinal cord. (From Meyer PR: Surgery of Spine Trauma. New York, Churchill Livingstone, 1989 (Fig. 14–10); with permission.)

The key feature in the production of neurologic compromise in traumatic injury of the lower cervical spine is spinal cord or nerve root compression occurring ventrally secondary to either bony compression from fragments of a vertebral body fracture (Fig. 6–5) or by intervertebral disk herniation or stretching of the spinal cord by means of translatory movement between vertebral segments due to ligament disruption and spine instability (Fig. 6–6). Vascular and direct mechanisms (e.g., gunshot wounds) also have a role. Although the identification of bony fracture may be the most obvious finding on radiography, its true significance lies as an indicator of ligament disruption.

In the lower cervical spine (segments C3–7), a three-column arrangement of the articulating bony elements provides a basis for considering mechanisms of injury (Fig. 6–7).

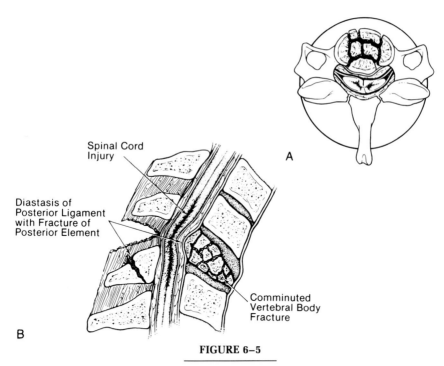

FIGURE 6–5

A, Superior view of vertebral process showing comminuted vertebral body fracture with resultant narrowing of the neural canal and spinal cord compression. B, Lateral view of cervical spinal column demonstrating spinal cord compression secondary to comminuted vertebral body fracture. (From Meyer PR: Surgery of Spine Trauma. New York, Churchill Livingstone, 1989 (Fig. 15–45b); with permission.)

The concept of a three-column model of spinal injury was originally proposed for thoracolumbar injuries (Table 6–3). This convention can be applied to the cervical spine as well, with the anterior column considered to comprise the anterior half of the vertebral body including the anterior longitudinal ligament and the anterior half of the intervertebral disk. The middle column comprises the posterior half of the intervertebral disk, the posterior portion of the vertebral body, and the posterior longitudinal ligament. The vertebral arches, which consist of the spinous process, laminae, and facet joints, make up the posterior column. Ligaments of the anterior, middle, and posterior columns contribute flexibility and strength to the configuration.

The facet joint articulations of the cervical spine permit 4 degrees of motion, including flexion, extension, lateral bending, and rotation, while acting as a stop-check to prevent translatory movements through the intervertebral disk space. Unilateral facet disloca-

tions correlate with a 25% loss of spinal canal cross-sectional area, whereas bilateral facet dislocations produce a 50% canal compromise (Fig. 6–8).[35] The application of unanticipated high-force loads exceeds the ability of the posterior ligamentous complex of the facets, laminae, and spinous processes to prevent translatory movements. The single force that consistently results in neurologic injury from such translatory movements is flexion. Flexion forces applied to the cervical spine frequently result in subluxation or dislocations of one or both facets (Fig. 6–9). Other directional forces of injury in the cervical spine in order of frequency of occurrence include vertical or axial compression, rotation and extension, and lateral bending. Generally, a combination of these forces is present during injury.

At the Midwest Regional Spinal Injury Center, the majority of patients (44.3%) treated for cervical spine injuries have sustained either an axial load or combined flexion load injury. This is seen radiographi-

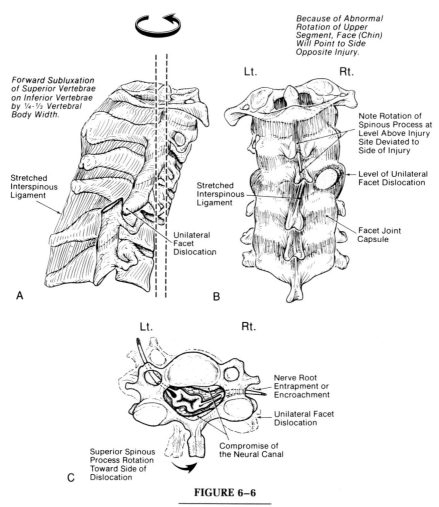

Because of Abnormal
Rotation of Upper
Segment, Face (Chin)
Will Point to Side
Opposite Injury.

Forward Subluxation
of Superior Vertebrae
on Inferior Vertebrae
by 1/4 - 1/3 Vertebral
Body Width.

Lt.   Rt.

Note Rotation of
Spinous Process at
Level Above Injury
Site Deviated to
Side of Injury

Stretched
Interspinous
Ligament

Level of Unilateral
Facet Dislocation

Stretched
Interspinous
Ligament

Facet Joint
Capsule

Unilateral
Facet
Dislocation

A   B

Lt.   Rt.

Nerve Root
Entrapment or
Encroachment

Unilateral Facet
Dislocation

Superior Spinous
Process Rotation
Toward Side of
Dislocation

Compromise of
the Neural Canal

C

FIGURE 6–6

Pathologic consequences of unilateral facet dislocation: lateral (A), posterior (B), and overhead transverse (C) views. (From Meyer PR: Surgery of Spine Trauma. New York, Churchill Livingstone, 1989 (Fig. 15–41); with permission.)

cally as either a "wedge" compression fracture or a "teardrop" fracture of the vertebral body. In this group of patients, 45.8% (1187 of 2589) sustained either a complete or partial neurologic injury (Table 6–4).

THORACIC SPINE (T1–10) INJURY

The thoracic spine is composed of 12 vertebral bodies to which the rib cage directly attaches, providing a protective envelope for the heart, esophagus, trachea, lungs, and great vessels. The rib cage imparts a stiffness to the thoracic spine 2.5 times that of the ligamentous spine alone. The typical thoracic vertebra (Fig. 6–10) surrounds a neural canal that is smaller than that found in either the cervical or lumbar spine. This correlates with the finding that the incidence of significant neurologic deficit following trauma to the thoracic vertebral column is higher than that with injury to other areas of the spine. At the Midwest Regional Spine Injury Center, 63% of such injuries are neurologically complete, 27% are incomplete, and 10% are intact. Acute spinal cord injuries in the thoracic spine can be divided into those resulting from injuries of the T1 through T10 vertebral segments and those occurring at the thoracolumbar junction (T11–L2). This distinction

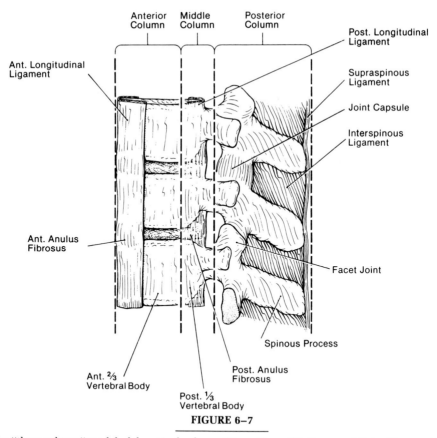

Anterior Column   Middle Column   Posterior Column

Post. Longitudinal Ligament

Ant. Longitudinal Ligament

Supraspinous Ligament

Joint Capsule

Interspinous Ligament

Ant. Anulus Fibrosus

Facet Joint

Spinous Process

Ant. ⅔ Vertebral Body

Post. Anulus Fibrosus

Post. ⅓ Vertebral Body

FIGURE 6–7

The "three column" model of the spinal column. (From Meyer PR: Surgery of Spine Trauma. New York, Churchill Livingstone, 1989 (Fig. 19–14); with permission.)

TABLE 6–3

COLUMN THEORY OF SPINE CONSTRUCTION AND STABILITY

TWO-COLUMN THEORY (HOLDSWORTH)	THREE-COLUMN THEORY (DENIS)

Posterior bone-ligament complex
  Posterior laminar arch
  Supraspinous ligament
  Interspinous ligament
  Posterior lateral capsule
  Ligamentum flavum
	Same*

	Middle column*
	  Posterior longitudinal ligament
	  Posterior annulus fibrosus
	  Posterior vertebral body wall

Anterior column
  Anterior vertebral body
  Anterior longitudinal ligament
  Anterior annulus fibrosus
	Same

* Disruption of any two indicates instability.

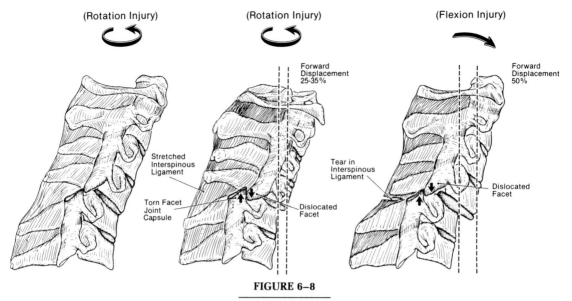

(Rotation Injury) (Rotation Injury) (Flexion Injury)

Forward
Displacement
25-35%

Forward
Displacement
50%

Stretched
Interspinous
Ligament

Tear in
Interspinous
Ligament

Torn Facet
Joint
Capsule

Dislocated
Facet

Dislocated
Facet

FIGURE 6–8

The anatomic and pathologic consequences of rotary injuries to the cervical spine include degrees of facet joint dislocation. (From Meyer PR: Surgery of Spine Trauma. New York, Churchill Livingstone, 1989 (Fig. 15–39); with permission.)

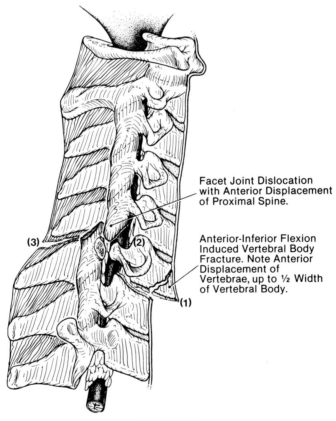

Facet Joint Dislocation
with Anterior Displacement
of Proximal Spine.

Anterior-Inferior Flexion
Induced Vertebral Body
Fracture. Note Anterior
Displacement of
Vertebrae, up to ½ Width
of Vertebral Body.

(3) (2) (1)

FIGURE 6–9

Anatomic consequences of bilateral facet dislocation. Bilateral facet dislocations are secondary to flexion-distraction injuries and result in three-column instability: disruption of the anterior (1) and posterior (2) longitudinal ligaments and tear or fracture through posterior structures (3). (From Meyer PR: Surgery of Spine Trauma. New York, Churchill Livingstone, 1989, (Fig. 15–43); with permission.)

TABLE 6–4

BIOMECHANICAL FORCE BY EXTENT (CERVICAL* SPINE), NORTHWESTERN UNIVERSITY ACUTE SPINE INJURY CENTER, 1972–1990

BIOMECHANICAL FORCE	TOTAL	COMPLETE		INCOMPLETE		INTACT		MISSING	
		NO.	%	NO.	%	NO.	%	NO.	%
Axial	69	13	18.8	20	29.0	36	52.2	0	0.0
Flexion	716	249	34.8	308	43.0	152	21.2	7	1.0
Axial with flexion	748	290	38.8	307	41.0	145	19.4	6	0.8
Rotation	125	42	33.6	57	45.6	23	18.4	3	2.4
Extension	824	271	32.9	354	43.0	193	23.4	6	0.7
Odontoid	135	9	6.7	27	20.0	98	72.6	1	0.7
Other	839	246	29.3	396	47.2	188	22.4	9	1.1
Totals†	3456	1120	32.4	1469	42.5	835	24.2	32	0.9

* C1–7 fractures.
† Totals represent actual number of injuries. Patients may have multiple injuries.

between the T1–10 segments and the thoracolumbar junction is both anatomic and fundamental because the thoracolumbar junction represents a transition zone not only in bony anatomy but in terms of transition from the spinal cord to the nerve roots of the cauda equina (Fig. 6–11).

The change in bony anatomical characteristics is a function of the orientation of the facet joints. In the upper thoracic spine, the orientation of the facet joints is such that a nearly unhindered rotation of one vertebral process on another can occur (Fig. 6–12). Consequently, few rotational injuries occur in this area, although it is associated with a higher incidence of axial load injuries. Toward the thoracolumbar junction, the change in facet joint orientation (Fig. 6–12) is such that an abrupt change in stiffness between the flexible upper thoracic spine and the relatively inflexible lower thoracic spine gives rise to an area of high-stress concentration at the thoracolumbar junction.

In the upper thoracic spine (T1–T10), the

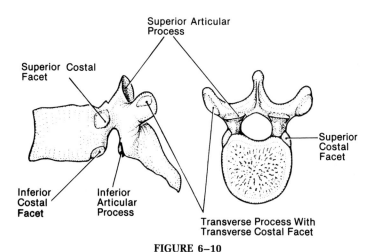

FIGURE 6–10

Prominent anatomic landmarks of a typical thoracic vertebra. (From Meyer PR: Surgery of Spine Trauma. New York, Churchill Livingstone, 1989 (Fig. 16–25); with permission.)

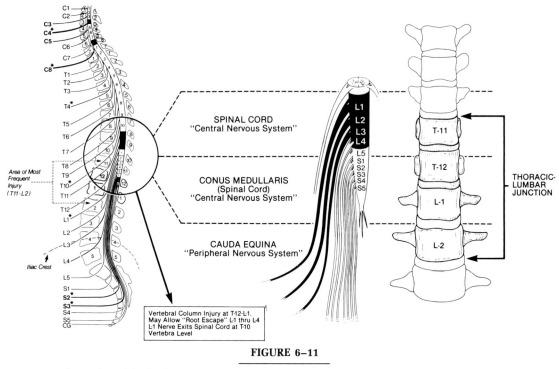

FIGURE 6–11

Relationship of the lumbar plexus and conus medullaris to the thoracolumbar spine. (From Meyer PR: Surgery of Spine Trauma. New York, Churchill Livingstone, 1989 (Fig. 18–1); with permission.)

inherent stability and rigidity imparted by the ribs, sternum, and vertebral column complex protects against the effect of perpendicular forces. However, the upper thoracic spine is vulnerable to axial (compression) and flexion loads, which produce a wedge or burst-type fracture pattern with associated anterior angulation (kyphosis) (Fig. 6–13). In our series (Table 6–5), 57.8% of patients with upper thoracic spine axial load injuries had complete neurologic injury whereas 15.9% were intact. The fracture pattern follows direct vertical loading of the spine, either from above by being hit by a falling object or from below after falling from a height and landing on the foot or buttocks. Neurologic injury of the spinal cord occurs with retropulsion of bone from the posterior vertebral body wall into the canal, producing a compromise of greater than 50%. The thoracic spinal cord is particularly at risk for vascular injuries. This predisposition is based on the tenuous "watershed" vascular supply of the spinal cord between T4 and T11, which is dependent on perfusion of the anterior and posterior spinal

arteries from the cervical region above and from the artery of Adamkiewicz from the thoracolumbar spine below, with a variable number of segmental vessels serving as a supplement to this region.

The normal kyphotic configuration of the proximal thoracic spine produces a slight degree of anatomic flexion. Flexion forces added to this configuration by motor vehicle accidents can produce vertebral body compression also leading to spinal cord compression. Torsional or rotational injuries of the upper thoracic spine produce severe disruption of all three columns of the spine (Fig. 6–14), with crushing, stretching, and shearing stresses imparted to the spinal cord, resulting in a complete permanent injury.

THORACOLUMBAR SPINE (T11–L2) INJURY

The thoracolumbar spine is the second most frequently injured area of the spine (Table 6–6). The biomechanical basis behind

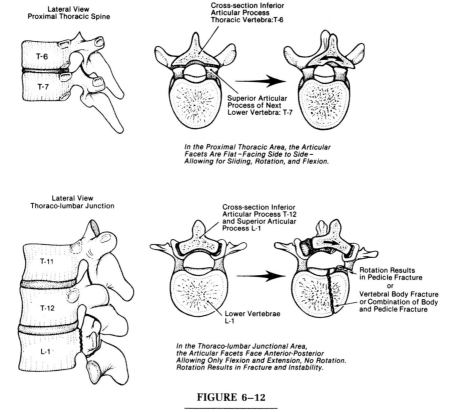

Lateral View
Proximal Thoracic Spine

T-6

T-7

Cross-section Inferior
Articular Process
Thoracic Vertebra:T-6

Superior Articular
Process of Next
Lower Vertebra: T-7

*In the Proximal Thoracic Area, the Articular
Facets Are Flat –Facing Side to Side –
Allowing for Sliding, Rotation, and Flexion.*

Lateral View
Thoraco-lumbar Junction

T-11

T-12

L-1

Cross-section Inferior
Articular Process T-12
and Superior Articular
Process L-1

Lower Vertebrae
L-1

Rotation Results
in Pedicle Fracture
or
Vertebral Body Fracture
or Combination of Body
and Pedicle Fracture

*In the Thoraco-lumbar Junctional Area,
the Articular Facets Face Anterior-Posterior
Allowing Only Flexion and Extension, No Rotation.
Rotation Results in Fracture and Instability.*

FIGURE 6–12

In the upper thoracic spine (*top*, T6–T7), the mediolateral and oblique vertical alignment of the facet joints allows freedom of motion in flexion, extension, and rotation. In the thoracolumbar spine (*bottom*, T12–L1), note that the inferior facet T12 is "locked" in by the cupped, lateral constraint produced by the superior facet at L1. Rotary injuries at this level result in fractures of the pedicle, the vertebral body, or both, owing to the lack of freedom of motion. (From Meyer PR: Surgery of Spine Trauma. New York, Churchill Livingstone, 1989 (Fig. 16–2); with permission.)

this is the transition at the T11 to L2 region from an area of rigid fixation provided by the rib cage to the more mobile lumbar spine. The transition from terminal spinal cord (conus medullaris) to cauda equina also occurs at this level, accounting for incompleteness or absence of neurologic injury in the majority of patients (Table 6–7). The increasing width of spinal canal between T11 and L2 also aids in mitigating the neurologic effects of bony injury.

Falls from heights (e.g., ladders, scaffolding), motor vehicle accidents, and gunshot wounds are the principal causes of injury. The biomechanical forces of injury involved include axial loading, flexion, other (gunshot wounds), rotation, and direct (Table 6–8). Axial loading and flexion produce compression or burst fractures of the vertebral bodies.

Neurologic compromise follows with encroachment of fracture fragments or disk material or both into the spinal canal.

LOWER LUMBAR SPINE (L3–5) AND SACRUM INJURIES

In the lower lumbar spine, falls from heights (e.g., scaffolding, suicide attempts), which produce axial loading, vertebral body burst-type fractures, account for the primary mechanism of injury, followed by flexion or flexion-distraction (lap or seatbelt) injuries and gunshot wounds. Sacral fractures often involve direct force and do not produce a particular pattern. Fractures of the lower lumbar spine produce complete neurologic injury in only a fraction of individuals, with

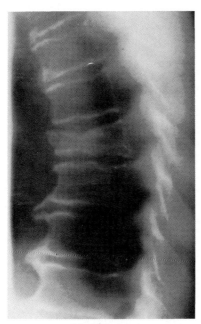

FIGURE 6–13

Thoracic "wedge" fracture with greater posterior than anterior body height loss leading to an increased kyphosis.

incomplete injuries being the rule (Table 6–9).

MANAGEMENT OF SPINAL INJURIES

Forty-three percent of patients who sustain acute traumatic spinal cord injuries also sustain trauma to other areas of the body. Therefore, initial evaluation of the trauma victim at the accident scene should include assessment of the ABCs—airway, breathing, and circulation. During airway assessment, trauma to the face should raise the suspicion of cervical spine injury, although its absence does not rule it out. Ventilatory difficulties can also be indicative of cervical cord injury. In any spinal injury, the cervical spine should be immobilized (Fig. 6–15) and the victim transported to an appropriate medical facility for definitive assessment and management.

On arrival to the emergency room an immediate, rapid, but thorough physical and neurologic examination should be performed. Guidelines for the level of neurologic involvement are indicated in Table 6–10 and Figure 6–16. Because an estimated 5% to 10% of neurologic injury after spinal cord trauma occurs after the patient has come under medical care (Rogers[37]), continued caution and vigilance must be maintained until further radiographic evaluation can be performed.

TABLE 6–5

BIOMECHANICAL FORCE BY EXTENT (THORACIC* SPINE), NORTHWESTERN UNIVERSITY ACUTE SPINE INJURY CENTER, 1972–1990

BIOMECHANICAL FORCE	TOTAL	COMPLETE		INCOMPLETE		INTACT		MISSING	
		NO.	%	NO.	%	NO.	%	NO.	%
Flexion	130	81	62.3	35	26.9	14	10.8	0	0.0
Axial with flexion	315	182	57.8	79	25.1	50	15.9	4	1.3
Rotation	8	6	75.0	1	12.5	1	12.5	0	0.0
Extension	126	75	59.5	31	24.6	20	15.9	0	0.0
Other	149	104	69.8	31	20.8	14	9.4	0	0.0
Totals†	728	448	61.5	177	24.3	99	13.6	4	0.6

* T1–10 fractures.
† Totals represent actual number of injuries. Patients may have multiple injuries.

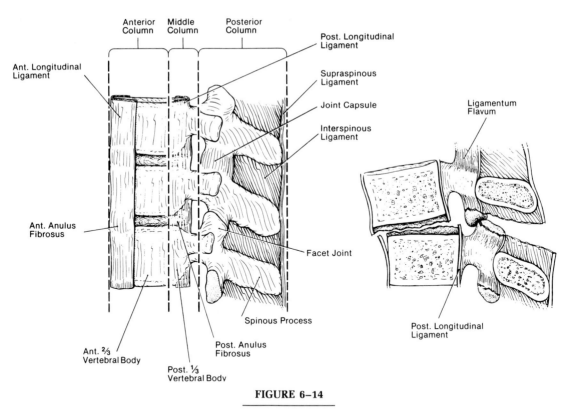

FIGURE 6–14

Diagrammatic representation of "three column" disruption. Loss of any two results in instability.

Every accident victim should be assumed to have a spinal cord injury until proven otherwise. Fractures of the thoracic spine, the cervicothoracic junction, and the thoracolumbar junction are frequently missed. Therefore, all cervical vertebrae and the first thoracic vertebra should be visualized on anteroposterior and lateral projection views, including an anteroposterior open mouth view of the odontoid process. Based on the physical and neurologic findings, the remainder of the radiographic examination is then tailored to the requirements for elucidating suspected areas of pathology using conventional polytomography, computed tomographic (CT) scanning, or magnetic resonance imaging (MRI).

TREATMENT OF SPINAL CORD INJURY

A major objective in the treatment of patients with traumatic spinal cord injury is the preservation of the functional and anatomic continuity of the spinal cord by recognizing mechanical neural compression or stretch and relieving it by means of restoring spinal alignment, removing bony fracture fragments or herniated disk material, and reestablishing spinal stability by the appropriate technique. When successfully achieved, these maneuvers help to mobilize the patient as quickly as possible so that rehabilitation can be begun.

Restoring Spinal Alignment: Closed Reduction with Skeletal Traction

Radiographic confirmation of spinal fracture/dislocation necessitates restoration of spinal alignment—the most effective method of spinal cord decompression. In cervical spine injuries, the best method of achieving this is by institution of spinal traction. This is most effectively performed with the transfer of the patient to a fracture bed or frame, such as the Stryker wedge frame (Fig. 6–17).

TABLE 6–6

FRACTURE TYPE BY EXTENT (THORACOLUMBAR* FRACTURES), NORTHWESTERN UNIVERSITY ACUTE SPINE INJURY CENTER, 1972–1990

FRACTURE TYPE	TOTAL	COMPLETE		INCOMPLETE		INTACT		MISSING	
		NO.	%	NO.	%	NO.	%	NO.	%
Body-axial compression—burst	328	49	14.9	137	41.8	141	43.0	1	0.3
Body-anterior compression—wedge	220	71	32.3	73	33.2	76	34.5	0	0.0
Lamina fracture—unilateral	125	20	16.0	65	52.0	40	32.0	0	0.0
Dislocation	107	53	49.5	42	39.3	12	11.2	0	0.0
Transverse process fracture—unilateral	75	18	24.0	34	45.3	23	30.7	0	0.0
Pedicle fracture—unilateral	59	18	30.5	22	37.3	19	32.2	0	0.0
Facet fracture—unilateral	53	22	41.5	20	37.7	11	20.8	0	0.0
Subluxation—unilateral	33	13	39.4	11	33.3	9	27.3	0	0.0
Spinous process fracture	32	7	21.9	12	37.5	13	40.6	0	0.0
Facet lock—bilateral	18	7	38.9	9	50.0	2	11.1	0	0.0
Chance fracture	17	2	11.8	6	35.3	9	52.9	0	0.0
Lamina fracture—bilateral	13	3	23.1	7	53.8	3	23.1	0	0.0
Subluxation—bilateral	8	2	25.0	3	37.5	3	37.5	0	0.0
Slice/plate fracture	8	0	0.0	3	37.5	5	62.5	0	0.0
Facet lock—unilateral	8	3	37.5	4	50.0	1	12.5	0	0.0
Spondylolisthesis	7	1	14.3	2	28.6	4	57.1	0	0.0
Transverse process fracture—bilateral	5	1	20.0	2	40.0	2	40.0	0	0.0
Facet fracture—bilateral	5	2	40.0	2	40.0	1	20.0	0	0.0
Disrupted/herniated disk	4	0	0.0	3	75.0	1	25.0	0	0.0
Post longitudinal ligament disruption	3	1	33.3	1	33.3	1	33.3	0	0.0
Pedicle fracture—bilateral	3	1	33.3	1	33.3	1	33.3	0	0.0
Interspinous ligament disruption	1	1	100.0	0	0.0	0	0.0	0	0.0
Body-cervical compression—teardrop	1	0	0.0	0	0.0	1	100.0	0	0.0
Totals†	1133	295	26.0	459	40.5	378	33.4	1	0.1

* T11–L2 fractures.
† Totals represent actual number of injuries. Patients may have multiple injuries.

TABLE 6–7

GROSS LEVEL OF SPINE INJURY VS. INJURY EXTENT, NORTHWESTERN UNIVERSITY ACUTE SPINE INJURY CENTER, 1972–1990

GROSS LEVEL	TOTAL	COMPLETE		INCOMPLETE		INTACT		MISSING	
		NO.	%	NO.	%	NO.	%	NO.	%
Atlanto-occipital	84	9	10.7	26	31.0	47	56.0	2	2.4
Cervical	1896	546	28.8	827	43.6	504	26.6	19	1.0
Thoracic	450	268	59.6	124	27.6	54	12.0	4	0.9
Thoracolumbar	650	173	26.6	253	38.9	223	34.3	1	0.2
Lumbar	109	2	1.8	65	59.6	42	38.5	0	0.0
Sacral	11	0	0.0	11	100.0	0	0.0	0	0.0
None/unknown	298	4	1.3	32	10.7	137	46.0	125	41.9
Totals	3498	1002	28.6	1338	38.3	1007	28.8	151	4.3

TABLE 6–8

BIOMECHANICAL FORCE BY EXTENT (THORACOLUMBAR* SPINE),
NORTHWESTERN UNIVERSITY ACUTE SPINE INJURY CENTER, 1972–1990

BIOMECHANICAL FORCE	TOTAL	COMPLETE		INCOMPLETE		INTACT		MISSING	
		NO.	%	NO.	%	NO.	%	NO.	%
Flexion	124	43	34.7	51	41.1	30	24.2	0	0.0
Axial with flexion	548	120	21.9	210	38.3	217	39.6	1	0.2
Rotation	8	3	37.5	4	50.0	1	12.5	0	0.0
Extension	201	42	20.9	95	47.3	64	31.8	0	0.0
Other	260	90	34.6	103	39.6	67	25.8	0	0.0
Totals[†]	1141	298	26.1	463	40.6	379	33.2	1	0.1

* T11–L2 fractures.
[†] Totals represent actual number of injuries. Patients may have multiple injuries.

Skeletal tongs, such as Gardner-Wells tongs (Fig. 6–18), are applied. The general rule is to use 5 lb of weight per level of injury. For example, in a bilateral facet dislocation of the C5–6 level, 25 to 30 lb of weight is initially used. During the application of weight for closed reduction by cervical traction, careful monitoring of the neurologic examination and serial radiographs to prevent overdistraction are essential.

TABLE 6–9

LUMBAR VS. SACRAL NEUROLOGIC EXTENT OF INJURY, NORTHWESTERN UNIVERSITY ACUTE SPINE INJURY CENTER, 1972–1990

	LUMBAR		SACRAL	
	NO.	%	NO.	%
Complete	2	1.8	0	0.0
Incomplete	65	59.6	11	100.0
Intact	42	38.5	0	0.0
Totals	109	100.0	11	100.0

Surgical Treatment: Surgical Decompression and Stabilization

Surgical management of spinal cord injury is indicated for definitive stabilization of cervical spine fracture/dislocations reduced by cervical traction (closed reduction), for reduction (open reduction) of cervical spine fracture/dislocations not amenable to reduction by cervical traction, to reduce and stabilize unstable fracture/dislocations at other levels of the spine, and to decompress the spinal cord, nerve roots, or both at any level of the spine.

Figure 6–19 demonstrates a bilateral facet dislocation of the cervical spine at the C6–7 level. This injury is extremely unstable because it involves all three columns of the spine; although it might be reduced by closed reduction, it would not be expected to remain reduced because of the extensive disruption of all spinal ligaments. Therefore, after closed reduction by cervical traction, the patient is brought to the operating room where posterior cervical wiring and fusion are performed (see Fig. 6–19). The process of wiring the dislocated facets together forms a posterior tension band holding the alignment of the cervical spine in anatomic position until

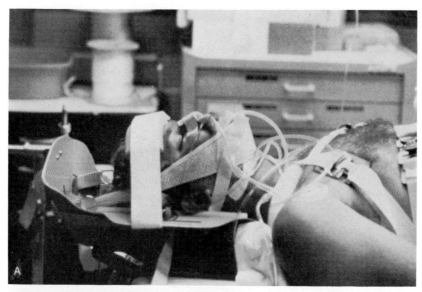

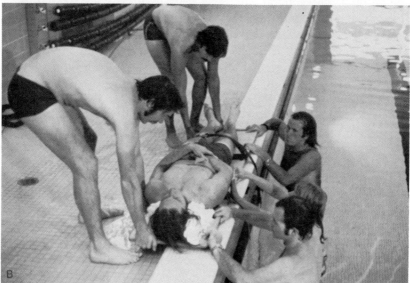

FIGURE 6–15

Examples of cervical spine immobilization in the emergency room (A) and in the field (B). (From Meyer PR: Surgery of Spine Trauma. New York, Churchill Livingstone, 1989 (Fig. 2–8); with permission.)

TABLE 6–10

NEUROLOGICAL FUNCTION: LEVEL OF INTACTNESS

MOTOR-SENSORY RESPONSE	INTACT LEVEL
Motor	
Diaphragm	C3,4,5
Shrug shoulders	C4
Deltoids (and flex elbows)	C5
Extend wrist	C6
Extend elbow/flex wrist	C7
Abduct fingers	C8
Active chest expansion	T1–12
Hip flexion	L2
Knee extension	L3–4
Ankle dorsiflexion	L5–S1
Ankle plantarflexion	S1–2
Sensory	
Anterior thigh	L2
Anterior knee	L3
Anterolateral ankle	L4
Dorsum great-second toe	L5
Lateral side of foot	S1
Posterior calf	S2
Perianal sensation (perineum)	S2–5

bony fusion can take place over approximately 3 months.

Anterior surgical stabilization of the cervical spine by means of intervertebral body spinal fusion is indicated when excision of a retropulsed vertebral body or herniated disk (as seen on MRI) is necessary to decompress the neural canal or to otherwise restore stability of the anterior column after compression fractures of the vertebral body (Fig. 6–20). The cervical spine is approached from the right side with a plane of dissection developed between the sternocleidomastoid muscle and carotid laterally and the trachea and esophagus medially. After identification of the appropriate level, removal of the fracture fragments is performed (Fig. 6–21). An iliac bone graft is then obtained and fashioned to fit the defect into which it is placed (Fig. 6–22). We use a metallic plate secured by screws into the vertebral body above and below the graft to ensure its placement (Figs. 6–23 and 6–24).

In patients with unstable thoracic and thoracolumbar spine injuries, the mainstay of surgical treatment has been the use of the Harrington distraction rod technique. This technique utilizes two ratcheted rods that fit into hooks above and below the injured segment. The rods can then be distracted to bring the spine back to normal alignment. A bone graft around the rods maintains this alignment. An alternative to this technique is the Luque rod, a system which comes in the form of either L-shaped rods or rectangles (Figs. 6–25 and 6–26). Luque rod instrumentation is excellent for use in fractures of the anterior vertebral column (wedge compression fractures).

Use of Orthotic Devices in Spinal Trauma

A wide variety of orthotic devices exists for use in spinal injury. The devices vary significantly in regard to their design, construction, and ability to achieve the goal of maintenance of the position of the spine. By controlling the position of the spine, orthotic devices assist in mitigating pain caused by muscle spasm and in reducing motion of disrupted osseous and ligamentous structures to promote their healing, and serve as a postoperative adjunct.

Cervical orthotic devices (Fig. 6–27) run the gamut from soft collars, which provide minimal support, to the rigid halo skeletal fixation device with vest. The soft collar provides little limitation of motion of the spine. The Philadelphia collar provides more support and limitation of flexion and extension. No collar can safely provide secure maintenance of cervical spinal alignment. The sterno-occipitomandibular immobilization (SOMI) brace provides three-point fixation at the shoulder-sternum, occiput, and mandible to better restrict motion (Fig. 6–28). The SOMI brace can be used as a postoperative adjunct in selected internal fixation procedures and in some nondisplaced fractures of the cervical spine. The halo orthosis provides the most secure control of motion of the cervical spine, particularly from the occiput through C3. Therefore, it is particularly useful for fractures involving C1–2, including odontoid fractures (type I), and is the most appropriate means of immobilization after

Text continued on page 133

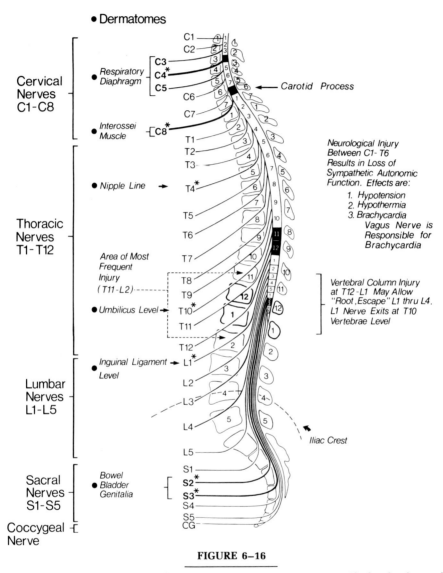

FIGURE 6–16

Spinal nerves. Asterisks indicate the primary innervating nerves or specific levels of neurologic importance.

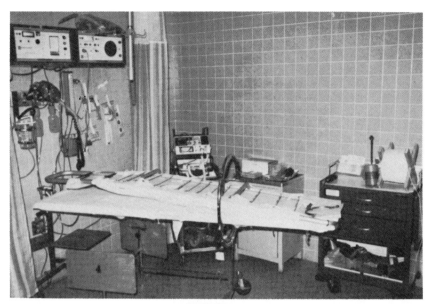

FIGURE 6–17

Stryker wedge frame, utilized both on the ward and in the operating room, allows rotation to prone and supine positions with maintenance of skeletal traction.

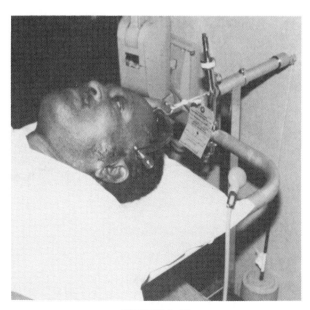

FIGURE 6–18

Detail of Gardner-Wells tongs. Applied to the skull, they permit skeletal traction for reduction or protective maintenance of alignment.

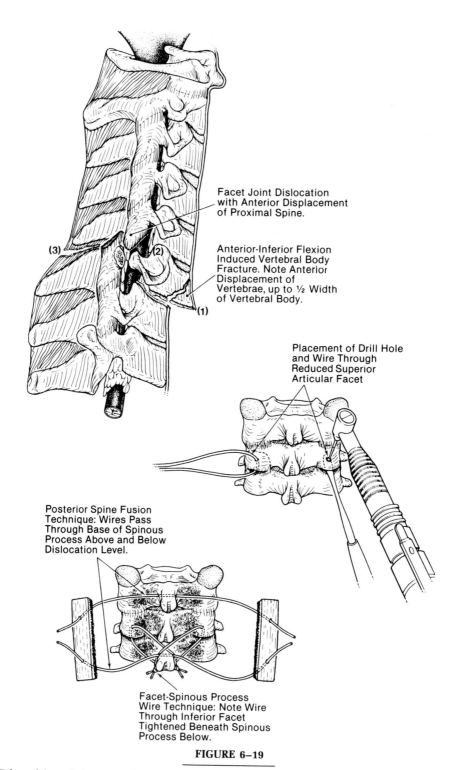

Facet Joint Dislocation with Anterior Displacement of Proximal Spine.

Anterior-Inferior Flexion Induced Vertebral Body Fracture. Note Anterior Displacement of Vertebrae, up to ½ Width of Vertebral Body.

Placement of Drill Hole and Wire Through Reduced Superior Articular Facet

Posterior Spine Fusion Technique: Wires Pass Through Base of Spinous Process Above and Below Dislocation Level.

Facet-Spinous Process Wire Technique: Note Wire Through Inferior Facet Tightened Beneath Spinous Process Below.

FIGURE 6–19

Bilateral facet dislocation in an unstable three-column injury. Stabilization with spinous process and facet wiring is demonstrated. (From Meyer PR: Surgery of Spine Trauma. New York, Churchill Livingstone, 1989 (Fig. 15–45c); with permission.)

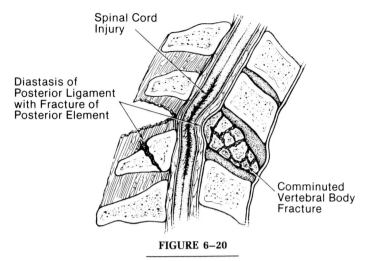

FIGURE 6–20

Lateral view of cervical spinal column, demonstrating spinal cord compression. (From Meyer PR: Surgery of Spine Trauma. New York, Churchill Livingstone, 1989 (Fig. 15–45); with permission.)

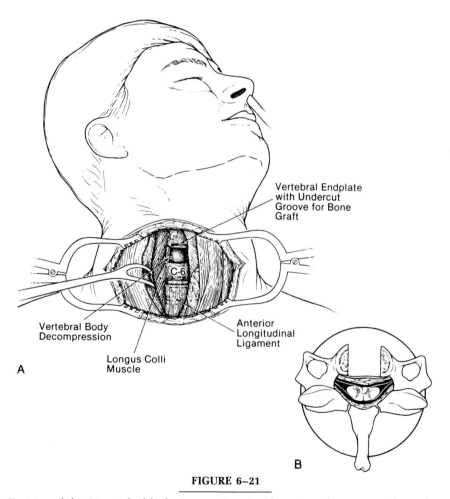

FIGURE 6–21

A, Excision of the C5 vertebral body (corporectomy) and creation of grooves on the undersurface of the C4 vertebral body and the superior surface of C6 for bone graft insertion are shown. *B*, Superior view showing removal of the central aspect of the affected vertebral body, allowing for decompression of the neural canal without complete excision of the vertebral body. (From Meyer PR: Surgery of Spine Trauma. New York, Churchill Livingstone, 1989 (Fig. 15–7); with permission.)

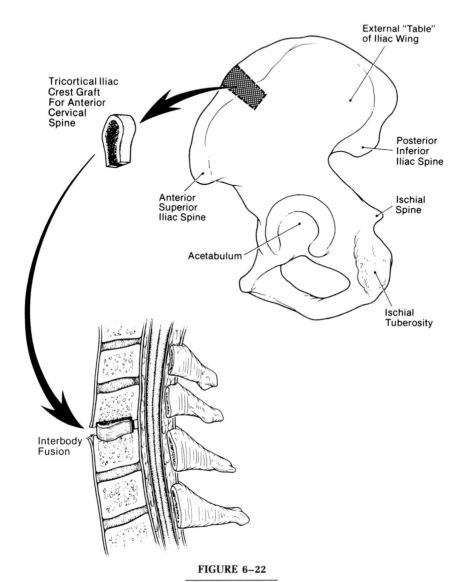

Tricortical Iliac
Crest Graft
For Anterior
Cervical
Spine

External "Table"
of Iliac Wing

Posterior
Inferior
Iliac Spine

Ischial
Spine

Anterior
Superior
Iliac Spine

Acetabulum

Ischial
Tuberosity

Interbody
Fusion

FIGURE 6–22

Anterior interbody inlay bone graft after excision of intervertebral disk. (From Meyer PR: Surgery of Spine Trauma. New York, Churchill Livingstone, 1989 (Fig. 15–8); with permission.)

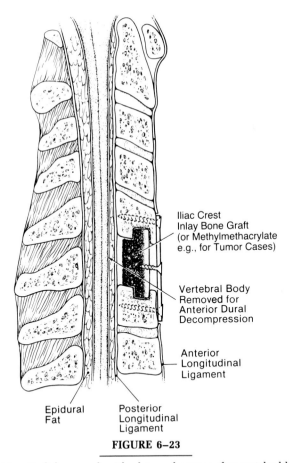

Iliac Crest
Inlay Bone Graft
(or Methylmethacrylate
e.g., for Tumor Cases)

Vertebral Body
Removed for
Anterior Dural
Decompression

Anterior
Longitudinal
Ligament

Epidural
Fat

Posterior
Longitudinal
Ligament

FIGURE 6–23

Anterior (inlay or tricortical) bone graft with plate and screws after vertebral body corporectomy for neural canal decompression. Cortical screws are usually 18 to 20 mm long. (From Meyer PR: Surgery of Spine Trauma. New York, Churchill Livingstone, 1989 (Fig. 15–9); with permission.)

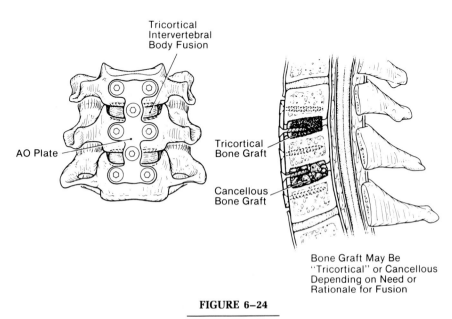

Tricortical
Intervertebral
Body Fusion

AO Plate

Tricortical
Bone Graft

Cancellous
Bone Graft

Bone Graft May Be
"Tricortical" or Cancellous
Depending on Need or
Rationale for Fusion

FIGURE 6–24

Modification of Robinson-Southwick anterior fusion technique using AO plate and screws for internal stabilization.

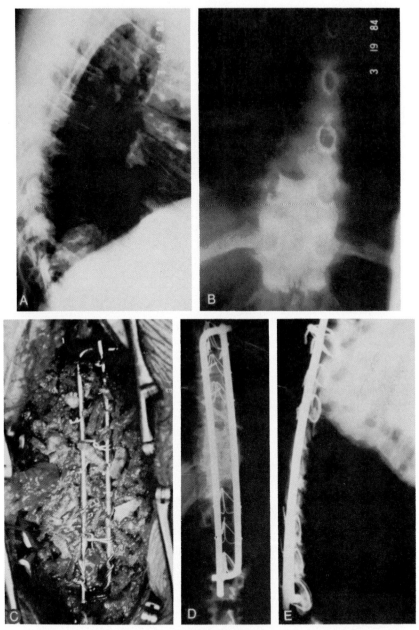

FIGURE 6–25

A and B, Anteroposterior (AP) and lateral radiographs of thoracic spine demonstrating Chance
fracture through T10. On AP view a horizontal fracture through the pedicles bilaterally is easily
identified. This fracture results from flexion distracton forces. C, Operative view of L-shaped Luque
segmental instrumentation and transverse wires to assist in maintenance of vertical alignment.
Note extent of spine fusion. D and E, AP and lateral radiographs of thoracic spine demonstrate
improved alignment with L-shaped Luque segmental rods.

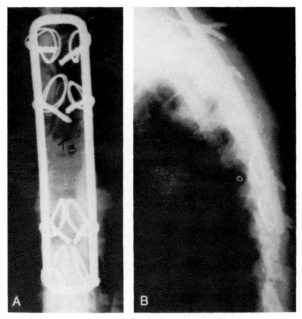

FIGURE 6–26

Anteroposterior (AP) (*A*) and lateral (*B*) views of rectangular Luque rods and postoperative alignment of the thoracic spine in a patient with axial load-flexion fracture dislocation of T3 on T4.

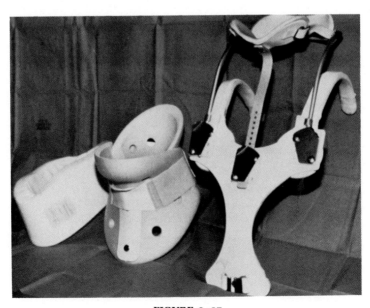

FIGURE 6–27

Cervical orthotic devices.

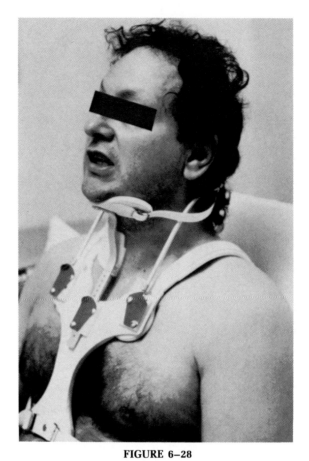

FIGURE 6–28

Sterno-occipitomandibular immobilizer (SOMI) orthosis.

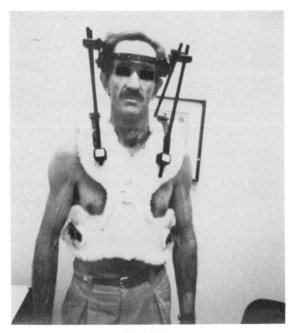

FIGURE 6–29

Halo orthosis.

130

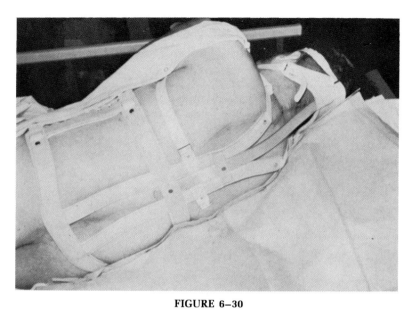

FIGURE 6–30

Knight-Taylor orthosis with cervical extension.

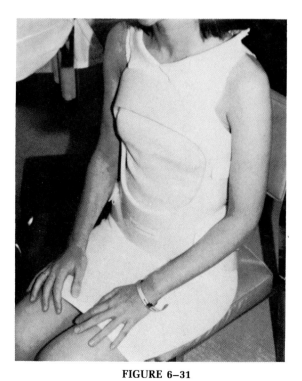

FIGURE 6–31

Thoracolumbosacral orthosis.

TABLE 6–11

INJURY TYPE BY EXTENT, NORTHWESTERN UNIVERSITY ACUTE SPINE INJURY CENTER, 1972–1990

INJURY TYPE	TOTAL	COMPLETE		INCOMPLETE		INTACT		MISSING	
		NO.	%	NO.	%	NO.	%	NO.	%
Jefferson	30	5	16.7	5	16.7	20	66.7	0	0.0
Anterior arch	2	0	0.0	1	50.0	1	50.0	0	0.0
Posterior arch	25	6	24.0	9	36.0	10	40.0	0	0.0
Type I odontoid	10	1	10.0	2	20.0	7	70.0	0	0.0
Type II odontoid	92	7	7.6	18	19.6	66	71.7	1	1.1
Type III odontoid	38	3	7.9	8	21.1	27	71.1	0	0.0
Hangman's	71	2	2.8	10	14.1	59	83.1	0	0.0
Lateral mass	13	2	15.4	6	46.2	5	38.5	0	0.0
Body–cervical compression—teardrop	130	41	31.5	59	45.4	28	21.5	2	1.5
Atlantoaxial subluxation	3	1	33.3	0	0.0	1	33.3	1	33.3
Body–anterior compression—wedge	900	362	40.2	330	36.7	203	22.6	5	0.6
Body–axial compression—burst	768	224	29.2	302	39.3	236	30.7	6	0.8
Body–compression—split fracture	13	5	38.5	6	46.2	2	15.4	0	0.0
Body–compression rotation—shear	2	1	50.0	0	0.0	1	50.0	0	0.0
Slice/plate fracture	18	1	5.6	6	33.3	11	61.1	0	0.0
Spinous process fracture	248	90	36.3	89	35.9	69	27.8	0	0.0
Transverse process fracture—unilateral	137	38	27.7	55	40.1	44	32.1	0	0.0
Transverse process fracture—bilateral	12	2	16.7	5	41.7	5	41.7	0	0.0
Lamina fracture—unilateral	577	205	35.5	248	43.0	122	21.1	2	0.3
Lamina fracture—bilateral	126	46	36.5	63	50.0	15	11.9	2	1.6
Pedicle fracture—unilateral	256	84	32.8	107	41.8	65	25.4	0	0.0
Pedicle fracture—bilateral	13	6	46.2	6	46.2	1	7.7	0	0.0
Facet fracture—unilateral	390	146	37.4	160	41.0	81	20.8	3	0.8
Facet fracture—bilateral	21	11	52.4	7	33.3	3	14.3	0	0.0
Chance fracture	26	3	11.5	10	38.5	13	50.0	0	0.0
Subluxation—unilateral	475	113	23.8	235	49.5	121	25.5	6	1.3
Subluxation—bilateral	82	21	25.6	26	31.7	35	42.7	0	0.0
Facet lock—unilateral	141	51	36.2	62	44.0	25	17.7	3	2.1
Facet lock—bilateral	106	56	52.8	44	41.5	6	5.7	0	0.0
Dislocation	528	263	49.8	209	39.6	53	10.0	3	0.6
Spondylolisthesis	46	5	10.9	25	54.3	16	34.8	0	0.0
Anterior longitudinal ligament disruption	12	4	33.3	4	33.3	4	33.3	0	0.0
Post longitudinal ligament disruption	53	16	30.2	23	43.4	14	26.4	0	0.0
Interspinous ligament disruption	10	1	10.0	7	70.0	2	20.0	0	0.0
Cord contusion	22	1	4.5	18	81.8	3	13.6	0	0.0
Cord sever/cut	1	1	100.0	0	0.0	0	0.0	0	0.0
Disrupted/herniated disk	20	2	10.0	14	70.0	4	20.0	0	0.0
Nerve root injury	5	0	0.0	4	80.0	1	20.0	0	0.0
Spine unstable/spondylolysis	4	0	0.0	1	25.0	3	75.0	0	0.0
Osteoarthritis erosion/degenerative	25	1	4.0	14	56.0	10	40.0	0	0.0
Spinal stenosis—congenital	7	2	28.6	3	42.9	2	28.6	0	0.0
Spinal stenosis—degenerative	21	3	14.3	15	71.4	3	14.3	0	0.0

TABLE 6–11

INJURY TYPE BY EXTENT, NORTHWESTERN UNIVERSITY ACUTE SPINE INJURY CENTER, 1972–1990 *Continued*

INJURY TYPE	TOTAL	COMPLETE		INCOMPLETE		INTACT		MISSING	
		NO.	%	NO.	%	NO.	%	NO.	%
Abscess	2	0	0.0	1	50.0	1	50.0	0	0.0
Infection—bone—osteomyelitis	10	0	0.0	6	60.0	3	30.0	1	10.0
Infection—soft tissue	1	0	0.0	1	100.0	0	0.0	0	0.0
Tumor—malignant	4	0	0.0	2	50.0	2	50.0	0	0.0
Metastases	4	0	0.0	3	75.0	0	0.0	1	25.0
Avulsion—chip	63	10	15.9	25	39.7	27	42.9	1	1.6
Spondylosis/osteophytes	51	4	7.8	33	64.7	14	27.5	0	0.0
Foreign body—bullet	206	143	69.4	56	27.2	6	2.9	1	0.5
Foreign body—other	1	0	0.0	1	100.0	0	0.0	0	0.0
Other	158	22	13.9	76	48.1	58	36.7	2	1.3
None/unknown	6	5	83.3	0	0.0	1	16.7	0	0.0
*Totals**	5985	2016	33.7	2420	40.4	1509	25.2	40	0.7

*Totals represent actual number of injuries. Patients may have multiple injuries.

operative internal reduction and fixation techniques (Fig. 6–29).

Immobilization of the thoracic spine necessitates control of the closest adjacent motion segment. Therefore, patients with upper thoracic vertebral injuries require adjacent cervical spine immobilization. This can be accomplished with a cervical extension on a Knight-Taylor orthosis (Fig. 6–30). In the lower thoracic spine or thoracolumbar junction, the thoracolumbosacral orthosis (Fig. 6–31) provides immobilization of vertebral compression fracture without neurologic involvement or can be used as an adjunct to surgical decompression with internal reduction and fixation.

RECOVERY OF FUNCTION AFTER ACUTE SPINAL CORD INJURY

Acute spinal cord injury remains one of the most devastating and frustrating injuries of the nervous system. The care of patients with such injuries and the understanding of its natural history have advanced significantly with the advent of multidisciplinary-multispecialty centers specifically designed for its treatment. For example, at the Midwest Regional Acute Spine Injury Center, we have observed a change in the pattern of injury with an increase in the number of incomplete injuries (Table 6–11). The surgical management of acute spinal cord injury in terms of stabilization of the spine has advanced significantly. Further work is necessary to mitigate the effects of neurologic injury.

REFERENCES

1. Alker GJ, Young SO, Leslie EV, et al: Postmortem radiology of head and neck injuries in fatal traffic accidents. Radiology 114:611–617, 1975.
2. Allen BL Jr: Recognition of injuries to the lower cervical spine. In The Cervical Spine Research Society Editorial Committee (eds): The Cervical Spine, ed 2. Philadelphia, JB Lippincott, 1989, p 287.
3. Bauer RD, Errico TJ: Cervical spine injuries. In Errico TJ, Bauer RD, Waugh T (eds): Spinal Trauma. Philadelphia, JB Lippincott, 1991, pp 95–96.
4. Beatson TR: Fractures and dislocations of the cervical spine. J Bone Joint Surg Br 45:21–35, 1963.
5. Bedbrook GM: Some pertinent observations on the pathology of traumatic spinal paralysis. Paraplegia 1:215–227, 1963.
6. Bohlman HH: Acute fractures and dislocations of the cervical spine: An analysis of 300 hospitalized patients and review of the literature. J Bone Joint Surg Am 61:1119–1142, 1979.
7. Bracken MB, Shepard MJ, Collins WF, et al: A randomized clinical trial of methylprednisolone and naloxone used in the initial treatment of acute spinal cord injury. Results of the Second National Acute

Spinal Cord Injury Study. N Engl J Med 322:1405–1411, 1990.

8. Burke DC, Tiong TS: Stability of the cervical spine after conservative treatment. Paraplegia 13:191–202, 1975.

9. Cheshire DJE: The stability of the cervical spine following the conservative treatment of fractures and fracture-dislocations. Paraplegia 7:193–203, 1969.

10. Cybulski GR, Penn RD, Jaeger RJ: Lower extremity functional neuromuscular stimulation in cases of spinal cord injury. Neurosurgery 15:132–146, 1984.

11. Denis F: Spinal instability as defined by the three-column spine concept in acute spinal trauma. Clin Orthop 189:65–76, 1984.

12. DeVivo MJ, Fine PR, Maetz HM, et al: Prevalence of spinal cord injury. A re-estimation employing life table techniques. Arch Neurol 37:707–708, 1980.

13. Dommisse GF: The blood supply of the spinal cord. J Bone Joint Surg Br 56:225–235, 1974.

14. Fidler MW, Plasmans CMT: The effect of four types of support on the segmental mobility of the lumbosacral spine. J Bone Joint Surg Am 65:943–947, 1983.

15. Fielding JW, Cochran GVB, Lawsing JF III, et al: Tears of the transverse ligament of the atlas: A clinical and biomechanical study. J Bone Joint Surg Am 56:1683–1691, 1974.

16. Fielding WJ, Hawkins RJ: Atlanto-axial rotary fixation. J Bone Joint Surg Am 59:37–44, 1977.

17. Forsyth HF: Extension injuries of the cervical spine. J Bone Joint Surg Am 46:1792–1797, 1964.

18. Forsyth HF, Alexander E, Davis C, et al: The advantages of early spine fusion in the treatment of fracture-dislocations of the cervical spine. J Bone Joint Surg Am 41:17–36, 1959.

19. Frymoyer JF, Stokes IA: Biomechanics of spinal trauma. In Dickson RA (ed): Spinal Surgery. Science and Practice. London, Butterworths, 1990, pp 264–268.

20. Hadley MN: Spinal orthoses. In Cooper PR (ed): Management of Posttraumatic Spinal Instability. Park Ridge, Ill, American Association of Neurological Surgeons, 1990, pp 51–63.

21. Hohl M: Normal motions in the upper portion of the cervical spine. J Bone Joint Surg Am 46:1777–1779, 1964.

22. Holdsworth FW: Review article: Fracture, fracture-dislocations of the spine. J Bone Joint Surg Am 52:1534–1551, 1970.

23. Johnson RM, Hart DL, Simmons EF, et al: Cervical orthoses: A study comparing their effectiveness in restricting cervical motion in normal subjects. J Bone Joint Surg Am 59:332–339, 1977.

24. Johnson RM, Owen JR, Hart DL, et al: Cervical orthoses: A guide to their selection and use. Clin Orthop 154:34–45, 1981.

25. Kraus JF, Franti CE, Riggins RS, et al: Incidence of traumatic spinal cord lesions. J Chron Dis 28:471–492, 1975.

26. Lantz SA, Schultz AB: Lumbar spine orthosis wearing. I. Restriction of gross body motions. Spine 11:834–837, 1986.

27. Lazorthes G, Gouaze A, Zadeh JO, et al: Arterial vascularization of the spinal cord: Recent studies of the anastomotic substitution pathways. J Neurosurg 35:253–262, 1971.

28. Levine AM, Edwards CC: The management of traumatic spondylolisthesis of the axis. J Bone Joint Surg Am 67:217–226, 1985.

29. Lind B, Sihlbom H, Nordual A: Halo-vest treatment of unstable traumatic cervical spine injuries. Spine 13:425–432, 1988.

30. Meyer PR Jr: Cervical spine: Overview and conservative management. In Meyer PR Jr (ed): Surgery of Spine Trauma. New York, Churchill Livingstone, 1989, pp 341–395.

31. Meyer PR Jr: Fractures of the lumbar and sacral spine: Conservative and surgical management. In Meyer PR Jr (ed): Surgery of Spine Trauma. New York, Churchill Livingstone, 1989, pp 717–821.

32. Meyer PR Jr: Fractures of the thoracic spine: T1 to T10. In Meyer PR Jr (ed): Surgery of Spine Trauma. New York, Churchill Livingstone, 1989, pp 525–571.

33. Meyer PR Jr: Indications: Anteroposterior surgical approach to the thoracolumbar spine. In Meyer PR Jr (ed): Surgery of Spine Trauma. New York, Churchill Livingstone, 1989, pp 625–715.

34. Meyer PR, Rosen JS, Hamilton BB, et al: Fracture dislocation of the cervical spine: Transportation, assessment and immediate management. In: Instructional Course Lectures, American Academy of Orthopaedic Surgeons, vol XXV. St. Louis, Mosby, 1976, pp 171–183.

35. Reid DC: Spinal trauma—general principles and cervical injuries. In Dickson RA (ed): Spinal Surgery Science and Practice. London, Butterworths, 1990, p 300.

36. Reiss SJ, Raque GH Jr, Shields CB, et al: Cervical spine fractures with major associated trauma. Neurosurgery 18:327–330, 1986.

37. Rogers WA: Fractures and dislocations of the cervical spine. J Bone Joint Surg 39:341–376, 1957.

38. Schneider RC, Kahn EA: Chronic neurological sequelae of acute trauma to the spine and spinal cord: II. The syndrome of chronic anterior spinal cord injury or compression. Herniated intervertebral discs. J Bone Joint Surg Am 41:449–456, 1959.

39. Sonntag VKH, Douglas RA: Management of spinal cord trauma. Neurosurg Clin North Am 1:729–750, 1990.

40. Steel HH: Anatomical and mechanical consideration of the atlanto-axial articulation. J Bone Joint Surg Am 50:1481–1482, 1968.

41. Stover SL, Fine PR: The epidemiology and economics of spinal cord injury. Paraplegia 25:225–228, 1987.

42. Stover SL, Fine PR: Spinal Cord Injury. The Facts and Figures. Birmingham, University of Alabama, 1986.

43. Taylor AR, Blackwood W: Paraplegia in hyperextension cervical injuries with normal radiographic appearance. J Bone Joint Surg Br 30:245–248, 1948.

44. White AA III, Panjabi MM: Clinical Biomechanics of the Spine, ed 2. Philadelphia, JB Lippincott, 1990.

45. Wortzman G, Dewar FP: Rotary fixation of the atlantoaxial joint: Rotational atlantoaxial subluxation. Radiology 90:479–487, 1986.

46. Yarkony GM, Roth EJ, Heinemann AW, et al: Benefits of rehabilitation for traumatic spinal cord injury. Multivariate analysis in 711 patients. Arch Neurol 44:93–96, 1987.

CHAPTER 7

The Clinical Diagnosis of Disorders of the Spinal Cord

Robert M. Woolsey, M.D.
Robert R. Young, M.D.

The diagnosis of disorders of the spinal cord utilizes the usual principles of neurologic diagnosis. With data from the history and physical examination, it is possible to ascertain which tracts and nuclei of the spinal cord are not functioning in a normal manner and the level at which this is occurring.

It has been estimated that there are only 30 disorders of the spinal cord, approximately half of which are commonly encountered. These 30 disorders can be segregated into nine spinal cord syndromes on the basis of five cardinal symptoms and signs.

Using only clinical skills, neurologists are usually able to diagnose a spinal cord disorder accurately or at least to arrive at a differential diagnosis including only two or three alternatives. At this juncture, but not before, it is appropriate to employ expensive ancillary diagnostic procedures, such as somatosensory or motor evoked potential studies and magnetic resonance imaging (MRI) procedures, to confirm the diagnosis.

THE FIVE NEUROLOGIC ABNORMALITIES SEEN IN SPINAL CORD DISEASE

Pain

Three types of pain occur in patients with spinal cord disease.[71] The most common variety, local pain, occurs over the site of a spinal cord lesion. The cord is surrounded by a ring

135

of bone and ligaments, all of which, except the ligamentum flavum, are pain sensitive.[54] Pain arising from these structures is most intense over the vertebral column at the level of the involved spinal element but may spread in less intense form into the paravertebral areas. With involvement of cervical or lumbar vertebrae, pain can extend into the shoulders or hips.[44, 51] Pain directly over the site of a spinal cord abnormality also can be mediated by the nervi vasorum of pial blood vessels[17] or can arise from involvement of intrinsic spinal cord pain pathways.[52] Acute severe pain developing over minutes is seen with vertebral fracture,[27] spinal hemorrhage,[68] spinal infarction,[58] and disk herniation.[19] Local pain developing over hours, days, or weeks occurs in patients with epidural abscess[5] or tumor[12] and transverse myelitis.[57] Pain can evolve over weeks, months, or even years in patients with spondylosis,[26] syringomyelia,[40] spinal cord glioma,[61] and intradural extramedullary tumor.[37]

When caused by a process within the spinal canal, radicular pain rarely occurs without associated local pain. Because of the tendency of local pain to extend into the paravertebral areas and proximal extremities, it can be difficult to distinguish this local pain from radicular pain.[44, 51] Radicular pain seldom extends into the terminal sensory distribution of a nerve root, that is, the fingers, toes, or midline of the chest and abdomen.[73] Paresthesias are more likely to extend to the terminal nerve territory and have greater localizing value than radicular pain.[73]

Diffuse aching or burning pain occasionally occurs in patients with spinal cord disease. Although its exact pathogenesis is poorly understood, it seems to be related to destructive lesions of spinal cord pain pathways.[13] This "central" or "funicular" pain is most frequently seen in patients with spinal cord injury. It is usually a late development, occurring months after other cord symptoms. The pain tends to occur in the buttocks, feet, and legs regardless of the site of spinal cord injury and is associated with significant impairment of pain perception in the involved areas.[52]

Motor Abnormalities

Some type of motor abnormality is present in practically all disorders of the spinal cord. The presence of clinically obvious weakness probably reflects cessation of function of more than 50% of descending motor pathways or more than 50% of anterior horn cells.[9, 48] Sudden weakness in its most severe form, paralysis, can be caused by spinal cord trauma,[27] infarction,[58] and hemorrhage.[69] Progressive weakness evolving over hours, days, or weeks is seen in transverse myelitis,[57] epidural tumor,[12] and epidural abcess.[5]

In more slowly evolving processes involving the motor systems, loss of dexterity and "fatigability" of movement precedes weakness.[30] Hands become clumsy and gait becomes unsteady.[10, 68] With worsening of the spinal cord damage, weakness and spasticity become evident. Of these components of the "upper motor neuron" syndrome, spasticity probably contributes the least to functional disability.[21, 36] This type of progressive motor deficit is seen in patients with spinal multiple sclerosis,[38] the myelopathy of cervical spondylosis,[26] intradural extramedullary tumors,[37] spinal gliomas,[61] arteriovenous malformations,[2] herniated thoracic disks,[41] acquired immunodeficiency syndrome (AIDS) myelopathy,[53] subacute combined degeneration of the spinal cord due to vitamin B_{12} deficiency,[35] amyotrophic lateral sclerosis,[42] arachnoiditis,[1] radiation myelopathy,[55] and the primarily spinal forms of spinocerebellar degeneration.[22]

In myelopathies involving anterior horn cells, such as amyotrophic lateral sclerosis, intramedullary spinal cord tumors, syringomyelia, and compressive lesions of the anterior aspect of the spinal cord, weakness is associated with muscle atrophy and fasciculations. These findings are prominent when the cervical spinal cord is involved at almost any level. Why lesions located well above the lower cervical segments produce atrophy and fasciculations in intrinsic hand muscles is poorly understood, although the phenomenon is well known.[25] With lesions of the cauda equina, which involve axons of motor neurons, or of the lumbar spinal cord, atrophy and fasciculations are sometimes not as evident as with cervical lesions,[34, 50] probably due to concealment of muscle by subcutaneous fat in the legs. Also, intrinsic foot muscle weakness causes less functional impairment than intrinsic hand muscle weakness and, therefore, is not noticed by the patient.

Sensory Abnormalities

A great many terms, many odd and unpronounceable, have been used to describe abnormal sensory phenomena. Because no standardized nomenclature exists, a precise definition of terms must be included in any discussion of disturbed sensation.

Paresthesias are "positive" sensory manifestations produced by malfunctioning, but not destroyed, sensory nerve roots or spinal cord sensory pathways. "Tingling," "buzzing," and "pins and needles" sensations arise from abnormal discharge patterns in dorsal root or dorsal column axons that convey tactile sensation. Sensations of warmth, cold, and itch, which are less common, indicate involvement of the dorsal horn or spinothalamic tract axons that convey pain and temperature sensations.[39]

Paresthesias of nerve root origin tend to be most evident in the distal distribution of a dermatome, i.e., the fingers and toes, and, therefore, have greater localizing value than pain that is poorly localized in general and that is manifest in the more proximal distribution of the nerve root.[73] Paresthesias in both feet and legs can indicate involvement of the cauda equina or of the dorsal columns.[28,49] Compressive lesions in the upper half of the cervical spinal cord can cause paresthesias that involve the hands only.[24]

Lhermitte's sign is a type of paresthesia arising from irritation of the dorsal columns of the cervical spinal cord. Patients usually describe the sensation as resembling an electric shock extending from the neck down the midline of the back and sometimes into the extremities as well.[32] The sensation usually lasts only a few seconds and is usually evoked by flexion of the neck. Although most commonly seen in patients with multiple sclerosis, it occurs in many other conditions involving the cervical spinal cord.[32]

"Negative" symptomatology, usually described by patients as a numbness or "deadness," indicates that they are conscious of a lack of sensation in some part of the body. These symptoms are probably indicative of a dorsal column lesion, because patients with anterolateral cordotomy do not experience them,[63] nor do patients with the Brown-Séquard syndrome experience such symptoms on their analgesic side.[29] These symptoms may actually be a type of paresthesia because patients with complete spinal cord lesions who have total loss of all sensation below the level of their injury deny experiencing sensations of numbness or deadness.

Patients with dorsal column lesions occasionally complain that parts of the neurologic examination, such as the evocation of the plantar response by stroking the foot, the bending of the digits to test position sense, and the testing of pain sensation with a pin, are unusually painful and unpleasant.[49]

The difficulty of performing a satisfactory sensory examination is well known to every practicing neurologist; however, the following findings on sensory examination strongly suggest a lesion of the spinal cord or cauda equina:

1. Loss of position and vibratory sense in the feet with preserved ankle jerks (dorsal cord syndrome [Fig. 7–1]).

2. Bilateral loss of position and vibratory sensation in the feet with a definite level of pinprick loss on the abdomen or chest (thoracic cord lesion).

3. Bilateral segmental sensory loss, i.e., sensory loss in the hands and forearms, not in median or ulnar nerve distribution, with normal sensation in the legs and trunk and in the upper arms and neck (central cord syndrome [Fig. 7–2]).

4. Loss of pinprick sensation on one side of the body with loss of position and vibration sensation on the other (Brown-Séquard syndrome [Fig. 7–3]).

5. Loss of pinprick sensation over the legs

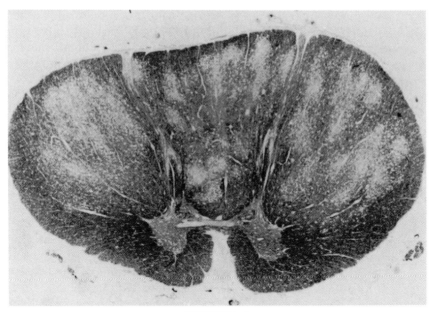

FIGURE 7–1

Dorsal cord syndrome due to subacute combined degeneration of the spinal cord in a patient with pernicious anemia.

and trunk with normal sensation in the perianal area (intramedullary or anterior extramedullary compression of the spinal cord).

6. Loss of pinprick sensation in the perianal area and in the upper part of both posterior thighs (conus medullaris or L5–S1 cauda equina lesion).

7. Loss of pinprick sensation on the legs and trunk with normal position and vibration sense in the toes and fingers (anterior cord syndrome [Fig. 7–4]).

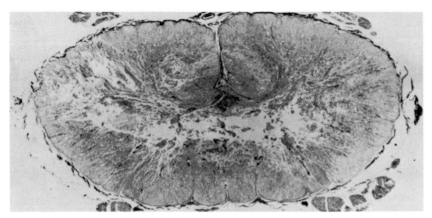

FIGURE 7–2

Central cord syndrome due to central spinal cord necrosis resulting from a hyperextension injury of the cervical spine.

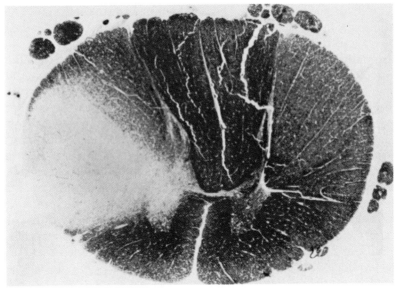

FIGURE 7–3

Brown-Séquard syndrome resulting from multiple sclerosis. The lesion is incomplete pathologically although all of the clinical features of the syndrome were present.

Abnormalities of Reflexes and Muscle Tone

Spinal cord lesions that produce paralysis over a short time course, i.e., minutes to days, such as trauma, infarction or hemorrhage, and transverse myelitis, usually produce the phenomena of spinal shock with areflexia, atonia, and nonresponsiveness to plantar stimulation. This is usually ascribed to the sudden withdrawal of facilitative influences descending from cerebral and brain stem structures to spinal segmental interneuronal pools or anterior horn cells.[15] Although the bulbocavernosus reflex returns almost immediately, tendon reflexes and muscle tone do not return for several weeks and then become exaggerated. More slowly progressive lesions

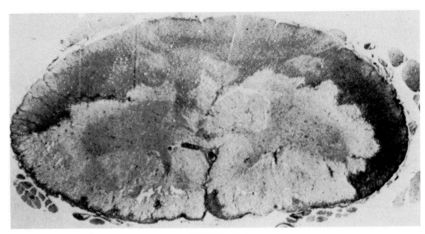

FIGURE 7–4

Anterior cord syndrome due to spinal cord infarction caused by occlusion of the anterior spinal artery by fibrocartilaginous embolus. (From Moossy J: Vascular disease of the spinal cord. *In* Joynt RJ (ed): Clinical Neurology, vol 3. Philadelphia, JB Lippincott, 1990, p 6; with permission.)

are associated with increased muscle tone and tendon reflexes from the onset.[10]

Tendon reflexes are depressed bilaterally in the lower extremities in patients with compressive lesions of the cauda equina.[50] Unilateral loss of a single tendon jerk may be a sign of spinal root or cord disease. Of course, loss of a single tendon reflex might occur with a mononeuropathy, although this would be unusual because the individual peripheral nerves mediating the tendon jerks are rarely involved by processes producing mononeuropathy. Intrinsic disease of the cervical cord is usually associated with loss of some or of all upper extremity tendon reflexes.[40]

Lower extremity or lower and upper extremity reflex hyperactivity is eventually seen in almost all spinal cord diseases. The finding of a reflex level is particularly important. Hyperactive reflexes in the legs with normal reflexes in the arms usually indicate that the patient has a lesion of the thoracic or upper lumbar spinal cord. Hyperactive lower extremity and finger flexor reflexes with a normal biceps reflex suggest a lesion of the lower cervical spinal cord. Hyperactivity of all lower and upper extremity reflexes with a normal "jaw jerk" indicates disease of the upper cervical spinal cord.

An extensor plantar response may be the earliest sign of spinal cord disease. On the other hand, the plantar response may be flexor even in the presence of other signs of an upper motor neuron lesion.[66] Other superficial reflexes that can be abolished by a lesion at or rostral to their spinal segment include the anal reflex (S2–4), the cremasteric reflex (L1–2/T10–12), the lower abdominal reflex (T10–12), and the upper abdominal reflex (T7–10).[12] The superficial reflexes are thought to have a spinocerebrospinal pathway as well as a purely segmental one, which may account for their loss in suprasegmental lesions.[18] However, interruption of a descending facilitative pathway to the segmental spinal interneurons mediating a reflex is a more likely explanation.

Bladder Symptoms

Except in the instance of lesions involving the conus medullaris[3] or the sacral roots of the cauda equina at the junction of the lumbar and sacral spine,[31] bladder dysfunction is not an early symptom of spinal cord disease. The most convincing and reliable symptom of neurogenic bladder dysfunction is urinary incontinence. Lesions of the cauda equina and acute and subacute myelopathies (spinal shock) are associated with flaccid bladder paralysis, which causes urinary retention and overflow incontinence. More slowly progressive myelopathies cause a small "spastic bladder." Decreased compliance and hyperactive detrusor stretch reflexes cause symptoms of urgency, frequency, and incontinence. Retention, urgency, or frequency without incontinence is usually symptomatic of a urologic problem, such as infection.[65]

NINE SPINAL CORD SYNDROMES

The five neurologic abnormalities indicative of spinal cord disease occur in different combinations and exhibit different tempos of evolution, but these combinations and permutations can be grouped into nine syndromes that encompass virtually all spinal cord diseases. Whenever trauma is mentioned in connection with these syndromes, it should be interpreted as having produced a persistent static deficit following an acute event. A complete description of the following individual conditions is given in the chapters on acute nontraumatic myelopathies, chronic nontraumatic myelopathies, and spinal cord injury (see Chapters 4, 5, and 6).

Paraplegia or Quadriplegia with Local Pain, Altered Reflexes, Nonselective Sensory Loss, and Loss of Bladder Function (Complete Cord Syndrome)

1. Acute disorders (occurring over minutes): These conditions are usually associated with areflexia (spinal shock). Spinal cord infarction spares dorsal column function as the brunt of the ischemia falls on the anterior two-thirds of the spinal cord.[58] Spinal cord trauma

is indicated by a history of severe injury to the neck or back and considerable local pain at the site of the spinal fracture or dislocation.[27] Spinal hemorrhage and acute disk herniation compressing the spinal cord[41, 60] are rare.

2. Subacute disorders (occurring over hours, days, or weeks): Those disorders that evolve over hours or 1 or 2 days, such as transverse myelitis (including multiple sclerosis),[57] are usually associated with areflexia. Those that come on more slowly may show hyperreflexia. Spinal epidural tumor[12] and spinal epidural abscess[5] are characterized by significant early local and radicular pain. Reflexes are usually hyperactive, and extensor plantar responses are ordinarily present. When the syndrome evolves more slowly, bladder symptoms are a later feature.

Chronic Spastic Paraplegia or Quadriplegia with Gait Ataxia (Evolving Over Months or Years)

3. Disorders without sensory abnormalities: causes include amyotrophic lateral sclerosis,[42] primary lateral sclerosis,[74] myelopathy of cervical spondylosis,[26] and familial spastic paraplegia.[7] Bladder symptoms are absent or of minor significance.

4. Disorders with loss of position and vibratory sensation (dorsal cord syndrome [see Fig. 7–1]): causes include arachnoiditis,[1] spinal multiple sclerosis,[38] the myelopathy of cervical spondylosis,[26] arteriovenous malformation,[2] subacute combined degeneration of the spinal cord,[35] meningioma and schwannoma,[37] spinal cord glioma,[61] vacuolar myelopathy,[53] spinocerebellar degeneration,[22] and spinal cord injury. Bladder symptoms are a late occurrence.

5. Disorders with loss of pain sensation bilaterally (anterior cord syndrome [see Fig. 7–4]) or unilaterally (Brown-Séquard syndrome [see Fig. 7–3]):

causes include meningioma or schwannoma,[37] myelopathy of cervical spondylosis,[26] radiation myelopathy,[55] and spinal cord injury.

Chronic Atrophic Paralysis of the Hands (Evolving Over Months or Years)

6. Disorders with segmental sensory loss involving pain only (central cord syndrome [see Fig. 7–2]) or all sensory modalities: sensory loss usually begins in a gauntlet distribution and spreads proximally into a shawl distribution. The causes include intrinsic spinal cord tumors,[61] syringomyelia,[40] and spinal cord injury.[59]

7. Disorders without sensory loss: Amyotrophic lateral sclerosis,[42] cervical spondylosis,[25] and extrinsic tumors of the upper cervical spinal cord[64] are causes.

Paraplegia with Low Back Pain, Areflexia, "Saddle Anesthesia," and Loss of Bladder Function (Cauda Equina Syndrome)

8. An acute cauda equina syndrome can be caused by lumbosacral spinal fractures,[33] a ruptured lumbar disk,[31, 34] and AIDS-related acute lumbosacral polyradiculopathy.[62]

9. A subacute or chronic cauda equina syndrome may be the result of a ruptured lumbar disk[31, 34] arachnoiditis,[1] lumbar spinal stenosis,[28] and tumors involving the cauda equina.[50]

Figure 7–5 presents the nine spinal cord syndromes in algorithmic form.

Differential Diagnosis

Because both Guillain-Barré syndrome and acute transverse myelitis can produce a rapidly evolving areflexic quadriparesis, differentiating the two can sometimes be difficult. The following features can be helpful. Back

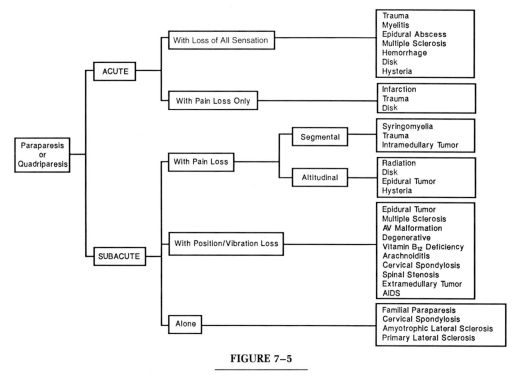

FIGURE 7–5

The nine spinal cord syndromes in algorithmic form. The term *loss* is used to mean either decreased or absent sensation. *Segmental* pain loss refers to an area of pain loss with normal pain sensation above and below the affected area. *Altitudinal* pain loss means a level below which pain is decreased. *Paresis* is used to mean either weakness or paralysis.

pain is rare in Guillain-Barré syndrome,[45] whereas it occurs in approximately a third of patients with transverse myelitis.[57] Patients with Guillain-Barré syndrome rarely show loss of pinprick sensation,[45] whereas a pinprick level is seen in most patients with transverse myelitis.[57] Generalized areflexia is usually seen in the Guillain-Barré syndrome,[4, 43] whereas reflexes are normal above the level of cord involvement in patients with transverse myelitis.[57] Loss of bladder function is rare in the Guillain-Barré syndrome[4] but is seen in three quarters of patients with transverse myelitis.[57] Cranial nerve involvement, usually of the seventh nerve but frequently of the tenth as well, is seen in most patients with Guillain-Barré syndrome[43, 46] and does not occur in patients with transverse myelitis.

Acute occlusion of the terminal aorta can cause ischemia of the proximal sciatic and femoral nerves or of the cauda equina, producing paresis, sensory loss, and reflex depression of the lower extremities.[8, 11] Rarely, the spinal cord itself may be involved.[20] Pale cold skin and the loss of pulses in the legs are constant features of aortic occlusion[11] and serve to differentiate it from primary disorders of the spinal cord and cauda equina.

Very rarely, occlusion of an anterior cerebral artery that gives rise to both callosomarginal arteries can cause bilateral infarction of the paracentral lobule, resulting in acute paraplegia with loss of bowel and bladder control,[16] as might occur with spinal cord infarction. However, sensory loss in cortical infarction is restricted to position sense with intact pain perception, which is the exact reverse of the sensory findings in spinal cord infarction.[58]

Whether chronic cerebral paraplegia,[72] Bruns' ataxia, and gait apraxia[47] are the same or different disorders is not completely clear. However, various conditions that involve the medial superior posterior portion of the frontal lobe bilaterally can produce a syndrome of gait ataxia, paraparesis, lower extremity hyperreflexia, and extensor plantar responses. Patients with these syndromes are always demented to some degree and have a paratonic rigidity and bilateral grasp reflexes.[47]

Patients with normal pressure hydrocephalus have gait ataxia and may complain of bilateral leg weakness, paresthesias, and urinary incontinence.[23] Unlike patients with gait ataxia due to spinal cord disease, in whom the ataxia is due to spastic paraparesis or position sense loss or both, patients with normal pressure hydrocephalus show little evidence of spasticity, weakness, or sensory loss in the lower extremities, although extensor plantar responses may be present.[23]

In 1889 Charcot[14] described a triad of findings characteristic of hysterical paraplegia consisting of (1) an untenable pattern of sensory loss, (2) normal tendon reflexes and plantar responses, and (3) normal bowel and bladder function. These criteria have proved to be remarkably reliable.[6] Factitious paraplegia is more commonly a manifestation of malingering than of hysteria. The neurologic features of the two conditions are the same. The distinction between hysteria and malingering is based solely on the patient's awareness of the simulation of disability. The diagnosis of factitious paraplegia should be based entirely on the neurologic findings.[56, 67] This diagnosis should never be made on the basis of psychological criteria alone.[70]

REFERENCES

1. Adams RD, Victor M: Principles of Neurology, ed 5. New York, McGraw-Hill, 1993, pp 1099–1100.
2. Aminoff MJ, Logue V: Clinical features of spinal vascular malformations. Brain 97:197–210, 1974.
3. Anderson NE, Willoughby EW: Infarction of the conus medullaris. Ann Neurol 21:470–474, 1987.
4. Asbury AK: Diagnostic considerations in Guillain-Barré syndrome. Ann Neurol 9 (suppl):1–5, 1981.
5. Baker AS, Ojemann RG, Swartz MN, et al: Spinal epidural abscess. N Engl J Med 293:463–468, 1975.
6. Baker JHE, Silver JR: Hysterical paraplegia. J Neurol Neurosurg Psychiatry 50:375–382, 1987.
7. Bickerstaff ER: Hereditary spastic paraplegia. J Neurol Neurosurg Psychiatry 13:134–145, 1950.
8. Bolduc ME, Clayson S, Madras PN: Acute aortic thrombosis presenting as painless paraplegia. J Cardiovasc Surg 30:506–508, 1989.
9. Bucy PC, Keplinger JE, Siqueira EB: Destruction of the pyramidal tract in man. J Neurosurg 21:385–398, 1964.
10. Burke D: Spasticity as an adaptation to pyramidal tract injury. Adv Neurol 47:401–423, 1988.
11. Busuttil RW, Keehn G, Milliken J, et al: Aortic saddle embolus. Ann Surg 197:698–706, 1983.
12. Byrne TN, Waxmann SG: Spinal Cord Compression: Diagnosis and Principles of Management. Philadelphia, FA Davis, 1990, pp 156–157.
13. Cassinari V, Pagni CA: Central Pain: A Neurosurgical Survey. Cambridge, Harvard University Press, 1969.
14. Charcot JM: Diseases of the Nervous System, vol III [translator Savill T]. London, The New Sydenham Society, 1989, p 374.
15. Creed RS, Denny-Brown D, Eccles JC, et al: Reflex Activity of the Spinal Cord. London, Oxford University Press, 1932, p 154.
16. Critchley M: The anterior cerebral artery and its syndromes. Brain 53:120–165, 1930.
17. Crosby EC, Humphrey T, Lauer EW: Correlative Anatomy of the Nervous System. New York, MacMillan, 1962, p 574.
18. DeJong RN: The Neurologic Examination, ed 4. Hagerstown, MD, Harper & Row, 1979, p 449.
19. DePalma AF, Rothman RH: The Intervertebral Disc. Philadelphia, WB Saunders, 1970, pp 191–192.
20. Dickson AP, Lum SK, Whyte AS: Paraplegia following saddle embolism. Br J Surg 71:321, 1984.
21. Duncan GW, Shahani BT, Young RR: An evaluation of baclofen treatment for certain symptoms in patients with spinal cord lesions. Neurology 26:441–446, 1976.
22. Eadie MJ: Hereditary spastic ataxia. In Vinken PJ, Bruyn GW (eds): Handbook of Clinical Neurology, vol 21. Amsterdam, North-Holland Publishing, 1975, pp 365–375.
23. Fisher CM: Hydrocephalus as a cause of disturbances of gait in the elderly. Neurology 32:1358–1363, 1982.
24. Good DC, Couch JR, Wacasar L: "Numb, clumsy hands" and high cervical spondylosis. Surg Neurol 22:285–291, 1984.
25. Goodridge AE, Feasby TE, Ebers GC, et al: Hand wasting due to mid-cervical spinal cord compression. Can J Neurol Sci 14:309–311, 1987.
26. Gregorius FK, Estrin T, Crandall PF: Cervical spondylotic radiculopathy and myelopathy. Arch Neurol 33:618–625, 1976.
27. Guttmann L: Spinal Cord Injuries: Comprehensive Management and Research. Oxford, Blackwell Scientific Publications, 1973, p 124.
28. Hall SH, Bartleson JD, Onofrio BM: Lumbar spinal stenosis: Clinical features, diagnostic procedures, and results of surgical treatment in 68 patients. Ann Intern Med 103:271–275, 1985.
29. Head H: Studies in Neurology. London, Oxford University Press, 1920, pp 398–432.
30. Holmes G: Introduction to Clinical Neurology, ed 2. Edinburgh, Churchill Livingstone, 1952, p 27.
31. Jennett WB: A study of 25 cases of compression of the cauda equina by prolapsed intervertebral discs. J Neurol Neurosurg Psychiatry 19:109–116, 1956.
32. Kanchandani R, Howe JG: Lhermitte's sign in multiple sclerosis: A clinical survey and review of the literature. J Neurol Neurosurg Psychiatry 45:308–312, 1982.
33. Kaufer H, Hayes JT: Lumbar fracture-dislocations. A study of 21 cases. J Bone Joint Surg Am 48:712–730, 1966.
34. Kostuik JP, Harrington I, Alexander D, et al: Cauda equina syndrome and lumbar disc herniation. J Bone Joint Surg Am 68:386–391, 1986.
35. Kunze K, Leitenmaier K: Vitamin B_{12} deficiency and subacute combined degeneration of the spinal cord. In Vinken PJ, Bruyn GW (eds): Handbook of Clinical

Neurology, vol 28. Amsterdam, North-Holland Publishing, 1976, pp 141–198.

36. Landau WM, Weaver RA, Hornbein TF: Fusimotor nerve function in man. Differential nerve block studies in normal subjects and in spasticity and rigidity. Arch Neurol 3:10–23, 1960.

37. Levy WJ Jr, Bay J, Dohn D: Spinal cord meningioma. J Neurosurg 57:804–812, 1982.

38. Liebowitz U, Halpern L, Alter M: Clinical studies of multiple sclerosis in Israel. V. Progressive spinal syndromes and multiple sclerosis. Neurology 17:988–992, 1967.

39. Lindblom U, Ochoa J: Somatosensory function and dysfunction. In Asbury AK, McKhann GM, McDonald WI (eds): Diseases of the Nervous System, ed 2. Philadelphia, WB Saunders, 1992, p 222.

40. Logue W, Edwards MR: Syringomyelia and its surgical treatment—An analysis of 75 patients. J Neurol Neurosurg Psychiatry 44:273–284, 1981.

41. Love JG, Schorn VG: Thoracic-disk protrusions. JAMA 191:627–631, 1965.

42. MacKay RP: Course and prognosis in amyotrophic lateral sclerosis. Arch Neurol 8:117–127, 1963.

43. Marshall J: The Landry-Guillain-Barré syndrome. Brain 86:55–66, 1963.

44. McCall IW, Park WM, O'Brien JP: Induced pain referral from posterior lumbar elements in normal subjects. Spine 4:441–446, 1979.

45. McFarland HR, Heller GL: Guillain-Barré disease complex. Arch Neurol 14:196–201, 1966.

46. Merritt HH: A Textbook of Neurology, ed 6. Philadelphia, Lea & Febiger, 1979, p 757.

47. Meyer JS, Barron DW: Apraxia of gait: A clinicophysiological study. Brain 83:261–284, 1960.

48. Mulder DW: The clinical limits of amyotrophic lateral sclerosis. In Rowland LP (ed): Human Motor Neuron Disease. New York, Raven Press, 1982, pp 15–21.

49. Nathan PW, Smith MC, Cook AW: Sensory effect in man of lesions of the posterior columns and of some other afferent pathways. Brain 109:1003–1041, 1986.

50. Norstrom CW, Kernohan JW, Love JG: One hundred primary caudal tumors. JAMA 178:1071–1077, 1961.

51. O'Brien JP: Mechanisms of spinal pain. In Wall PD, Melzack R (eds): Textbook of Pain. Edinburgh, Churchill Livingstone, 1984, p 242.

52. Pagni CA: Central pain due to spinal cord and brain stem damage. In Wall PD, Melzack R (eds): Textbook of Pain. Edinburgh, Churchill Livingstone, 1984, p 481–495.

53. Petito CK, Navia BA, Cho ES, et al: Vacuolar myelopathy pathologically resembling subacute combined degeneration in patients with acquired immunodeficiency syndrome. N Engl J Med 312:874–879, 1985.

54. Posner JB: Back pain and epidural spinal cord compression. Med Clin North Am 71:185–204, 1987.

55. Reagan TJ, Thomas JE, Colby MY Jr: Chronic progressive radiation myelopathy. JAMA 203:106–110, 1968.

56. Riddoch G: Differential diagnosis of functional and organic nervous disorders. Br Med J 2:499–503, 1934.

57. Ropper AH, Poskanzer DC: The prognosis of acute and subacute transverse myelopathy based on early signs and symptoms. Ann Neurol 4:51–59, 1978.

58. Sandson TA, Friedman JH: Spinal cord infarction: Report of 8 cases and review of the literature. Medicine 68:282–292, 1989.

59. Schneider RC, Cherry G, Pantek H: The syndrome of acute central cervical spinal cord injury. J Neurosurg 11:546–577, 1954.

60. Scoville WB: Types of cervical disk lesions and their surgical approaches. JAMA 196:479–481, 1966.

61. Slooff JL, Kernohan JW, MacCarty CS: Primary Intramedullary Tumors of the Spinal Cord and Filum Terminale. Philadelphia, WB Saunders, 1964, pp 16–19, 59.

62. So YT, Olney RK: Acute lumbosacral polyradiculopathy in acquired immunodeficiency syndrome: Experience in 23 patients. Ann Neurol 35:53–58, 1994.

63. Sweet WH, Poletti CE: Operations in the brain stem and spinal canal with an appendix on open cordotomy. In Wall PD, Melzack R (eds): Textbook of Pain. Edinburgh, Churchill Livingstone, 1984, pp 615–631.

64. Symonds CP, Meadows SP: Compression of the spinal cord in the neighborhood of the foramen magnum. Brain 60:52–84, 1937.

65. Tanagho EA, Schmidt RA: Neuropathic bladder disorders. In Tanagho EA, McAninch JW (eds): Smith's General Urology, ed 12. Norwalk, CT, Appleton & Lange, 1988, pp 435–451.

66. Van Gijn J: The Babinski sign and the pyramidal syndrome. J Neurol Neurosurg Psychiatry 41:865–883, 1978.

67. Walshe FMR: Diagnosis of hysteria. Br Med J 2:1451–1454, 1965.

68. Walshe FMR: Diseases of the Nervous System, ed 11. Baltimore, Williams & Wilkins, 1979, p 19.

69. Wisoff HS: Spontaneous intraspinal hemorrhage. In Wilkins RH, Rengachary SS (eds): Neurosurgery. New York, McGraw Hill, 1985, pp 1500–1504.

70. Woolsey RM: Hysteria: 1875–1975. Dis Nerv Syst 37:379–386, 1976.

71. Woolsey RM: Chronic pain following spinal cord injury. J Am Paraplegia Soc 9:39–41, 1986.

72. Yakovlev PI: Paraplegia in flexion of cerebral origin. J Neuropathol Exp Neuro 13:267–281, 1954.

73. Yoss RE, Corbin KB, MacCarty S, et al: Significance of symptoms and signs in localization of involved root in cervical disc protrusion. Neurology 7:673–683, 1957.

74. Younger DS, Chou S, Hays AP, et al: Primary lateral sclerosis: A clinical diagnosis reemerges. Arch Neurol 45:1304–1307, 1988.

CHAPTER 8

Neurophysiology of Spinal Cord Injury

Jeremy M. Shefner, M.D., Ph.D.

Many processes that affect the spinal cord are diffuse or multifocal; that is, clinical and electrophysiologic abnormalities in affected patients are a product of disease at multiple levels. The most obvious example of such a disease is multiple sclerosis. Within a given myotome or dermatome, clinical signs may reflect damage to white matter tracts either at or anywhere rostral to that level; electrophysiologic findings depend on the exact distribution of pathologic lesions as well. Focal processes, on the other hand, affect the spinal cord in a more clear-cut way, with characteristic abnormalities noted at the level of injury or disease and as specific findings seen caudal to the level of the lesion. The clearest example of such a process is traumatic spinal cord injury; other focal processes include extrinsic cord compression from spondylosis, neoplasia, infection, vascular malformation, or hematoma or infarction. Syringomyelia is another example of a focal process with characteristic signs at and below the level of the pathologic process. Although most of the data in the subsequent discussion are from the spinal cord injury literature, most are generalizable to patients with any focal spinal cord lesion.

ABNORMALITIES ABOVE THE LESION

The most obvious sequelae of focal spinal injury are seen at and below the level of injury. When motor unit firing patterns were studied in muscles innervated by myotomes just rostral to the injury site, no clear abnormalities in rate of firing were found.[57] However, when discharge intervals were analyzed for individual motor units in biceps muscles of patients with C6 and/or C7 injuries, subtle changes were noted.[58] In particular, the variability between successive interspike intervals was significantly increased in approximately 50% of motor units studied, despite the fact that muscle was clinically normal in strength. Thus, variability of motor unit firing rate is affected by spinal lesions just caudal to the motor neurons being studied. The increased variability could be due to altered sensory input to motor neurons, or could reflect a more complex interaction between sensory input and feedback from muscle groups that have been rendered paretic by the spinal cord lesion. The increased variability of firing rate seems to depend on the level of spinal injury; when interspike interval variability was studied in arm muscles of patients with thoracolumbar lesions, no abnormalities were found.[12]

A more rostral change in neural processing can also be documented in response to spinal cord injury. With the newly developed technique of cortical motor stimulation using focal magnetic fields, the somatotopic arrangement of human motor cortex can be mapped noninvasively. Levy and colleagues[35] performed this mapping in three normal subjects and in two patients with chronic spinal cord injury at about the C5 level. When recordings were made over the biceps muscle in normal subjects, stimulation of only a very restricted area of motor cortex was effective in producing a response. However, in quadriplegic patients for whom the biceps was among the few muscles remaining under voluntary control, stimulation of a wide area of motor cortex resulted in a response in the contralateral biceps. This result implies that some type of cortical remodeling may occur in adults after output pathways are transected.

ABNORMALITIES AT THE LEVEL OF THE LESION

Spinal cord injury produces a region of cell death within the traumatized portion of the spinal cord; this is called the *injury zone.* The injury zone is of variable length in the rostral-caudal dimension, encompassing at least one and often more segments. In addition, within any single segment, injury may be patchy and incomplete. The electrophysiologic sequelae of such an injury can be predicted from a basic knowledge of electromyography (EMG). Immediately after the injury, EMG study of muscles innervated by nerve roots coming from the injury zone is nonrevealing; no motor units can be voluntarily evoked in plegic muscles, and there are no signs of denervation. In paretic muscles, a reduced number of normal-appearing motor units can be recorded, sometimes making difficult the distinction between an upper motor neuron lesion and a lower motor neuron lesion. With upper motor neuron lesions, strong voluntary effort results in a reduced number of motor units being activated, with firing rates of individual units being lower than expected for the subjective effort. However, with a lower motor neuron lesion, although a reduced number of motor units are available, they are able to fire at rapid rates. Thus, in the latter circumstance, strong voluntary effort produces fewer than expected numbers of motor units firing very rapidly.

Within 2 to 3 weeks, signs of denervation in the form of fibrillation potentials and positive sharp waves become apparent.[16] These potentials reflect spontaneous activity in single muscle fibers that have lost contact with surviving motor axons. The timing of the occurrence of fibrillations depends on motor axon length; initially, they may only be seen in paraspinal muscles, appearing in distal extremity muscles approximately 1 to 2 weeks later. While fasciculations can be seen, they are not a prominent part of this electrophysiologic picture.

With incomplete lesions, signs of reinnervation can be seen after approximately 1 to 3 months. An increase in the number of prolonged, polyphasic motor units is a relatively early finding.[16] In the first 6 months to 1 year after injury, the size and number of phases of motor units progressively increase, often associated with a measurable increase in muscle strength.[37] Thus, the slow improvement often seen in the first year after spinal cord injury may be due at least in part to terminal sprouting of surviving motor neurons to re-innervate denervated muscle fibers. This sprouting can sometimes result in striking dysfunctional connections; for example, several reports have been made of arm-diaphragm synkinesis following high cervical injury.[6, 54] In such cases, visible muscle contractions can be observed in arm muscles in synchrony with the respiratory pattern.

Even in patients with complete cervical lesions, the presence of surviving motor units within the injury zone can usually be documented. Using the motor unit counting method developed by McComas and coworkers,[38] Brandstater and Dinsdale[7] evaluated the total number of motor units in thenar and hypothenar muscles after spinal cord injuries from C5–6 to C7–8. In the patients with C5–6 lesions, total numbers of motor units were reduced in intrinsic hand muscles in six of nine patients tested. With lower lesions, reduced motor unit counts were seen in virtually every patient. These data suggest that loss of motor axons is present at least three to four levels below the most rostral damaged segment. Yang and colleagues[60] also used motor unit counting techniques to evaluate number of motor units in the thenar muscles after cervical spinal cord injury. They studied 11 patients with remote spinal cord injury at or rostral to the C5–6 level. There was great variability in motor unit counts, with a few patients having normal numbers of motor units and others having greatly reduced numbers. Those with the most reduced numbers of motor units also had units that were greatly enlarged and prolonged, consistent with the idea that a reduced number of axons were innervating a greater than normal number of muscle fibers. Both of the studies just mentioned show that the injury zone in traumatic spinal cord lesions can be of variable length, with most patients showing evidence of anterior horn cell death in at least three to four myotomes.

Variability in the rostral-caudal extent of the injury zone in cervical spinal cord injuries was emphasized in a recent study by Berman and others.[4] Electromyography and upper extremity nerve conduction studies were performed on 15 patients with high cervical (C5 or above) lesions. In most of these patients, the highest density of fibrillation potentials was seen in intrinsic hand muscles innervated by C8 and/or T1 nerve roots. Motor nerve conduction studies showed either small or absent motor evoked potentials, despite normal sensory function. These results suggest that severe loss of motor neurons occurs at spinal levels from two to five levels caudal to the clinical level, and demonstrate that the damage caused by injury is distributed over a significantly greater area than was previously appreciated.

The different segmental innervation of muscles supplied by the dorsal and ventral rami is well demonstrated in patients with complete cervical spinal cord lesions. Gough and Koepke[24] compared the most caudal level of voluntary paraspinal EMG activity with the ventral ramus sensory and motor levels. They found that the sensory and motor levels from ventral rami correlated well with the bony injury measured radiographically, but paraspinal activity was noted two to three segments more caudal. Donovan and Bedbrook[17] confirmed these results and also found that sensory function in the distribution of the dorsal rami was preserved from one to six segments below that seen in anterior dermatomes. Thus, it appears that paraspinal muscles, as well as the skin overlying them, are innervated by spinal segments up to six levels rostral to the bony level.

ABNORMALITIES BELOW THE LEVEL OF THE LESION

Lower Motor Neuron Abnormalities

Our current understanding of the relationship between the spinal cord and peripheral sensory and motor neurons would suggest that in segments clearly caudal to the site of injury, EMG and nerve conduction studies should be within normal limits. Obviously, with complete spinal cord transection there is no volitional movement caudal to the lesion, so that evaluation of motor unit morphology is impossible with routine techniques. However, as motor axons should not be interrupted, no evidence of denervation in the form of fibrillation potentials or fasciculations should be expected. Similarly, motor and sensory nerve conduction studies should not be affected by a remote rostral spinal lesion.

One possible reason for exceptions to the expectations just mentioned would be the presence of multiple entrapment or compression neuropathies, which are frequently seen in any population of immobile patients. The progressive loss of muscle bulk seen in many spinal cord–injured patients increases the risk of multiple nerve compressions. There is abundant evidence that focal peripheral nerve lesions are frequent in the spinal cord–injured population. Studies of sural nerve conduction have revealed abnormalities in 15% to 66% of patients.[16, 27] Another study found reduced upper extremity sensory potentials in 36% of patients with cervical spine injuries.[7] In an extensive study of multiple lower extremity sensory nerves, Blaik and co-workers[5] found that 10 of 10 patients studied had at least one abnormal response, with most having multiple sensory nerves affected. The asymmetrical and multifocal nature of the abnormalities suggested that they were not the result of an underlying generalized peripheral or central process.

Many studies have also provided evidence for focal slowing of motor conduction at common sites of entrapment in patients with spinal cord injury. Ulnar neuropathies at the elbow were found in more than 30% of patients with chronic cervical injuries.[31] Prolonged median distal motor latencies suggesting entrapment in the carpal tunnel have been reported in up to 63% of patients,[1] with another study reporting either an ulnar or median nerve lesion in 67% of hands studied.[13] Thus, multiple compressive neuropathies appear to be the rule rather than the exception in patients with chronic spinal cord injury.

In addition to the frequent incidence of entrapment neuropathies in patients with spinal cord lesions, a number of reports have suggested that generalized lower motor neuron damage below the level of injury is a frequent sequela of spinal cord trauma. Fi-

brillations in the legs of patients with cervical lesions were noted in from 50% to 100% of patients studied.[7, 11, 16, 40, 44, 51, 55] Biopsies of muscles innervated by spinal segments caudal to the site of injury showed neurogenic atrophy,[43] and motor unit counts of intrinsic foot muscles have been found to be reduced after cervical injury.[27] However, the etiology of this apparent denervation is unclear. As noted earlier, spinal cord–injured patients are at risk for multiple compression neuropathies, which could cause local denervation in multiple muscles. Hunter and Ashby[27] found reduced motor units in abductor hallucis in patients with normal sural nerve potentials, and argued that the reduction in motor units could therefore not be due to local nerve compression. However, while fewer than 200 motor axons project to the abductor hallucis in normal subjects, there are more than 6000 myelinated fibers in the sural nerve.[8] In addition, the normal variability of sural nerve sensory action potential amplitudes is much greater than that of the motor potential derived from abductor hallucis. Thus, a mild to moderate reduction in axons present in the sciatic nerve could cause a significant reduction in motor unit counts without reducing the sural nerve action potential amplitude below the normal range. In summary, while denervation clearly occurs in muscles innervated by segments caudal to the site of spinal cord injury, the etiology of this denervation may be related to local compression of peripheral nerves.

Autonomic Changes

The entire sympathetic nervous system is isolated from the brain in patients with complete cervical lesions. This isolation is thought to have relevance for the syndrome of autonomic dysreflexia, in which stimuli such as bladder distension or pressure sores can result in increased sympathetic output and bouts of severe hypertension. Using microneurography, the activity of sympathetic axons after spinal cord injury has been studied directly.[52, 53] Spontaneous activity of sympathetic fibers was decreased in patients as compared with that of normal subjects. An increase in vesical pressure to a level that caused significant increases in blood pressure caused only small responses in sympathetic outflow fibers. However, after a stimulus below the level of injury, sympathetic responses were often prolonged. In addition, responses in sympathetic fibers were often coupled with discharges in nerves to skeletal muscle, suggesting a generalized activation of autonomic and non-autonomic fibers. Thus, while there appears to be no generalized increase in sympathetic tone below the level of spinal cord injury, the ability of the sympathetic nervous system to provide a specific and time-limited response is impaired. These findings may be relevant to the syndrome of autonomic dysreflexia, in which the ability of the sympathetic nervous system to make localized responses to specific stimuli is impaired.

F Wave Abnormalities

F waves result from antidromic activation of motor neurons, which produces an orthodromic response in a fraction of the originally stimulated axons. Although the F response does not involve a synapse, its amplitude and persistence are affected by changes in the level of excitability of motor systems.[20, 22, 47] In patients with hemiplegia from acute strokes, both F wave amplitude and persistence were decreased from normal levels.[22] However, in a population of patients with chronic spasticity, including some with spinal lesions, the relative F wave amplitude compared with the direct motor response was increased.[21] This implies that in such patients a greater number of motor axons produce F responses than under normal conditions, and presumably represents an increase in the baseline level of excitability of the motor neuron.

In addition to reflecting changes in the general level of activation of the motor system, F wave abnormalities can be a sensitive indicator of localized damage to motor neurons such as is produced by syringomyelia, a common consequence of cervical spine injury. Prolongation of F wave latency and decreased persistence have both been associated with

post-traumatic syringomyelia.[18, 45] In cases in which large cavities are present, F wave latencies have returned toward normal after surgical decompression.

H Reflex Changes

The H reflex is elicited by stimulating Ia afferent fibers and recording the compound motor action potential from a homonymous muscle; this reflex arc is mediated monosynaptically and oligosynaptically. The H reflex can be seen with stimulation of multiple nerves in upper or lower extremities, but it is recorded most frequently from the soleus muscle with stimulation of the tibial nerve in the popliteal fossa. As this response is the electrophysiologic equivalent of the ankle jerk, it is not surprising that its amplitude varies with time after spinal cord injury. Immediately after injury, patients are areflexic; this is the syndrome known as spinal shock. Within the first 24 hours, areflexia is associated with an inability to elicit H reflexes.[10] Thereafter, H reflexes become progressively easier to elicit. As the lesion becomes chronic, deep tendon reflex hyperactivity is seen, and both H reflex amplitude and the ratio of H reflex amplitude to the amplitude of the supramaximal direct motor response (H/M ratio) are increased.[36, 49, 56] However, considerable variability exists and often a clinical impression of increased spasticity is not correlated with increased amplitude of the H reflex. Some conditions that increase spasticity (e.g., bladder distension) have been shown to increase H reflex amplitude.[42]

In recent years, investigators have used various stimuli to modify the H reflex in an attempt to understand the mechanisms that underlie spasticity, both from spinal and intracranial lesions. In the late 1960s it was noted that muscle vibration causes a clear reduction in the amplitude of monosynaptic tendon reflexes.[32, 33, 46] The amount of reflex inhibition is maximized when vibration parameters are picked that selectively stimulate Ia afferents. The suppressive effect of vibration is present even when subjects are required to maintain a constant level of muscle force, so that postsynaptic influences on the motor neuron are minimized.[28] In addition, vibration still reduces the amplitude of H reflexes when the amount of cutaneous stimulation caused by the vibratory stimulus is minimized.[15] For these reasons, it is felt that vibration suppresses monosynaptic reflexes through a presynaptic inhibitory mechanism, with the most important input being Ia afferent fibers.

In patients with a complete spinal cord lesion, vibration can suppress reflexes at segments below the lesion,[3] indicating that supraspinal influences are not required. However, many studies have demonstrated alterations in the level of inhibition with different kinds of upper motor neuron lesions. In chronic lesions, vibration is less effective at suppressing the H reflex than in normal subjects.[9, 14, 28, 50, 56] However, in more acute cerebral lesions, vibration-induced suppression is either absent or actually enhanced,[2] indicating that the level of activation of presynaptic inhibitory pathways may vary in a complex way after injury.

By combining stimuli that activate antagonist and agonist muscles in sequence, reciprocal inhibitory pathways have also been shown to modulate the H reflex.[39] For example, the H reflex recorded from the soleus muscle can be modified by a previous stimulus to the peroneal nerve, which contains afferent fibers from antagonist muscle stretch receptors. In spastic patients, the effects of such reciprocal inhibition have been shown to be reduced.[34, 59]

Other segmental spinal circuits have also been shown to be altered by a rostral spinal lesion. One pathway of potential importance for patients with spinal cord lesions is the recurrent inhibitory pathway involving Renshaw cells.[30] The Renshaw cell is well situated to affect behavior of alpha motor neurons, but its primary role in motor outflow is as yet undefined. It is monosynaptically activated by collaterals from alpha motor neurons, and feeds back to inhibit the pool of homonymous neurons. In addition, Renshaw cells inhibit the Ib inhibitory interneuron responsible for reciprocal inhibition of antagonist muscles. Thus, Renshaw cell activity can potentially inhibit the firing of homonymous motor neurons and disinhibit antagonist mo-

tor neurons. One hypothesis regarding the role of recurrent inhibition in motor control is that Renshaw cell activity selectively inhibits early-firing, low-threshold motor neurons at a time when higher-threshold units are being recruited.[19, 23] However, other studies have suggested that recurrent inhibition may act to modulate the level of activity of the entire motor neuron pool.[26]

A noninvasive technique for evaluating Renshaw cell activity in patients has been described by Hultborn, Katz, and Pierrot-Deseilligny and colleagues.[25, 29, 41] The method involves analysis of H reflex amplitudes in response to a paired stimulus. The first stimulus in the pair evokes an H reflex in motor neurons, while the second stimulus supramaximally stimulates both sensory and motor fibers. Because of collision between orthodromically and antidromically conducting action potentials within a single motor axon, the reflex response to the second stimulus represents the activity of motor neurons that have fired twice in rapid succession. Thus, the response to the second stimulus may be altered by Renshaw cell firing induced by the motor neuron activation caused by the first stimulus.

Initial reports of Renshaw cell activity studied in this fashion in patients with upper motor lesions suggested that the amount of recurrent inhibition was quite variable. At rest, 13% of spastic patients showed reduced recurrent inhibition.[30] However, in the majority of patients, no evidence for a decrease of recurrent inhibition was noted at rest, and in a substantial number of patients, inhibition might even have been increased. One possible reason for this variability may have been the variability of the patient population; patients evaluated for this study had a wide variety of neurologic lesions producing spasticity.

Renshaw cell activity has recently been studied in a group of patients with spasticity due to cervical spinal cord injuries. In this group, Renshaw cell activity was reliably increased, with the level of activity correlated to the amount of spasticity.[48] Patients with severe limb stiffness showed the clearest increase in recurrent inhibition, while patients whose spasticity was characterized more by flexor spasms had more variable levels of Renshaw cell activity. In patients with clearly increased recurrent inhibition, treatment with the partial alpha$_2$-adrenergic agonist clonidine often produced dramatic clinical reduction in muscle tone; activity in recurrent inhibitory pathways was markedly reduced in concert with the reduction in spasticity. In patients with spasticity due to cervical spinal cord injuries, therefore, Renshaw cell activity may be extremely important in generating increased muscle tone.

SUMMARY

A focal spinal cord injury produces a host of electrophysiologic abnormalities, most of which reflect either local spinal cord destruction or the functional disconnection of rostral and caudal portions. Routine EMG/nerve conduction studies are most useful to investigate the deficits that result from local cord damage, and have demonstrated that the injury zone most often extends over at least three to four myotomes. EMG studies of muscles innervated by more caudal myotomes have also reported abnormalities, but the extent to which these reflect primary changes of spinal cord injury is uncertain. Electrophysiologic studies of spinal cord function caudal to the site of injury have shown alterations in autonomic output and changes in the level of excitability of reflex pathways. These changes may provide insight into the mechanisms that underlie the development of spasticity.

REFERENCES

1. Aljure J, Eltorai I, Bradley WE, et al: Carpal tunnel syndrome in paraplegic patients. Paraplegia 23: 182–186, 1985.
2. Ashby P, Verrier M: Neurophysiologic changes in hemiplegia: Possible explanation for the initial disparity between muscle tone and tendon reflexes. Neurology 26:1145–1151, 1976.
3. Ashby P, Verrier M: Neurophysiological changes following spinal cord lesions in man. Can J Neurol Sci 2:91–100, 1975.
4. Berman SA, Foo D, Tun C, et al: Denervation within the injury zone in spinal cord injury. J Am Paraplegia Soc 14:187, 1991.
5. Blaik A, McGarry J, Daura R: Peripheral neuropathy

6. in spinal cord injured patients. Electromyogr Clin Neurophysiol 29:469–472, 1989.
6. Blazek BW, Rodriguez AA: Arm diaphragm synkinesis after spinal cord injury. Muscle Nerve 13: 870, 1990.
7. Brandstater ME, Dinsdale SM: Electrophysiological studies in the assessment of spinal cord lesions. Arch Phys Med Rehabil 57:70–74, 1976.
8. Buchthal F, Rosenfalck A: Evoked action potentials and conduction velocity in human sensory nerves. Brain Res 3:2–122, 1966.
9. Burke D, Ashby P: Are spinal "presynaptic" inhibitory mechanisms suppressed in spasticity? J Neurol Sci 15:321–326, 1972.
10. Cadilhac J, Georgesco M, Benezech J, et al: Potential évoqué cerebral somethesique et réflexe d'Hoffman dans les lésions médullaires aiguës intérêt physiolpathologique et pronostic. EEG Clin Neurophysiol 43:160–167, 1977.
11. Campbell JW, Herbison GJ, Chen YT, et al: Fibrillations in acute and chronic spinal cord injured patients. Presented at the 35th annual meeting of the American Paraplegia Society, Las Vegas, 1989.
12. Davey NJ, Ellaway PH, Friedland CL, et al: Motor unit discharge characteristics and short term synchrony in paraplegic humans. J Neurol Neurosurg Psychiatr 53:764–769, 1990.
13. Davidoff G, Werner R, Waring W: Compressive mononeuropathies in chronic paraplegia. Presented at the 36th annual meeting of the American Paraplegia Society, Las Vegas, 1990.
14. Delwaide PJ: Electrophysiological analysis of the mode of action of muscle relaxants in spasticity. Ann Neurol 17:90–95, 1985.
15. Delwaide PJ: Human monosynaptic reflexes and presynaptic inhibition. In Desmedt JE (ed): New Developments in Electromyography and Clinical Neurophysiology, vol 3. Basel, S Karger, 1973, pp 508–522.
16. Di Benedetto M: Electrodiagnostic phenomena observed in patients with spinal cord lesions. Electromyogr Clin Neurophysiol 17:205–220, 1977.
17. Donovan WH, Bedbrook GM: Sensory and motor activity in the posterior primary rami following complete spinal cord injury. Arch Phys Med Rehabil 61:133–138, 1980.
18. Dyro FM, Rossier AB: Electrodiagnostic abnormalities in 15 patients with post traumatic syringomyelia: Pre and post operative studies. Paraplegia 23:233–242, 1985.
19. Eccles JC, Eccles RM, Iggo A, et al: Electrophysiological studies on Renshaw cells. J Physiol (Lond) 159:461–479, 1961.
20. Fisher MA: F response analysis of motor disorders of central origin. J Neurol Sci 62:13–22, 1983.
21. Fisher MA: F/M ratios in polyneuropathy and spastic hyperreflexia. Muscle Nerve 11:217–222, 1988.
22. Fisher MA, Shahani BT, Young RR: Assessing segmental excitability after acute rostral lesions: I. The F response. Neurology 28:1265–1271, 1978.
23. Friedman WA, Sypert GW, Munson JB, et al: Recurrent inhibition in type identified motoneurons. J Neurophysiol 46:1349–1359, 1981.
24. Gough JG, Koepke GH: Electromyographic determination of motor root levels in erector spine muscles. Arch Phys Med Rehabil 47:9–11, 1966.
25. Hultborn H, Pierrot-Deseilligny E: Changes in recurrent inhibition during voluntary soleus contractions in man studied by an H-reflex technique. J Physiol (Lond) 297:229–251, 1979.

26. Hultborn H, Pierrot-Deseilligny E: Input-output relations in the pathway of recurrent inhibition to motoneurones in the cat. J Physiol (Lond) 297:267–287, 1979.

27. Hunter J, Ashby P: Secondary changes in segmental neurons below a spinal cord lesion in man. Arch Phys Med Rehabil 64:702–705, 1984.

28. Iles JE, Roberts RCA: Presynaptic inhibition of monosynaptic reflexes in the lower limbs of subjects with upper motoneuron disease. J Neurol Neurosurg Psychiatr 49:937–944, 1986.

29. Katz R, Pierrot-Deseilligny E: Facilitation of soleus-coupled Renshaw cells during voluntary contraction of pretibial flexor muscles in man. J Physiol (Lond) 355:587–603, 1984.

30. Katz R, Pierrot-Deseilligny E: Recurrent inhibition of alpha motoneurons in patients with upper motor neuron lesions. Brain 105:103–124, 1982.

31. Krasilovsky G: Nerve conduction studies in patients with cervical spinal cord injuries. Arch Phys Med Rehabil 61:204–209, 1980.

32. Lance JW, De Gail P, Neilson PD: Tonic and phasic spinal cord mechanisms in man. J Neurol Neurosurg Psychiatr 29:535–544, 1966.

33. Lance JW, Neilson PD, Tassinari CA: Suppression of the H reflex by peripheral vibration. Proc Aust Assoc Neurol 5:45–49, 1968.

34. Levin M, Chapman CE: Inhibitory and facilitatory effects from the peroneal nerve onto the soleus H reflex in normal and spinal man. EEG Clin Neurophysiol 67:468–478, 1987.

35. Levy WJ, Amassian VE, Traad M, et al: Focal magnetic coil stimulation reveals motor cortical system reorganized in humans after traumatic quadriplegia. Brain Res 510:130–134, 1990.

36. Little JW, Halar EM: H reflex changes following spinal cord injury. Arch Phys Med Rehabil 66:19–22, 1985.

37. Little JW, Moore D, Brooke M, et al: Electromyographic evidence for motor axon sprouting in recovering upper extremities of acute quadriplegics. Presented at the 35th annual meeting of the American Paraplegia Society, Las Vegas, 1989.

38. McComas AJ, Fawcett PRW, Campbell MJ, et al: Electrophysiological estimation of number of motor units within a human muscle. J Neurol Neurosurg Psychiatr 34:121–131, 1971.

39. Mizuno Y, Tanaka R, Yanagisawa N: Reciprocal group I inhibition on triceps surae motoneurones in man. J Neurophysiol 34:1010–1017, 1971.

40. Onkelinx A, Chantraine A: Electromyographic study of paraplegia patients. Electromyogr Clin Neurophysiol 15:71–81, 1975.

41. Pierrot-Deseilligny E, Bussel B, Held JP, et al: Excitability of human motoneurones after discharge in a conditioning reflex. EEG Clin Neurophysiol 40:279–287, 1976.

42. Porter RW, Krell M: Alterations in the H reflex in paraplegia induced by bladder distention. Paraplegia 14:105–114, 1976.

43. Reske-Nielsen E, Harmsen A, Ovesen N: Pathological study of muscle biopsies from the legs in patients with fractures of the cervical spine. In Serratrice G, Roux H (eds): Advances in Neuromuscular Diseases. Paris, Expansion Scientifique, 1971, pp 509–520.

44. Rosen JS, Lerner IM, Rosenthal AM: Electromyography in spinal cord injury. Arch Phys Med Rehabil 48:271–273, 1969.

45. Rossier AB, Foo D, Shillito J, et al: Posttraumatic cervical syringomyelia: Incidence, clinical presentation, electrophysiological studies, syrinx protein and results of conservative and operative treatment. Brain 108:439–461, 1985.

46. Rushworth G, Young RR: The effect of vibration on tonic and phasic reflexes in man. J Physiol (Lond) 185:63P–64P, 1966.

47. Schiller HH, Stålberg E: F response studies with single fiber EMG in normal subjects and spastic patients. J Neurol Neurosurg Psychiatr 41:45–53, 1978.

48. Shefner JM, Berman SA, Sarkarati M, et al: Recurrent inhibition is increased in patients with spinal cord injury. Neurology 42:2162–2168, 1992.

49. Shemesh Y, Rozin R, Ohry A: Electrodiagnostic investigation of the motor neuron and spinal reflex arc (H-reflex) in spinal cord injury. Paraplegia 15:238–274, 1977.

50. Somerville J, Ashby P: Hemiplegic spasticity: Neurophysiologic studies. Arch Phys Med Rehabil 59:592–596, 1978.

51. Spielholz NI, Sell GH, Goodgold J, et al: Electrophysiological studies in patients with spinal cord injuries. Arch Phys Med Rehabil 53:558–562, 1972.

52. Stjernberg L, Blumberg H, Wallin BG: Sympathetic activity in man after spinal cord injury: Outflow to muscle below the lesion. Brain 109:695–715, 1986.

53. Stjernberg L, Wallin BG: Sympathetic neural outflow in spinal man: A preliminary report. J Auton Nerv Syst 7:313–318, 1983.

54. Swift TR, Leshner RT, Gross JA: Arm diaphragm synkinesis: Electrodiagnostic studies of aberrant regeneration of phrenic motor neurons. Neurology 30:339–344, 1980.

55. Taylor RG, Kewalramani LS, Fowler WM: Electromyographic findings in lower extremities of patients with high spinal cord injury. Arch Phys Med Rehabil 55:16–23, 1974.

56. Taylor S, Ashby P, Verrier M: Neurophysiological changes following traumatic spinal lesions in man. J Neurol Neurosurg Psychiatr 47:1102–1108, 1984.

57. Wiegner AW, Davies L, Cynn M, et al: Single motor unit discharge patterns in patients with spinal cord injury. Presented at the 36th annual meeting of the American Paraplegia Society, Las Vegas, 1990.

58. Wiegner AW, Wierzbicka MM, Davies L, et al: Discharge properties of single motor units in patients with spinal cord injuries. Muscle Nerve 16:661–671, 1993.

59. Yanagisawa N, Tanaka R, Ito A: Reciprocal Ia inhibition in spastic hemiplegia of man. Brain 99:555–574, 1976.

60. Yang JF, Stein RB, Jhamandas JT: Motor unit numbers and contractile properties after spinal cord injury. Ann Neurol 28:496–502, 1990.

CHAPTER 9

Motor and Somatosensory Evoked Potentials in Spinal Cord Disorders

Lynette Kiers, M.B.B.S., F.R.A.C.P.
Keith H. Chiappa, M.D.

MOTOR EVOKED POTENTIALS

The motor evoked potential (MEP), which is generated by stimulation of the motor cortex through the intact skull, provides the clinical neurophysiologist with a method to examine alterations in the function of central motor pathways in diseases affecting the motor system. This was initially achieved using an electrical stimulator,[1] but for clinical purposes the more recently developed magnetic stimulator is preferable because the technique is essentially painless.[2] Responses obtained by transcranial stimulation are produced primarily by activity in direct, fast-conducting corticospinal pathways.[3, 4] Other descending pathways with monosynaptic and/or polysynaptic connections with the spinal cord (e.g., reticulospinal tract) may be activated by the cortical stimulus and may contribute to the later phases of the compound motor action potential. Studies of single motor unit behavior[5] have shown that a single cortical stimulus can produce multiple descending motor volleys in corticospinal tracts. Therefore, asynchronous activation of a population of spinal motoneurons results in complex, polyphasic electromyographic (EMG) waveforms.

By placing the magnetic or electrical stimulator over the spinal enlargements, it is also possible to activate the cervical or lumbar nerve roots. Excitation of lower motor neurons probably occurs at or very near the site of emergence of their axons from the cord,[6, 7] although a number of studies have suggested that excitation occurs at the site where the nerve roots exit the intervertebral foramen.[8, 9]

It is possible to obtain estimates of central motor conduction times (CMCT) by subtracting the peripheral motor latency from spinal cord to muscle from the latency of the EMG response evoked by transcranial scalp stimulation. Peripheral motor latency can be calculated indirectly from F-wave latencies using the following formula:

$$(F + M - 1)/2$$

where F = minimum F-wave latency; M = distal motor latency; and 1 msec is the estimate of F-wave turnaround time. Alternate estimates can be obtained using cervical and/ or lumbar stimulation (Fig. 9–1). CMCT re-

flects propagation of the impulses along fast-conducting pyramidal axons.[3, 10, 11] Increases in CMCT have been reported to occur in many neurologic conditions, including multiple sclerosis,[12–16] motor neuron disease,[17–19] cervical spondylosis,[16, 20, 21] and some types of spinocerebellar degeneration.[22, 23]

Transcutaneous electrical stimulation has also been used to obtain measurement of the motor conduction velocity in the human spinal cord. Snooks and Swash[24] stimulated the spinal cord and cauda equina at C6, L1, and L4 vertebral levels and recorded from puborectalis (S4 myotome) and tibialis anterior (L5 myotome). Latencies between C6 and L1, and between L1 and L4 represented conduction times from C6 to the conus medullaris and to the rostral portion of the motor roots in the cauda equina, respectively. Measurement of the interelectrode distances allowed for calculation of motor conduction velocity, although it is recognized that the measured length of the spinal cord from C6 to T12 is some 13% less than the surface measurement of interspinous distances.[25]

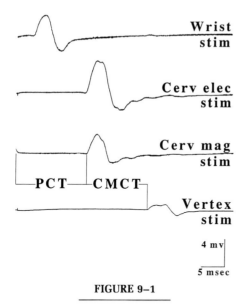

FIGURE 9–1

Recordings from surface electrodes over the abductor pollicis brevis muscle in a normal subject following median nerve electrical stimulation at the wrist, cervical electrical stimulation (C7 needle electrode), cervical magnetic stimulation (C7 spine level), and vertex magnetic stimulation (at rest). Note the low-amplitude motor evoked potential following vertex magnetic cortical stimulation in a relaxed muscle. Additional activation of ulnar innervated thenar muscles following cervical electrical stimulation accounts for the greater compound muscle action potential amplitude than that following supramaximal median nerve stimulation. PCT = peripheral conduction time; CMCT = central motor conduction time.

Multiple Sclerosis

Multiple sclerosis (MS) may present as either an acute or subacute myelopathy in young adults or as a chronic progressive spinal cord disease late in adult life. Multiple sclerosis has been studied extensively using both electrical and magnetic cortical and spinal stimulation.

In 1985, Mills and Murray[15] reported marked prolongation of central conduction times in eight patients with clinically definite MS, all of whom had severe pyramidal weakness and leg spasticity. No correlation was found between the degree of central motor slowing and the degree of pyramidal motor involvement as judged on clinical grounds. Thompson and co-workers[16] studied eight patients with clinically definite MS and noted, in addition to marked prolongation of CMCT, an increase in variability in the latency of responses from trial to trial. Caramia and colleagues[26] studied 49 patients with MS and found abnormal MEPs in 51/94 tested arms (54%). Alterations of median nerve somatosensory evoked potentials (SEPs) were found in 36 arms (38%). In clinically unaffected arms, MEPs were abnormal in 40% and SEPs in 27%. In a further study of 34 patients with MS,[22] CMCT prolongation, increased thresholds or absent responses, and low-amplitude, dispersed, polyphasic MEPs were found. Hess and others[12, 13] studied 83 patients with definite, probable, and possible MS and found that either the CMCTs to upper limb muscles were prolonged or the amplitude of the response with cortical stimulation was reduced in 60/83 patients (72%). Central motor conduction abnormalities were seen in 7/39 limbs with no physical signs. In 7/49 sides with low-amplitude responses, CMCT was normal. In the same group of patients, pattern shift visual evoked potentials (VEPs), median SEPs, and brain stem auditory evoked potentials (AEPs) were abnormal in 54/81 cases (67%), 36/61 cases (59%), and 24/61 cases (39%), respectively. For each evoked potential modality, some patients had abnormal central motor conduction and a normal sensory evoked potential result. Magnetic resonance imaging (MRI) findings were abnormal in 83% of patients tested. In one of the two cases in which MRI was normal, central motor conduction was abnormal.

Both Hess and co-workers[13] and Ingram and co-workers[27] reported an association between prolonged CMCT and clinical findings of hyperreflexia and brisk finger flexion jerks; the latter group also found a correlation with functional motor disability in 20 patients. Increased CMCT to tibialis anterior was associated with extensor plantar responses in 16/17 feet.

Snooks and Swash[24] studied motor conduction velocities in the spinal cord of five patients with MS, all with corticospinal signs in the legs. Transcutaneous electrical stimulation of the spinal cord and cauda equina at C6, L1, and L4 vertebral levels was performed, recording from puborectalis or tibialis anterior muscles. In 4/5 patients, motor conduction velocities between C6 and L1 were slowed, but cauda equina conduction was normal.

In summary, abnormalities of central motor conduction in patients with MS are characterized by markedly prolonged CMCT,

slowing of spinal cord motor conduction velocity, and low-amplitude dispersed responses to scalp stimulation. Occasionally, low-amplitude responses or increased latency variability are the only abnormalities that are seen. These abnormalities are compatible with the physiologic effects of demyelination in the central nervous system, namely slowing of conduction, conduction block, and temporal dispersion of descending volleys. Generally, the MEP abnormalities are well correlated with clinical deficits.

Cervical Myelopathy

Central motor conduction times are often prolonged in patients with cervical spondylosis and myelopathy, provided the recording is being done from muscles innervated by spinal motor neurons below the level of the lesion. Thompson and co-workers,[16] using percutaneous electrical cortical stimulation, studied five patients with cervical spondylosis and myelographically proven cord compression at C3–4 in one and C5–6 in four. Prolonged latencies to thenar muscles were found in four patients and absent responses in one. When recording was done from biceps, CMCT was prolonged in only the patient with C3–4 compression. EMG responses were small and of increased duration. In all patients, peripheral conduction times were normal, implying involvement of central motor pathways. In a previous study,[28] three patients with cervical myelopathy who had prolonged MEP latencies to thenar muscles all had normal median SEPs; two had normal tibial SEPs.

Berardelli and others[21] studied seven patients with cervical spondylosis and myelographic signs of cervical cord compression. Electrical stimulation of the motor cortex was performed, recording from biceps, thenar muscles, and tibialis anterior with surface electrodes. Cortical MEPs in the upper limbs were always delayed in at least one muscle. Cortical MEPs in tibialis anterior were absent in three patients and delayed in four.

In contrast to previous studies, in which prolongation of CMCT was noted in patients with *severe* cervical spondylosis and definite spinal cord compression, Maertens de Noord-hout and colleagues[20] assessed the usefulness of magnetic cortical stimulation in detecting *early* dysfunction of central motor pathways. Sixty-seven patients were studied, 44 with radiologic evidence of cord compression and 23 with root compression. Thirty-four patients (51%) had upper motor neuron signs. MEPs to cortical stimulation were abnormal in 84% of patients with radiologic signs of cord compression and in 22% of those without. Median nerve SEPs were altered in only 25% of patients. The frequency of MEP alterations correlated with upper motor neuron signs. In 5/44 patients (11%) with radiologic evidence of cord compression, subclinical cord compression was disclosed by cortical stimulation. The authors suggest that in some patients lesions can be detected at a preclinical stage with a sensitivity that exceeds that of SEP. By recording responses from selected muscles, it may be possible to determine the segmental level of the cord compression.

Di Lazzaro and colleagues[29] used magnetic stimulation of the motor cortex and cervical spine to study 24 patients with cervical spondylotic myelopathy documented by MRI. Compound muscle action potentials (CMAPs) were recorded from the biceps and the thenar muscles to study central motor pathways of two different myotomes, C5–6 and C8–T1. Central motor conduction was abnormal in all 24 patients to thenar muscles and in 5 patients to biceps brachii. A significant correlation was found between CMCT abnormalities to thenar muscles and clinical signs of long motor tract involvement ($P = 0.013$, χ^2 test). All patients with upper cervical cord compression (C2–4) showed an abnormal CMCT to both biceps and thenar muscles. Patients with lower cervical compression (C4–6) had abnormal thenar CMCT but normal biceps CMCT. Patients with multilevel compression of the cervical cord had abnormal CMCT to thenar muscles but normal CMCT to biceps. However, the mean value of biceps CMCT was significantly greater than that in control subjects, suggesting a slight involvement of central motor pathways for proximal upper limb muscles. The direct correlation between radiologic and electrophysiologic findings in patients

with single compression levels suggests that in these cases, mechanical cord compression is the most important factor in the pathogenesis of myelopathy.

In summary, in patients with cervical myelopathy, the CMCT is usually prolonged when recording is performed from muscles innervated by spinal neurons below the level of the lesion. Low-amplitude prolonged-duration EMG responses are often found in upper extremity muscles and responses in lower extremity muscles are absent or delayed. MEP abnormalities can identify lesions at a preclinical stage in some cases.

Motor Neuron Disease

In motor neuron disease (MND), corticospinal and corticobulbar tract degeneration is combined with varying degrees of lower motor neuron degeneration. Lower motor neuron function can be assessed using conventional electromyography, but a direct neurophysiologic test has not been previously available to evaluate impairment of the corticospinal tract. Using either percutaneous electrical or magnetic cortical and spinal stimulation, a number of abnormalities have been identified. These include (1) increased thresholds or absence of response to scalp stimulation; (2) mild prolongation of CMCTs, primarily involving spinal conduction times; and (3) low-amplitude poorly defined EMG responses.

Berardelli and colleagues[18] studied 20 patients with amyotrophic lateral sclerosis (ALS). In 4 patients, stimulation of one or both hemispheres failed to elicit cortical MEPs in both biceps and thenar muscles. In 2 patients, cortical MEPs were absent in the thenar muscles and delayed in the biceps, and in 8 patients they were delayed in at least one muscle. In 11/15 patients with abnormal cortical MEPs, cervical MEPs were also delayed, which is attributed to the loss of anterior horn cells and large myelinated fibers. However, in these patients, an abnormality of central motor conduction was also present because the slowing of conduction was out of proportion to the peripheral slowing. Cortical MEPs were absent in the patients with the most severe pyramidal signs, but the same patients also showed a greater degree of amyotrophy.

Ingram and Swash[17] studied 12 patients with motor neuron disease, 6 of whom had definite clinical signs of corticospinal tract involvement. In addition to electrical cortical stimulation, spinal cord motor conduction velocity was calculated. Prominent and often asymmetrical slowing of central motor conduction was demonstrated in 7/12 patients with recording performed from lower limb muscles; these findings were most marked in the spinal cord and correlated with clinical features of corticospinal involvement. Of 8 patients studied with scalp stimulation, with recording performed from upper limb muscles, 3 had absent responses to at least one of the muscles. Evidence of subclinical involvement of central motor pathways was found in 5 patients. In general, it was more difficult to excite motor pathways (cortical and cervical) in the patients with MND than in control subjects.

Hugon and colleagues[19] studied 13 patients with different forms of MND and found abnormal CMCTs to upper extremities in 10 patients and slowed CMCTs to lower extremities in all, even those without clinical pyramidal signs. In patients with pyramidal tract involvement, the prolongation of CMCT was generally proportional to the severity of the neurologic impairment.

Caramia and others[26] studied 9 patients with ALS. Twelve of 18 tested arms showed an altered MEP; it was totally absent in 8 arms with moderate prolongation of CMCT in the remaining 4. In a further study[22] of 7 patients with ALS, CMCT was prolonged in 6/14 upper limbs and in 12/14 lower limbs. Three of 4 patients with primary lateral sclerosis had increased thresholds and prolonged CMCT both for upper and lower limb MEPs. Thompson and colleagues[16] reported small, poorly defined EMG responses following electrical cortical stimulation in 4 patients with MND. Estimates of central conduction times were normal or at the upper limit of the normal range. Absence of EMG responses to cortical stimulation in a particular muscle was found in 3 patients, despite the ability of the patient to voluntarily activate the muscle.

Barker and others[30, 31] found normal mean magnetic CMCTs in 5 patients with MND. Triggs and co-workers[32] studied 8 patients with MND, 6 with clinical features of ALS and 2 with a syndrome suggesting primary lateral sclerosis. Elevated thresholds for magnetic cortical stimulation were found in 3 patients and absence of MEPs was seen in 5. In 6 patients, silent periods could be obtained in muscles without preceding MEPs, suggesting different susceptibilities of excitatory and inhibitory pathways to pathophysiologic processes in MND.

In summary, the relative inexcitability of the central motor pathways in MND probably reflects a reduction in the size and number of excitatory postsynaptic potentials (EPSPs) generated by the cortical stimulus as a result of motor cell loss. This finding correlates with clinical evidence of upper motor neuron involvement, but may also indicate subclinical involvement of corticospinal pathways in patients apparently presenting with "pure" lower motor neuron syndromes. The prolongation of CMCT reflects loss of large-diameter fast-conducting pyramidal neurons.

Traumatic Spinal Cord Lesions

In spinal cord injury, the lesions responsible for the major clinical deficit (i.e., paralysis) are inaccessible to conventional electrophysiologic tests. The spinal cord lesion at the level of the injury may be diffuse, involving all major ascending and descending tracts and neuronal systems, or it may be partial, involving only a portion of the cord. Numerous animal studies have been performed to evaluate the reproducibility and possible prognostic utility of MEPs in spinal cord injury.[33-35]

Levy and others[33] studied the MEP elicited by transcranial electrical stimulation in a series of 30 cats subjected to a standard injury to the thoracic cord (T6) by the Allen weight drop test. The MEPs were recorded above (T3) and below (T11) the injury and from the sciatic nerves. The peripheral nerve response was the most sensitive to injury, disappearing immediately on weight drop. The MEP spinal cord signal below the lesion showed both a latency increase and an amplitude decrease after impact. In all 17 animals in whom ambulation was regained, peripheral nerve signals returned either at or immediately before the time of ambulation. The MEP spinal cord signal below the lesion as a percentage of that above the lesion was a significant correlate of current ambulation recovery (r = 0.55). It was concluded that evaluation of SEP and MEP spinal cord signals may have prognostic value in animals and perhaps in humans.

Fehlings and colleagues[34] studied MEPs from normal and spinal cord–injured rats (lesion at C8) using direct cortical stimulation and recording from microelectrodes in the cord. Four rats had complete transection and six had clip compression injuries of varying degrees. Cord transection and severe compression injury abolished the MEP distal to the lesion, whereas the less severe compression injuries resulted in a latency shift and amplitude decrement of the MEP peaks.

Simpson and Baskin[35] studied SEPs and MEPs following blunt spinal cord injury in the rat. Animals subjected to a 50 g/cm impact on the spinal cord showed no change in SEP waveforms, but all components of the MEP were greatly attenuated and accompanied by very weak or no movement to noxious stimuli. A spectrum of clinical recovery correlated closely with return and normalization of the amplitude of the MEP. The eventual degree of clinical and MEP improvement correlated well with the degree of histologic damage that was present.

A number of clinical studies have also been undertaken in patients with acute and chronic spinal cord injury. Gianutsos and coworkers studied five quadriplegic patients at 6 to 12 months following traumatic spinal cord injury (levels C3–4 to C6–7) using percutaneous electrical stimulation of the motor cortex and recording from biceps brachii and abductor pollicis brevis muscles. In all five patients, latencies to muscles for which innervation originated above the lesion (biceps brachii) were in the normal range, whereas latencies to muscles for which innervation originated below the lesion (abductor pollicis brevis) were prolonged. Of particular interest was the finding in three patients that electromyographic signals could be elicited in muscles that showed no voluntary motor activity below the spinal cord lesion. This indicates the presence of functioning fibers that traverse the injured portion of the spinal cord, which is consistent with postmortem studies in which continuity of the white matter of the spinal cord was noted in patients who had been completely paralyzed during life, according to clinical criteria.[37, 38] The prolonged latencies of the MEPs suggest transmission through slowly conducting fibers.

Thompson and colleagues[28] compared electrical stimulation of the motor cortex with cortical SEPs in three patients with cervical cord trauma. Absent, low-amplitude, or prolonged latency responses were recorded from both upper and lower limb muscles with segmental innervation below the level of the lesion. Furthermore, two patients had abnormal MEPs with normal cortical SEPs, demonstrating abnormal conduction in the descending motor pathways without detectable involvement of the ascending sensory pathways.

Cohen and others[39] studied the induction of leg paresthesias by magnetic stimulation of the brain in seven patients with thoracic (T9–12) spinal cord injury and in four normal subjects. In three of the patients, all with complete lesions at T9, stimulation evoked sensations that lasted up to 10 seconds, which were referred to different parts of the legs and toes. The closer the site of stimulation was to the midline, the more distal were the sensations felt by the patients. It was concluded that portions of the cortical representation areas for body parts that undergo deafferentation as a result of complete spinal cord injury can remain related to those body parts for up to several years. These patients showed the lowest degree of motor reorganization in muscles proximal to the lesion.

Macdonell and Donnan[40] studied 25 patients (16 quadriplegic, 8 paraplegic, and 1 with suspected cervical cord injury) within 6 hours of acute spinal cord injury to determine whether MEPs could be used to predict motor recovery. MEPs were recorded from abductor digiti minimi, biceps, flexor hallucis brevis, and tibialis anterior muscles on each side. In no patient were MEPs obtained, either at rest or during contraction in any muscle, without preceding clinical or EMG evidence of voluntary activation. This was found to be the case even for muscles in which motor recovery occurred after initial paralysis. The authors concluded that magnetically evoked MEPs do not add to the clinical and EMG evaluation of completeness of the motor injury.

Although central nervous system neurons are not capable of replicating, reorganization of synaptic connections has been demonstrated in animal models following peripheral nerve lesions,[41] amputation,[42] spinal cord transection,[43] and reversible limb deafferentation by local anesthesia.[44] Reorganization of the motor system in human patients after injury has been reported by several groups. Levy and co-workers[45] used a figure-eight magnetic coil for focal stimulation of the motor cortex of two adult paraplegics with traumatic spinal injury and three normal adults. The patients had been injured approximately 2 years previously and biceps and deltoid were the most caudally located muscles that were spared. MEPs were elicited in these muscles from a much wider area of scalp than in the normal subjects. Topka and colleagues[46] studied magnetic MEPs in six patients with complete spinal cord injuries at low thoracic levels (2 to 20 years after injury) and eight healthy subjects. Stimuli were delivered using either a circular or figure-eight coil and EMG was recorded bilaterally from abdominal wall muscles at three levels using surface electrodes. Amplitudes were expressed as a percentage of the largest M-response obtained by direct (electrical or magnetic) stimulation over the spine of the ventral roots (T5–12). Magnetic stimulation at rest activated a larger fraction of the motor neuron pool and evoked MEPs with shorter latencies from a larger number of scalp positions in muscles immediately rostral to the level of the spinal cord injury than in corresponding muscles in control subjects. The MEPs associated with activation were not significantly different in the two groups. These results suggested enhanced excitability of motor pathways targeting muscles rostral to the level of spinal transection, which reflects reorganization of motor pathways either within cortical motor representation areas or at the level of the spinal cord. Possible mechanisms for such reorganization include increased efficacy of preexisting synapses, collateral sprouting of axons, and disinhibition of longer-latency pathways secondary to reduced afferent input. Using regional anesthetic block to induce transient deafferentation of the forearm, Brasil-Neto and colleagues[47] found a gradual increase in biceps MEP amplitude (the muscle immediately proximal to the block) during anesthesia and a return to preanesthetic levels within 20 minutes after anesthesia was ended. The speed of the changes described in this report strongly suggested an unmasking of previously existing but physiologically "inactive" connections as the likely mechanism underlying motor modulation.

In summary, although studies of MEPs in animals with traumatic spinal cord injury suggested possible prognostic value, this has not been borne out in human studies of acute spinal cord injury. Furthermore, the demonstration that clinically complete lesions may not be electrophysiologically complete adds limited prognostic data, as these remaining functional fibers do not appear to be of clinical significance. The demonstration of motor cortical system reorganization after traumatic spinal cord injury in humans may be useful in directing the emphasis of rehabilitation programs.

Miscellaneous Spinal Cord Diseases

RADIATION MYELOPATHY. Snooks and Swash[24] and Mills and co-workers[23] each found central motor conduction delays in one patient with radiation myelopathy.

SPINOCEREBELLAR DEGENERATION. Caramia and others[22] found increased thresholds for thenar MEPs or absent foot responses in three patients with spinocerebellar degeneration. Mills and colleagues[23] found a normal CMCT in one patient.

HEREDITARY SPASTIC PARAPLEGIA. Thompson and co-workers[16] found only mildly delayed scalp-to-leg latencies with normal-amplitude responses on one side of each of two patients with hereditary spastic paraparesis despite the presence of severe spasticity.

Berardelli and others[21] and Mills and colleagues[23] found increased latencies to upper extremity muscles in single patients with hereditary spastic paraplegia.

SYRINGOMYELIA. Nogués and co-workers[48] studied MEPs from upper and lower limb muscles to transcranial and spinal stimulation in 13 patients with syringomyelia. Prolonged central motor conduction times or absent motor responses in upper or lower limb muscles were found in 10 patients. Two of five patients undergoing surgery improved clinically and showed reduction in CMCT after surgical treatment. Caramia and colleagues[26] reported prolonged CMCT with normalization after surgery in a single patient with a syringomyelic cyst that extended the entire length of the cervical spinal cord.

Caramia and others[26] found prolonged CMCTs in seven patients with a variety of spinal cord lesions (foramen magnum meningioma, disk protrusions, intramedullary tumor, anterior spinal artery infarction, syringomyelia) and in one patient with subacute combined degeneration of the spinal cord.

SOMATOSENSORY EVOKED POTENTIALS

Short-latency SEPs can be recorded after electrical stimulation of peripheral sensory nerve fibers. The close relationship between SEP waveforms and the anatomy of sensory tracts allows precise localization of conduction defects. The stimulus intensity employed excites only the largest-diameter myelinated fibers in the peripheral nerve (cutaneous, subcutaneous, and intramuscular somatesthetic and proprioceptive fibers, and motor axons of equivalent diameter). Cell bodies of sensory axons of the large-fiber sensory system lie in the dorsal root ganglia; their central processes travel rostrally in ipsilateral posterior columns of the spinal cord and synapse in the dorsal column nuclei at the cervicomedullary junction. Second-order fibers cross to the opposite side shortly after origination and travel through the medial lemniscus to the primary receiving nucleus of the thalamus, the ventroposterolateral nucleus. Third-order fibers continue from thalamus to frontoparietal sensorimotor cortex. SEPs can reasonably be considered to be generated from volleys traversing the large-fiber sensory system (posterior columns and medial lemnisci) and, possibly, the spinocerebellar tracts.[49] Based on results from microneurography experiments, Burke and Gandevia[50] suggested that the dominant afferent input for lower limb mixed nerve SEPs consists of group I muscle afferents.

The diphasic positive-negative waveform recorded at the Erb's point electrode (EP) following stimulation of a peripheral nerve of the upper limb is generated by the ascending volley in motor and sensory fibers as it approaches and passes through the brachial plexus. The N11 potential is generated postsynaptically in the gray matter of the cervical cord (dorsal horns) from axon collateral input up to two levels above and below the root entry level, and by the ascending volley in the posterior columns (cuneate tract). The P/N13 potential of the neck is generated in the central cord gray matter (dorsal horns), scalp P13 in dorsal column nuclei, and scalp P14 in the medial lemniscus in the medulla and low pons. The negative activity appearing 16 to 19 msec after stimulation (N19) is generated in the thalamus, and the subsequent positivity (P22) is generated in the parietal sensory cortex.

Following stimulation of a peripheral nerve in the lower limb, the initial component of the waveform recorded from the lower lumbar region (LP) is generated by the afferent volley in the cauda equina. The second component of LP is generated in the root entry zone/dorsal horns of the lower spinal cord. The negative activity seen at 30 to 34 msec following stimulation of the posterior tibial nerve at the ankle presumably is generated in the thalamus. The subsequent positive activity at 36 to 38 msec (N/P37) is generated in the parietal sensory cortex (Fig. 9–2).

Cervical Myelopathy

Few patients with cervical spondylosis have associated myelopathy, and relatively little correlation exists between the severity

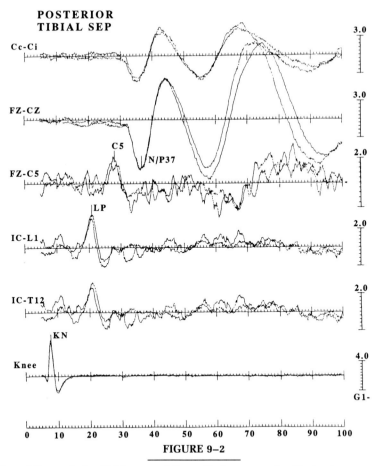

POSTERIOR TIBIAL SEP

FIGURE 9–2

Stimulation of the posterior tibial nerve at the ankle in a normal subject using a recommended recording montage. Cc refers to the central scalp area overlying the primary sensory cortex in the parietal lobe contralateral to the limb stimulated and Ci refers to the same area ipsilateral to the limb stimulated; C5, T12, and L1 are at the spinous processes, and the knee potential is derived from electrodes 5 cm apart vertically in the popliteal fossa. Each trace is the average of 1000 stimuli with two repetitions superimposed. Calibrations are in microvolts. Relative negativity of G1 caused a downward trace deflection. IC = iliac crest.

of radiologic spondylosis and the presence or severity of myelopathy. SEPs may, therefore, have an application in the detection of posterior column involvement.

In 1985, Yu and Jones,[51] using median, ulnar, and tibial nerve stimulation, studied 34 patients with cervical spondylosis: 15 with myelopathy, 6 with combined radiculopathy and myelopathy, 6 with radiculopathy, and 7 with nonspecific neck pain. SEP abnormalities, particularly with lower limb stimulation, were strongly correlated with myelopathy but not with radiculopathy. With myelopathy, SEPs were more sensitive to sensory pathway involvement than was clinical sensory testing. Significantly, 6/21 patients

with clinical myelopathy had abnormal tibial SEPs but no radiologic evidence of cord compression, suggesting that ischemia may be a significant factor in the development of myelopathy. Abnormalities of at least one SEP were detected in 2/6 patients (33%) with radiculopathy alone; in 1 the abnormal SEP was consistent with subclinical posterior column involvement.

Veilleux and Daube[52] confirmed the high sensitivity of tibial SEPs compared with median SEPs in 37 patients with cervical myelopathy. However, they suggested that ulnar SEPs were the most sensitive, perhaps related to the fact that tibial N20–P37 interpeak latencies were calculated in only 24 patients, and 30 patients had bilateral tibial nerve stimulation, which would prevent detection of interside differences. Restuccia and co-workers[53] studied 17 patients with cervical spondylotic myelopathy and found abnormal median, ulnar, and common peroneal nerve SEPs in 41%, 71%, and 100% of cases, respectively. They reported latency delay or absence of the cervical N13 or scalp far-field P14 response following upper limb stimulation, and absence or latency delay of the P27 response following common peroneal nerve stimulation. Abnormalities of the scalp far-field P14 response evoked by upper limb stimulation correlated with joint and touch sensation impairment, but not with radiologic findings; this may therefore be a reliable marker of dorsal column impairment.

Yiannikas and co-workers[54] studied 68 patients with cervical radiculopathy and/or myelopathy. In 22 patients with clinical and radiologic features of spinal cord compression, 15 (68%) had abnormal median SEPs and 21 (95%) had abnormal results with tibial or peroneal studies. The abnormalities noted were a low-amplitude or absent P/N13 and N19, a prolonged EP–P/N13 conduction time, an increase in central conduction time, and low-amplitude scalp responses from the lower limb.

Restuccia and others[55] have advocated use of a noncephalic reference montage (C6 spinous process to anterior neck) to permit selective analysis of the N13 potential, which reflects the response of dorsal horn neurons to inputs from large myelinated fibers. This has been shown to uncover abnormal cervical SEPs in patients with focal cervical cord lesions and preserved dorsal column function. These researchers studied 11 patients with MRI evidence of cervical spondylosis, all of whom had clinical evidence of bilateral pyramidal tract involvement but no posterior column involvement. Normal scalp SEPs (P14, N20) were found in all patients, reflecting normal activity of the dorsal column system up to the parietal cortex, whereas segmental cervical cord dysfunction was manifested by an abnormal spinal N13 potential in 95% of radial, 90% of median, and 54% of ulnar SEPs. The abnormality consisted exclusively of an absent or reduced N13 spinal response.

In summary, in patients with cervical spondylosis, SEP abnormalities, particularly those detected after tibial nerve stimulation, are a highly sensitive indicator of myelopathy. Use of a noncephalic reference montage permits selective analysis of the N13 potential and increases diagnostic sensitivity in patients with clinically preserved dorsal column function.

Traumatic Spinal Cord Injury

A number of studies have used SEPs in spinal cord trauma.[56–61] In 377 patients who underwent median and posterior tibial SEP study, a good correlation was found between the severity of the spinal cord injury and the SEP. During the acute phase, patients with complete functional spinal cord transection had no recordable SEPs over the scalp when lower extremity nerves were stimulated. Median and ulnar SEPs were present or absent depending on the segmental level of the spinal cord lesion.

In patients with incomplete lesions, responses to posterior tibial nerve stimulation were present and depended largely on the integrity of the posterior columns as judged by clinical examination. In some patients with apparently complete lesions, SEPs were present, which suggested some residual spinal cord function. Early persistence and progressive normalization of the SEP may antedate clinical evidence of improvement. The abnormalities described have included a reduction of amplitude and latency shifts of the early scalp components. Young[59] suggested that in the acute phase (1 week), amplitude changes predominated with little latency change, but in the more chronic phase (6 weeks), the SEP showed both amplitude and latency changes. Perot and Vera[56] reported transient abnormalities in SEPs 3 to 6 days following injury that were inconsistently associated with clinically detectable changes in the patient's status. This was thought to be related to spinal cord edema.

Sedgwick and colleagues[57] recorded spinal cord potentials (C2, C7, L1, and L4) in patients with traumatic paraplegia and quadriplegia. A normal lumbar N14 potential was found in patients with spinal cord lesions (partial or complete) several segments rostral to the generator segments (T10 or above), implying that dorsal horn neurons were able to respond normally to an incoming volley. An unexpected finding was of minor abnormalities of cervical potentials in patients with lesions at T5 and below. These included increased delay between N11 and N13 compared with that seen in controls. With high-level cervical lesions, the early cervical potentials were sometimes still present, but the later potentials were absent or, in partial lesions, delayed.

Dorfman and co-workers studied 23 patients with incomplete localized spinal cord lesions of varying etiologies. They used a calculation for indirect spinal somatosensory conduction velocity (SSCV) based on SEP latency. The leg-to-arm (L : A) ratio was defined as the amplitude ratio of the cortical response following tibial nerve stimulation to that following median nerve stimulation on the same side of the body. In 8/46 sides, tibial SEPs were unrecordable. Of the remaining 38 sides, spinal SSCV was abnormally slow in 20 and the L : A ratio was abnormally low in 20. Serial postoperative studies in 4 cases documented an increase in the spinal SSCV and L : A ratio following spinal decompression.

In a subsequent study, Chen and others[62] examined 36 patients with cervical spinal cord injuries and obtained clinical and electrophysiologic data on the same day within 2 weeks after injury. Ulnar and tibial SEP grading was based on the presence or absence of the cortical evoked potential (CEP), the amplitude of the early cortically generated waveform (P22 or P37), and the interpeak latency across the lesion site. Motor index score, pinprick sensory score, and joint position score were also calculated. Mean ulnar and tibial SEP grade had the strongest individual relationship with outcome ($R^2 = 0.75$; $P < 0.0001$), and mean SEP improvement over a 1-week interval during the first 3 weeks after injury was associated with motor index score improvement over a 6-month period. SEPs had a unique role in predicting outcome for patients with neurologically incomplete injuries because such patients with absent cortical responses had a significantly poorer outcome than did patients with responses, even though the two groups could not be differentiated on the basis of early clinical neurologic examinations.

Occasional studies have cast doubt on the ability of SEPs to predict recovery. McGarry and others[63] found that of 25 spinal cord–injured patients, 9 with normal CEP latencies were paraplegic, whereas 8 with prolonged CEP latencies had "useful ambulation." York and colleagues[64] found no relationship between the presence of a CEP or its amplitude, consistency, or latency in the early stages following injury and recovery from spinal cord injury. Both studies, however, focused on later, less reproducible CEP waveforms, including those that occurred after P22 (with upper limb stimulation) or P37 (with lower limb stimulation).

The value of performing early SEPs in patients with traumatic spinal cord lesions remains controversial. Abnormalities of median and posterior tibial SEPs correlate with the severity of spinal cord injury. In some patients, SEPs may be present despite clinically complete lesions, and progressive normalization of the SEP may antedate clinical improvement. Quantitative grading of SEP abnormalities, as performed by Chen and others,[62] suggests that mean ulnar and tibial SEP grades are more useful in predicting outcomes than are clinical motor or sensory scores, particularly in patients with incomplete lesions.

Motor System Disorders

Motor system disorders include a group of degenerative diseases with variable expression of involvement of motor neurons and their axons in cortex, brain stem, and spinal cord. A number of reports of both clinical and pathologic involvement of the sensory system have been made. Previous studies of SEPs in MND have shown conflicting results.[65–68]

Cascino and colleagues[65] found normal median SEPs in 29/30 patients with MND. Care was taken to exclude patients with cervical spondylosis or other compressive lesions.

Four patients were excluded on the basis of spinal cord compression on myelography and 16 further patients had normal myelograms. No statistical group tendency toward abnormalities in the EP-P/N13, P/N13-N19, and EP-N19 interpeak latencies was manifested in patients when compared with controls. Only 1/18 patients had definite central sensory conduction abnormalities following tibial stimulation. In addition, 4 patients had peripheral abnormalities and 4 had abnormalities that did not allow differentiation of central from peripheral defects. Oh and others[66] also reported normal median nerve cervical and cortical SEPs in 21/22 patients with ALS. In contrast, Matheson and co-workers[67] reported abnormal median SEPs in 11/32 patients. However, in 8/11 patients, the abnormality was only in absolute N13 latency (N19 was normal, EP was not measured) and, therefore, may have been caused by peripheral lesions. Twenty of 32 patients were found to have abnormal lower extremity SEPs, of which 13 were attributed to defects in central conduction based on normal H-reflexes (LP was not measured). The H-reflexes were performed with knee stimulation and, therefore, 30 to 40 cm of peripheral sensory nerve was not evaluated. Other studies have not adequately distinguished central and peripheral abnormalities or excluded coexisting cervical compression or inadequate tibial nerve stimulation as the cause of apparently delayed scalp potentials.

Subramanium and Yiannikas[68] studied 27 patients with MND. Abnormal median SEPs were found in 8/27 patients, all of whom had normal myelograms. The abnormalities consisted of delayed N9 potentials (1 patient), prolonged N9–P/N13 (2 patients), and P/N13–N19 (5 patients), as well as dispersion of the thalamocortical potential (1 patient). Comparison of a group of 8 patients with MND and normal myelograms with an age-matched control group showed no difference in peripheral conduction (normal N9 latency), but a prolongation was present of N9–P/N13 and P/N13–N19 conduction in the group with MND. Three of 21 patients had abnormal tibial SEPs and normal myelograms. One patient had unilaterally absent N20, 1 had bilaterally absent N20 and delayed cortical responses, and 1 had bilaterally dispersed cortical potentials in the presence of normal spinal potentials. Thus, the conduction deficit may have been peripheral in 2 patients.

Caramia and colleagues[26] reported abnormal median SEPs (absent cortical N20–P25 complex) in 3/18 tested arms of 12 patients with ALS.

In summary, the frequency of SEP abnormalities in MND remains a point of contention. However, significant SEP central conduction abnormalities are likely to be due to concurrent disease and should prompt consideration of diagnoses other than MND.

Syringomyelia

SEP abnormalities correlate well with loss of joint and cutaneous sensations due to circumscribed lesions of the cervical cord, posterior thalamus, and parietal cortex. Traditionally they have been thought not to reflect function in the spinothalamic pathways and have therefore not been viewed as a useful investigation in patients with syringomyelia.

Veilleux and Stevens[69] studied SEPs in 10 patients with syringomyelia; 7 patients had abnormal tibial SEPs, 3 patients had abnormal median SEPs, and 7/9 patients had abnormal ulnar SEPs. The authors noted that median and ulnar SEPs were usually normal in the presence of a dissociated sensory loss, and were usually abnormal (ulnar more frequently than median) when all sensory modalities were impaired; abnormalities of tibial SEPs were related to impaired proprioceptive sensation in the lower extremities.

Anderson and colleagues[70] studied 9 patients with syringomyelia and dissociated sensory loss. Six patients had abnormally low amplitude or absent cervical potentials following median and ulnar nerve stimulation, but did not have abnormal latencies. The abnormalities of cervical potentials were significantly asymmetrical in 5/6 cases, with the more abnormal findings corresponding to the side with greater clinical involvement. Six patients had abnormal central conduction times, all of whom had cerebellar tonsillar herniation at the foramen magnum.

Nogués and others[48] studied 13 patients with syringomyelia that had been confirmed by MRI, 7 of whom had an associated Chiari type I anomaly. Eight of 13 patients showed either unilateral or bilateral abnormal CCT findings, and 4 showed abnormal latencies or an absent cervical N14 after median nerve stimulation. Three patients showed N20 abnormalities. The N40 latencies after tibial nerve stimulation were normal in 4 patients and prolonged or unobtainable in 7.

Restuccia and Mauguière[71] studied median nerve SEPs in 24 patients with syringomyelia documented by CT scan or MRI. Cervical N13 was recorded using a C6 anterior cervical montage, which cancels the potentials generated above the foramen magnum and enhances the amplitude of N13. Scalp far-field and early cortical SEPs were recorded using a noncephalic reference electrode. The N13/N9 amplitude ratio was used as an index to quantify N13 amplitude. Absent or reduced N13 was observed in 40 median SEPs (83%) in conjunction with normal P14 and N20 in 30 SEPs (63%). Dissociated loss of the cervical N13 was identified as the most conspicuous SEP feature in syringomyelia. A significant correlation was found between abnormal N13 and loss of pain and temperature sensations, whereas P14 abnormalities correlated well only with loss of joint and touch sensations. Posterior neck N13 negativity elicited by electrical stimulation of the median nerve is thought to have a fixed transverse generator in the lower cervical cord, and reflects the response of dorsal horn neurons to non-noxious inputs. Abnormalities of N13 cervical potentials in patients with syringomyelia suggest that it is an indicator for central cervical cord lesions.

Urasaki and others[72] and Emerson and co-workers,[73] using a noncephalic reference and an expanded montage (including anterior cervical and lateral neck recording electrodes), identified abnormalities of spinal N13/P13 components that were not evident using a standard montage in 3 patients with syringomyelia.

In summary, patients with cervical cord syrinxes may show abnormalities in median nerve SEPs, indicating a lesion in the upper cervical cord with relative sparing of lower limb SEPs. The differential involvement presumably results from involvement of the lesion with the root entry zone (collateral) portion of the spinal cord rather than the dorsal columns. Detection of abnormalities of the cervical N13 response is increased by use of a noncephalic reference montage.[71–73]

Multiple Sclerosis

Small and colleagues[74] studied median SEPs recorded over the cervical spine (C2, C7) in 126 patients with MS. Abnormalities of cervical N14 were found in 59% of patients, increasing to 69% of those in the definite diagnostic category. Reduction of amplitude or absence of the response was much more common than was latency prolongation. Abnormal cervical SEPs were often found in the absence of relevant clinical signs, suggesting the presence of clinically silent cervical spinal cord plaques.

Turano and co-workers[75] studied 31 patients with definite or suspected MS who presented with a cervical cord syndrome. SEPs were recorded following median and posterior tibial nerve stimulation using cephalic and noncephalic reference electrodes. SEPs were abnormal in 67.7% of patients, whereas MRI showed cervical cord lesions in 74.2% and intracranial lesions possibly involving the somatosensory pathways in 64.5% of patients. A significant correlation was found between abnormalities of cervical (N13) and cortical (N20) potentials following median nerve stimulation and MRI abnormalities involving the ipsilateral or posterior half of the cervical cord. The N13 potential, recorded from the low cervical region, using a supraglottal reference, was most frequently abnormal in patients with MRI lesions at C6 or 7, whereas P14, recorded between the scalp and a clavicle reference, was most often affected by lesions at C1 or the cervicomedullary junction. The N9–N20 interpeak latency and the absolute P40 latency to tibial nerve stimulation were significantly correlated with the length of abnormalities in the ipsilateral cervical cord seen on MRI. No significant correlation was observed between SEP abnormalities and brain MRI lesions, which might have possibly involved the intracranial somatosensory pathways.

Ropper and co-workers[76] studied SEP abnormalities in 12 consecutive patients with inflammatory acute transverse myelopathy (ATM) that was not associated with other features of MS. All 9 patients tested with median SEPs had normal findings, as the lesions were below cervical levels that mediated that response. Five of 6 patients tested with peroneal SEPs had abnormal findings.

In patients with MS, a peculiar SEP abnormality has been reported, consisting of absence of P/N13 with preservation of N19–P22 and a normal brachial plexus to N19 interpeak latency. The pathophysiologic source of this finding and its relation to SEP generators remain unclear.

In summary, upper and lower extremity SEPs are useful for detection of clinically silent cervical spinal cord plaques with potentials from the lower limb showing a higher abnormality rate, presumably as a result of the greater length of involved white matter. When lower limb testing is normal, upper limb SEPs may still be abnormal. The most frequent abnormalities are reduction or absence of the cervical N13 potential or prolon-

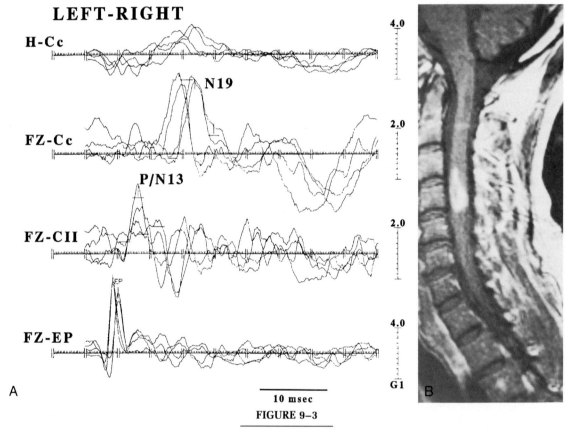

FIGURE 9–3

Median nerve somatosensory evoked potentials (SEPs) and magnetic resonance imaging (MRI) scan in a 45-year-old man with a 1-month history of progressive bilateral hand and foot numbness and paresthesias with associated clumsiness of the hands. *A,* Superimposed median nerve SEPs from both sides of the patient. The SEP following right median nerve stimulation shows a long duration, low-amplitude, asynchronous P/N13, with prolongation of the EP–P/N13 interpeak latency. The left median SEP is normal, as are both tibial SEPs. The findings suggest an abnormality of the large fiber sensory pathways between the mid–brachial plexus and lower medulla (see Fig. 9–2 for electrode derivations); CII was at the second spinous process, EP was at Erb's point, H = hand. Calibration in microvolts. Each trace is the average of 512 stimuli with two replicated superimpositions. *B,* The T2-weighted MRI scan shows a bright lesion with gadolinium enhancement at the level of C4. A cranial T2-weighted MRI (not shown) revealed multiple bright lesions in the periventricular white matter bilaterally, consistent with demyelination.

gation of the EP–P/N13 interpeak latency following median nerve stimulation (Fig. 9–3) and prolongation of the N20–N/P37 interpeak latency following tibial nerve stimulation.

Friedreich's Ataxia

Jones and colleagues[77] studied 22 patients with Friedreich's ataxia. They found marked attenuation of the brachial plexus potential, but N9 and P/N13 latencies were normal. The N19 latency was delayed in all patients but two, in whom it could not be recognized. This study provided evidence of a central conduction disturbance in SEPs. Mastaglia and others[78] studied 8 patients, all with abnormal P/N13 and N19 components. Trojaborg and co-workers[79] studied 10 patients, 5 with abnormal P/N13 to N19 interpeak latencies. Noel and Desmedt[80] reported dispersed initial scalp negativity at latencies normal for N19.

Hereditary Spastic Paraparesis

Of 7 patients with hereditary spastic paraparesis, Mastaglia and colleagues found abnormal P/N13 components in 3 and delayed, reduced amplitude N19 latencies in 2. Trojaborg and others[79] studied 13 patients with spastic paraplegia, 4 of whom had abnormal SEPs (all but 1 had normal central conduction times from the upper limb). Thomas and colleagues[81] studied median SEPs in 18 patients with hereditary spastic paraplegia and normal peripheral nerve conduction studies. P/N13 was absent in 6 patients and was reduced in amplitude in the remainder.

CONCLUSION

In patients with acute and chronic spinal cord injury, MEPs and SEPs are complimentary tests that provide information regarding functional integrity of both anterolateral and posterior afferent and efferent pathways. In acute traumatic spinal cord injury, the role of evoked potentials in predicting neurologic outcome remains controversial. SEPs appear to be more useful than MEPs, particularly in incomplete lesions, although the number of studies with MEPs is limited. With other spinal cord disorders, evoked potentials assist in lesion localization and, in contrast to imaging studies, reflect the functional integrity of spinal cord pathways. Furthermore, lesions may be detected at a subclinical stage using evoked potentials.

REFERENCES

1. Merton PA, Morton HB: Stimulation of the cerebral cortex in the intact human subject. Nature 285:227, 1980.
2. Barker AJ, Jalinous R, Freeston IL: Non-invasive stimulation of human motor cortex. Lancet 2: 1106–1107, 1985.
3. Rothwell JC, Thompson PD, Day BL, et al: Motor cortex stimulation in intact man: I. General characteristics of EMG responses in different muscles. Brain 110:1173–1190, 1987.
4. Hess CW, Mills KR, Murray NMF: Responses in small hand muscles from magnetic stimulation of the human brain. J Physiol 388:397–419, 1987.
5. Day BL, Rothwell JC, Thompson PD, et al: Motor cortex stimulation in intact man: II. Multiple descending volleys. Brain 110:1191–1209, 1987.
6. Cros D, Chiappa KH, Gominak S, et al: Cervical magnetic stimulation. Neurology 40:1751–1756, 1990.
7. Macdonell RAL, Cros D, Shahani BT: Lumbosacral nerve root stimulation comparing electrical with surface magnetic coil techniques. Muscle Nerve 15:885–890, 1992.
8. Epstein CM, Fernandez-Beer E, Weissman JD, et al: Cervical magnetic stimulation: The role of the neural foramen. Neurology 41:677–680, 1991.
9. Maccabee PJ, Amassian VE, Eberle LP, et al: Measurement of the electric field induced into inhomogeneous volume conductors by magnetic coils: Application to human spinal neurogeometry. Electroencephalogr Clin Neurophysiol 81:224–237, 1991.
10. Rossini PM, Di Stefano E, Stanzione P: Nerve impulse propagations along central and peripheral fast conducting motor and sensory pathways in man. Electroencephalogr Clin Neurophysiol 60:320–334, 1985.
11. Rothwell JC, Thompson PD, Cowan JMA, et al: A method of monitoring function in corticospinal pathways during scoliosis surgery with a note on motor conduction velocities. J Neurol Neurosurg Psychiatry 49:251–257, 1986.
12. Hess CW, Mills KR, Murray NMF: Measurement of central motor conduction in multiple sclerosis by magnetic brain stimulation. Lancet 2:355–358, 1986.
13. Hess CW, Mills KR, Murray NMF, et al: Magnetic brain stimulation: Central motor conduction studies in multiple sclerosis. Ann Neurol 22:744–760, 1987.
14. Cowan JMA, Dick JPR, Day BL, et al: Abnormalities in central motor pathway conduction in multiple sclerosis. Lancet 2:304–307, 1984.

15. Mills KR, Murray NMF: Corticospinal tract conduction time in multiple sclerosis. Ann Neurol 18:601–605, 1985.
16. Thompson PD, Day BL, Rothwell JC, et al: The interpretation of electromyographic responses to electrical stimulation of the motor cortex in diseases of the upper motor neuron. J Neurol Sci 80:91–110, 1987.
17. Ingram DA, Swash M: Central motor conduction is abnormal in motor neuron disease. J Neurol Neurosurg Psychiatry 50:159–166, 1987.
18. Berardelli A, Inghilleri M, Formisano R, et al: Stimulation of motor tracts in motor neuron disease. J Neurol Neurosurg Psychiatry 50:732–737, 1987.
19. Hugon J, Lubeau M, Tabarand F, et al: Central motor conduction in motor neuron disease. Ann Neurol 22:544–546, 1987.
20. Maertens de Noordhout A, Remade JM, Pepin JL, et al: Magnetic stimulation of the motor cortex in cervical spondylosis. Neurology 41:75–80, 1991.
21. Berardelli A, Inghilleri M, Priori A, et al: Electrical stimulation of motor cortex in patients with motor disturbances. In Rossini PM, Marsden CD (eds): Neurology and Neurobiology: vol 41. Non-invasive Stimulation of Brain and Spinal Cord. New York, Alan R. Liss, 1988, pp 219–230.
22. Caramia MD, Cicinelli P, Paradiso C, et al: "Excitability" changes of muscular responses to magnetic brain stimulation in patients with central motor disorders. Electroencephalogr Clin Neurophysiol 81:243–250, 1991.
23. Mills KR, Murray NMF, Hess CW: Magnetic and electrical transcranial brain stimulation: Physiological mechanisms and clinical applications. Neurosurgery 20:164–168, 1987.
24. Snooks SJ, Swash M: Motor conduction velocity in the human spinal cord: Slowed conduction in multiple sclerosis and radiation myelopathy. J Neurol Neurosurg Psychiatry 48:1135–1139, 1985.
25. Desmedt JE, Chevon G: Spinal and far-field components of human somatosensory evoked potentials to posterior tibial nerve stimulation analyzed with oesophageal derivations and noncephalic reference recording. Electroencephalogr Clin Neurophysiol 56:635–651, 1983.
26. Caramia MD, Bernardi G, Zarola F, et al: Neurophysiological evaluation of the central nervous impulse propagation in patients with sensorimotor disturbances. Electroencephalogr Clin Neurophysiol 70:16–25, 1988.
27. Ingram DA, Thompson AJ, Swash M: Central motor conduction in multiple sclerosis: Evaluation of abnormalities revealed by transcutaneous magnetic stimulation of the brain. J Neurol Neurosurg Psychiatry 51:487–494, 1988.
28. Thompson PD, Dick JPR, Asselman P, et al: Examination of motor function in lesions of the spinal cord by stimulation of the motor cortex. Ann Neurol 21:389–396, 1987.
29. Di Lazzaro V, Restuccia D, Colosimo C, et al: The contribution of magnetic stimulation of the motor cortex to the diagnosis of cervical spondylotic myelopathy: Correlation of central motor conduction to distal and proximal upper limb muscles with clinical and MRI findings. Electroencephalogr Clin Neurophysiol 85:311–320, 1992.
30. Barker AT, Freeston IL, Jalinous R, et al: Clinical evaluation of conduction time measurements in central motor pathways using magnetic stimulation of human brain. Lancet 1:1325–1326, 1986.
31. Barker AT, Freeston IL, Jalinous R, et al: Magnetic stimulation of the human brain and peripheral nervous system: An introduction and the results of an initial clinical evaluation. Neurosurgery 20:100–109, 1987.
32. Triggs WJ, Macdonell RAL, Cros D, et al: Motor inhibition and excitation are independent effects of magnetic cortical stimulation. Ann Neurol 32:345–351, 1992.
33. Levy WJ, McCaffrey M, Hagichi S: Motor evoked potential as a predictor of recovery in chronic spinal cord injury. Neurosurgery 20:138–142, 1987.
34. Fehlings M, Tator CH, Dean Linden R, et al: Motor evoked potentials recorded from normal and spinal cord-injured rats. Neurosurgery 20:125–130, 1987.
35. Simpson RK, Baskin DS: Corticomotor evoked potentials in acute and chronic blunt spinal cord injury in the rat: Correlation with neurological outcome and histological damage. Neurosurgery 20:131–137, 1987.
36. Gianutsos J, Eberstein A, Ma D, et al: A noninvasive technique to assess completeness of spinal cord lesions in humans. Exp Neurol 98:34–40, 1987.
37. Kakulas BA, Bedbrook GM: A correlative clinico-pathological study of spinal cord injury. Proc Aust Assoc Neurol 6:123–132, 1969.
38. Kakulas BA, Bedbrook GM: Pathology of injuries of the vertebral spinal cord with emphasis on microscopic aspects. In Vinken PJ, Bruyn GW (eds): Handbook of Clinical Neurology: vol 25. Injuries of the Spine and Spinal Cord, part 1. Amsterdam, Elsevier–North Holland, pp 27–42, 1976.
39. Cohen LG, Topka H, Cole RA, et al: Leg paresthesias induced by magnetic brain stimulation in patients with thoracic spinal cord injury. Neurology 41:1283–1288, 1991.
40. Macdonell RAL, Donnan GA: Cortical motor evoked potentials in acute spinal cord injury. Neurology 43(suppl 2):262, 1993.
41. Wall JT, Cusick CG: Cutaneous responsiveness in primary somatosensory (S-1) hindpaw cortex before and after partial hindpaw deafferentation in adult rats. J Neurosci 4:1499–1515, 1984.
42. Pons TP, Garraghty PE, Ommaya AK, et al: Massive cortical reorganization after sensory deafferentation in adult macaques. Science 252:1857–1860, 1991.
43. McKinley PA, Jenkins WM, Smith, JL, et al: Age-dependent capacity for somatosensory cortex reorganization in chronic spinal cats. Dev Brain Res 31:136–139, 1987.
44. Metzler J, Marks PS: Functional changes in cat somatic sensory-motor cortex during short-term reversible epidermal blocks. Brain Res 177:379–383, 1979.
45. Levy WJ, Amassian VE, Traad M, et al: Focal magnetic coil stimulation reveals motor cortical system reorganized in humans after traumatic quadriplegia. Brain Res 510:130–134, 1990.
46. Topka H, Cohen LG, Cole RA, et al: Reorganization of corticospinal pathways following spinal cord injury. Neurology 41:1276–1283, 1991.
47. Brasil-Neto JP, Cohen LG, Pascual-Leone A, et al: Rapid reversible modulation of human motor outputs after transient deafferentation of the forearm: A study of transcranial magnetic stimulation. Neurology 42:1302–1306, 1992.
48. Nogués MA, Pardal AM, Merello M, et al: SEPs and

CNS magnetic stimulation in syringomyelia. Muscle Nerve 15:993–1001, 1992.

49. Chiappa KH: Evoked Potentials in Clinical Medicine, ed 2. New York, Raven, 1990.

50. Burke D, Gandevia SC: Muscle afferent contribution to the cerebral potentials of human subjects. *In* Cracco RQ, Bodis-Wollner I (eds): Frontiers of Clinical Neuroscience: vol 3. Evoked Potentials. New York, Alan R. Liss, pp 262–268, 1986.

51. Yu YL, Jones SJ: Somatosensory evoked potentials in cervical spondylosis: Correlation of median, ulnar and posterior tibial nerve responses with clinical and radiological findings. Brain 108:273–300, 1985.

52. Veilleux M, Daube JR: The value of ulnar somatosensory evoked potentials (SEPs) in cervical myelopathy. Electroencephalogr Clin Neurophysiol 68:415–423, 1987.

53. Restuccia D, Di Lazzaro V, Lo Monaco M, et al: Somatosensory evoked potentials in the diagnosis of cervical spondylotic myelopathy. Electromyogr Clin Neurophysiol 32:389–395, 1992.

54. Yiannikas C, Shahani BT, Young RR: Short-latency somatosensory evoked potentials from radial, median, ulnar and peroneal nerve stimulation in the assessment of cervical spondylosis. Arch Neurol 43:1264–1271, 1986.

55. Restuccia D, Di Lazzaro V, Valeriani M, et al: Segmental dysfunction of the cervical cord revealed by abnormalities of the spinal N13 potential in cervical spondylotic myelopathy. Neurology 42:1054–1063, 1992.

56. Perot PL, Vera CL: Scalp-recorded somatosensory evoked potentials to stimulation of nerves in the lower extremities and evaluation of patients with spinal cord trauma. Ann NY Acad Sci 388:359–368, 1982.

57. Sedgwick EM, El-Negamy E, Frankel H: Spinal cord potentials in traumatic paraplegia and quadriplegia. J Neurol Neurosurg Psychiatry 43:823–830, 1980.

58. Dorfman LJ, Perkash I, Bosley TM, et al: Use of cerebral evoked potentials to evaluate spinal somatosensory function in patients with traumatic and surgical myelopathies. J Neurosurg 52:654–660, 1980.

59. Young W: Correlation of somatosensory evoked potentials and neurological findings in spinal cord injury. *In* Tator CH (ed): Early Management of Acute Spinal Cord Injury. New York, Raven, pp 153–165, 1982.

60. Cracco RQ: Spinal evoked responses: Peripheral nerve stimulation in man. Electroencephalogr Clin Neurophysiol 35:379–386, 1973.

61. Spielholz NI, Benjamin MV, Engler G, et al: Somatosensory evoked potentials and clinical outcome in spinal cord injury. *In* Popp AJ (ed): Neural Trauma. New York, Raven, pp 217–222, 1979.

62. Chen Li, Houlden DA, Rowed DW. Somatosensory evoked potentials and neurological grades as predictors of outcome in acute spinal cord injury. J Neurosurg 72:600–609, 1990.

63. McGarry J, Friedgood DL, Woolsey R, et al: Somatosensory evoked potentials in spinal cord injuries. Surg Neurol 22:341–343, 1984.

64. York DH, Watts C, Raffensberger M, et al: Utilization of somatosensory evoked cortical potentials in spinal cord injury: Prognostic limitations. Spine 8:832–839, 1983.

65. Cascino GD, Ring SR, King PJL, et al: Evoked potentials in motor system diseases. Neurology 38:231–238, 1988.

66. Oh SJ, Sunwoo IN, Kim HS, et al: Cervical and cortical somatosensory evoked potentials differentiate cervical spondylotic myelopathy from amyotrophic lateral sclerosis (abstract). Neurology 35(suppl 1):147–148, 1985.

67. Matheson JK, Harrington HJ, Hallett M: Abnormalities of multimodality evoked potentials in amyotrophic lateral sclerosis. Arch Neurol 43:338–340, 1986.

68. Subramanium JS, Yiannikas C: Multimodality evoked potentials in motor neuron disease. Arch Neurol 47:989–994, 1990.

69. Veilleux M, Stevens C: Syringomyelia: Electrophysiological aspects. Muscle Nerve 10:449–458, 1987.

70. Anderson NE, Frith RW, Synek VM: Somatosensory evoked potentials in syringomyelia. J Neurol Neurosurg Psychiatry 49:1407–1410, 1986.

71. Restuccia D, Mauguière F: The contribution of median nerve SEPs in the functional assessment of the cervical spinal cord in syringomyelia. Brain 114:361–379, 1991.

72. Urasaki E, Wada S, Kadoya C, et al: Absence of spinal N13-P13 and normal scalp far-field P14 in a patient with syringomyelia. Electroencephalogr Clin Neurophysiol 71:400–404, 1988.

73. Emerson RG, Pedley TA: Effect of cervical spinal cord lesions on early components of the median nerve somatosensory evoked potential. Neurology 36:20–26, 1986.

74. Small DG, Matthews WB, Small M. The cervical somatosensory evoked potential (SEP) in the diagnosis of multiple sclerosis. J Neurol Sci 35:211–224, 1978.

75. Turano G, Jones SJ, Miller DH, et al: Correlation of SEP abnormalities with brain and cervical cord MRI in multiple sclerosis. Brain 114:663–681, 1991.

76. Ropper AH, Miett T, Chiappa KH: Absence of evoked potential abnormalities in acute transverse myelopathy. Neurology 32:80–82, 1982.

77. Jones SJ, Baraitser M, Halliday AM: Peripheral and central somatosensory nerve conduction defects in Friedreich's ataxia. J Neurol Neurosurg Psychiatry 43:495–503, 1980.

78. Mastaglia FL, Black JL, Edis R, et al: The contribution of evoked potentials in the functional assessment of the somatosensory pathway. Clin Exp Neurol 15:279–298, 1978.

79. Trojaborg W, Bottcher J, Saxtrup O: Evoked potentials and immunoglobulin abnormalities in multiple sclerosis. Neurology 31:866–871, 1981.

80. Noel P, Desmedt JE: The somatosensory pathway in Freidreich's ataxia. Acta Neurol Belg 76:271, 1976.

81. Thomas PK, Jeffreys JGR, Smith IS, et al: Spinal somatosensory evoked potentials in hereditary spastic paraplegia. J Neurol Neurosurg Psychiatry 44:243–246, 1981.

CHAPTER 10

Segmentally Specific Somatosensory Evoked Potentials

Michael J. Aminoff, M.D., F.R.C.P.

Somatosensory evoked potentials (SEPs) are usually elicited by electrical stimulation of a mixed nerve, such as the median or ulnar nerve at the wrist, the peroneal nerve at the knee, or the tibial nerve at the ankle (see also Chapter 9). Responses recorded over the spine and scalp reflect the integrity of fibers that traverse two or more different roots and enter the cord at different levels, because the stimulated nerve trunks are polysegmental. Attempts have been made to improve the segmental specificity of the stimulus by applying it to cutaneous nerves or to the skin in the territory of individual dermatomes in the hope that the resulting SEPs would be of particular value in the recognition of isolated root lesions or discrete lesions in the somatosensory pathways within the spinal cord.

Responses to the stimulus are recorded in the same manner as when a mixed nerve trunk is stimulated. Responses are thus recorded with surface or needle electrodes over the scalp and spine and in the limb that is stimulated. There is no unanimity as to the optimal recording montage, particularly for responses elicited by lower limb stimulation, although a committee of the American Electroencephalographic Society has recently reviewed the issue and made certain recommendations.[1] Recordings over the scalp should generally include both a bipolar and referential recording montage. Specific technical details are provided elsewhere.[5] A relatively broad bandpass is used for recording purposes (e.g., 10–3000 Hz). Several different factors influence the number of trials to be averaged, but often between 500 and 2000 trials are necessary for recording responses to stimulation of the upper limbs and as many as 4000 trials when the lower limbs are stimulated. At least two averages are always obtained to ensure that the findings are replicable.

As with SEPs elicited by nerve trunk stimulation, responses are assessed with regard to the presence of certain specific components and to the latency and interpeak latency of these components. Response latency is influenced by limb length, height, and age, and these factors must be taken into account in determining the bounds of normality in healthy control subjects. Furthermore, normal variation of absolute and interpeak latency dictates that the responses of individual patients should not be regarded as abnormal unless they exceed by 3 SD or more the mean values for normal subjects of similar age and height or limb length. Response amplitude and morphology are of lesser importance in evaluating SEP findings.

SEGMENTALLY SPECIFIC SEPs IN THE EVALUATION OF RADICULOPATHY

Attempts have been made to identify compressive root lesions using cerebral responses elicited with nerve trunk stimulation. There have thus been reports that peroneal- or tibial-derived SEPs are abnormal in patients with lumbosacral root lesions, even though abnormalities would not be expected in patients with isolated radiculopathies because these nerves are derived from several segments. The normal function of fibers traversing an unaffected root should lead to an SEP of normal configuration and latency, so that abnormalities are not found. This conforms with our own experience with the peroneal-derived SEP, which has been normal in every patient with an isolated L5 or S1 root lesion whom we have studied.[4]

Cutaneous Nerve Stimulation

Eisen and Elleker[7] elicited SEPs by stimulating several different cutaneous nerves in the upper and lower limbs and published normal values for the responses obtained, emphasizing the segmental specificity of this approach. In the upper limbs for example, the musculocutaneous nerve was stimulated in the forearm as a means of evaluating the C5 segment, the median nerve fibers in the thumb for C6, the adjoining surfaces of the second and third digits for C7, and the ulnar nerve fibers in the fifth digit for C8. In the lower limbs, L2 was evaluated by stimulating the lateral femoral cutaneous nerve in the thigh, L3 and L4 by stimulating the saphenous nerve at the knee and ankle, respectively, L5 by stimulating the superficial peroneal nerve at the ankle, and S1 by stimulating the sural nerve at the ankle. Eisen and associates[8] also assessed the utility of this and other electrophysiologic techniques in the evaluation of 36 patients with radiculopathies. The yield from SEPs was disappointing (57%) in comparison with needle electromyography (EMG) (75%). Moreover, the latency of the SEP was rarely prolonged, the most common abnormalities being a reduction in amplitude or an altered configuration. Abnormalities of morphology are difficult to quantify, which limits the utility of this parameter.

Perlik and associates[12] subsequently used a similar approach to evaluate 30 patients with low back pain and unilateral radicular symptoms. Three patients with normal computed tomographic (CT) scans of the lumbosacral spine and normal electrophysiologic studies were excluded from further analysis. Among the remaining 27 patients, all of whom had abnormal lumbosacral CT scans, 21 had abnormalities in the SEP elicited by cutaneous nerve stimulation. Six of these 21 patients also had clinical signs and other electrophysiologic abnormalities indicative of root dysfunction, whereas the remaining 15 patients had neither a clinical deficit nor any electrophysiologic abnormality other than the SEP changes. Based on these findings, Perlik and colleagues concluded that the SEPs elicited by cutaneous nerve stimulation were an important means of evaluating root injury in patients with low back pain, especially when there was no associated clinical deficit to indicate root involvement. The most common abnormality in their experience was a delay in the SEP recorded over the scalp. This is surprising because it would be expected that any conduction delay in the short compressed segment of the somatosensory pathway under study would be obscured by the normal conduction velocity along the much greater length of the uncompressed portion. In some patients a delay was found in the latency of the lumbar potential, but this particular component was not recorded with sufficient reliability to make it a useful indicator of pathology, and, similarly, the interval between the lumbar potential and the responses recorded over the scalp could not be used reliably for this purpose.

To study dorsal root function more directly, Seyal and associates[18] recorded SEPs at the lumbar root entry zone following stimulation of cutaneous nerves in the legs. In particular, they recorded a reproducible negativity over the lumbar spine in every instance following stimulation of the saphenous (L3/4), superficial peroneal (L5), and sural nerves (S1) in 60 limbs of 30 normal subjects and found that latency correlated significantly with lower limb length. Because the responses so obtained are not state-dependent and would not be affected by lesions within the brain or rostral portions of the spinal cord, they believed that they would be more helpful than the scalp-recorded responses in the evaluation of patients with suspected radiculopathies. Furthermore, it was anticipated that focal compressive radiculopathies would be more likely to lead to latency abnormalities of these spinal SEPs than of the scalp-recorded responses because the total conduction distance is shorter and the proportion occupied by the compressed segment is therefore relatively greater. In a subsequent study of 20 patients with lumbosacral radiculopathy and radiologic abnormalities, spinal SEPs were abnormal (absent, markedly attenuated, or delayed) in 10 patients, in 3 of whom the EMG examination was normal.[19] By contrast, the scalp-recorded SEP was abnormal in only 20% of patients who had appropriate radiologic abnormali-

ties, a value considerably lower than that claimed by Perlik and co-workers[12] but similar to the value we obtained for dermatomally elicited SEPs (discussed later).

Thus, the role of SEPs elicited by cutaneous nerve stimulation in the evaluation of radiculopathies is unclear, but the preponderance of evidence suggests that the scalp-recorded responses have a low diagnostic yield and are unlikely to be helpful in most patients, whereas the responses recorded over the spine are likely to be more sensitive but are harder to record reliably.

Dermatomal Stimulation

SEPs elicited by dermatomal stimulation are also segmentally specific. Considerable variation exists in the dermatomal charts published by different investigators, but comparison of these maps permits the definition of certain areas that are generally agreed to lie within the territory of particular dermatomes. Electrical stimulation in such areas at an intensity two to three times the sensory threshold elicits responses that can be recorded with facility over the spine and scalp. Such dermatomally elicited SEPs have been used particularly to evaluate patients with root disease. Because the responses can be recorded with greater facility over the scalp than over the spine, attention has been directed primarily to the scalp-recorded responses.[3, 4, 6, 9, 10]

Interest in the use of dermatomal SEPs was aroused by early reports that more than 90% of patients with surgically verified L5 or S1 root lesions had abnormal responses elicited by stimulation in the appropriate dermatome.[13] Unfortunately, however, evaluation of the reliability of these findings is prevented by lack of normal data and failure of the original investigators to indicate how their criteria for abnormality were selected. Accordingly, my colleagues and I undertook an independent study of the clinical utility of dermatomal SEPs in the diagnosis of lumbosacral radiculopathies.[3, 4] We first recorded responses over the scalp to L5 or S1 stimulation in 32 normal subjects, obtaining a positive–negative–positive complex at the vertex with reference to either the midfrontal region or the contralateral C3′–4′ electrode placement (Fig. 10–1). The amplitude and latency of the initial positive peak were then determined. In general, latency values are about 5 to 10 msec greater than when SEPs are elicited by mixed nerve stimulation, due at least in part to the more proximal stimulation site with nerve trunk stimulation and to activation of fast-conducting group I muscle afferents in the latter context. Based on the findings in normal subjects, criteria for abnormality were defined by an interside difference in latency exceeding 3 SD for the segmental level under study, an absolute latency value deviating from our usual height-latency regression line by more than 3 SE, or a response that was absent or markedly attenuated unilaterally. We subsequently studied patients with an isolated L5 or S1 root lesion but found that the dermatomal SEPs were

abnormal only in approximately 25% of instances and were much less helpful than needle EMG. As might have been expected, the most common abnormality was loss of the response, although occasionally there was a prolongation in latency of the initial positive peak (see Fig. 10–1).

A subsequent study performed in England by Katifi and Sedgwick[9] suggested that dermatomal SEPs were of more value than we had recognized. Their recording technique and normative data were very similar to our own.[10] They claimed, however, that their SEP findings enabled them to predict correctly the presence of lumbosacral root compression in 19 of 20 patients with surgically confirmed prolapsed intervertebral disk or canal stenosis. The criteria that they employed for abnormality were less stringent than ours, consisting of a departure from normal mean latency values of 2 rather than 3 SD. Further-

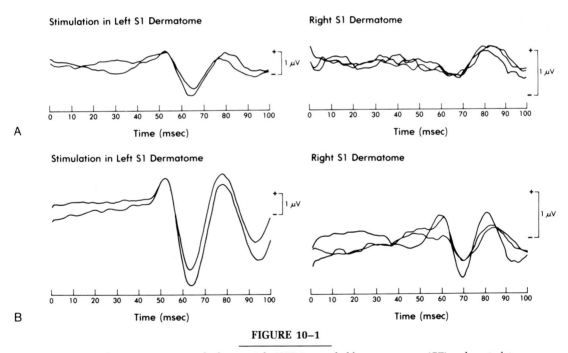

FIGURE 10–1

Dermatomal somatosensory evoked potentials (SEPs) recorded between vertex (CZ) and contralateral C3′ or C4′ electrodes to stimulation in the S1 dermatome on either side in two patients. Two or three trials, each the average of 512 responses, have been superimposed. An upward deflection indicates positivity at the CZ electrode. The response to stimulation in the left S1 territory is normal and shows a positive–negative–positive complex at the vertex. In A there is loss of the first positive component of the response to stimulation in the right S1 dermatome; in B a prolonged response latency is evident with right S1 stimulation. These findings suggest right S1 radiculopathy in each case. (From Aminoff MJ, Goodin DS, Barbaro NM, et al: Dermatomal somatosensory evoked potentials in unilateral lumbosacral radiculopathy. Ann Neurol 17:171–176, 1985; with permission.)

more, they made numerous comparisons between the findings in their patients and those in normal subjects, thereby increasing the risks of obtaining false-positive results. This complicates the interpretation of their study because many patients had bilateral or multilevel disease. Closer inspection of their published findings indicates that they correctly identified 25 of the 34 roots involved at operation but, in addition, incorrectly identified another 12 roots that were not compressed when visualized at surgical exploration (which was the gold standard used for reference).[2] When this is taken into account, they were able to predict accurately and completely the operative findings on the basis of dermatomal SEP studies in only 4 of their 20 patients, a yield similar to our own and one that is discouragingly low.

Dermatomal SEPs have been equally disappointing in the evaluation of cervical radiculopathies. Schmid and colleagues[14] examined 28 patients with unilateral sensory and motor deficits from cervical root lesions using this electrophysiologic approach. They found that with segmental stimulation, 72% of patients had false-negative findings on the symptomatic side and 22% had positive findings on the incorrect (asymptomatic) side. They therefore concluded that segmental stimulation would be unhelpful in the electrophysiologic evaluation of patients with cervicobrachialgia of unknown origin.

More recently, Slimp and colleagues[20-23] in Seattle have undertaken a large study to evaluate more fully the utility of dermatomal SEPs. They obtained normative data for dermatomes C4–8, T2, T6, T8, T10, T12, and L2–S1 and, for clinical purposes, regarded as abnormal any latency values that exceed 3 SD from the normal mean. Their findings suggest that dermatomal SEPs are useful in recognizing definite or probable spinal stenosis but are of more limited or little use in the recognition of isolated radiculopathies. More specifically, of 26 patients with clinical and radiographic evidence of lumbar spinal stenosis, 25 (96%) had abnormal dermatomal SEPs bilaterally, whereas only 15 (59%) had bilateral electromyographic abnormalities.[20]

Thus, the role of dermatomal SEPs in the evaluation of isolated radiculopathies appears to be limited by low sensitivity when stringent criteria for abnormality are used and by reduced specificity when less rigid criteria are employed. Preliminary studies suggest, however, that the technique may be useful in the evaluation of spinal stenosis.

SEGMENTALLY SPECIFIC SEPs IN THE EVALUATION OF CORD LESIONS

Experience with segmentally specific SEPs in the evaluation of cord lesions has been more limited. In contrast to the findings in cervical radiculopathy (in which SEPs occasionally reveal focal neurologic involvement but in only one or a few neighboring segments), SEP abnormalities in cervical myelopathy are more common, more severe, and more extensive. However, it is not possible to distinguish reliably between root or cord involvement underlying any SEP changes.[15] Similarly, the cause of cord pathology cannot be distinguished by the SEP findings.

Schramm and co-workers[17] have reported their experience with dermatomal SEPs in the evaluation of patients with cord pathology of diverse etiology (other than space-occupying lesions). Their methodology and criteria for abnormality are not entirely clear, and they appear to have relied to some extent on subjective qualitative criteria (involving alterations in waveform morphology and amplitude) when evaluating the responses recorded. Nevertheless, they found that recording segmentally specific SEPs from several different levels was of greater utility than simply recording SEPs elicited by stimulating the major nerve trunks in the limbs, despite the expense and time involved. Abnormalities could be focal, lateralized, generalized, or suggestive of cord transection because of bilateral polysegmental involvement below a specified level. Further, the SEP findings sometimes suggested a sensory level that was several segments more rostral than the clinical sensory level or indicated a transverse myelopathy in patients with only lateralized clinical sensory loss. In other words, SEP findings often revealed more extensive involvement of the cord than was apparent clinically.

In a subsequent study, Schramm and colleagues[16] recorded segmentally specific SEPs before and after removal of spinal space-occupying lesions. The most common SEP finding was that associated with a transverse myelopathy, and this corresponded to the clinical findings. After operation, there was both clinical and electrophysiologic improvement in 21 of 32 patients (67%); in the remaining patients, there was a discrepancy between clinical and SEP changes so that, for example, among 4 patients who improved clinically, the SEP either deteriorated or remained unchanged, and in 4 patients whose conditions deteriorated clinically, the SEP either improved or remained unchanged. This suggests that SEP findings do not provide a reliable prognostic guide to the outcome of operation.

Segmentally specific SEPs also have been used to localize the posterior column sensory level in patients with quadriplegia from cervical cord trauma. Sensory branches of the musculocutaneous (C5, C6), median (C7, C8), and ulnar (C8) nerves were stimulated, and the cortically generated responses were recorded over the scalp. In 8 of 10 patients tested, there was a direct linear relationship of SEP abnormalities with clinically determined posterior column sensory level, whereas in the remaining 2 patients the SEP findings suggested a higher level than was evident clinically.[11] However, the role of this approach in the management of patients with acute cord injuries remains to be explored, as does any advantage of the technique over SEPs elicited by nerve trunk stimulation. In this regard, Toleikis and Sloan[24] studied 496 patients with acute spinal injury and emphasize that SEPs elicited by dermatomal stimulation may permit the identification of spared neural function beyond that evident clinically or on SEPs derived from major nerve trunks, and the recognition of areas of neurologic involvement at or around the level of a spinal fracture despite the lack of any gross neurologic abnormality.[24] Although it may be true that dermatomal SEPs sometimes provide information that cannot be obtained more easily by clinical examination, standard electrophysiologic techniques, and imaging studies, it remains to be shown that this added information is of practical relevance in influencing patient management.

CONCLUSION

Recording of segmentally specific SEPs is an intuitively appealing approach to the electrophysiologic investigation of patients with radiculopathies or discrete lesions of central somatosensory pathways in the spinal cord. It is time-consuming to record these responses, however, and the findings have generally been of little practical relevance. Depending on the clinical context in which they are recorded and the criteria of abnormality adopted, segmentally specific SEPs have had either a low sensitivity or low specificity or have provided information that does not influence patient management. Preliminary studies suggest that they may have a more important role in the evaluation of spinal stenosis.

REFERENCES

1. American Electroencephalographic Society: Guidelines on evoked potentials: standards for short latency somatosensory evoked potentials. J Clin Neurophysiol 11:66–73, 1994.
2. Aminoff MJ, Goodin DS: Dermatomal somatosensory evoked potentials in lumbosacral root compression. J Neurol Neurosurg Psychiatry 51:740–741, 1988.
3. Aminoff MJ, Goodin DS, Barbaro NM, et al: Dermatomal somatosensory evoked potentials in unilateral lumbosacral radiculopathy. Ann Neurol 17:171–176, 1985.
4. Aminoff MJ, Goodin DS, Parry GJ, et al: Electrophysiologic evaluation of lumbosacral radiculopathies. Electromyography, late responses, and somatosensory evoked potentials. Neurology 35:1514–1518, 1985.
5. Chiappa KH (ed): Evoked Potentials in Clinical Practice, ed 2. New York, Raven Press, 1990.
6. De Meirsman J, Steemans I: Dermatome-evoked action potentials at L5 and S1. Medica Physica 9:273–279, 1986.
7. Eisen A, Elleker G: Sensory nerve stimulation and evoked cerebral potentials. Neurology 30:1097–1105, 1980.
8. Eisen A, Hoirch M, Moll A: Evaluation of radiculopathies by segmental stimulation and somatosensory evoked potentials. Can J Neurol Sci 10:178–182, 1983.
9. Katifi HA, Sedgwick EM: Evaluation of the dermatomal somatosensory evoked potential in the diagno-

sis of lumbo-sacral root compression. J Neurol Neurosurg Psychiatry 50:1204–1210, 1987.

10. Katifi HA, Sedgwick EM: Somatosensory evoked potentials from posterior tibial nerve and lumbo-sacral dermatomes. Electroencephalogr Clin Neurophysiol 65:249–259, 1986.

11. Louis AA, Gupta P, Perkash I: Localization of sensory levels in traumatic quadriplegia by segmental somatosensory evoked potentials. Electroencephalogr Clin Neurophysiol 62:313–316, 1985.

12. Perlik S, Fisher MA, Patel DV, et al: On the usefulness of somatosensory evoked responses for the evaluation of lower back pain. Arch Neurol 43:907–913, 1986.

13. Scarff TB, Dallman DE, Toleikis JR, et al: Dermatomal somatosensory evoked potentials in the diagnosis of lumbar root entrapment. Surg Forum 32:489–491, 1981.

14. Schmid UD, Hess CW, Ludin HP: Somatosensory evoked potentials following nerve and segmental stimulation do not confirm cervical radiculopathy with sensory deficit. J Neurol Neurosurg Psychiatry 51:182–187, 1988.

15. Schramm J: Clinical experience with the objective localization of the lesion in cervical myelopathy. In Grote W, Brock M, Clar HE, et al (eds): Advances in Neurosurgery, vol 8. Berlin, Springer-Verlag, 1980, pp 26–32.

16. Schramm J, Assfalg B, Brock M: Segmentally evoked preoperative and postoperative somatosensory potentials in spinal tumors. In Nodar RH, Barber C (eds): Evoked Potentials: II. Proceedings of the Second International Evoked Potentials Symposium. London, Butterworths, 1984, pp 406–412.

17. Schramm J, Oettle GJ, Pichert T: Clinical application of segmental somatosensory evoked potentials (SEP): Experience in patients with non-space occupying lesions. In Barber C (ed): Evoked Potentials. Proceedings of an International Evoked Potentials Symposium held in Nottingham, England. Lancaster, MTP Press, 1980, pp 455–464.

18. Seyal M, Palma GA, Sandhu LS, et al: Spinal somatosensory evoked potentials following segmental sensory stimulation. A direct measure of dorsal root function. Electroencephalogr Clin Neurophysiol 69:390–393, 1988.

19. Seyal M, Sandhu LS, Mack YP: Spinal segmental somatosensory evoked potentials in lumbosacral radiculopathies. Neurology 39:801–805, 1989.

20. Slimp JD, Robinson LR, Kraft GH, et al: Somatosensory evoked potentials in cord and root disease. Western J Med 153:433, 1990.

21. Slimp JC, Rubner DE, Snowden ML, Stolov WC: Dermatomal somatosensory evoked potentials: cervical, thoracic, and lumbosacral levels. Electroencephalogr Clin Neurophysiol 84:55–70, 1992.

22. Snowden ML, Haselkorn JK, Kraft GH, et al: Dermatomal somatosensory evoked potentials in the diagnosis of lumbosacral spinal stenosis: comparison with imaging studies. Muscle Nerve 15:1036–1044, 1992.

23. Stolov WC, Slimp JC: Dermatomal somatosensory evoked potentials in lumbar spinal stenosis. Syllabus, AAEE/AEEGS Joint Symposium, 1988, pp 17–22.

24. Toleikis JR, Sloan TB: Comparison of major nerve and dermatomal somatosensory evoked potentials in the evaluation of patients with spinal cord injury. In Barber C, Blum T (eds): Evoked Potentials: III. The Third International Evoked Potentials Symposium. Boston, Butterworths, 1987, pp 309–316.

CHAPTER 11

Neuroimaging of the Spinal Cord

Jack O. Greenberg, M.D.

Use of magnetic resonance imaging (MRI) for diagnosis of spinal disease continues to expand. In most imaging centers, examinations of the spine outnumber brain studies, reflecting not only that back pain is a very common problem[8] but also that definitive diagnosis is no longer deterred by the discomfort and morbidity formerly associated with myelography.

As Oldendorf[31] described in *The Quest for an Image of the Brain*, physicians have also searched for better ways to obtain images of the spine with little discomfort or risk to the patient. Conventional radiography and myelography, the only approaches possible until the early 1970s, have been almost completely replaced by computed tomography (CT) and by MRI. Rapid advances in MRI technology continue to improve the images of the spine and shorten the time needed to do an examination.

The major advance has been improved surface coils. Modern coils and sequence optimization increase signal-to-noise ratio and shorten scanning times. An increased signal-to-noise ratio permits smaller voxel elements and, hence, greater spatial resolution. Methods of eliminating flow artifact, such as refocusing, saturation pulses, and cardiac gating, further improve image quality. Partial flip angle imaging (also called "gradient echo") has improved contrast and produces the desirable myelographic effect (bright cerebrospinal fluid) in shorter time and over a greater extent of the spine. Three-

177

dimensional techniques yield artifact-free complex three-dimensional anatomy of great interest to the neurologist and neurosurgeon.[28]

Initial limitations of MRI, such as thick slices, poor spatial resolution, and long imaging times, have been eliminated. In general, MRI has replaced CT as the neuroimaging method of choice for the evaluation of spine disorders. High-resolution spine images, once the product only of high-field magnets, are now routinely obtained with mid-field scanners in comparable acquisition times. Complete spine studies are now performed in less than 30 minutes.

TECHNICAL CONSIDERATIONS

The spine is first studied with sagittal T1-weighted scans (short TR and TE). These have high signal-to-noise ratios, excellent spatial resolution, and display excellent anatomic detail. At times, the diagnosis of spinal disease is obvious from this first series, permitting the rest of the study to be altered in accordance with the findings. Sagittal gradient recalled (flip angle) sequences with flow compensation are performed next. These produce a myelographic effect that is most useful to show extradural disease, although intramedullary lesions can be seen as well. Axial views then cover the area of lesion detected in the sagittal views. Flip angle axials are usually used for imaging of the cervical spine and proton density spin echo axials for the lumbar spine. With cervical coils, the cervical and thoracic spine to T4 are visualized. In the lumbar area, it is advisable to begin with a body coil (low power) 5-mm T1-weighted study, which displays the spine from T8 to the coccyx and includes a segment of the cord and the conus medullaris. Spinal cord tumors, osteomyelitis, and metastatic disease can be missed in patients with back pain when a small field of view surface coil or a routine CT scan is used to rule out a disk problem (Fig. 11–1). The latter consists only of axial views through L3–4, L4–5, and L5–S1. Surface coil imaging visualizes the spine from L1 to the coccyx. The T1 locator permits the imager to determine where to put the surface coil for high-resolution imaging with a small field of view. A 5-mm double-echo sagittal surface coil study is helpful to determine tissue type (e.g., scar, fluid, tumor). The surface coil will increase the signal-to-noise ratio three- to five-fold. With surface coil imaging, a resolution of 1.25 mm (instead of 0.95 mm) produces excellent quality images in half the time (utilizing a 256 by 128 matrix instead of a 256 by 256 one).[30]

PHYSICAL BASIS OF THE MAGNETIC RESONANCE SIGNAL IN THE SPINAL CORD

The water content of white and gray matter in the spinal cord is similar to that of white and gray matter in the brain. In the brain, gray matter has 12% more free water than white matter and, therefore, has longer relaxation times (T1 and T2) than white matter. Myelin in the white matter also influences magnetic resonance difference between gray and white matter. The membrane lipids of myelin shorten T2 relaxation, causing a lower signal in white than in gray matter.

Similar to lesions in the brain, most abnormalities of the spinal cord cause an increase in free water leading to a low signal on T1-weighted images and a high signal on T2-weighted images along with distorted anatomy.[9]

The signal from the cord reflects water content and relaxation times of gray and white matter. The boundaries of the cord are best seen on high-resolution, flow-compensated, sagittal and axial MRI scans. T1-weighted images show high contrast between cord and cerebrospinal fluid and have the least artifact from cerebrospinal fluid flow.[9]

Cortical bone appears black because of a paucity of mobile hydrogen protons. Cancellous bone has a high fat content and on T1-weighted studies and early echoes of T2 it produces images that are bright. The contrast between cortical and cancellous bone permits excellent anatomic detail. Vertebral bodies, pedicles, facets, and lamina appear as high-signal cancellous bone framed by a thin margin of low-signal cortical bone. On T2-weighted studies fat signal diminishes, and the distinction is not as marked.[30]

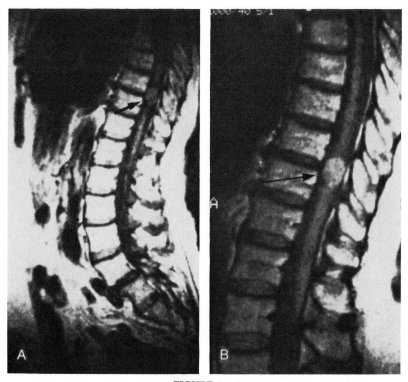

FIGURE 11–1

A, Patient presented with back pain. MR was ordered to rule out disk. 5 mm body locator T1 study. Note round meningioma at T9–10 level (*arrow*). A computed axial tomographic scan performed at the lumbar level missed this lesion. *B,* A 5 mm surface coil proton density study. Tumor is brighter and more obvious.

CONTRAST AGENTS

Paramagnetic contrast agents enhance proton relaxation parameters. Increased signal occurs by shortening T1 relaxation. In addition, these agents also shorten T2 relaxation, an effect that leads to loss of signal. If the concentration of the contrast agent is too large, this effect can override the T1 shortening and cause loss of signal.

In 18 of 30 patients with spinal cord lesions[42] (e.g., tumors, angiomas, myelitis, Wegener's disease), studies with gadolinium–diethylenetriamine penta-acetic acid (Gd-DTPA) were more informative than those without Gd-DTPA. In these patients the T2-weighted spin echo images were not as good as the T1-weighted studies with contrast. Cerebrospinal fluid pulsations often caused artifacts making it difficult to separate the lesion from healthy tissue and cerebrospinal fluid. Both cerebrospinal fluid and lesions led to a

high signal on T2-weighted spin echo studies, again making them difficult to interpret. T1 with Gd-DTPA enhanced the lesion alone. Occasionally, some delayed scans showed greater signal, especially in patients with ependymomas. In patients with intramedullary lesions with cysts (three of four ependymomas, two of six astrocytomas, and two of two hemangioblastomas), Gd-DTPA demonstrated the solid part of the tumor in two ependymomas and in both hemangioblastomas, which helped the surgeon immensely. Patchy enhancement or no enhancement permitted the diagnosis of a low-grade glioma.[42]

Stimac and others[40] utilized Gd-DTPA and short inversion time recovery (STIR) in 20 patients. Gd-DTPA was most helpful in demonstrating intradural tumors, and STIR was most effective in demonstrating extradural tumors and bone metastases. Gd-DTPA can increase signal in bone tumors, causing the postenhanced study to be the same signal as normal bone. Therefore, all patients should have a preenhanced T1 study.

Sze and colleagues[41] reported on 26 patients with intramedullary disease of the spinal cord. They found that contrast could (1) localize a tumor nidus and separate it from edema, (2) localize more active parts of gliomas for biopsy or removal, and (3) possibly differentiate active plaques of multiple sclerosis from inactive ones.

Leptomeningeal spread of tumor, such as lymphoma, breast, or small cell carcinoma of lung (the three most common), can be well visualized by Gd-DTPA when the unenhanced study is not clear.[4]

SPINAL TUMORS

Until the mid-1980s, myelography was the primary mode of investigation in patients suspected of having spinal tumors.[38] Visualization of the subarachnoid space and negative shadows of the cord margins provided a sensitive technique from which originated the useful classification of extradural or intradural extramedullary/intramedullary tumors. Postmyelographic CT provided an additional plane of imaging with superior in-plane contrast resolution.

Magnetic resonance imaging has supplanted CT myelography as the method of choice for the evaluation of spinal tumors. It is noninvasive, has superior multiplanar capabilities for accurate localization, and has unequaled contrast resolution.

The frequency of spinal tumors at various levels of the spinal canal is roughly proportional to the number and length of segments at that level. Only 1% of primary spinal cord tumors involve multiple, separate levels, a finding that should suggest the possibility of neurofibromatosis.[21]

SPECIFIC TUMORS

Intradural

INTRAMEDULLARY. Approximately 90% of intramedullary tumors are gliomas represented mostly by ependymomas, astrocytomas, and oligodendrogliomas.

EPENDYMOMA. This lesion (Fig. 11–2) is the most common glial tumor in adults (65%), especially in the conus medullaris and filum terminale, although any portion of the spinal cord can be involved. MRI findings for all types of intramedullary gliomas are similar, demonstrating fusiform enlargement of the spinal cord over one or several segments by a soft tissue mass of normal or slightly decreased signal intensity on T1 study and high-signal intensity on T2 study that represents both tumor and edema. Cysts may be present. In one series,[39] 38% of astrocytomas and 46% of ependymomas demonstrated syringomyelic cavities at autopsy.

ASTROCYTOMAS. These lesions (Fig. 11–3) represent 30% of intramedullary glial tumors.[39] Seventy-five percent of cord astrocytomas occur in the thoracic-cervical region. They usually extend over 2 vertebral segments but, occasionally, can span 10 or more segments. Unlike ependymomas, there is rarely a cleavage plane between the tumor and cord substance.

HEMANGIOBLASTOMAS. These lesions are uncommon benign tumors of vascular origin. They are frequently confused with vascular malformations or other vascular tumors.

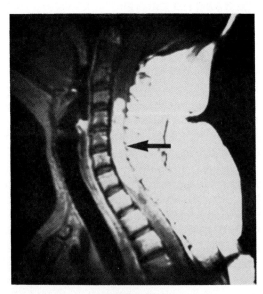

FIGURE 11–2

T1 study with gadolinium revealing an anaplastic ependymoma (*arrow*) in a 40-year-old woman. Tumor was isointense with cord on noncontrast study. The cystic cavity is seen above and below the tumor.

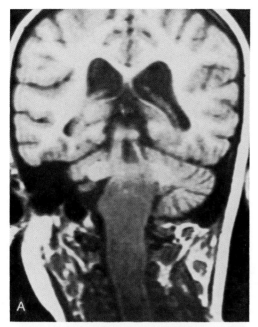

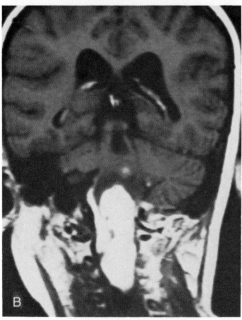

FIGURE 11–3

A, A 5 mm coronal T1 noncontrast study demonstrating an astrocytoma of the cervical cord growing into the medulla. *B*, Same patient after contrast (gadolinium) was given.

They are composed of endothelial cells forming vascular channels separated by lipid-rich cells of obscure nature.[37] They occur primarily in the cervical-thoracic and thoracic-lumbar regions and are often multiple. MRI is extremely helpful because of its ability to image not only the spinal cord but also the posterior fossa structures. On T1-weighted scans a fusiform enlargement of the cord is revealed with multiple or single cysts. On T2-weighted scans there is marked hyperintensity over several segments. Abnormal vascularity is seen as focal or serpiginous areas of low-signal flow-voids. With contrast (Gd-DTPA), there is marked enhancement. In many instances, the tumor nodule is visualized (Fig. 11–4).

OLIGODENDROGLIOMA. This lesion of the spinal cord represents 2.5% of intramedullary glial tumors. MRI experience with this tumor is limited.

METASTATIC INTRAMEDULLARY DISEASE. This is rare, occurring in only 1% to 2% of patients with spinal tumors.

DEVELOPMENTAL TUMORS. Epidermoids, dermoids, lipomas, and teratomas demonstrate a characteristic MRI appearance: high-signal intensity mass on T1-weighted images, which is less intense on T2-weighted scans, frequently seen in conjunction with tethered cord or some form of lipomyelomeningocele[2] (Fig. 11–5). In 5% of normal subjects, prominent high-signal fat is seen on a T1-weighted study of the conus.

Dermoid and epidermoid tumors are cystic lesions lined by single or stratified squamous epithelium. Dermal appendages (hair follicles, sweat glands and sebaceous glands) are found only in dermoid cysts. These constitute 1% to 2% of intraspinal tumors in all age groups and 10% of intraspinal tumors in those younger than 15 years. Both dermoid and epidermoid tumors occur throughout the entire spinal axis in both extramedullary and intramedullary compartments but are more common in the conus medullaris/filum terminale/cauda equina region[1] (Fig. 11–6).

EXTRAMEDULLARY. This group of lesions represents 55% of primary intraspinal tumors. Schwannomas and neurofibromas are two types of nerve sheath tumors. The term schwannoma (neurinoma) applies to benign isolated nerve sheath tumors arising from Schwann cells. Neurofibromas are often multiple, occurring in the context of von Recklinghausen's disease. They include hyperplasia of Schwann cells and fibroblastic supporting elements that separate individual nerve fibers.

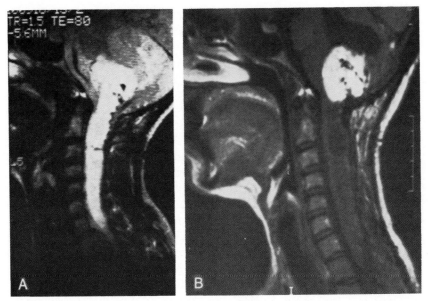

FIGURE 11-4

A, A 5 mm sagittal T2 study (no contrast) demonstrating a hemangioblastoma from the cerebellum to C7 cord. High signal denotes tumor and low signal denotes flow voids from abnormal vessels. The patient had von Hippel-Lindau Syndrome. *B,* T1 sagittal postgadolinium scan performed after the cervical cord portion of the tumor has been surgically removed. Cerebellar portion enhances vividly. Note abnormal vessels in tumor. Syrinx present in cord at C2–3.

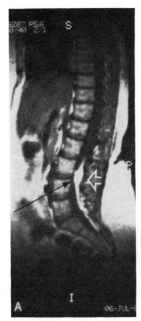

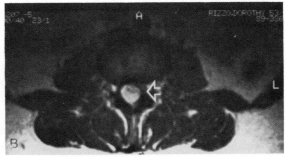

FIGURE 11-5

A, A 5 mm T1 sagittal body coil study demonstrating a lipoma from L3 to S2 (high signal posterior to thecal sac) (*arrow*). *B,* A 5 mm axial T1 scan at L3–4 interspace. Note lipoma compressing thecal sac (comma-shaped structure isointense to muscle to the left of high signal lipoma) (*arrow*).

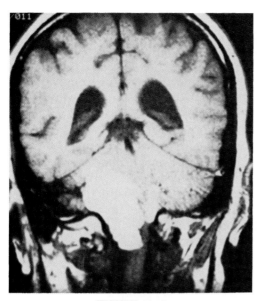

FIGURE 11–6

T1 coronal scan demonstrating a large high signal lesion in the posterior fossa extending through the foramen magnum on the right. This proved to be a dermoid cyst.

NEURINOMAS. These lesions represent 29% of intraspinal tumors and are the most common extramedullary lesions. They are most common in the cervical and thoracic spine. Most neurinomas are extramedullary intra-

dural, 10% are intradural and extradural, and 11% are strictly extradural.

MRI is particularly helpful in the diagnosis of these lesions because the entire spine can be imaged and multiple tumors seen. Neurinomas present as soft tissue masses isointense on T1, usually with displacement of the spinal cord. They have high signals on T2-weighted images. Neurofibromas enhance vividly with Gd-DTPA. Occasionally, syringomyelic cavities occur in the spinal cord secondary to these lesions and are readily demonstrated by MRI (Fig. 11–7).

MENINGIOMA. This lesion is the second most common intradural-extramedullary tumor, representing 25% of all primary intraspinal tumors. MRI demonstrates an isointense signal on T1 and occasionally on T2 also, although instances of hyperintensity have occurred on T2-weighted studies. Similar to neurinomas, meningiomas displace the cord and widen the subarachnoid space. Gadolinium-DTPA–enhanced T1-weighted scans show marked enhancement of the tumor (Fig. 11–8).

EMBRYONAL TUMORS. Epidermoids, dermoids, lipomas, and teratomas have been discussed previously and are typically intradural in location.

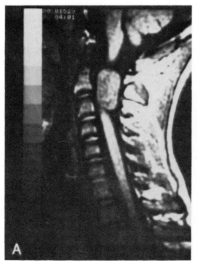
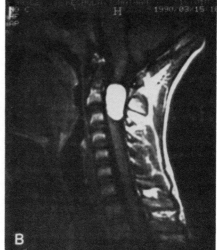

FIGURE 11–7

A, T1 sagittal noncontrast study demonstrating a large isointense lesion growing through the neural foramen at C2. This was a neurofibroma in a 16-year-old boy. *B,* Sagittal T1 study with contrast demonstrating a vividly enhancing neurofibroma.

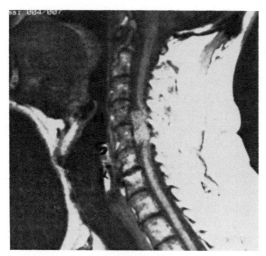

FIGURE 11–8

T1 sagittal noncontrast study in a 66-year-old man with compressive myelopathy. A large isointense meningioma is noted at C4–5.

INTRADURAL-EXTRAMEDULLARY METASTATIC DISEASE (DROP METASTASES). These lesions usually develop from primary intracranial neoplasms of childhood by subarachnoid seeding. Medulloblastomas, ependymomas, malignant gliomas, and germinomas are the usual tumor types presenting with drop metastases. Metastases from outside the nervous system, such as from lung, breast, and melanoma, can also seed the subarachnoid space. Without contrast they can remain relatively inconspicuous as nonspecific subtle filling of the subarachnoid space or thickening of the nerve roots in the cauda equina. The use of contrast in this type of lesion is mandatory (Fig. 11–9).

Extradural

Extradural tumors include primary or metastatic benign and malignant neoplasms involving the vertebrae, adjacent soft tissue, nerve roots, and dura. These lesions account for approximately 30% of all spinal neoplasms. Primary benign soft tissue tumors include a small number of extradural meningiomas, neurinomas, and developmental tumors that have been described previously.

METASTATIC. These extradural lesions present as focal areas of hypointensity in verte-brals bodies on T1-weighted images. The tumor replaces fat, causing a low signal in the vertebral body. On T2 studies the same part of the vertebral body becomes bright. These lesions can narrow the bony canal and cause cord compression. The thoracic spine is most frequently involved, followed by the lumbosacral and cervical regions.

The hallmark on MRI examination is multiple foci of low signal intensity in vertebral bodies on T1-weighted sagittal images (Fig. 11–10). Collapse and destruction of the vertebral body sparing the adjacent disk spaces are common. Epidural invasion and spinal cord compression are clearly seen on unenhanced T1 studies. Gadolinium contrast usually increases the conspicuousness of epidural lesions, but at times, vertebral body involvement can be obscured as low-intensity lesions become isointense with enhancement. STIR and water and fat suppression sequences can be used to increase the sensitivity of MRI examinations in patients with metastatic spine disease.[10]

Multiple myeloma is another form of metastatic disease of the spine. It has a peculiar

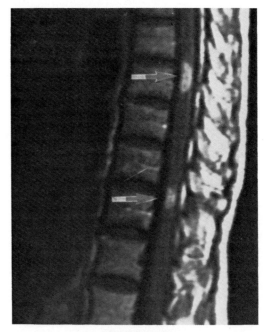

FIGURE 11–9

Sagittal postcontrast T1 study demonstrating drop metastases at two levels (*arrows*). Noncontrast study was normal.

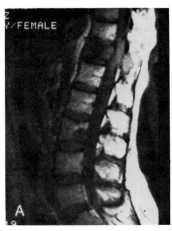
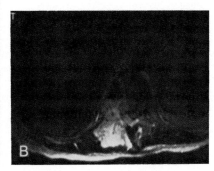

FIGURE 11–10

A, T1 noncontrast study in a 40-year-old woman with breast cancer and back pain. Note the marrow replacement at T12 and partially at L3 posteriorly. There is also cord compression at T12 from tumor and there is tumor in the posterior elements. *B,* Axial T2 (noncontrast) study demonstrates tumor that is brighter than on T1 and involves the pedicle and soft tissues. Note compression of cord by epidural tumor.

"salt-and-pepper" appearance (Fig. 11–11) and represents 34% of malignant bone tumors. Multiple myeloma preferentially involves the thoracic spine, followed by the lumbar, cervical, and sacral regions.[32]

Bone Tumors

HEMANGIOMA. Vertebral hemangiomas are slow-growing benign lesions that are seen in 11% of spines at autopsy and are only rarely symptomatic. They are collections of thin-walled blood vessels or sinuses lined by endothelium interspersed among bony trabeculae and adipose tissue.[29] They are most common in the thoracic spine and have a distinct appearance on MRI. A mottled increased signal intensity is evident on T1-weighted studies secondary to adipose tissue interspersed among thickened bony trabeculae. On T2-weighted images interosseous and extraosseous tumors demonstrate increased signal intensity related to the cellular components of the tumor (Fig. 11–12). Rarely, they may enlarge and cause cord compression.[22]

CHORDOMA. These lesions are rare malignant bone tumors derived from remnants of the notochord. They are usually found in the sacral-coccygeal area, basosphenoid region, and vertebral bodies.[7] Chordomas are isoin-

tense on T1-weighted images and hyperintense on T2 images. They usually present in adults as expansile, destructive lesions.

OSTEOSARCOMA. This is the most common primary malignant bone tumor (excluding

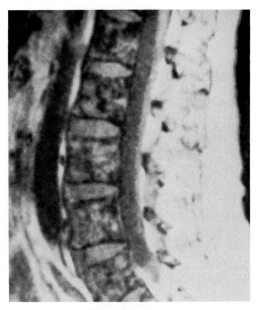

FIGURE 11–11

T1 sagittal spine (noncontrast) scan demonstrating marrow replacement (*dark lesions*) and the typical "salt-and-pepper" appearance of multiple myelomas. (Courtesy of Roger G. Schnell, M.D., F.A.A.N.)

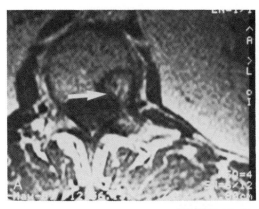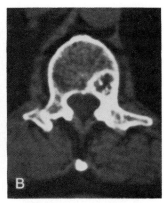

FIGURE 11–12

A, T1 axial noncontrast scan in an elderly man with prostatic cancer. The lesion retains high signal intensity and is a hemangioma of bone (*arrow*). *B,* A computed tomographic scan through the same lesion seen in *A* shows an osteolytic lesion with thick sclerotic margins indicating slow growth. Several rounded densities are seen within the lesion representing thickened trabeculae; this is the characteristic appearance of a hemangioma.

myeloma). Osteosarcomas arise at the growing ends of long bones. They present with pain, neurologic deficit, and a paraspinal soft tissue mass seen on radiography. They can be osteolytic, osteoblastic, or mixed. On T1-weighted images there is a paraspinal mass of low-signal intensity extending through the vertebral body into the epidural space. On T2-weighted images, hyperintensity is evident (Fig. 11–13).

CHONDROSARCOMAS. These lesions are malignant bone tumors related to neoplastic car-

tilage often extending from the medial ends of the ribs.[7] On MRI they are slightly hyperintense relative to vertebral marrow and often similar to muscle. They are typically hyperintense on T2-weighted scans.

GIANT CELL TUMORS. These lesions can be either malignant or benign and may represent as many as 5% of bone tumors. They are most common in the sacral region. They appear as destructive infiltrating lesions of low and high signal on T1-weighted and T2-weighted scans, respectively, and may be contiguous with a paraspinal mass.

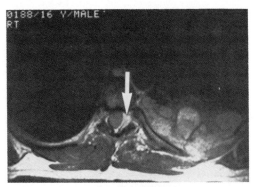

FIGURE 11–13

Axial proton density view through T6 in a 16-year-old boy with progressive cord compression, which proved to be due to an osteogenic sarcoma of the rib growing into the spinal canal and compressing the cord (*arrow*). The bubbly appearance of the high-signal structure denotes tumor growing out of the rib. (Courtesy of Carl Ellenberger, M.D.)

INFECTION

Symptoms arising from spinal infection can mimic those of neoplasm or degenerative disease. Spinal infection is frequently an insidious disorder and can remain undiagnosed for a long period. Changes on plain film take days to weeks to become manifest. In the past, the one diagnostic test that gave the highest yield was the radionuclide scan. Although sensitive and specific, radionuclide scanning can take hours to days to perform and may be equivocal. CT can add further information when bony and soft tissue components are present. MRI has a high sensitivity for infection in either bone or soft tissue and can detect such infections even when radiographic and isotope scans are normal. In one study, MRI had a sensitivity of 96%, a specificity of 93%, and an accuracy of 94% in 37 patients suspected of having vertebral osteomyelitis.[24]

Osteomyelitis of the spine and disk space produces characteristic changes in the vertebrae and disks on MRI (Fig. 11–14). Decreased signal intensity of the vertebral bodies and the intervertebral disk space with obliteration of the disk margins and the adjacent end plates occurs on T1-weighted images. In contrast, metastasis to the spine usually leaves the end plates intact. Increased signal intensity in the vertebral bodies adjacent to the disk, as well as increased signal intensity in the disk itself, occurs on T2-weighted images. This pattern clearly distinguishes disk space infection from neoplasm. MRI is positive early in the course of disk space infection, and in some patients may be the only abnormality found after obtaining a bone scan, gallium scan, CT, or plain film. It is also useful in the follow-up of disk space infection, because eventually the vertebral

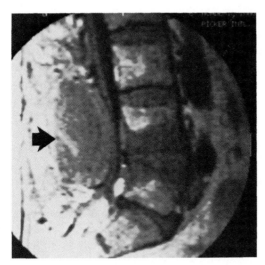

FIGURE 11–14

T1 sagittal spine (noncontrast) scan demonstrating low signal replacing marrow at L4 and L5. The end plates are destroyed, indicating the presence of discitis and osteomyelitis. The low signal behind the thecal sac compressing it is a huge epidural abscess (*arrow*). On T2 these lesions (abscess, discitis, and osteomyelitis) were bright. This proved to be secondary to staphylococcal infection. The bone scan was normal early in the course when the magnetic resonance imaging scan was positive.

body and disk return to normal signal intensity with successful treatment.

Epidural infections result from extension of vertebral osteomyelitis (Fig. 11–15). Differentiation of degenerative disease and tumor from vertebral osteomyelitis is easier by MRI than by radionuclide studies or plain films. Degenerated disks have decreased signal intensity on T2-weighted images, whereas infected disks have high-signal intensity. Severe degenerative disease can produce changes similar to vertebral osteomyelitis on plain films and radionuclide studies. On MRI, degenerative disk disease may lead to decreased signal intensity within the adjacent vertebral bodies on T1-weighted images and increased signal intensity on T2-weighted images (type 1 degenerative marrow changes). However, the disk space is not involved and is clearly distinguished from the vertebral body end plate on T1-weighted images. Involvement of extravertebral osseous or soft tissue structures is better appreciated with radionuclide studies, because these are generally whole body examinations.

On MRI, tuberculous spondylitis may resemble tumor rather than infection, because it may spare the disk space and not produce abnormally increased signal on T2-weighted images. Both tuberculosis and fungal infections can produce large paraspinal soft tissue masses preferentially involving the posterior elements. The lack of disk involvement is thought to be due to a lack of proteolytic enzymes in mycobacteria.[5]

RHEUMATOID ARTHRITIS

Rheumatoid arthritis produces synovial inflammation, which results in destruction of subchondrial bone and cartilage by the pannus. Subluxation and dislocation can result from laxity of joint capsules and ligaments. In 60% to 70% of patients with rheumatoid arthritis, symptoms related to the cervical spine develop during the course of their illness. A variety of subluxations can occur at the atlantoaxial joint and are easily identified by MRI. MRI is as accurate as tomography in evaluating the atlantodental interval, dens erosion, osteophytes, and the various C1–2

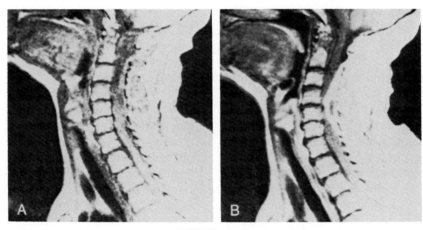

FIGURE 11–15

A, Precontrast T1 sagittal view of cervical spine in a 73-year-old woman with fever and cord signs. No definite abnormality was seen. B, Contrast scan of same patient as in A demonstrates large epidural abscess posterior to and compressing spinal cord from C2 to C6.

subluxations. Pannus is found behind the dens as increased soft tissue material. Loss of the normal fat pad rostral to the dens suggests thickened ligaments or pannus. When brain stem symptoms are present, MRI consistently shows marked cranial-vertebral junction abnormalities.[3]

DEGENERATIVE DISEASE

Degenerative disorders of the spine are among the most common causes of complaints in the general population and are the leading cause of disability in the working years. Radiculopathies, myelopathies, and conus syndromes are the clinical presentations; all of these can be caused by either osseous or soft tissue structural abnormalities of the spine. CT is better for detecting osseous abnormalities, whereas MRI is the procedure of choice for soft tissue abnormalities.

Degenerative disk disease is a process that begins early in life, can be caused by several factors, and can be a part of normal aging. Disk degeneration and herniation remain among the leading causes of functional incapacitation. Many asymptomatic patients will have degenerative disk disease and, indeed, may have large asymptomatic disk herniations.[18, 20a] Clinical correlation is still the most important aspect in deciding treatment.

Plain films, myelography, CT, and MRI all have been used in the diagnosis of degenerative disk disease, and it is clear that MRI has become the dominant imaging modality.

Modic and co-workers[26] found 86.8% agreement between MRI and CT findings in all patients at 151 levels. There was 87.2% agreement between MRI and myelography. In surgical patients, 82.3% agreement was noted between MRI and surgical findings and 83% between CT and surgical findings. There was 71% agreement between myelography and surgical findings, 92.5% agreement between metrizamide CT and surgical findings, and 81% agreement between plain CT and surgical findings. When MRI and CT were used jointly, combined results agreed with surgical findings in 92.5% of patients. All disks were normal on MRI when they were normal on CT and myelography.

MRI is as accurate as CT and slightly more accurate than myelography in evaluating lumbar disk disease and canal stenosis.[25] Combined results of MRI and CT are as accurate as those of CT and myelography. MRI is much better than myelography for detecting lateral disk herniations, which are missed regularly with the latter (Fig. 11–16). Another advantage of MRI is that the spine can be seen above and below a block (Fig. 11–17), whereas myelography does not give information distal to a block. Modic and colleagues[25]

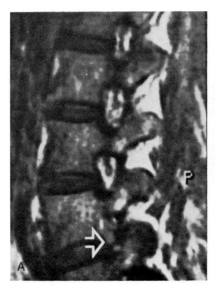
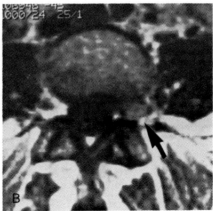

FIGURE 11–16

A, T1 lateral spine scan demonstrating a large structure (*arrow*) beneath and compressing the nerve root at L4–5 on the right. It is isointense with nerve root. *B,* Axial 5 mm cut. Note large lateral disk herniation (*arrow*).

concluded that a technically accurate MRI is equivalent to CT and myelography in the diagnosis of lumbar spinal canal stenosis and herniated nucleus pulposus. A disagreement ranging from 17% to 29% with the surgical findings still occurs when any of the three modalities is used alone. The disagreement is most apparent in the evaluation of lumbar stenosis. CT and MRI can be complementary studies, but MRI is an important alternative to myelography. Although CT is superior in providing definition of osseous abnormalities, MRI is capable of showing cortical bone disruption and distortion of facet articular surfaces in two planes and is excellent for detecting nerve root canal stenosis. When a T1-weighted image is used, the relatively low-intensity nerve roots can easily be distinguished from the surrounding fat in the neural foramina. Images with more T2 weighting increase the contrast differentiation between the herniated disk and the cerebrospinal fluid. More lateral herniations of the disk can be identified by distortion of the epidural fat on parasagittal images, and these can all be correlated easily with the axial images.

Changes in water content are probably responsible for the loss of signal in the disk in degenerative disease. All degenerated disks are not herniated, but almost all herniated disks have degenerated. The exception is the acute herniated disk, which retains high signal intensity. Hypertrophic facet joints and bony overgrowth are clearly appreciated, but the distinction between hypertrophy of the ligamentum flavum and overgrowth of corti-

FIGURE 11–17

From a 60-year-old patient who is paraplegic after a fall. Note huge disk extrusion compressing cord at C6–7 (*arrow*) on this T1-unenhanced sagittal scan.

cal bone is difficult because of the similar hypointensity.[27]

Modic and others[26] studied cervical radiculopathy. They found that MRI findings agreed with surgical findings 74% of the time. The findings on CT with metrizamide agreed with surgical findings 85% of the time, and the findings on myelography agreed with surgical findings 67% of the time. When MRI and CT with metrizamide were used together, the findings agreed 90% of the time with surgical findings, and when CT with metrizamide was used with myelography, the findings agreed with surgical findings 92% of the time. MRI is as good for determining the level of disease as CT with metrizamide but not as useful in specifying disease type. With CT, there is good resolution of bone vs. soft tissue. The advantage of MRI is that the whole cervical canal can be seen, including high signals with gliosis, hematoma, and other intrinsic processes. Osteophyte signal can vary depending on whether fat is present in the marrow of the osteophyte. If a low-signal osteophyte protrudes into the spinal fluid and the spinal fluid has low intensity as on a T1-weighted study, the osteophyte will be invisible. Another problem with MRI of the cervical spine is that oblique foramina are difficult to visualize. Oblique imaging in MRI of the cervical spine has solved this problem.

DEMYELINATING DISEASE OF THE SPINAL CORD

Multiple sclerosis affects white matter in the brain and spinal cord with almost equal frequency. Before the availability of MRI, plaques were occasionally seen in the brain with CT, but there was no way of directly imaging plaques in the spinal cord. Anecdotal reports demonstrated cord swelling on myelography and CT and, in one patient, with intravenous contrast enhancement on CT.[6] MRI can image subtle changes in water content and proton relaxation time and permits identification of multiple sclerosis plaques in a manner unmatched by any other imaging modality.

When a spinal cord lesion is seen in a patient in whom multiple sclerosis is suspected

on a clinical basis, MRI of the brain should be performed. High signals in the white matter of the brain in a distribution typical of multiple sclerosis confirm the diagnosis (Fig. 11–18). Given a typical clinical history, supporting neurologic examination, and lesions in the brain and cord typical of multiple sclerosis, no further studies are necessary. Collagen vascular disease, Lyme disease, infection, immune myelitis, and tumor should be ruled out with appropriate studies as necessary.

Techniques

The best protocols for imaging multiple sclerosis in the cord are flow-compensated T2-weighted spin echo images in the sagittal plane. With high field magnets, it may be necessary to perform cardiac gating, but with mid-field magnets this has not been necessary. T2-weighted images are sensitive to increases in water content that accompany the perivenular inflammation and edema in the acute lesions of multiple sclerosis. Acute and chronic lesions both give high signals relative

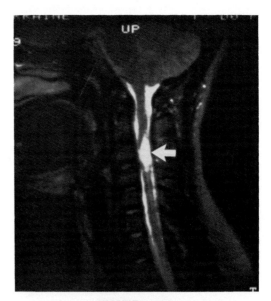

FIGURE 11–18

From a 27-year-old woman with subacute myelopathy. This T2 study demonstrates a large high signal area at C3 (*arrow*). Brain magnetic resonance imaging revealed the classic picture of multiple sclerosis. (Courtesy of Carl Ellenberger, M.D.)

to that given by the normal cord.[20] Axial flip angle images are useful in helping to locate plaques and in correlation with what is seen on the sagittal views. T1-weighted studies are usually not helpful in spinal cord multiple sclerosis, although at times, swelling is noted with acute lesions. Occasionally we have found contrast agents useful in spinal cord multiple sclerosis. A possible explanation is that acute plaques in multiple sclerosis enhance (and chronic lesions do not) because of leaky endothelium and blood-cord barrier breakdown.[20] Enhancement in cerebral lesions seems to correlate with active symptoms.[17] Some acutely enhancing cerebral lesions may resolve completely on follow-up MRI after steroid therapy, and in some patients, this has occurred spontaneously without steroid therapy. This suggests that the acute inflammatory phase of this disease may not always progress to permanent demyelination or gliosis.[33] This same phenomenon has not been demonstrated in the spinal cord.

MRI shows lesions in the spinal cord in 75% to 86% of patients with clinically suspected multiple sclerosis of the spinal cord. In a series by Maravella and co-workers,[23] lesions were seen in the cervical spinal cord in 48% of patients with or without myelopathic symptoms. Typical periventricular cerebral lesions of multiple sclerosis were seen in 81% of patients with myelopathic symptoms and positive spinal MRIs in one series.[11]

In patients with myelopathy, spinal cord lesions can present with normal findings on MRI of the brain and, conversely, brain lesions can present with normal findings on a spinal cord study. The rate of true negative findings on MRI studies of the spinal cord is not precisely known because pathologic material is not available from most of the patients with multiple sclerosis who have undergone imaging.[11]

VASCULAR DISEASES

Arteriovenous Malformations

Two types of arteriovenous malformations of the spinal cord are seen: intradural and dural. Intradural malformations are usually obvious on MRI, especially if they are large (Fig. 11–19). They are often associated with arterial or venous aneurysms and can present as a subarachnoid hemorrhage.[36] MRI findings in intramedullary spinal cord arteriovenous malformations are quite prominent. Glomus and juvenile types of intradural arteriovenous malformations have a nidus that is in the parenchyma of the spinal cord, and the appearance is similar to that seen with an arteriovenous nidus. Multiple serpiginous signal voids are seen. Signal voids are areas with rapid blood flow through abnormal vessels. High signal on T1-weighted images may represent methemoglobin from a previous hemorrhage, and low signal on either T1-weighted or T2-weighted or flip angle studies usually represents hemosiderin from previous hemorrhages. Abnormal gliotic tissue can be seen as high signal on T2-weighted studies. Small intradural arteriovenous malformations can be difficult to detect or to differentiate from low-flow (cryptic) arteriovenous malformations. Intravenous gadolinium can be helpful in detecting the nidus or the draining vessels.[12]

Dural arteriovenous malformations have a nidus located near a nerve root sleeve and are found in the dura itself.[19] They may be so small that they are not seen on MRI. There are no areas with signal voids. Dural arteriovenous malformations are detected by noting their secondary effects, i.e., enlarged draining veins on the dorsal surface of the spinal cord and cord enlargement related to congestion secondary to elevated venous pressure. Gadolinium may demonstrate slow flow in abnormal veins.

Cryptic vascular malformations are vascular lesions in the brain that are not seen on angiography. They also can be seen in the spinal cord and include thrombosed arteriovenous malformations, cavernous hemangiomas (cavernomas) (Fig. 11–20), capillary telangiectasia, and venous angiomas. Venous angiomas have a characteristic large draining vein that can be seen on MRI. The other three lesions are difficult to differentiate. Cavernomas have multiloculated, hemorrhagic cysts similar to those seen in the brain. If such lesions are seen in the spinal cord, a scan of the brain may demonstrate similar lesions

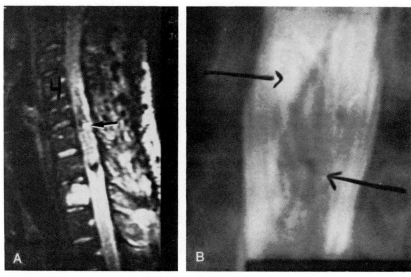

FIGURE 11–19

A, T2 sagittal spine image demonstrates multiple low signals in the spinal cord from C4 to C7, which represent serpiginous vessels and hemosiderin from a previous bleed. The high signal in center of the lesion (*arrow*) represents methemoglobin. *B,* Myelogram demonstrates the arteriovenous malformation of cord (*arrows*).

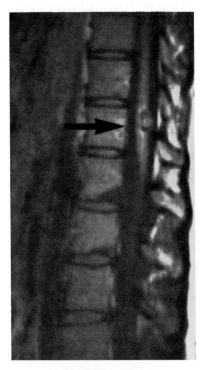

FIGURE 11–20

T1 noncontrast sagittal view demonstrating a lesion in the conus with high signal intensity inside and outside (methemoglobin) and a dark area between these two areas (hemosiderin). This is a cavernous angioma (*arrow*).

because 25% of such patients have multiple arteriovenous malformations.[19] MRI findings in cavernoma are similar to those in chronic hematoma. On T1 study there is a central area of isointensity or hyperintensity surrounded by a ring of low signal that represents hemosiderin. Occasionally, on T2-weighted scans the central portion becomes bright and the outer signal is low. Flip angle studies accentuate the low signal of the hemosiderin. Small additional lesions may be seen in the spinal cord when the flip angle study is used; it may demonstrate multiple areas of low signal.[19]

The MRI findings in cord infarction are similar to those in brain infarction, i.e., low signal on a T1 study and high signal on T2. Occasionally, the lesion can be enhanced by gadolinium (Fig. 11–21).

EPIDURAL HEMORRHAGE

Epidural hemorrhage is rare[34, 44] but MRI can enable the physician to make this important diagnosis quickly. The MRI findings are those of acute hemorrhage in the first few days. On T1-weighted images, the extradural lesion will have high signal intensity, al-

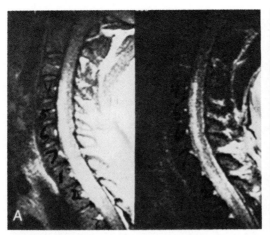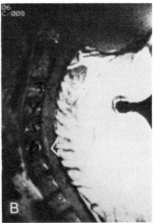

FIGURE 11–21

A, Proton density on left and T2 on right. High signal of anterior cord extends from C4 to T2. This is a spinal infarction secondary to anterior spinal artery thrombosis. *B,* T1 sagittal view with gadolinium demonstrating enhancement at C6 not seen on unenhanced T1 study—spinal cord infarction (*arrow*).

though occasionally it may have intermediate signal due to methemoglobin. On T2-weighted scans the appearance will depend on the age of the hemorrhage. In the acute stage it may be low signal because of the desoxyhemoglobin or high signal because of high proton density or high water content.[16] All of the changes seen in the evolution of blood breakdown on high field MRI scanning are diagnosed easily with mid-field magnets utilizing flip angle studies (Fig. 11–22).

CONGENITAL ANOMALIES

The fact that in many infants the spine can be imaged in one sequence makes MRI extremely helpful in the treatment of the infant

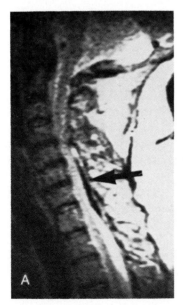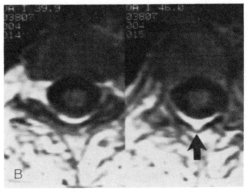

FIGURE 11–22

A, T2 sagittal cervical spine image following neck trauma. Large black lesion (*arrow*) is an epidural clot that is chronic (hemosiderin). *B,* Image from the same patient after surgical removal of epidural clot. High signal area dorsal to cord on this T1-unenhanced axial study (*arrow*) indicates methemoglobin related to surgery.

with anomalies such as Chiari's malformation, meningomyelocele, tethered cord, and syringomyelia. MRI can also demonstrate spinal dysraphism, such as failures of segmentation, duplications of spinal cord, and scoliosis.[2]

Frequently, the imager is asked to determine whether a patient with one congenital anomaly, such as a meningomyelocele, has other associated lesions, such as Chiari's malformation with obstructive hydrocephalus, syringomyelia, diastematomyelia, or tethering of the cord. When imaging for congenital spine lesions, the physician should include the base of the skull and the entire spine.

Plain radiography can diagnose the Klippel-Feil syndrome. At times, however, associated anomalies are seen with this entity that can be diagnosed easily by MRI. These include syringobulbia, syringomyelia, spina bifida, lipoma, hemivertebrae, and diastematomyelia.[35]

The most common and serious congenital anomaly of the spine is the defect in neural and posterior bony elements known as spina bifida. A high association exists between this defect and other anomalies such as tethered spinal cord, sacral lipoma, diastematomyelia, and syringomyelia.[14] These anomalies may manifest clinically later in life. Any patient with spina bifida occulta in whom neurologic symptoms develop should have further investigations for these occult anomalies. One single sagittal sequence can diagnose Chiari's malformation, hydrosyringomyelia, tethered cord, and diastematomyelia in the same patient (Fig. 11–23).

The Chiari I malformation is not usually associated with spina bifida or hydrocephalus but is commonly associated with hydrosyringomyelia of the cervical and thoracic spinal cord (Fig. 11–24). This anomaly can remain asymptomatic into adulthood and can present with upper extremity sensory symptoms. All patients with cervical hydrosyringomyelia who do not have a Chiari malformation should undergo investigation for a spinal cord tumor including contrast MRI. The hydrosyringomyelia should always be fully imaged throughout the spinal cord with sagittal and axial MRI because the neurosurgeon needs to know the full extent of the syrinx.

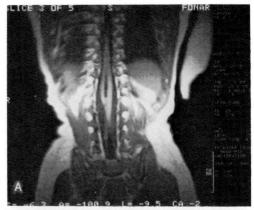

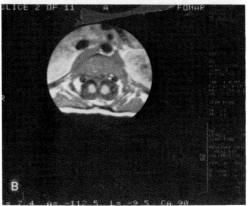

FIGURE 11–23

A, Coronal T1 study through the lower thoracic cord in a child with diastematomyelia. B, Axial view of same subject demonstrates a midline septum and split cord on T1 study. (Courtesy of George W. Privett, Jr., M.D.)

Hydromyelia is dilatation of the central canal of the spinal cord. Syringomyelia refers to dissections from the central canal into the spinal cord. On MRI it is difficult to differentiate between these two entities, and the term *hydrosyringomyelia* may be appropriate (Fig. 11–25).

The diagnosis of tethered cord has occurred more frequently since the utilization of MRI. The tethered spinal cord lies below the L3 level. At times, a thickening in the filum terminale can be seen, which is a normal variant. Occasionally the tethered cord may terminate in a lipoma or a dermal sinus. All of these features are clearly seen on MRI (Fig. 11–26).

Duplications of the spinal cord include diastematomyelia and diplomyelia. The latter is extremely rare and refers to a true duplication

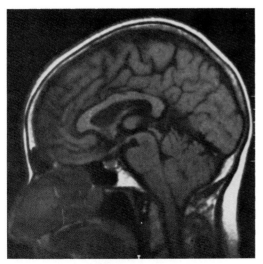

FIGURE 11–24

Sagittal T1 study demonstrates tonsillar invasion of foramen magnum—Chiari I malformation without a syrinx.

of the whole spinal cord. A more common defect is diastematomyelia in which there is splitting or only partial duplication of the spinal cord, with each half having its own dorsal and ventral roots, often in association with a bony or fibrous spur that divides the cord. This spur may result in tethering.[43]

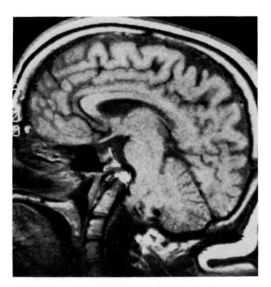

FIGURE 11–25

T1-unenhanced study demonstrates basilar invagination. Note fat pad of dens (high signal) approaching the pons, platybasia, and a large syrinx in this 24-year-old man.

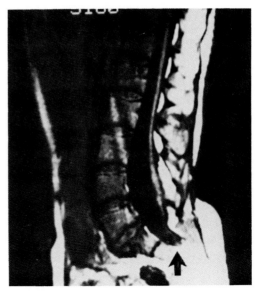

FIGURE 11–26

From a 24-year-old woman with calf atrophy, gait disorder, and areflexia. Scan demonstates cord tethered at S2 (*arrow*).

Intraspinal enterogenous cyst is a rare finding. Fifty-three cases have been reported in the world literature since this was first described in 1934 as an *intestinoma*.[13] This lesion is a cyst lined by columnar mucin-secreting epithelium, usually without cilia, similar to that of the gastrointestinal tract. An endodermal rest lies between the primitive notochord and the neuroectoderm and forms a cystic mass. Intraspinal enterogenous cysts usually occur in patients younger than 40 years with a 2:1 male-to-female preference. The most common location is in the cervical spine extending over two to three segments and is intradural-extramedullary typically anterior to the spinal cord (Fig. 11–27). Fifty percent of these cysts are associated with other congenital anomalies, such as spina bifida, fused vertebrae, hemivertebrae, or anterior spina bifida. MRI reveals low signal on T1-weighted images and high signal on T2-weighted images.[13]

CONCLUSION

Magnetic resonance imaging is the imaging procedure of choice for the evaluation of spi-

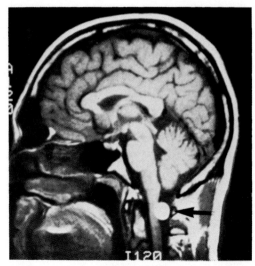

FIGURE 11–27

Sagittal T1 study in a 32-year-old man with progressive myelopathy. The high signal round structure compressing the cord at C1–2 is a neuroenteric cyst with highly proteinacious fluid (*arrow*).

nal disease. Centers wherein the rates of myelography have not decreased are those without access to MRI. CT is excellent for detecting osseous abnormalities, but reformated sagittal and coronal scans do not compare with those of MRI. The ability to see the entire cord in its length has made the diagnosis of spinal disease easier. With new software permitting faster scans and new coil designs, MRI has come of age in evaluating spinal disease.

REFERENCES

1. Alves AM, Norrell H: Intramedullary epidermoid tumors of the spinal cord. Int Surg 54:239, 1970.
2. Barnes PD, Lester PD, Yamanashi WS, et al: Magnetic resonance imaging in infants and children with spinal dysraphism. AJNR 7:465, 1986.
3. Beltram J, Caudill JL, Herman L, et al: Rheumatoid arthritis: MR imaging manifestations. Radiology 165:153, 1987.
4. Berns D, Blaser S, Ross J, et al: MR imaging with Gd-DTPA in leptomeningeal spread of lymphoma. J Comput Assist Tomogr 12:499, 1988.
5. Chapman M, Murray RO, Stokes DJ: Tuberculosis of the bones and joints. Semin Roentgenol 14:266, 1979.
6. Coin CH, Hucks-Follis A: Cervical computed tomography in multiple sclerosis with spinal cord involvement. J Comput Assist Tomogr 3:421, 1979.
7. Dakin DC: Bone Tumors: General Aspects and Data on 6,221 Cases. Springfield, Ill, Charles C Thomas, 1978, pp 329–343.
8. Editorial: Progress in back pain. Lancet 1:977, 1981.
9. Enzmann DR, Delapaz RL, Rubin JB: Magnetic Resonance of the Spine. St. Louis, Mosby–Year Book, 1990, pp 110–114.
10. Enzmann DR, Delapaz RL, Rubin JB: Magnetic Resonance of the Spine. St. Louis, Mosby–Year Book, 1990, pp 301–402.
11. Enzmann DR, Delapaz RL, Rubin JB: Magnetic Resonance of the Spine. St. Louis, Mosby–Year Book, 1990, pp 423–434.
12. Enzmann DR, Delapaz RL, Rubin JB: Magnetic Resonance of the Spine. St. Louis, Mosby–Year Book, 1990, pp 521–526.
13. Enzmann DR, Delapaz RL, Rubin JB: Magnetic Resonance of the Spine. St. Louis, Mosby–Year Book, 1990, pp 231–232.
14. Flannigan-Sprague B, Modic MT: The pediatric spine: Normal anatomy and spinal dysraphism. In Modic MT, Masaryk TJ, Ross JS (eds): Magnetic Resonance Imaging of the Spine. Chicago, Year Book Medical Publishers, 1989, pp 240–256.
15. Garland H, Greenberg JO, Harriman D: Infarction of the spinal cord. Brain 89:645, 1966.
16. Gomori JM, Grossman RI, Hackney DB, et al: Variable appearance of subacute intracranial hematomas on high-field spin-echo MR. AJNR 8:1019, 1987.
17. Gonzalez-Scarano F, Grossman RI, Galetta S, et al: Multiple sclerosis disease activity correlates with gadolinium-enhanced magnetic resonance imaging. Ann Neurol 21:300, 1987.
18. Greenberg JO, Schnell RG: Magnetic resonance imaging of the lumbar spine in asymptomatic adults. J Neuroimaging 1:2, 1991.
19. Griffen C, De La Paz R, Enzmann DR: Magnetic resonance appearance of slow flow vascular malformations of the brainstem. Neuroradiology 29:512, 1987.
20. Grossman RI, Lisak RP, Macchi PJ, et al: MR of acute experimental allergic encephalomyelitis. AJNR 8:1045, 1987.
20a. Jensen MC, Brant-Zawadzki MN, Obuchowski N, et al: Magnetic resonance imaging of the lumbar spine in people without back pain. N Engl J Med 331:69–73, 1994.
21. Kernohan JN, Sayre GP: Tumors of the central nervous system. In National Research Council, Atlas of Tumor Pathology. Washington, DC, Armed Forces Institute of Pathology, 1952.
22. Lare DJD, Reizine D, Bard M, et al: Vertebral hemangiomas: Radiologic evaluation. Radiology 161:182, 1986.
23. Maravella KR, Weinreb JC, Suss R, et al: Magnetic resonance demonstration of multiple sclerosis plaques in the spinal cord. AJNR 5:685, 1984.
24. Modic MT, Feiglin DH, Piraino DW, et al: Vertebral osteomyelitis: Assessments using MR. Radiology 157:157, 1985.
25. Modic MT, Masaryk T, Baumphrey F, et al: Lumbar herniated disc disease and canal stenosis. AJNR 7:709, 1986.
26. Modic MT, Masaryk TJ, Mulopulos GP: Cervical radiculopathy: Prospective evaluation with surface coil MR imaging, CT with methcyanide and metrizamide myelography. Radiology 161:753, 1985.
27. Modic MT, Masaryk T, Paushter D: Magnetic resonance imaging of the spine. Radiol Clin North Am 24:229, 1986.
28. Modic MT, Ross JR: Morphology symptoms and causality. Radiology 175:619, 1990.
29. Murray RO, Jacobson HG: Radiology of Skeletal Dis-

orders, ed 2. New York, Churchill Livingstone, 1977, p 578.

30. Norman D: MRI of the central nervous system. In Brant-Zawadski M, Norman D (eds): MRI of the Central Nervous System. New York, Raven Press, 1987, pp 289–328.

31. Oldendorf WH: The Quest for an Image of the Brain. New York, Raven Press, 1980.

32. Onofrio BM, Svien HJ: Solitary and multiple vertebral myelomas. In Vinken PJ, Bruyn GW (eds): Handbook of Clinical Neurology, vol 20. Tumors of the Spine and Spinal Cord. New York, Elsevier-North Holland, 1976, pp 9–18.

33. Poser CM, Kleefield J, O'Reilly GV, et al: Neuroimaging and the lesion of multiple sclerosis. AJNR 8:549, 1987.

34. Post MJD, Seminar DS, Quencer RM: CT diagnosis of spinal epidural hematoma. AJNR 3:190, 1982.

35. Roaf R: Scoliosis, spondylodysplasia, and other spine malformations. In Vinken PJ, Bruyn GW (eds): Handbook of Clinical Neurology, vol 32. Congenital Malformations of the Spine and Spinal Cord. Amsterdam, North-Holland 1986, pp 131–158.

36. Rosenblum B, Oldfield EH, Doppman JL, et al: Spinal arteriovenous malformations: A comparison of dural arteriovenous fistulas and intradural AVM's in 81 patients. J Neurosurg 67:795, 1987.

37. Russell DS, Rubinstein CJ: Pathology of Tumors of the Nervous System. Baltimore, Williams & Wilkins, 1989.

38. Shapiro R: Tumors, Myelography. Chicago, Year Book Medical Publishers, 1984, pp 345–421.

39. Sloof JL, Kernohan JW, Macarty JB: Primary Intramedullary Tumors of the Spinal Cord and Filum Terminale. Philadelphia, WB Saunders, 1964.

40. Stimac GK, Porter B, Olson D, et al: Gadolinium-DTPA-enhancing MR imaging of spinal neoplasms. AJNR 9:839, 1988.

41. Sze G, Krol G, Zimmerman RD, et al: Intramedullary disease of the spine: Diagnosis using Gd-DTPA-enhanced MR imaging. AJNR 9:847, 1988.

42. Valk J: Gd-DTPA in MR of spinal lesions. AJNR 9:345, 1988.

43. Wolf A, Tubman DE, Seljeskog EL: Diastematomyelia of the cervical cord with tethering in an adult. Neurosurgery 21:94, 1987.

44. Zilkha A, Irwin GAL, Fagelman D: Computed tomography of spinal epidural hematoma. AJNR 4:1073, 1983.

CHAPTER 12

Neurogenic Urinary Tract Infection

Samuel L. Stover, M.D.
L. Keith Lloyd, M.D.
Ken B. Waites, M.D.
Amie B. Jackson, M.D.

Spinal cord pathologic lesions often lead to neurologic deficits that affect the coordinated control of the bladder, which frequently results in incomplete bladder emptying that predisposes to bacteriuria. The roles of bacteriuria, intravesical pressure, and the possible alteration of host defense mechanisms in the development of renal failure are still uncertain. Because advances in urologic management have lessened the incidence and severity of renal complications, renal failure is no longer the leading cause of death following spinal cord injury. However, renal function is often compromised, and alterations in upper urinary tract morphology and physiology secondary to infection are common.[28, 49, 61] As prevention and treatment strategies have advanced, sepsis rather than renal failure has become the more common cause of death relating to the urinary tract.[8]

The following terms and definitions are used throughout this chapter and are selected because of their general acceptance in recent medical literature:[56]

- Asymptomatic bacteriuria: Bacteriuria without clinical symptoms.

- Colonization: Bacteriuria without tissue invasion.

- Urinary tract infection: Microbial invasion of any of the tissues of the urinary tract.

- Uncomplicated urinary tract infection: Community-acquired cystitis without structural or neurologic abnormalities.

- Complicated urinary tract infection: Presence of any underlying condition making therapy less effective, i.e., neurogenic bladder, large residual urine volumes, renal parenchymal disease, tumors, stones, and structural abnormalities.
- Relapse: The recurrence of bacteriuria from infection with the same organism within a defined interval after treatment.
- Reinfection: Isolation of a new pathogen within a defined interval after treatment.

When a common terminology base is not used, the results of research and treatment are often confusing. Bacteriuria is not necessarily synonymous with urinary tract infection. When urine cultures are positive, the question of colonization vs. true infection remains. Without precise methods of determining the extent and location of tissue invasion, some terms remain vague and need to be considered in regard to their relationship to the source of the specimen, method of collection, bacterial colony count, and other associated laboratory findings. Unfortunately, the terminology in this chapter is also sometimes confusing, because the terms and definitions used from referenced articles follow the use described in that literature.

PATHOPHYSIOLOGY AND PATHOGENESIS

The pathologic status of the entire urinary tract after spinal cord injury is dependent on the status of the bladder. Neurologic damage and the need for bladder instrumentation result in impairment of the normal anatomic and physiologic defense mechanisms responsible for eliminating bacteria and maintaining sterility of this system. Normally, the physical barrier of the urethra, urine flow, various antibacterial enzymes and antibodies, and toxic or antiadherence effects mediated by bladder mucosal cells limit spread and multiplication of bacteria in the urinary tract.[1, 3, 30, 56]

The type of neurogenic bladder that develops after spinal cord injury depends on the location of the neurologic lesion and the length of time after injury. Immediately following injury, a state of spinal shock develops in which there is absent or markedly diminished reflex activity for varying periods. During this time, some reflex activity may be present in the sacral segments, whereas reflex activity in the bladder detrusor muscle may be absent. Days to weeks later, detrusor reflex activity may return in patients in whom the injury was to the spinal cord, whereas reflex activity to the detrusor almost never returns in an injury of the conus medullaris or cauda equina. Under such abnormal neurologic conditions, in which there is complete or partial denervation or unrestrained reflex activity, the lower urinary tract is typically affected. Lower tract involvement is frequently a precursor to upper tract involvement. Bladder pathophysiology after denervation is affected secondarily by derangement of smooth muscle and neural tissue of the bladder wall, which occurs if there is overdistension, chronic infection, or both.[34, 44] Therefore, the goals of bladder management after spinal cord injury are to establish and maintain unrestricted urine flow from the kidneys and to maintain urine sterility and bladder continence, ultimately preserving renal function.

With normal bladder emptying, a natural washout effect eliminates the vast majority of all bacteria that may be present. Those remaining may be adherent to the bladder epithelium or located in the film of urine that covers the mucosa. If the bladder is emptied frequently and adequately, residual organisms do not have a chance to multiply before washout occurs. However, in the neurogenic bladder, stagnant residual urine frequently remains for long periods of time, permitting large colony counts to be attained.[42] Mucosal ischemia associated with obstructed high-pressure voiding and poor bladder wall compliance can also facilitate tissue invasion.[31, 34] The presence of vesicoureteral reflux secondary to elevated bladder pressures facilitates access of urinary pathogens to the kidneys, leading to serious complications such as pyelonephritis, septicemia, and renal faliure.[49]

The distal urethra is colonized by skin flora dominated by gram-positive cocci and diphtheroids. Lactobacilli are common in females. Under normal circumstances, the remainder of the urinary tract is sterile.[56] Colonization of the urethra by urinary pathogens in individuals with neurogenic bladder dysfunction precedes the spread of bacteria to the bladder and from which point pathogens have the potential to spread to other parts of the urinary tract.[39] This is enhanced by catheterization, which is often necessary to maintain adequate bladder drainage. However, bacteriuria frequently occurs even in patients free of indwelling catheters as a result of neurologic deficits and their secondary effects.

Moloney and others[39] observed that in patients with spinal cord injury who retain the normal, predominantly, gram-positive skin flora, urinary tract infections do not develop. Although these investigators do not specifically address the question of why normal skin flora are replaced by urinary pathogens in some persons but not in others, possible explanations that merit further investigation include the prior or current use of antibacterial soaps and systemic antibiotics, the extent and technique of bladder instrumentation, catheter care, and the level and degree of neurologic impairment. Fawcett and colleagues[15] compared the bacterial skin flora of hospitalized patients with spinal cord injury with that of healthy nonhospitalized controls. Diverse gram-negative bacilli, which were often multidrug resistant, were present in the patients within 2 to 3 days after admission but were rarely isolated from controls. In several patients, urinary tract infections developed with the same bacterial species that were isolated from the skin. Antibacterial soaps selectively active against gram-positive bacteria were used on the patient group and may have influenced these results. Sanderson and Rawal[50] found that organisms causing urinary tract infections in patients with spinal cord injury were also recoverable from the immediate environment, thus stressing the importance of proper handwashing and skin disinfection by both patients and staff to avoid cross-contamination and further spread of infection.

The presence of Enterobacteriaceae and other organisms, such as Pseudomonas, Acinetobacter, and Enterococcus species on the skin of patients with spinal cord injury is presumed to be due to spread from a fecal reservoir, although the natural history and epidemiology of individual bacterial colonization can be complex and is incompletely understood.[41] Despite the preponderance of anaerobic colonic flora, anaerobes are relatively uncommon as urinary pathogens.[30] Donovan and co-workers[13] used plasmid DNA analysis to assess the source of Klebsiella pneumoniae urinary tract infections in patients with spinal cord injury undergoing intermittent catheterization and confirmed the premise that this organism is spread from feces to urine. In spinal cord injury, a large percentage of urinary tract infections are polymicrobial. Both the precise identity of the urinary pathogens and the antibiogram are unpredictable, further complicating management strategies. The actual percentage of urinary isolates belonging to individual bacterial species can vary considerably among institutions and can change spontaneously even in the absence of intervention.

For bacteria to produce disease in the urinary tract they must gain access, attach, and colonize the uroepithelium (to prevent their being washed out in the urine), multiply, survive, evade host defenses, and induce a host inflammatory response leading to tissue damage. The ability of a given bacterial strain to accomplish these tasks depends on virulence, inoculum size, and the integrity of host defenses.[52] Certain bacterial strains are more capable of colonizing the urinary tract and of producing disease than others, even in the absence of underlying anatomic or physiologic derangements.[48, 60] These organisms have evolved potent virulence factors that permit them to evade or survive the usual host defenses. One of the bacterial virulence factors most important to the clinician is the multiantimicrobial resistance exhibited by many bacteria found in the hospital or chronic care environment. The most important mechanism for antimicrobial resistance is the extrachromosomal resistance transfer plasmid that can confer simultaneous resistance to multiple classes of antimicrobial agents enzymatically.[30]

The molecular biology of virulence factors, adherence properties in particular, in the pathogenesis of urinary tract infection has become more clearly understood and has been the subject of intensive research and reviews.[6, 19, 20, 48, 59] Evidence of the role of bacterial adherence in the pathogenesis of urinary tract infection in catheterized patients in the non–spinal-cord-injury population is provided by the observation that the development of bacteriuria in recently catheterized patients is preceded by a significant increase in bacterial adherence to uroepithelial cells.[48] Limited information is available regarding attachment defense mechanisms in the urinary tract. The uromucoid lining of the bladder can bind *Escherichia coli* and impair its attachment to uroepithelial cells, but the protective role of this substance remains theoretical. Oligosaccharides secreted by the host can also prevent bacterial adherence and detach adherent bacteria from the bladder epithelium.[24]

Montgomerie and Morrow[41] measured serum antibodies in 28 patients with spinal cord injury before and after the development of bacteriuria during their hospital rehabilitation. After bacteriuria was detected, a fourfold or greater increase in IgG or IgA antibodies or both against the infecting strain of *Pseudomonas aeruginosa* isolated from the urine of each patient was found in 9 patients (33%). This increase was significantly associated with leukocytosis and was thought to be indicative of tissue invasion by this microorganism. Intermittent catheterization might have predisposed to local inflammation and tissue invasion of the bladder or urethra or both in this population, as renal involvement was probably not present. Such a rise in serum antibody titer aids the opsonophagocytic clearance of organisms but frequently does not occur with localized infections that involve only the bladder.[52] Local antibodies can also inhibit attachment of bacteria to uroepithelial cells in patients with pyelonephritis.[48] Uropathogenic bacteria often synthesize antiphagocytic capsules and other means of eluding interaction with host immune defenses.[20]

Bacterial growth alone, even in the kidney, does not necessarily culminate in tissue destruction and scarring. If followed by penetration of the epithelium, colonization will result in neutrophil chemotaxis, inflammation, desquamation of the surface epithelium, and, possibly, scarring and functional loss. Although it is beneficial in the sense that it facilitates clearance of the organisms, inflammation seems to be a prerequisite for necrosis and renal scarring.[19]

Although many other bacterial virulence factors exist,[19, 20, 30, 48, 52, 58–60] urease activity is of particular importance in patients with spinal cord injury. *Proteus* may be the best known genus for its association with urolithiasis secondary to precipitation of calcium phosphate and magnesium ammonium phosphate under the alkaline conditions induced by urea hydrolysis. *Pseudomonas, Serratia, Morganella, Providencia, Klebsiella, Staphylococcus,* and *Ureaplasma* species and *E. coli* can also produce urease[30] and result in renal stone formation.

CLINICAL EVALUATION

Signs and symptoms, such as frequency, urgency, nocturia, and dysuria, in persons with neurologic deficits are dependent on the level and extent of neurologic impairment and are often unreliable as diagnostic criteria. A large majority of persons with spinal cord injury who have bacteriuria can remain completely asymptomatic. Chills and spiking fevers with or without nausea and vomiting are often considered to be signs of acute pyelonephritis, but these signs do not always confirm an infection in either the upper or lower urinary tract. Other clinical parameters that can be indicative of a urinary tract infection in patients with spinal cord injury are increased sweating, abdominal discomfort, costovertebral angle pain or tenderness, increased muscle spasticity, and foul-smelling urine. Deresinski and Perkash[11] found that symptoms were present in a minority of subjects, with the most common symptom being vague, such as unexplained sweating suggestive of autonomic dysreflexia. The presence or absence of symptoms as well as pyuria can be poorly predictive of the urine culture results.[11] Any person with neurologic deficits who has fever of undetermined origin should undergo a careful physical examination of all body systems including an examination for bladder distension and scrotal pathologic lesions. The existence of fever along with bacteriuria does not automatically imply that the fever is the result of a urinary tract infection, and other sources of fever also must be ruled out.

LABORATORY DIAGNOSIS OF URINARY TRACT INFECTION

Urinalysis

A complete urinalysis should be performed whenever a urinary tract infection is suspected. Turbid, malodorous urine with a dense precipitate can reflect pyuria and infection but also can be normal. Urine pH ranges from approximately 4.6 to 8 and is usually not of major diagnostic significance. Infection with urease-producing bacteria resulting in alkaline urine can increase the risk of calculogenesis.[30]

Several biochemical tests are available that screen indirectly for infection, many of which can be performed at the bedside in inpatients or even by patients at home without resorting to time-consuming and costly laboratory tests. Because these relatively new tests offer some degree of identification of the likely presence of a urinary tract infection, appropriate intervention can be initiated if necessary. Some of the tests include nitrate reduction, which is useful for detecting the presence of many gram-negative organisms, and reagent strips for detection of leukocyte esterase in persons with abnormal numbers of urinary leukocytes. The latter is of particular value when microscopic quantitation is not possible. Rapid information can be obtained from examination of gram-stained smears of unspun urine. The presence of two or more bacteria in gram-stained smears of unspun urine examined under an oil immersion lens ($\times 1000$) implies that bacteriuria is present ($\geq 10^5$ colony-forming units [cfu]/mL). Measurement of pyuria by microscopic examination and enumeration of leukocytes with a high-power field are poorly reproducible. Observer bias, lack of standardization of the thickness of the film beneath the coverslip, and varying volumes of resuspension all contribute to this poor reproducibility. A rule of thumb often quoted is that one leuko-cyte per low-power ($\times 100$) microscopic field reflects the presence of three leukocytes per cubic millimeter. Counting the number of leukocytes per cubic millimeter in unspun urine in a hemocytometer is the most accurate method for assessing urinary tract inflammation, although this is rarely practiced in clinical laboratories. Casts are molds of renal tubules composed of inspissated protein and often admixed with cellular components. Leukocyte casts are definitive evidence of an inflammatory reaction in the kidney and are thus potentially of considerable significance in patients with spinal cord injury.

Given the fact that it is possible with reasonable accuracy to assess the degree of inflammation (pyuria) in urine samples, provided that appropriate techniques are employed, the significance of its presence, particularly in the asymptomatic patient, is controversial. Stamm[54] observed that a count of equal to or greater than 10 leukocytes per cubic millimeter of urine occurs in fewer than 1% of asymptomatic, nonbacteriuric patients without spinal cord injury but in more than 96% of symptomatic patients with significant bacteriuria. Hooton et al[23] further stressed the importance of pyuria as a marker for invasive disease in patients with spinal cord injury by suggesting that the risk of upper urinary tract involvement increases as the leukocyte excretion rate increases above a certain level.

Peterson and Roth[47] reviewed the records of 32 patients with spinal cord injury who had indwelling catheters and who were admitted to a rehabilitation hospital to assess the significance of pyuria diagnosed at the time of admission in relation to the incidence of unexplained febrile episodes during a hospitalization period of up to 75 days. They found that 22 patients with 50 or fewer white blood cells per high-power field had an incidence of 3 to 22 febrile episodes, whereas the second group with more than 50 white blood cells per high-power field, had an incidence of 6 to 10 febrile episodes. The difference in the incidence of fever in the two groups was statistically significant. These results were interpreted to mean that patients with spinal cord injury with indwelling catheters and gross pyuria may be at risk for increased morbidity secondary to untreated urinary tract infections. Because this was a retrospective study, patients were not actually tested for the presence of pyuria at the time of the febrile episodes, which would have been useful for further clarification of the strength of association of these variables. Anderson and Hsieh-Ma[5] showed that the presence and degree of pyuria in 156 hospitalized patients with spinal cord injury undergoing intermittent catheterization, in whom daily urine cultures and quantitation of leukocytes in uncentrifuged urine were performed was influenced by the type of organism isolated from urine. Gram-positive bacteria produced minimal white cell response, even in high colony counts. However, gram-negative and fungal organisms elicited much greater pyuria.

Clearly, much is unknown about the significance of pyuria as a predictor of bacteriuria or various urologic complications in any patient population with spinal cord injury, especially catheter-free outpatients. The definition of what constitutes significant pyuria is controversial, as is the definition of significant bacteriuria. In a study of male patients with spinal cord injury, Deresinski and Perkash[11] found that pyuria with a leukocyte count of 10 or more cells per cubic millimeter was predictive of bacteriuria as determined by a culture of bladder urine by suprapubic aspiration and was thought to be predictive of true bladder infection rather than simple colonization. The absence of pyuria, however, did not exclude infection. There was a poor correlation between pyuria and absolute numbers of organisms and the presence of symptoms related to urinary tract infection. Pyuria in conjunction with negative cultures in persons without spinal cord injury suggests the presence of fastidious organisms, such as mycobacteria, anaerobes, or mycoplasms or inflammation due to some other noninfecting process.[30] Gribble et al[17] found that estimates of pyuria from catheter urine obtained from patients with spinal cord injury undergoing intermittent catheterization did not clearly separate bacteriuric from abacteriuric specimens, verified by suprapubic aspiration of urine for culture, thus reiterating the need for urine culture for ultimate determination of the presence of bacteriuria.

Urine Culture

The standard for diagnosis of urinary tract infection remains the quantitative urine culture in which appropriate bacteriologic media are used with antibiotic susceptibility testing. The importance of proper handling and refrigeration of the specimen when media inoculation cannot be performed immediately cannot be overemphasized. If the results are to be valid, urine specimens must be processed within 1 hour or refrigerated for not more than 24 hours before media are inoculated. Agar dip-slides have been described as a rapid, cost-effective means of screening urine specimens for bacteria in patients with spinal cord injury.[4]

The common aerobically growing gram-negative and gram-positive bacteria that are responsible for most urinary tract infections in patients with spinal cord injury are easily cultivated and identified using commercially available bacteriologic media and biochemical reagents. Only in specialized, unusual circumstances, such as in suspected mycobacterial infection, are additional techniques and reagents needed. The significance of a positive culture depends on the number and species of microorganisms isolated. Bacteriuria does not distinguish between washed-out contaminants originating from the distal urethra and actual multiplying pathogens from within the urinary tract. Lactobacilli, diphtheroids, and alpha-hemolytic streptococci should be considered contaminants unless they are recovered directly from bladder urine by suprapubic aspiration.[30]

The safest and usually the most practical means of assessing the bacteriologic status of the urinary tract is to collect a clean, midstream urine specimen and to perform quantitative cultures. Significant bacteriuria from voided urine has traditionally been defined as greater than or equal to 10^5 colonies/mL, with lesser numbers equated with contamination from the urethral or perineal flora.[30] However, symptomatic urinary tract infections, even septicemia, are known to occur in the presence of much lower bacterial counts verified by suprapubic aspiration than the standard 10^5 cfu/mL.[16, 57] Stamm[54] recommended lowering the threshold of significant bacteriuria to greater than or equal to 10^2 cfu/

mL for women with acute dysuria. There is definite validity in reconsidering these diagnostic standards, even in patients with spinal cord injury. Gribble et al[16] collected daily mid-stream urine cultures in 50 patients by intermittent catheterization that were paired with suprapubic aspirates to define the presence or absence of bacteriuria over an average period of 5 consecutive days. Low-level bacteriuria was frequently observed in conjunction with signs and symptoms attributable to urinary tract infection. They concluded that in this population, a criterion of greater than or equal to 10^2 colonies/mL of mid-catheter urine should be used for the diagnosis of significant bacteriuria. They did not address the subject of asymptomatic bacteriuria. Such differences in the standards for determination of what constitutes significant bacteriuria have led to continued confusion and make comparison of studies using different interpretive criteria difficult.

Urine specimens obtained by catheterization should be more reflective of the true bacteriologic status of bladder urine, yet there is always a risk, despite careful technique, of introducing organisms into the bladder through the catheter, resulting in infection. Patients may occasionally experience transient bacteremia with fever and chills after catheterization. Because of these risks, we no longer advocate obtaining a catheterized specimen during outpatient evaluation solely for microbiologic examination in asymptomatic patients with spinal cord injury.

Urine cultures from a patient with an indwelling catheter are indicated only when the patient is acutely ill or symptomatic with signs suggestive of possible sepsis. Routine cultures are not cost-effective, because the urinary tracts of all patients with indwelling catheters will eventually become colonized with one or several species of bacteria, usually in a number greater than 10^5/mL.[1] Species can unpredictably change at frequent intervals. If cultures are to be performed, specimens from an indwelling catheter must always be collected directly from the disinfected collection port or wall of the catheter with a sterile syringe and never from the drainage bag or by disconnecting the catheter from the collection tube.

Suprapubic aspiration, although much less commonly employed as a routine screening procedure for urinary tract infection, is sometimes used to clarify equivocal results obtained from voided specimens or to verify anaerobic bacteriuria. It is the most accurate method of assessing the true bacteriologic status of the bladder.

Many methods of localizing the source of bacteriuria by noninvasive procedures have been advocated over the years, including the bladder washout procedure, antibody coating, and determination of urinary lactic dehydrogenase. These procedures have not been demonstrated to be of value as clinical procedures either in determining tissue invasion or in localizing the infection in patients with spinal cord injury.[27, 30] Ureteral catheterization as a means of localizing infection cannot be recommended for most patients, because bacteria in the bladder or urethra could be introduced into the kidney. Therefore, the high-risk patient who might benefit from more intensive treatment remains unidentifiable until pathologic changes become evident. Currently, localization studies are considered to be research tools.[30]

COMPLICATIONS

The lower urinary tract is colonized by bacteria in most patients with spinal cord injury regardless of the bladder management method used. Urethritis is an infection of the periurethral glands, which in its milder forms may result only in urethral discharge. More severe urethritis can manifest with fever and induration around the urethra. Urethritis is usually secondary to an indwelling urethral catheter, and patients appear to be more prone to this complication early after spinal cord injury. If untreated, urethritis can result in periurethral abscess, although this is usually not seen unless it is accompanied by ventral urethral erosion at the penoscrotal angle. Urethral stricture can be a late sequela of urethritis. Infection in the posterior urethra can also result in prostatitis, which can be either acute or chronic in nature. Fortunately, acute prostatitis and prostatic abscess are uncommon, although chronic bacterial prostatis is thought to occur commonly in patients with spinal cord injury.[3] Chronic bacterial prostatitis usually is asymptomatic but makes the eradication of bacteriuria virtually impossible. Patients with urethritis may be susceptible to migration of the bacteria through the ejaculatory ducts and vas deferens, resulting in epididymitis. On cystographic examination, reflux of bladder urine can sometimes be observed into the seminal vesicles, vas deferens, and ejaculatory ducts. Epididymitis in the patient with spinal cord injury is almost always due to bacteria that have colonized the urinary tract. In this condition, cultures from the epididymis and urine are usually identical, and this may guide the choice of appropriate antibiotic therapy. Unfortunately, the lack of symptoms in early infection and the ultimate severity of bacterial infections can combine to produce orchitis and testicular abscess.

Bladder calculi are a common complication and are related both to infection and foreign bodies, e.g., urethral or suprapubic catheters. Bladder calculi are frequently seen early after spinal cord injury and are related primarily to the period of indwelling catheter drainage. When an indwelling catheter is present and colonization with urease-producing bacteria occurs, formation of bladder stones can be rapid. Polymicrobial infection should also alert the physician to the possibility of urinary tract calculi. Bladder stones generally are not a serious complication and usually can be managed with endoscopic removal. Bladder stones secondary to urease-producing organisms, however, are associated with a higher incidence of renal calculi.[12]

Renal calculi are perhaps the most serious of all upper urinary tract complications. Renal calculi develop in approximately 8% of patients with spinal cord injury, and 98% of these stones are infection-type stones resulting from urease-producing bacterial infection.[3, 12] Bacteria are bound within the interstices of the stones as they form, and it is difficult to achieve complete eradication of infection without removal of the stones from the kidney. Untreated calculi can progress to produce obstruction of the kidney, parenchy-

mal abscess (renal carbuncle), or perinephric abscess.[22] These more severe complications can be associated with septicemia and even death.

Vesicoureteral reflux might be more appropriately termed a lower urinary tract complication, although its major manifestations are seen in the kidney. Reflux occurs in 5% to 10% of patients with spinal cord injury and is a result of several factors, including obstructed high-pressure voiding, alterations of the morphologic characteristics in the bladder wall that result in a periureteral diverticulum with loss of the posterior support to the intramural ureter, and inflammation of the periureteral tissues, which makes them less pliable and also decreases the flap-valve effect of the intramural ureter.[25] Vesicoureteral reflux permits free reflux of bladder urine containing bacteria into the kidney. In high-pressure reflux, the colonized urine can even be forced intraparenchymally. Higher grades of reflux are usually associated with recurrent symptomatic pyelonephritis and declining renal function. Segmental or global renal atrophy can occur as a result of reflux. Early detection and appropriate changes in bladder management are necessary to minimize these deleterious effects.

Renal or perinephric abscess should be suspected when patients do not respond promptly to antibiotic therapy or in patients with known renal calculi. Confirmation is obtained by renal ultrasonography or abdominal CT scanning. Bacteremia in patients with spinal cord injury is frequently related to urinary tract infection, shown in one retrospective study to be responsible for 72.4% of all occurrences.[8] Urosepsis is frequently the result of urinary tract manipulations, including catheterization, endoscopy, or surgical procedures, although ascending infection into the upper tract and into the bloodstream can occur in the absence of any type of instrumentation.[8] Blood cultures should be obtained in any patient with such symptoms of toxic effects as spiking fever and chills when bacteremia is suspected. However, patients with spinal cord injury with urosepsis can present with minimal symptoms.[8] Urologic complications, including renal deterioration, can develop insidiously. Thorough urologic evaluations on a regular basis, including tests to measure renal function, are recommended for all patients with neurogenic bladder impairments.

TREATMENT

Treatment of asymptomatic bacteriuria remains controversial. Recent data suggest that there are few benefits and that treatment is often excessive.[11, 30, 32] Mohler et al[38] reported that treatment of asymptomatic urinary tract infections offered no advantage over placebo. Others also found that infection rates did not differ when asymptomatic urinary tract infections were treated or merely observed in patients with spinal cord injury.[35]

Bacteriuria associated with indwelling catheters should not be treated unless the patient is symptomatic. Because most patients with bladder management by intermittent catheterization, reflex voiding, or Credé maneuver have chronic asymptomatic bacteriuria, many clinicians believe that treatment should be reserved for those who become symptomatic.[32]

The presence of pyuria (greater than 10^4 white blood cells/mL urine) with bacteriuria is thought by some to be an important consideration in determining treatment, because this may be an indication of tissue invasion.[11] Others[55] do not advocate treatment of asymptomatic bacteriuria even in the presence of pyuria. The relationship or effect, if any, of prolonged urinary inflammation on the long-term status of the kidneys is not known.

There is little question as to the need for antibiotic treatment for the first episode of bacteriuria with or without pyuria or in the situation of acutely symptomatic infections. The value of continuing aggressive treatment for relapse or reinfection is less well established. This is especially true for asymptomatic bacteriuria, in which the value of repeated antibiotic treatment must be weighed against the development of resistant organisms.[7] Recurrent symptomatic urinary tract infections, however, require special consideration, and the patient must be reevaluated for inadequately treated infection, inadequate bladder emptying, obstruction, calculi, and compromised immune status. Relapses or reinfections are a problem either because the infecting organisms persist within protected renal or prostatic foci, resulting in resurgence after transient suppression, or because new organisms enter the urinary tract from the perineal-fecal reservoir.[62]

The benefits of either short-term or long-term therapy have not been demonstrated convincingly. Therefore, a 10-day course of antibiotics is generally considered acceptable. Stickler and Chawla[55] raised a pertinent issue regarding the potential benefits of a 6-week course of chemotherapy to permit time for damaged, inflamed tissues of the urinary tract to regenerate before exposing them to recolonization by bacteria. For acute symptomatic urinary tract infections, oral therapy guided by drug susceptibility testing is usually adequate unless nausea and vomiting prevent adequate fluid intake and oral treatment or serious upper tract involvement or bacteremia or both are suspected. Specific antibiotic therapy should be administered before any urinary operative procedure in an effort to minimize the risk of urosepsis. Although intravenous therapy is frequently used for acute episodes, the benefits of parenteral therapy over oral therapy have not been demonstrated clearly. It is important to remember that the pharmacodynamics of treatment can be altered in patients with spinal cord injury, requiring adjustment of drug dosage,[51] and that sustained urinary levels of antibiotics are more important than blood levels.

The diverse and often multi-drug resistant polymicrobial nature of urinary tract infections in patients with neurogenic bladder often precludes the use of many oral antibiotics available for treating uncomplicated urinary tract infections. Parenteral antimicrobial chemotherapy, with its expense and potential toxicity, is especially undesirable or unrealistic in many instances because these patients are commonly asymptomatic or only mildly to moderately uncomfortable and are optimally engaged in daily rehabilitative or vocational activities. The fluoroquinolones have greatly expanded and improved the ability to utilize oral therapy in the management of complicated urinary tract infections in a wide variety of settings, including those infections in persons with neurogenic bladder dysfunction. Studies of patients with spinal cord injury given oral ciprofloxacin[45] or norfloxacin[62] for urinary tract infections have been performed, with generally favorable short-term results. Activity against *Pseudomonas* species is perhaps the most significant advantage of the orally administered quinolones for treating complicated urinary tract infection in this population.[62] Clinical experience with the quinolones in patients with spinal cord injury is limited, and the extent to which the emergence of drug-resistant bacteria occurs as a result of their use is not yet known.

PREVENTION/PROPHYLAXIS

The prevention of colonization has been the primary goal in preventing urinary tract infection. Eliminating the indwelling catheter removes a foreign body nidus for bacterial colonization, and efficient bladder emptying causes the physical removal of bacteria from the bladder. Infection rates with reflex voiding and external condom catheter collection are similar to those with intermittent catheterization.[14] Low residual urine volumes are important in preventing bacterial multiplication and can also reduce the pressure within the bladder that is a contributor to vesicoureteral reflux and possibly to ischemic changes within the bladder wall that can impair local host defenses against infection.[31] Pharmacologic agents such as alpha-blockers can improve bladder emptying. Transurethral external sphincterotomy or bladder neck resection or both can reduce detrusor-sphincter dyssynergia and lead to smaller residual urine volume, which is often helpful in preventing recurrent symptomatic urinary tract infections.[46]

Clinical studies of the instillation of various antimicrobial agents into leg bags to prevent bacteriuria are inadequate. Various adjuvants bound to catheter polymers and catheters and tubing impregnated with antibiotics or heavy metals have also not been proved effective. Earlier studies suggested that infection could be decreased successfully with bladder instillation of abrasive or acidifying chemicals or both, such as hemiacidrin and chlorhexidine digluconate, as well as with antibiotic preparations such

as neomycin and polymyxin.[3, 26] The side effects of hematuria and allergic reactions along with questionable long-term efficacy leave doubt as to the benefits of these practices.[63] Analogs to uromucoid,[10] mannose-sensitive adherents,[24] P-fimbria receptors,[58] and transitional cell-secreted glycosaminoglycan[43] are uroepithelial cell receptorlike elements and inherent antiadherence substances that bind bacteria in vitro and that have been considered for bladder instillation. Effective intravesicular concentrations of these agents are difficult to achieve, limiting in vivo application. Furthermore, microorganisms have multiple mechanisms for adherence, and blocking just one site may be inadequate. The difficulty of attempting to inhibit all antiadherence receptors is obvious when multiple bacterial strains are present.

Although numerous studies have been performed in which attempts have been made to determine the utility of systemic antibiotics to prevent or suppress urinary tract infection in persons with spinal cord injury,[2, 29, 35, 37, 38, 55] the methods of bladder management in these subjects have been varied, the definitions of significant urinary tract infection have been inconsistent, the numbers of patients studied often have been small, and several different antibiotic regimens have been utilized. The overall consensus appears to be that antimicrobial prophylaxis has no clearly beneficial effect on reducing the incidence of urinary tract infection following spinal cord injury. The effect of antimicrobial prophylaxis on long-term renal function has not been addressed systematically.

Commonly used systemic prophylactic antimicrobial agents such as trimethoprim, sulfamethoxazole, and nitrofurantoin can reduce the incidence of bacteriuria initially,[37] but studies addressing long-term efficacy reveal no significant effect on rates of bacteriuria[29] and symptoms.[38] In addition, the emergence of resistant strains of bacteria becomes a problem. Proponents of acidification using ammonium chloride, ascorbic acid, cranberry juice, or of alkalinization using sodium bicarbonate, oral citrate, and acetazolamide have not provided evidence of direct bacteriostatic activity that is clinically effective. Vaccination of high-risk groups prone to urinary tract infections is another systemic measure that may hold promise for future prophylaxis; however, several unresolved problems make it untenable in clinical practice at the present time.

THE ROLE OF BLADDER MANAGEMENT

Intermittent catheterization during the rehabilitation period after spinal cord injury has been shown to lower infection rates and has greatly reduced many of the complications associated with indwelling catheters, such as urethritis, penoscrotal abscess or fistula, and epididymitis.[19] However, a short period of indwelling catheter drainage following injury does not adversely affect the patient's long-term outlook.[33] Some maintain that a sterile intermittent catheterization technique reduces the incidence of infection,[2] whereas others have shown that the clean technique is more practical, especially after hospital discharge, and is not associated with increased complications.[35] Appreciation of the risks for catheter-associated urosepsis has prompted most clinicians to render patients with spinal cord injury free from indwelling urinary catheters on a long-term basis whenever possible. If this is not feasible, rigorous patient education on proper methods for intermittent catheterization or condom catheter care to reduce contamination is essential when these bladder management techniques are utilized.

Although there is no universal agreement on the most efficacious long-term management of the neurogenic bladder, it is generally agreed that a catheter-free status places the patient at the lowest risk for significant long-term urinary tract complications. Of those patients in whom reflex voiding develops but who require an external urine collecting device for control of incontinence, approximately 80% have chronic or recurrent bacteriuria.[33] Approximately one third of patients maintained on long-term intermittent catheterization remain free of urinary tract infection.[36] Patients who, at some phase, require both an external collecting device and periodic urethral catheterization appear to be at an even greater risk of developing a urinary

tract infection.[21] Cardenas and Mayo[9] found that patients who are catheterized by someone else are much more likely to experience at least one episode of bacteriuria with fever than those performing intermittent self-catheterization or even those using an indwelling catheter. No exact data exist concerning how frequently a medically important urinary tract infection develops in the outpatient setting in a catheter-free person with spinal cord injury, nor on the efficacy of antimicrobial therapy in eradicating infection or maintaining urine sterility. It is undetermined what effect the maintenance of sterile urine for longer intervals during the early stages of neurogenic bladder dysfunction will have on kidney status after 15 to 20 years.

The risk factors associated with various methods of bladder management in women have been difficult to ascertain because most female patients are managed by indwelling catheters. Some studies have found that there are no statistical differences in infection rates between women and men with spinal cord injury when matched by bladder management.[14]

Sotolongo and Koleilat[53] prospectively evaluated 56 patients with spinal cord injury undergoing condom catheter drainage within 6 months of injury for 5 years. They monitored bladder pressures and performed external sphincterotomies as needed and yearly imaging of the upper urinary tract. All patients had bacterial colonization of urine and were asymptomatic during the entire study period. No patient sustained deterioration of the urinary tract during the 5-year period. Therefore, it was concluded that asymptomatic bacteriuria is of no consequence to the integrity of the upper urinary tract when low pressures are operant during this interval. Whether this relationship holds true for longer periods following spinal cord injury is unproven.

SUMMARY

Even though renal failure secondary to the urologic complications of chronic or recurrent urinary tract infection has decreased markedly due to advances in diagnostic, preventive, and therapeutic measures, infection and its sequelae continue to be major problems in patients with spinal cord injury regardless of the bladder-emptying method employed. Although lower urinary tract complications have decreased with intermittent catheterization, the effects of increased intravesicular pressure, inflammation, and chronic bacterial colonization or invasion of the urinary tract on long-term renal function are still undetermined. Thorough evaluation of the urologic status on a regular basis in all patients with spinal cord injury is encouraged. Treatment of urinary tract infection should be guided by scientific data and drug susceptibilities of etiologic bacteria. The general consensus is that the presence of asymptomatic bacteriuria, particularly in the absence of pyuria, usually does not warrant antibiotic treatment, and that prophylaxis or suppression of infection with systemic antibiotics is not effective for any considerable length of time. Preservation of renal function is the ultimate goal of all bladder management strategies.

REFERENCES

1. Achong MR: Urinary tract infections in the patient with a neurogenic bladder. In Bloch RF, Basbaum M (eds): Management of Spinal Cord Injuries. Baltimore, Williams & Wilkins, 1986, p 164.
2. Anderson RU: Prophylaxis of bacteriuria during intermittent catheterization of acute neurogenic bladder. J Urol 123:364, 1980.
3. Anderson RU: Urinary tract infections in spinal cord injury patients. In Walsh PC, Gittes RE, Perlmutter AD, et al (eds): Campbell's Urology, vol 1, ed 5. Philadelphia, WB Saunders, 1986, p 888.
4. Anderson RU, Hatami-Tehrani G: Monitoring for bacteriuria in spinal cord-injured patients on intermittent catheterization. Dip-slide culture technique. Urology 14:244, 1979.
5. Anderson RU, Hsieh-Ma ST: Association of bacteriuria and pyuria during intermittent catheterization after spinal cord injury. J Urol 130:299, 1983.
6. Andriole VT: Urinary tract infections: Recent developments. J Infect Dis 156:865, 1987.
7. Bahnson RR: Urosepsis. Urol Clin North Am 13:627, 1986.
8. Bhatt K, Cid E: Bacteremia in the spinal cord injury population. J Am Paraplegia Soc 10:11, 1987.
9. Cardenas DD, Mayo ME: Bacteriuria with fever after spinal cord injury. Arch Phys Med Rehabil 68:291, 1987.
10. Chick S, Harber MJ, Mackenzie R, et al: Modified method for studying bacterial adhesion to isolated uroepithelial cells and uromucoid. Infect Immun 34:256, 1981.
11. Deresinski SC, Perkash I: Urinary tract infections in male spinal cord injured patients. Part II: Diagnostic value of symptoms and of quantitative urinalysis. J Am Paraplegia Soc 8:7, 1985.
12. DeVivo MJ, Fine PR, Cutter GR, et al: Risk of renal calculi in spinal cord injury patients. J Urol 131:857, 1984.
13. Donovan WH, Hull R, Cifu X, et al: Use of plasmid analysis to determine the source of bacterial invasion of the urinary tract. Paraplegia 28:573, 1990.
14. Erickson RP, Merritt JL, Opitz JL, et al: Bacteriuria during follow-up in patients with spinal cord injury. I: Rates of bacteriuria in various bladder-emptying methods. Arch Phys Med Rehabil 63:409, 1982.
15. Fawcett C, Chawla JC, Quoraishi A, et al: A study of the skin flora of spinal cord injured patients. J Hosp Infect 8:149, 1986.
16. Gribble MJ, McCallum NM, Schecter MT: Evaluation of diagnostic criteria for bacteriuria in acutely spinal cord injured patients undergoing intermittent catheterization. Diagn Microbiol Infect Dis 9:197, 1988.
17. Gribble MJ, Puterman ML, McCallum NM: Pyuria: Its relationship to bacteriuria in spinal cord injured patients on intermittent catheterization. Arch Phys Med Rehabil 70:376, 1989.
18. Guttmann L: Disturbances of the bladder and upper urinary tract. In Guttman L (ed): Spinal Cord Injuries—Comprehensive Management and Research, ed 2. Oxford, Blackwell Scientific Publications, 1976, p 331.
19. Harber MJ, Asscher AW: Virulence of urinary pathogens. Kidney Int 28:717, 1985.
20. Harber MJ, Topley N, Asscher AW: Virulence factors of urinary pathogens. Clin Sci 70:531, 1986.
21. Hirsh DD, Fainstein V, Musher DM: Do condom catheter collecting systems cause urinary tract infection? JAMA 242:340, 1979.
22. Holder CD, Craig CP: Complications of urinary tract infections. Hosp Pract 21:110C, 1986.
23. Hooton TM, O'Shaughnessy EJ, Clowers D, et al: Localization of urinary tract infection in patients with spinal cord injury. J Infect Dis 150:85, 1984.
24. Jarvinen AK, Sandholm M: Urinary oligosaccharides inhibit adhesion of E. coli onto canine urinary tract epithelium. Invest Urol 17:443, 1980.
25. King LR, Levitt SB: Vesicoureteral reflux, megaureter, and urethral reimplantation. In Walsh PC, Gittes RE, Perlmutter AD, et al (eds): Campbell's Urology, vol 2, ed 5. Philadelphia, WB Saunders, 1986, p 2031.
26. Krebs M, Halvorsen RB, Fishman IJ, et al: Prevention of urinary tract infection during intermittent catheterization. J Urol 131:82, 1984.
27. Kuhlemeier KV, Lloyd LK, Stover SL: Failure of antibody-coated bacteria and bladder washout tests to localize infection in spinal cord injury patients. J Urol 130:729, 1983.
28. Kuhlemeier KV, Lloyd LK, Stover SL: Long-term follow up of renal function after spinal cord injury. J Urol 134:510, 1985.
29. Kuhlemeier KV, Stover SL, Lloyd LK: Prophylactic antibacterial therapy for preventing urinary tract infections in spinal cord injury patients. J Urol 134:514, 1985.
30. Kunin CM: Detection, Prevention and Management of Urinary Tract Infections, ed 4. Philadelphia, Lea & Febiger, 1987.

31. Lapides J: Role of hydrostatic pressure and distension in urinary tract infection. *In* Kass EH (ed): Progress in Pyelonephritis. Philadelphia, FA Davis, 1965, p 578.

32. Lewis RI, Carron HM, Lockhart JL, et al: Significance of asymptomatic bacteriuria in neurogenic bladder disease. Urology 23:343, 1984.

33. Lloyd LK, Kuhlemeier KV, Stover SL: Initial bladder management in spinal cord injury: Does it make a difference? J Urol 135:523, 1986.

34. Lloyd-Davies RW, Henman F: Structural and functional changes leading to impaired bacterial elimination after overdistension of rabbit bladder. Invest Urol 9:136, 1971.

35. Maynard FM, Diokno AC: Urinary infection and complications during clean intermittent catheterization following spinal cord injury. J Urol 132:136, 1984.

36. McGuire EJ, Savastano JA: Long-term followup of spinal cord injury patients managed by intermittent catheterization. J Urol 129:775, 1983.

37. Merritt JLM, Erickson RP, Opitz JL: Bacteriuria during follow-up in patients with spinal cord injury. Part II: Efficacy of antimicrobial suppressants. Arch Phys Med Rehabil 63:413, 1982.

38. Mohler JL, Cowen DL, Flanigan RC: Suppression and treatment of urinary tract infection in patients with intermittently catheterized neurogenic bladder. J Urol 138:336, 1987.

39. Moloney PJ, Doyle AA, Robinson BL, et al: Pathogenesis of urinary tract infection in patients with acute spinal cord injury on intermittent catheterization. J Urol 125:672, 1981.

40. Montgomerie JZ, Guerra DA, Schick DG, et al: *Pseudomonas* urinary tract infection in patients with spinal cord injury. J Am Paraplegia Soc 12:8, 1989.

41. Montgomerie JZ, Morrow JW: *Pseudomonas* colonization in patients with spinal cord injury. Am J Epidemiol 108:328, 1978.

42. O'Grady F, Catell WR: Kinetics of urinary tract infection: II. The bladder. Br J Urol 38:155, 1966.

43. Parson CL, Pollen JJ, Anwar H, et al: Antibacterial activity of bladder surface mucin duplicated in rabbit bladder by exogenous glycosamine (sodium pentosanpolysulfate). Infect Immun 27:876, 1980.

44. Pearman JW: Pathological changes in the bladder muscle and nervous tissue due to overdistension and infection. *In* Pearman JW (ed): The Urological Management of the Patient Following Spinal Cord Injury. Springfield, IL, Charles C. Thomas, 1973, p 34.

45. Pedersen SS, Horbov S, Biering-Sorensen F, et al: Peroral treatment with ciprofloxacin of patients with spinal cord lesion and bacteriuria caused by multiply resistant bacteria. Paraplegia 28:41, 1990.

46. Perkash I, Giroux J: Prevention, treatment and management of urinary tract infection in neuropathic bladders. J Am Paraplegia Soc 8:15, 1985.

47. Peterson JR, Roth EJ: Fever, bacteriuria, and pyuria in spinal cord injured patients with indwelling urethral catheters. Arch Phys Med Rehabil 70:839, 1989.

48. Reid G, Sobel JD: Bacterial adherence in pathogenesis of urinary tract infections: Review. Rev Infect Dis 9:470, 1987.

49. Ruutu M, Lehtonen T: Urinary tract complications in spinal cord injury patients. Ann Chir Gynaecol 73:325, 1984.

50. Sanderson PJ, Rawal P: Contamination of the environment of spinal cord injured patients by organisms causing urinary tract infection. J Hosp Infect 10:173, 1987.

51. Segal JL, Gray DR, Gordon SK, et al: Gentamicin disposition kinetics in humans with spinal cord injury. Am Chir Gynaecol 73:325, 1984.

52. Sobel J, Kaye D: Urinary tract infections. *In* Gillenwater JY, Grayhack JT, Howard SS, et al (eds): Adult and Pediatric Urology, vol 1. Chicago, Year Book Medical Publishers, 1987, p 246.

53. Sotolongo JR, Koleilat N: Significance of asymptomatic bacteriuria in spinal cord injury patients on condom catheter. J Urol 143:979, 1990.

54. Stamm WE: Measurement of pyuria and its relation to bacteriuria. Am J Med 75(1B):53, 1983.

55. Stickler DJ, Chawla JC: An appraisal of antibiotic policies for urinary tract infections in patients with spinal cord injuries undergoing long-term intermittent catheterization. Paraplegia 26:215, 1988.

56. Stover SL, Lloyd LK, Waites KB, et al: Urinary tract infection in spinal cord injury. Arch Phys Med Rehabil 70:47, 1989.

57. Strand CL, Bryant JK, Sutton KH: Septicemia secondary to urinary tract infection with colony counts less than 10^5 cfu/ml. Am J Clin Pathol 83:619, 1985.

58. Svanborg-Eden C, Anderson B, Hagbergh L: Receptor analogues and anti-pili antibodies as inhibitors of bacterial attachment in vivo and in vitro. Ann NY Acad Sci 409:580, 1983.

59. Svanborg-Eden C, Hausson S, Jodal U, et al: Host-parasite interaction in urinary tract. J Infect Dis 157:421, 1988.

60. Svanborg-Eden C, Jodal U, Hanson LA, et al: Variable adherence to normal human urinary tract epithelial cells of *Escherichia coli* strains associated with various forms of urinary tract infection. Lancet 2:490, 1976.

61. Vaziri ND, Cesarior T, Mootoo K, et al: Bacterial infections in patients with chronic renal failure: Occurrence with spinal cord injury. Arch Intern Med 142:1273, 1982.

62. Waites KB, Canupp KC, DeVivo MJ: Norfloxacin treatment of nosocomial urinary tract infection in patients undergoing intermittent catheterization following spinal cord injury. Curr Ther Res 48:503, 1990.

63. Warren JW, Platt R, Thomas RJ, et al: Antibiotic irrigation and catheter-associated urinary tract infections. N Engl J Med 299:5670, 1978.

CHAPTER 13

The Urinary Bladder in Spinal Cord Disease

Michael E. Mayo, M. B. B. S.,
F. R. C. S.
William E. Bradley, M. D.

ANATOMY AND PHYSIOLOGY OF THE URINARY BLADDER

The neural innervation of the human urinary bladder is complex, and the contributions of many areas of the central nervous system to bladder control are undefined and unexplored. With the significant scarcity of normal human data on bladder innervation, a considerable effort has been made to fill in the gaps by use of an experimental animal model.[33] This has resulted in a free application of findings from animal studies to the problems of understanding human urinary bladder function. Also, since the mid-1980s, a shift has been taking place in the selection of the animal being studied, from the domesticated cat to the laboratory rat. The gap in the knowledge base of human function has been made larger by this change.

Differences between animal and human bladder innervation and function include an unknown voiding habitus in the animal, a lissencephalic brain in the rat (in contrast to the gyrencephalic brain in humans), a much greater accentuation of limbic system representation in the rat, differing spinal cord segmentation in the rat, and a quadruped posture in the animal that renders the bladder an abdominal viscus. Lack of cognitive interaction with the animal renders an event such as detrusor reflex contraction an uninterpretable occurrence. A key element in the human cystometrogram is the volitional attempt by the patient to suppress a detrusor reflex contraction. Inability to suppress a detrusor reflex contraction is a common indication of suprasacral interruption of bladder innervation and is termed *detrusor hyperreflexia*. Selection of a laboratory animal to model such an event can only be regarded as inappropriate.

This discussion of anatomy and physiology of human bladder function is confined to human studies. Animal studies are reported as indicators of organization but are not offered as evidence on their own. To further support this position, it is wise to evaluate the benefits and disadvantages of animal research to the understanding of human bladder function in cases in which this has been done. An early and prominent investigator of bladder function who utilized the cat model was F. J. F. Barrington, whose laboratory work was performed at University College Hospital, London. Barrington, a British urologist, was influenced by early pioneers in physiology and neurosurgery, Sherrington and Horsley. Barrington used the new techniques of intercollicular decerebration and the new stereotaxis instrument introduced by Horsley and Clarke to define the contribution of the brain stem to contraction of the urinary detrusor. The experiments extended from 1914 to 1941[14–17] and revealed the contribution of spinal cord and peripheral innervation of the urinary detrusor and urethra to voiding. Results of these experiments have strongly influenced the interpretation of clinical data including the results of cystometry. Briefly, Barrington described a series of seven interrelated reflexes in the cat that promote evacuation of intravesical contents. These reflexes are described in the following text.

1. Reflex 1 is a brain-stem reflex consisting of long-routed pelvic visceral afferent impulses from the urinary detrusor muscle to neurons localized in the dorsolateral gray matter of the pontine tegmentum. After synapsing in this nucleus, activity descends to the lateral gray matter of the sacral spinal cord. This was Barrington's first and most significant description of a reflex. Activation of this reflex provided for the initial event of voiding: contraction of the urinary detrusor. This reflex has been utilized to interpret cystometric data as well as to predict the result of interrup-

tion at various levels of the central neuraxis. Unfortunately, no direct evidence exists for a similar reflex pathway in humans. Although the animal data have been accepted without question, it is unlikely that, lacking significant changes in our ability to trace brain-stem reflexes in humans, this reflex path will ever be documented.

2. Reflexes 2 and 7 provide a facilitatory effect of flow of urine through the urethra on detrusor contraction. These reflexes have been demonstrated not to be present in humans.

3. In reflex 4, urine flow through the urethra produces urethral relaxation. This reflex has not been confirmed in humans.

4. Reflex 3 is mediated by afferent and efferent impulses in the hypogastric nerve. It has been determined to have little significance in humans.

5. Finally, it has been pointed out that relaxation of the striated sphincter muscle, which occurs during urine flow through the urethra, is a result of detrusor contraction. Barrington visualized this event as a urethral reflex.

Review of Barrington's original studies and of the plethora of reports that have emanated from animal research laboratories in succeeding years has raised the question, "How valuable or relevant is animal research to the understanding of human bladder function?" The results to this time, particularly in the laboratory rat, would make an affirmative answer doubtful. The lack of similarity of neuroanatomic organization (particularly in the rat) and the lack of capability for cognitive interaction will continue to mandate that animal experimentation be two-tiered: (1) to confirm the original animal experiments and (2) to undertake to confirm whether the results apply to humans.

These conclusions suggest that greater emphasis in urinary bladder research should be placed on human studies. This approach has been impeded by lack of neurologic sophistication on the part of the urologist, by the lack of extensive development of electrodiagnostic techniques for the study of bladder innervation, and by the limited use of magnetic resonance imaging (MRI) studies of the central nervous system in affected patients. To elicit the full value of MRI in bladder innervation studies requires careful history-taking and a detailed physical and neurologic examination. This integrated examination is best performed by a physician who is skilled in clinical neurology and urology. In addition, research on the neurology of the human genitourinary system performed by such individuals should provide critical information on the neuroanatomy and physiology of human bladder function.

In the study of the effects of diseases of the nervous system on voiding, cystometry has been an early useful laboratory indicator.[69] Cystometry consists of filling the bladder with water or saline usually in a retrograde manner as is done for urethrography.[38] In early studies it was observed that bladder sensation could be tested, and that at an appropriate filling volume, a high-amplitude rise in pressure occurred, which was associated with a feeling of urgency. These high-amplitude pressure rises, which are a result of detrusor reflex contraction, can be voluntarily attenuated in normal individuals.[35] By employing the concept of Barrington's first reflex, it was concluded that the pressure rise represented activation of a spinobulbospinal reflex from bladder afferent nerves to the pontine gray matter. All subsequent attempts to define the influence of lesions in the nervous system on urination used cystometry, the interpretation of which was based on the cystometrogram and whether the subjects could suppress the reflex on command. As mentioned earlier, inability to suppress the reflex was termed *detrusor hyperreflexia*, and absence of the reflex was termed *detrusor areflexia*. Subsequently, concurrent recording of electromyographic (EMG) activity of the external urinary sphincter has been added to the methodology.[37]

Cerebrocortical Innervation of the Urinary Bladder

Cerebrocortical innervation of the urinary bladder has been studied in patients with lesions of the cerebral cortex[11] using evoked potentials,[93, 94, 97] electroencephalography (EEG),[30] and transcranial magnetic stimulation.[68]

Patients with lesions of the frontal lobes demonstrate uncontrollable detrusor reflex contractions on cystometrogram, termed *detrusor hyperreflexia*. EEG responses to bladder filling in humans have also been reported.[30] These initial studies were performed with the limited resolution of the 10–20 system using 21 electrode positions. Further studies with increased numbers of electrode placements and quantitative assessment may provide evidence of a localized response to detrusor reflex activation. Innervation of the urinary detrusor muscle and external urinary sphincter has also been documented in humans by the evoked potential technique. Stimulation of the pelvic nerve innervation of the proximal urethra evoked diphasic responses at the cranial vertex. Stimulation of the dorsal nerve of the penis, the terminal sensory division of the pudendal nerve, and an analog to the afferent innervation of the external urinary sphincter, evoked a maximal response 2 cm posterior to the vertex. The latency of the pelvic nerve response was approximately two-thirds longer than that of the pudendal nerve.

Recording responses in the external urinary sphincter after transcranial magnetic stimulation of the cerebral cortex has also been reported.[68]

The Basal Ganglia

The most compelling evidence for innervation of the urinary bladder by the basal ganglia is the finding of their dysfunction and urinary incontinence in patients with Parkinson's disease.[137] Such patients may show a number of detrusor reflex abnormalities including detrusor hyperreflexia and detrusor areflexia.

The Limbic System

In animals, the limbic system has been reported to have an influence on the urinary bladder. No similar reports have come from patients with temporal lobe epilepsy or those who have undergone temporal lobectomy for seizures.

The Thalamus

Thalamic nuclei are probably involved in the relay of afferent impulses from both the urinary bladder and the urinary sphincter. However, no specific information about humans is available.

The Cerebellum and Bladder Function

Animal experiments trace pathways from the urinary detrusor and external urinary sphincter to the cerebellum.[40] No evidence of this kind has been reported in patients owing to the relative inaccessibility of the cerebellum to skin surface electrodes. Animal experiments have also demonstrated characteristic urinary detrusor reflex responses to removal of the anterior vermis. Unfortunately no similar responses have been reported in patients with acute cerebellar injuries. Effects of chronic cerebellar injury on bladder function are moderated by compensatory mechanisms in the central nervous system that follow this event.[65] Hence, clinical reports have been made of urinary bladder dysfunction in chronic cerebellar disease accompanied by a range of cystometric findings from detrusor hyperreflexia to detrusor areflexia.[116] Further evolution of evoked potential testing may help to clarify these results.[2]

Innervation of the Urinary Bladder by Pontine Nuclei

The role ascribed to pontine nuclei in urinary detrusor contraction has been heavily influenced by animal research. Beginning with Barrington, there have been many reports in the animal literature documenting his results and extending his work to include more precise localization of the neurons in these nuclei as well as in their connections. Their location in the dorsolateral pontine tegmentum has been confirmed many times, as

has the long routing of detrusor afferent pathways to this location.[39, 60] Impulses arise there and descend to neurons in the lateral gray matter of the sacral spinal cord, where synapses occur.

Unfortunately there is no confirmation of this mode of innervation in humans. With nonconfirmation of many of Barrington's other reflexes in humans, the whole question of applicability of the animal brain-stem innervation of the urinary detrusor to humans is unanswered. No evoked potential data for humans are on record and no correlative autopsy studies of human brain-stem lesions and bladder function have taken place.

Cystometric interpretation would be helped significantly by these data. The presence or absence of detrusor hyperreflexia could be confirmable by evoked potential studies, and the correlation of lesion site and nature of bladder dysfunction would constitute an advance in knowledge.

Ascending and Descending Spinal Tracts from the Pelvic and Pudendal Nuclei in the Conus Medullaris

Principal afferent and efferent spinal pathways from the urinary detrusor have been identified in humans.[139, 140] These tracts are localized to the posterior portions of the lateral columns. Location of the spinal tracts innervating the external urinary sphincter has not been identified in humans.

The Pelvic Detrusor and Pudendal Nuclei of the Conus Medullaris

The anatomy and physiology of the pelvic and pudendal nuclei in the sacral spinal cord of humans and their inflows and outflows have been tentatively identified.[44, 29, 149] Methods employed for this determination have included electrodiagnostic studies, neural blockade of spinal roots with local anesthesia, and postmortem examination of the sacral spinal cord. None of these studies has examined the question of sexual dimorphism (i.e., differences between neuronal populations based on gender). A significant number of animal studies using axonal and cellular tracers, such as horseradish peroxidase, have also been undertaken.

In human studies, sacral root blockade by injection of local anesthetic has demonstrated that the urinary detrusor is innervated from a longitudinal distribution of segments S3 and 4. Vertical displacement of one spinal segment may exist in a rostral or caudal direction, depending on the presence of prefixation or postfixation of the lumbosacral plexus.

Histologic examination of the sacral spinal cord in patients dying of Fabry's disease found exclusive accumulation of intraneuronal lipid in autonomic neurons.[168] Unfortunately these data are in conflict with those of previous studies, and resolution of the problem will require further study. Neurons of the pudendal nucleus were first identified by Onuf[146] as being located in the ventral gray matter. The longitudinal extent of this nucleus ranges from the first to the third sacral segments.

Pathways to and from the human pudendal nuclei have also been defined by evoked potential techniques. Connections from the urinary detrusor, the pudendal innervation of the urethra, and the dorsal nerve of the penis have been traced to pudendal motor neurons and axons that innervate the rectal sphincter. Bladder distension and reflex contraction have been observed to attenuate these responses. Spinal pathways from pudendal afferent impulses to the cerebral cortex have been traced by stimulation of the dorsal nerve of the penis. The descending path has been documented by transcranial magnetic stimulation of the motor cortex. The location and organization of pelvic and pudendal nuclei in the sacral spinal cord have been traced in extensive animal investigations. The extent to which this work applies to humans is the subject of future research.

Thoracolumbar Innervation of the Urinary Bladder

Whereas considerable evidence exists of thoracolumbar innervation of the urinary bladder in animals, human research has indicated that sympathetic innervation of the urinary detrusor muscle does not significantly affect bladder function.[117] Adrenergic endings have been demonstrated to be extensive in the proximal portion of the male urethra, but evidence that a functional role exists has not accumulated.

Central Nervous System Reflex Pathways and the Urinary Bladder

Animal studies have indicated a series of four interrelated reflexes of crucial significance in controlling urinary bladder function.[36] Only two of these reflex pathways (the third and fourth) have been confirmed in humans.

1. Reflex 1 consists of connections in both directions between the dorsolateral portion of the pontine tegmentum and the frontal cortex anterior to the sensory motor strip.

2. Reflex 2 consists of afferent activity from the urinary detrusor that ascends to the dorsolateral portion of the pontine tegmentum and then descends to synapse on autonomic neurons in the lateral column of the sacral gray matter.

3. Reflex 3 consists of detrusor afferent impulses that synapse on pudendal motor neurons in the ventral horn of the sacral gray matter.[29]

4. Reflex 4 consists of the supraspinal and segmental innervation of the external urinary sphincter.[93]

Peripheral Innervation of the Urinary Bladder

Many questions are unanswered concerning the peripheral innervation of the human urinary bladder. As with the central nervous system pathways, the tendency has been to fill in the gaps with experimental animal data.

In humans, innervation of the urinary detrusor consists of motor and sensory axons in the hypogastric nerves and pelvic nerve outflow from the sacral spinal cord. These two nerves course distally to plexuses that innervate the bladder and urethra. The pudendal nerves originate from the motor neurons in the ventral horn of the sacral gray matter and travel distally to innervate the external urinary sphincter.[85, 86]

Ganglia are present in two principal locations: in the mesh of connective tissue surrounding the bladder base and in the interstices of smooth muscle bundles of the urinary detrusor. In humans, neurons from these ganglia stain for acetylcholinesterase, and synaptic transmission is presumed to be cholinergic. No electrophysiologic data from human ganglionic transmission have appeared in the literature. Postganglionic axons and vesical afferent nerves provide dense innervation to individual smooth muscle cells of the urinary detrusor. Heavy axon accumulations are present that contain a specific form of axon varicosity with a specific type of synaptic vesicle. Gosling[86] has speculated that these represent a specialized form of sensory receptor.

In the urinary detrusor, many areas of close contact exist between axons with axon varicosities and individual smooth muscle cells. Small-diameter clear vesicles are seen in the axon varicosities that are presumed to be cholinergic. How smooth muscle contraction occurs and is coordinated in the human bladder is unknown. No in vivo, and only a few in vitro, electrophysiologic records exist from human urinary detrusor muscle cells.

Descriptions of muscle bundles from the human urinary detrusor and their organization in the area of the bladder neck are as individual and varied as the anatomists who have investigated the problem.[87] Individual groupings of smooth muscle cells in the human urinary detrusor form loops, or *arcades*, around the bladder neck. The effect of bladder contraction, therefore, is to separate these opposing arcades.

The bladder neck in the male, formed from the circular fibers described earlier, merges into the preprostatic urethra. The preprostatic and prostatic portions of the urethra are formed from circularly arranged smooth muscle fibers. As the urethra transits through the urogenital diaphragm, it acquires an external layer of striated muscle, the external urinary sphincter. Nerve endings in the preprostatic and prostatic urethra are principally adrenergic.

The female urethra, however, consists of longitudinal smooth muscle fibers from the urinary detrusor and is innervated by cholinergic axons. Fibers of the external urinary sphincter are thinner than in the male and are deficient posteriorly.

An extraordinary deficiency exists in our knowledge of human urinary bladder function. Whether this can be compensated for by animal research, particularly in the rat model, is doubtful. More attention should be paid to human investigation and studies of human voiding physiology in future research.

LABORATORY EVALUATION OF BLADDER FUNCTION IN SPINAL CORD DISEASE

The laboratory evaluation of a patient with suspected neurologic bladder disease is outlined in Table 13–1. At the first clinic visit, after the history and physical examination are complete, if the patient has a reasonably full bladder, a flow rate,[66, 88, 160, 163, 174] urine specimen, and postvoiding residual volume measurement can be obtained noninvasively, without resorting to catheterization. Postvoiding residual volume can be measured by

TABLE 13–1

LABORATORY EVALUATION OF URINARY BLADDER FUNCTION IN NEUROLOGIC DISEASE

Urinalysis and culture
Blood urea nitrogen and creatinine clearance
Uroflow and postvoid residual volume studies
Upper tract studies (e.g., ultrasound or excretory urogram)
Cystometry
Voiding cystourethrography
Sphincter electromyography
Urethral pressure profile
Electrodiagnostic studies of bladder and pelvic floor innervation
Videourodynamics
Transrectal ultrasound of voiding
Long-term (ambulatory) monitoring

a commercially available portable ultrasound machine,[53] which is accurate enough for clinical purposes. Symptomatic and asymptomatic bacteriuria are common with neurogenic bladder diseases,[70] and before invasive studies are undertaken it is prudent to at least obtain culture and sensitivity data; in most cases, it is wise to start treatment. Flow rates are easily obtained in most urology clinics and are reasonable screening tests for voiding obstruction and dysfunction, especially when combined with a postvoiding residual volume measurement. Maximum flow rates, flow pattern, and voided volume are the most useful parameters derived from a flow rate study. Laboratory screening tests of renal function, for example, blood urea nitrogen and serum creatinine assays, should be performed at the initial clinic visit.

Further studies can be planned individually. If lower tract symptoms are predominant and the risk of upper tract involvement is low, an ultrasound (Fig. 13–1) can be done as conveniently as a baseline examination. In patients with a risk for upper tract involvement, an excretory urogram should be done at an early stage if the serum creatinine level is less than 1.5 mg/dL. The term *excretory urogram* has replaced *intravenous pyelogram* because modern techniques show much more than a pyelogram of the collecting system. Renal tomograms taken in the first 2 to 3 minutes after injection of contrast usually show a clear nephrogram. If the creatinine level is greater than 1.5 mg/dL, ultrasound, renography, and a possible retrograde study should be considered. For evaluation of the lower urinary tract, cystometry[2, 6, 41, 42] can be performed in the clinical setting and may give significant information on which to base a treatment plan. However, if it is anticipated that voiding cystourethrography and sphincter EMG will be required, it is preferable to go straight to a videourodynamic study, which has the capability of combining pressure, EMG, flow, and radiologic images in

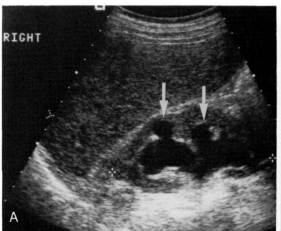

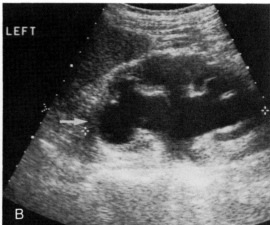

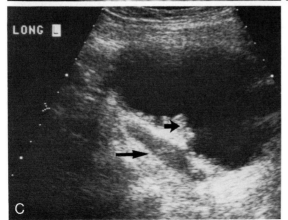

FIGURE 13–1

A, Ultrasound of the right kidney in a patient with C6 quadriplegia with increasing serum creatinine and very high bladder pressure. Hydronephrosis and dilated calyces (*arrows*) are present. *B,* Left kidney of the same patient also showing marked hydronephrosis and dilated calyces (*arrow*). *C,* Ultrasound of the bladder in the same patient showing an irregular bladder wall with marked trabeculation (*short arrow*). Dilated ureter is on the left (*long arrow*).

one study, with a printout of the combined data.[24, 26] Urethral pressure profiles in conjunction with sphincter EMG have application in studies of neurologic bladder disease,[5] but this is limited because maximum pressure is dependent on the degree of urethral (and thus reflex pelvic floor) stimulation.[128] Electrodiagnostic studies can reveal a subtle interruption of the sacral reflexes or denervation of the pelvic floor musculature.[29, 62, 96, 97, 151] Studies with further refinements using sensory evoked potentials may reveal unique information concerning the detrusor reflex and its control. Finally, a new technique of long-term "ambulatory" monitoring may be invaluable in patients whose symptoms are not reproduced by the laboratory studies mentioned.[21, 89, 173, 177] Patients who have difficulty with reflex voiding while sitting in a wheelchair and those with dysreflexia or unexplained incontinence are candidates for long-term monitoring.

Cystometry

This test, which is performed with a fast filling rate and uses carbon dioxide or water as the medium, gives information concerning bladder sensation, compliance, capacity, and the presence or absence of a detrusor contraction during bladder filling. During this test, the patient can either be instructed to suppress any tendency to void or be asked to allow spontaneous voiding when the desire occurs. With the former instruction, any detrusor contraction during filling is abnormal. In the latter circumstance, to test supraspinal control mechanisms the patient is asked to inhibit contraction; if the patient is unable to do so, the result is regarded as abnormal. Individuals who have intact bladder innervation will normally suppress urination when the bladder is filled under these circumstances. Patients with reflex neurogenic bladders due to suprasacral lesions are unable to suppress urination either when asked to do so during the filling phase or when the detrusor contraction occurs. It is probably easier to have patients suppress urination during

filling and then try to relax and void when the bladder reaches its capacity. Patients who are intact neurologically have difficulty trying to void or to produce a contraction when the bladder is filled with carbon dioxide. The main indication, therefore, for cystometrography is to test for the presence of a detrusor reflex in patients suspected of having a suprasacral lesion. As many neurologically intact patients exhibit apparent areflexia due to psychological inhibition, even with provocative testing (for example, with a change in position from supine to sitting, standing, or even walking in place), the test is of value only if results are positive for a detrusor reflex. Thus, confirming the presence of detrusor hyperreflexia in patients recovering from spinal shock or in patients with multiple sclerosis is helpful, but a finding of areflexia in a patient with a cauda equina lesion is not necessarily confirmation that the detrusor muscle is decentralized (i.e., disconnected from the central nervous system).

Any size catheter can be employed when carbon dioxide is used as a filling medium, as there is little resistance to flow and therefore no artifact from the pump. With water, it is better to use a two-channel catheter: one channel for inflow and the other to measure pressure (to eliminate the pressure head or pump artifact from the trace).

With a normal cystometrogram, an initial sensation of filling occurs at approximately 50% of capacity or reflex threshold; the latter should be approximately 300 to 600 mL. Two sensations are said to be present when the bladder is filled to capacity: the first is fullness in the lower abdomen and the second is a sense of urgency, which is appreciated in the perineum.[182] The rise in volume divided by the rise in pressure in the absence of a detrusor contraction (tonus limb) yields compliance, which should be greater than 10 mL/cm H_2O. The presence of a detrusor contraction and its suppression have already been discussed. A rise in bladder pressure owing to a detrusor contraction has to be distinguished from a rise due to transmitted abdominal pressure, and a separate measurement of intra-abdominal pressure (e.g., by a balloon placed in the rectum) is necessary to verify this.

Voiding Cystourography

This study is limited by the inability to know when the detrusor is contracting. For example, the bladder neck may be open as a result of either a detrusor contraction or impairment of bladder neck closure secondary to previous surgery. Reflux may occur at high or low pressures, so this differentiation cannot be made without simultaneous pressure measurements; voiding cystourography does indicate whether reflux is present. Voiding may be associated with a detrusor contraction, a rise in abdominal pressure due to straining, or a combination of both. It may cease because of detrusor failure or dyssynergia. All of this information may be lost without simultaneous pressure measurements.

Sphincter Electromyography

Sphincter EMG is performed by recording from one of several sites, using several different methods. EMG activity can be recorded from either the external urinary sphincter or the anal sphincter. In most patients it is easier to record from the anal sphincter, and it may be assumed that responses to bladder filling and emptying are similar for both sphincters.[29, 37] However, some authors have shown differences in responses from the anal and the periurethral sphincter in patients with neurologic disease.[27] Types of recording electrodes include EMG needles, wires, and ring electrodes mounted on an anal or urinary catheter. Ring electrodes on the catheter are placed in close apposition to the sphincter muscle. Either monopolar or bipolar recordings can be made. EMG signals are amplified and the output is fed to the recording pen of a strip-chart recorder, which is operating at the same time as the cystograph. An alternative method focuses on the pattern of EMG activity and consists of processing the EMG signals through a pulse counter or integrator[46] with the output recorded as an integral of sphincter activity.

The normal sphincter pattern consists of an increase in amplitude of the EMG signals with increased bladder filling.[124] On reflex detrusor contraction, either sphincter quiescence may be found (if voiding is permitted) or enhanced EMG activity may be seen when the patient is instructed to suppress the detrusor reflex. In patients with lesions of the corticospinal tract, loss of voluntary control of sphincter contraction and relaxation is associated with limb spasticity and extensor plantar responses. In this situation, the combined cystometric and sphincter EMG record demonstrates the pattern called detrusor-sphincter dyssynergia,[3] which consists of failure of the sphincter to relax (it often increases its activity) during detrusor contraction. Detrusor-sphincter dyssynergia is of particular importance in patients with suprasacral spinal cord injury because it can obstruct urinary flow.

In patients with cauda equina injuries associated with lower limb weakness, lax external urinary sphincters, sensory loss, and depressed or absent deep tendon reflexes, the sphincter EMG reveals a lack of response to bladder filling and to voluntary contraction or relaxation.

Urethral Pressure Profile

Urethral function can also be evaluated with the urethral pressure profile. In this test, a catheter that is perfused continually with water or carbon dioxide[5, 7] is withdrawn from the bladder at a constant velocity. As the catheter is withdrawn, the critical escape pressure is measured continually through perforations in the catheter. This same procedure can be performed using a microtip transducer mounted in the catheter.

This method yields a curve that shows urethral pressure (measured in centimeters of water) on the Y axis plotted against position in the urethra (measured in centimeters) on the X axis. Although this can be useful in neurologically intact patients with possible sphincter weakness (for example, after prostatectomy in males[125] and with stress incontinence in females[13, 159]), better methods are available for obtaining the same information (for example, by demonstrating leakage with coughing on videourodynamic studies).

With neurogenic bladders, the test can be used to determine the completeness of the sphincterotomy; again, alternate methods using video-urodynamic studies are available.

Electrodiagnostic Studies

Electrodiagnostic studies of innervation of the human lower urinary tract are in initial stages of development and application. These tests define the presence of an autonomic and somatic neuropathy that affects the urinary bladder, enhance information gained by cystometry and sphincter EMG, and delineate the connections of the pelvic and pudendal nuclei in the human conus medullaris.

Conus medullaris reflex pathways that are definable electrodiagnostically include those involved in the bulbocavernosus reflex and the urethroanal evoked response.[29, 151, 171] The latency and presence of the pudendal cortical evoked response document the anatomic integrity of this pathway.[96, 97] Measurement of the conduction velocity of the dorsal nerve of the penis ensures accurate interpretation of prolonged latencies in these evoked potentials.[109]

Bulbocavernosus reflex latency is measured by percutaneously stimulating the dorsal nerve of the penis and recording the EMG response evoked in the bulbocavernosus muscle. Simultaneous performance of cystometry in normal individuals demonstrates that the bulbocavernosus response is depressed when a detrusor contraction occurs. The pudendal cortical evoked response is obtained by percutaneously stimulating the dorsal nerve of the penis, which is the terminal sensory portion of the pudendal nerve. The response is maximal at a location posterior to the central vertex. Diabetes mellitus and other diseases that produce penile neuropathy are reflected in prolonged latencies in the conus medullaris pathways and in the pudendal cortical evoked response. Many of these patients also exhibit slowed nerve conduction velocity in the dorsal nerve of the penis.

Videourodynamic Studies

Videourodynamic studies and the long-term monitoring procedure discussed in the next section attempt to create more natural conditions in which to study "physiologic" filling and voiding in a particular patient.[26] Cystometry using carbon dioxide at a filling rate of 120 mL/minute is designed to stimulate the detrusor afferent nerves maximally so that a detrusor reflex is provoked. Conversely, the slower filling rates using liquid media may not be truly "physiologic," but with a small catheter and with the patient in a sitting or standing position, if appropriate, the chance of seeing a more typical voiding phase is maximized. If contrast agents are used as filling media and fluoroscopy is combined with pressure measurements, a maximum amount of information can be obtained from this study.

In practice, a 7F two-channel bladder catheter and an 8F rectal catheter are used. Rectal pressure is subtracted from bladder pressure electronically to arrive at a detrusor pressure. Surface EMG of the anal sphincter and flow rates, if appropriate, are determined and are combined with fluoroscopy of the lower urinary tract. The combined urodynamic and radiologic images are mixed on one screen and recorded on videotape. Spot films of critical events in the study are taken from the videotape at the end of the procedure (Figs. 13–2 and 13–3). In patients with neurologic lesions, filling rates of 50 mL/minute are used. The amount of radiation used may be of some concern to both patient and staff, but with modern equipment that uses an image intensifier and with the fluoroscopy time being limited to no more than 1 minute, the amount of radiation to the patient will be equivalent to that of a regular cystogram using standard x-ray films.

This study is most useful in assessing the failure of bladder emptying in patients with incomplete spinal cord lesions who have some voluntary control. It is essential in patients who may have a combination of neuropathy and mechanical obstruction from prostate enlargement. It is also useful to assess characteristics of detrusor contraction when selecting candidates for sphinctero-

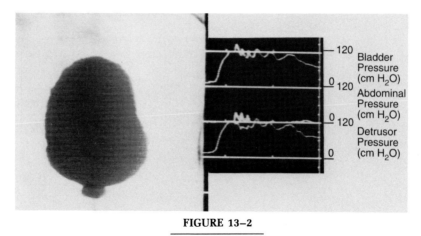

FIGURE 13–2

Hyperreflexic bladder in a female patient with a T6 complete spinal cord injury. Well-sustained detrusor contraction of greater than 120 cm H_2O is seen with closure of distal sphincter.

tomy. A spontaneous contraction at less than 200 mL of volume with a rise time of 20 seconds or less, a maximum pressure of 50 cm H_2O or more, and a duration of contraction of more than 60 seconds are desirable.[20] An assessment of bladder neck opening can also be obtained, and if opening pressure is more than 50 cm of H_2O, a bladder neck incision should be performed along with the distal sphincterotomy.

Ultrasound

Transrectal ultrasound, which was developed for imaging the prostate, can be used to visualize the posterior urethra during voiding.[143] It has the advantage of allowing continuous monitoring of the posterior urethra without exposure to radiation. However, the bladder wall cannot be evaluated and the presence or absence of ureteral reflux cannot be determined. Also, the rectal probe is large and is probably too uncomfortable in patients with anal sensation.

Long-Term (Ambulatory) Monitoring

With the introduction of microtip solid-state transducers and miniaturized digital recorders, monitoring of the lower urinary tract for 12 to 24 hours is now possible while patients undertake their normal daily activi-

ties.[21] To distinguish intra-abdominal pressure changes from true detrusor contractions, it is necessary to record rectal pressure. Also, with a sensor at the distal sphincter in the urethra, a decrease in intraurethral pressure in the presence of detrusor activity identifies the detrusor pressure change as a true detrusor reflex. However, the bladder catheters (although they are only 4F to 5F in diameter) may themselves alter lower urinary tract function. However, with natural filling rates and in patients undertaking normal daily activities, long-term monitoring promises to provide insights into some of the problems that it is not possible to address with more conventional studies (Figs. 13–4 and 13–5). Results reported to date indicate that compliance changes seen on standard cystometry are to a large extent artifacts of a fast filling rate, and upper tract dilation is related to phasic detrusor activity rather than to poor compliance.[177] However, further studies are needed to evaluate the invasiveness of this technique and to determine its clinical utility.

MANAGEMENT OF THE NEUROGENIC BLADDER IN PATIENTS WITH SPINAL CORD DISEASE

Few medical or surgical management strategies will restore bladder and urethral function to normal in patients with significant

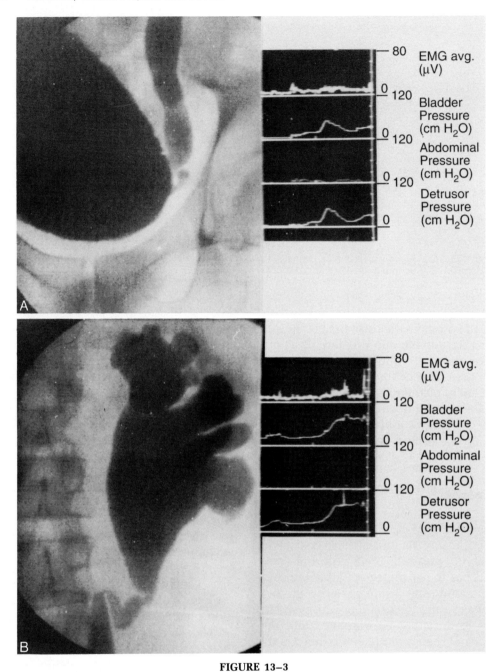

FIGURE 13–3

A, Hyperreflexic bladder of a male patient with T9 paraplegia shows vesicoureteral reflux with dilatation at a relatively low pressure (30 cm H_2O). B, Further, high-pressure contractions and a view of the left kidney in the same patient shows marked dilatation of the calyces and tortuosity of the ureter.

neurogenic bladder dysfunction. Goals of management are therefore more modest and can be stated simply as the creation of a reservoir of adequate capacity (500 to 600 mL) at low pressure (compliance greater than 10 mL/cm H_2O with no detrusor contractions during filling) that empties adequately (postvoiding residual volume less than 100 mL) at low pressure (less than 60 cm H_2O in males and less than 30 cm H_2O in females). Continence of urine with normal daily activities is also desirable, as is absence of such compli-

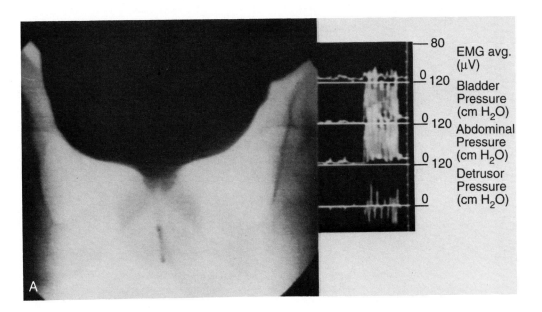

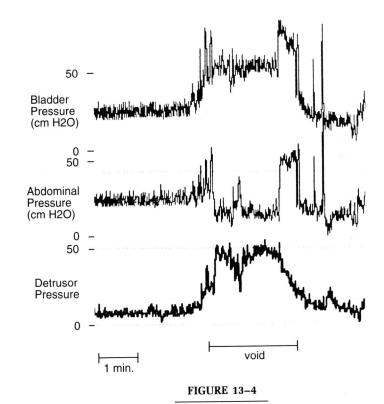

FIGURE 13–4

A, Attempted voiding in a patient with a possible cauda equina lesion. Patient tries to void by straining; high-amplitude pressure swings are seen on bladder and abdominal pressure tracings. In the lowest channel, however, which represents true detrusor or subtracted pressure, no evidence of detrusor contraction is present. B, Ambulatory long-term monitoring of abdominal and rectal pressures shows detrusor contraction of approximately 40 cm H_2O with voiding in the absence of abdominal straining. The diagnosis of true areflexia is sometimes difficult to make in the laboratory situation, and long-term monitoring often reveals a more normal pattern.

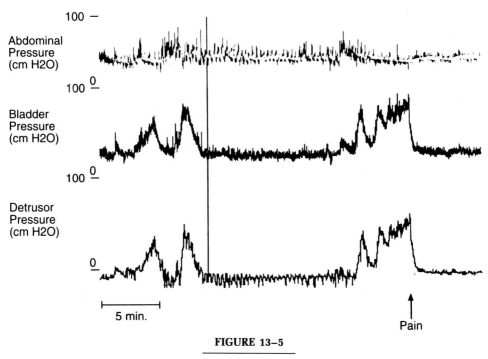

FIGURE 13–5

A 20-minute section of an 8-hour period of long-term monitoring in a patient with T12 paraplegia who was having autonomic dysreflexic symptoms and incontinence with intermittent catheterization and oxybutynin. The traces reveal intermittent detrusor contractions; the patient noted pain or dysreflexia with the second contraction.

cations as infections and stones. The case for reducing intravesical pressure in patients with neurologic bladder disease is well documented by several authors[77, 91, 165] who have shown that low pressure is associated with a reduced prevalence of upper tract deterioration.

Many factors influence the choice of management. Upper tract deterioration is probably the most important medical factor, influencing in particular the management of patients with chronic disabilities. With more recent lesions, or when the upper tracts are normal, management choices are dependent on such patient characteristics as age and mental status, stability of the neurologic disease, level of the lesion, degree of spasticity, gender, body habitus, and motivation and lifestyle. For elderly patients with cognitive impairment, therapy should be simple. Surgical management for patients with unstable disease, such as multiple sclerosis, is rarely recommended. Quadriplegics with lesions above the C6 level cannot do self-catheterization. Women with high paraple-

gia, severe spasticity of the lower limbs, and obesity have more difficulty than men doing self-catheterization. Motivation and lifestyle are perhaps the most important and most intangible factors to consider. A great deal can be achieved by an intelligent, motivated, and careful patient; the same achievement might be impossible for a patient who wants convenience and simplicity at the expense of increased risks.

When considering pharmacologic and surgical management, it is helpful to break down the basic abnormality into detrusor dysfunction and sphincter disorder (Tables 13–2 and 13–3). Detrusor and sphincter abnormalities may be further analyzed as a failure to store or a failure to empty.[180] For example, the detrusor may fail to store because of poor compliance or hyperreflexia and may fail to empty because of hypocontractility or areflexia. Similarly, a sphincter may fail to permit storage because of denervation at the conal or cauda equina level and may fail to allow emptying because of discoordinated activity (dyssynergia) or a failure to relax dur-

TABLE 13–2

PHARMACOTHERAPY OF THE LOWER URINARY TRACT

Detrusor problems	
Failure to store	Anticholinergic and musculotropic agents
	Calcium channel blockers
	Adrenergic antagonists
Failure to empty	Cholinergic agonists
Sphincter problems	
Failure to store	Adrenergic agonists
	Estrogens
Failure to empty	Adrenergic antagonists
	Muscle relaxants (possibly intrathecal)

ing voiding. Clearly a combination of both detrusor and sphincter abnormalities is often present, but a logical approach to management often involves manipulating one factor or the other. For example, a hyperreflexic detrusor with a dyssynergic distal sphincter and reflex incontinence could be managed by increasing detrusor storage capacity with anticholinergic agents and using clean intermittent self-catheterization to empty the bladder if the patient is paraplegic. However, in a quadriplegic patient whose lesion is above the C6 level, it might be better to treat failure to empty owing to sphincter dyssynergia by

TABLE 13–3

SURGICAL MANAGEMENT OF THE LOWER URINARY TRACT

Detrusor problems	
Failure to store	Augmentation cystoplasty
	Denervation
	Rhizotomy
	Ganglioneurectomy
	Detrusor transection
	Hyperdistension
Failure to empty	Electrical stimulation
	Intravesical stimulation
Sphincter problems	
Failure to store	Artificial sphincter
	Teflon or collagen periurethral injection
Failure to empty	Sphincterotomy (incision or stent)
	Intrathecal baclofen administration
	Botulinum toxin injection
	Prostatectomy
	Urinary diversion

performing sphincterotomy and using condom catheter drainage.

Medical

BEHAVIORAL

Many patients with conal or cauda equina lesions, detrusor areflexia, and pelvic floor denervation are able to learn to void using Valsalva's and Credé's maneuvers to effectively empty the bladder. This is usually most effective in women, but because of severe pelvic floor descent over time, stress incontinence often becomes a major problem. In paraplegics with a spastic pelvic floor, voiding by sphincter stretch to relax the pelvic floor and using Valsalva's maneuver was described some time ago,[113] but it has not achieved widespread application. It is based on the principle that a spastic striated muscle will relax when stretched gently. The patient has to be well-motivated and able and willing to transfer for voiding and must have adequate Valsalva pressure for voiding, with or without an abdominal binder. The patient also must have a sensory complete lesion, because the anal sphincter and pelvic floor are stretched digitally; once the sphincter relaxes, the patient strains to empty the bladder. This technique's failure to gain popularity is probably the result of its being more labor-intensive and inconvenient; it is more difficult to transfer for bladder emptying every 4 to 6 hours than to do self-catheterization in a wheelchair. Behavioral therapy using habit training, conditioning methods, and biofeedback is generally harmless but is very labor-intensive. Although these methods have achieved some success in neurologically intact patients with stress incontinence,[169] after prostatectomy,[49] and with urgency incontinence,[74, 176] they have limited application to patients with spinal cord disease.

CLEAN INTERMITTENT SELF-CATHETERIZATION

Since its introduction by Lapides in 1972,[63, 115] this technique has been employed extensively for patients with neurogenic bladder disease. The sphincter mechanism must have adequate baseline and reflex contractility to maintain continence with normal daily activities, and the bladder must have low pressure, either because of areflexia or because reflex activity has been suppressed by anticholinergic agents. Patients must restrict intake of fluids so that incontinence does not occur and so that the maximum bladder volume does not exceed 500 to 600 mL in the time between catheterizations. A few patients have some sensation of bladder fullness but most choose to self-catheterize on a schedule, such as every 4 to 6 hours during the daytime and 8 hours overnight. Use of this technique should be limited to well-motivated patients who have adequate dexterity. Men with lesions at the C7 level or below can usually manage alone but sometimes require a splint. Women have much more difficulty with urethral catheterization because of adductor spasms and poor trunk control; they often need to lie down to accomplish it.[104] The program is therefore of limited value in many patients with multiple sclerosis. Although family members and attendants can perform catheterizations for quadriplegic patients, the program restricts the activity of both patient and attendant and often breaks down. In fact, the yearly incidence of bacteriuria with fever was significantly higher in patients who were catheterized by others than even in those with indwelling catheters.[55] Although Lapides first used the technique in patients with bacteriuria due to chronic retention, it is safer to treat any bacteriuria before starting a program of self-catheterization. Catheters are usually reused and can be washed with soap and water and rinsed. Some patients attempt to sterilize them in boiling water for 10 minutes or in a microwave. If the latter method is used, the catheters must be placed in the microwave with a cup of water to act as a heat sink or the catheters may melt.

Potential problems with clean intermittent self-catheterization are trauma, urinary tract infection, bladder stones, and upper tract deterioration. Urethral trauma is surprisingly uncommon but does occur in men with spinal cord injury who have severe spasticity in muscles of the pelvic floor. Extra lubrication with 5 mL of water-soluble surgical lubricant, introduced with a syringe, normally resolves the problem. If it does not, 2% lidocaine (Xylocaine) urethral gel may help block some of the reflex activity provoked by the catheter. Changing the catheter from one with a straight tip to one with a curved tip (Coudé) may also help. Patients who have repeated urethral bleeding should undergo urethroscopy; if the mucosa is broken, a Foley catheter should be inserted for a week to allow healing. An actual false passage may need to be unroofed and then allowed to heal with an indwelling Foley catheter. Urinary tract infection is discussed later, but clean intermittent self-catheterization often controls the effects of chronic bacteriuria. Those who start with sterile urine often have development of bacteriuria, but symptoms and evidence of tissue invasion with significant pyuria are relatively less common.[8, 9] If patients have problems of infection, their technique should be carefully reviewed and more frequent catheterizations, with complete emptying of the bladder, should be stressed. If the average doubling time of bacteria is allowed, 100,000 organisms/mL may be present when urine is in the bladder for 6 to 8 hours.[145] Therefore, patients should perform a minimum of three catheterizations in 24 hours; if they experience recurrent urinary tract infections they should increase the number to five or six. Bladder stones are much less common with intermittent than with indwelling catheterization, but they develop around pubic hairs that are accidentally introduced with the catheter; patients should be warned of this possibility. Upper tract problems in patients using clean intermittent self-catheterization usually occur because of ureteral reflux or obstruction at the ureterovesical junction. The usual underderlying factors are poorly controlled reflex detrusor contraction or inadequate technique. Many mild to moderate degrees of reflux will cease with a well-performed catheterization program as long as the detrusor responds to anticholinergic agents. However, if reflux continues even with low bladder pressure, a regimen of prophylactic antibiotics can be tried; if this fails, surgical correction of the reflux may have to be considered.

Self-catheterization is appealing in its simplicity and effectiveness but it is not appropriate for all patients and requires a benign attitude toward bacteriuria. Whether this attitude is justified requires more long-term evaluation of the technique.

URINE COLLECTION DEVICES

Condom catheters in males with balanced bladders or ones that drain freely or with manual stimulation[54] in men who have had bladder neck ablation and sphincterotomy are often the only practical devices for urine collection in quadriplegic patients who are unable to do self-catheterization. Condom catheters should be changed once a day and the skin should be allowed to air dry. Problems with skin lacerations and urethral damage occur when condoms are too tight, and urinary tract infections occur from the high concentration of bacteria around the penile glans and meatus.[81, 108, 141] A combination of condom catheter drainage for incontinence and intermittent catheterization is likely to increase this risk of infection.

Indwelling catheters, either urethral or suprapubic, are frequently used either because other programs have failed or for reasons of patient preference and convenience. The bad reputation of indwelling catheters is perhaps unjustified. A large number of patients tolerate them well and show no significant difference in upper tract status when compared with patients using other methods of bladder management.[107] This is probably a result of better catheter materials and manufacturing methods. Important aspects of care include changing the catheter at least once a month, avoiding kinking and obstruction of the catheter, having a non-return valve in the drainage tube or collecting bag, having the patient drink copious fluids to dilute the urine and any sediment, controlling hyperreflexia with medication, and avoiding traction on the catheter, which may lead to meatal erosion or urethral trauma. Although the prevalence of squamous cell bladder cancer appears to be lower[22] than originally reported,[110] yearly cystoscopic examination is recommended after an indwelling catheter has been present for 10 years (earlier in high-risk patients).

Absorbent materials in protective garments, diapers, and underpants can be used in patients who have uncontrollable incontinence related to dementia associated with spinal cord disease or in patients with bladder neuropathy in whom trauma from an indwelling catheter is likely.

PHARMACOTHERAPY

Elegant and rational explanations of pharmacologic effects on voiding, largely inferred from findings in experimental animals, have appeared in reviews of treatment methods.[38] These reports, based on pharmacologic characteristics of synaptic and neuromuscular transmission involved in bladder innervation, have been employed to design pharmacotherapy for patients. Drugs can be administered orally, parenterally, or topically to the bladder mucosa. In most instances, it is assumed that the agents act at peripheral sites. Unfortunately, results of such therapy in patients with neurologic bladder disease have been frequently disappointing.

Several impediments exist to implementation of therapy. First, the premise of drug therapy is that neurologically impaired reflex control of the detrusor muscle can be restored with pharmacologic assistance. In patients with detrusor hyperreflexia, the aim of anticholinergic therapy is reflex suppression and increased bladder capacity. Unfortunately, these drugs produce increased residual urine volume and, frequently, urinary retention. In patients with detrusor areflexia, restoration of the detrusor reflex by pharmacotherapy is attained infrequently. A second difficulty is that drug compliance is a problem with many patients, except those in a supervised environment such as a hospital or nursing home. Side effects with drug administration are common and represent a third problem with pharmacotherapy. Anticholinergic drugs are poorly tolerated by the elderly.

Thus, pharmacotherapy has not proved to be particularly successful in humans, despite the rational conceptualization based on animal experiments and extensive clinical use. However, adjunctive use of anticholinergic drugs for suppression of detrusor hyperreflexia in combination with clean intermittent catheterization perhaps illustrates the most successful role for pharmacotherapy in patients with spinal cord disease.

CHOLINERGIC AGENTS. Evidence that peripheral innervation of the human urinary detrusor is cholinergically mediated is convincing. Hence, bethanechol, a cholinergic agonist,[179] has been employed extensively for the treatment of detrusor areflexia in such neurologic diseases as diabetic autonomic neuropathy. The pharmacokinetics of this drug remain unexplored, although clinical reports of its effectiveness abound. An oral dosage of several hundred milligrams a day has been suggested from its use in the clinical setting. However, lack of drug metabolism data, absence of randomized trials, and the impression that bethanechol is relatively ineffective in resuscitating an impaired detrusor reflex have discouraged continued use of the drug.

ANTICHOLINERGIC AGENTS. Anticholinergic agents have long been used for suppression of detrusor hyperreflexia. The principal example of this group of agents is propantheline bromide,[19] and its usual adult oral dosage is 15 to 30 mg every 4 to 6 hours. Other anticholinergic agents include emepromium chloride (100 mg every 8 hours) and oxybutynin chloride (5 mg three to four times daily). Oxybutynin acts on the cell membrane and should more correctly be called musculotropic. Intravesical administration is being tried in patients on an intermittent catheterization program. Although absorption occurs and the serum levels are similar to those following oral administration, the rate of absorption is slower, peak levels are reached later, and the drug is better tolerated with fewer side effects[123] when it is placed in the bladder. At present, there is no sterile form of the drug for administration, and a 5-mg pill is dissolved in sterile water for instillation in the drained bladder. Imipramine (25 mg three times a day) has found favor as an anticholinergic, often in combination with oxybutynin or propantheline. It is useful in some types of incontinence because of its alpha-adrenergic

agonist and central actions. Other proprietary medications containing hyoscyamine (0.125 to 0.25 mg three or four times a day) have also been used for their anticholinergic actions. All of these drugs tend to increase residual urine volume and are most useful when combined with clean intermittent self-catheterization.

ADRENERGIC AGENTS. Adrenergic agents have been prescribed for the treatment of voiding dysfunction. Phenoxybenzamine was reported early to be an effective alpha$_1$- and alpha$_2$-adrenergic receptor antagonist, useful in promoting voiding in patients with increased urethral smooth muscle tonus.[113] It has fallen into disfavor because of reported carcinogenic effects in laboratory animals.

Prazosin, an alpha$_1$-adrenergic receptor antagonist, has replaced phenoxybenzamine; it is given in small oral doses gradually increasing to 20 mg/day.[58, 98] Prazosin has to be taken twice daily and terazosin, also an alpha$_1$-adrenergic antagonist, can be used once a day. If the latter is taken at night, side effects are less troublesome. Postural hypotension, the most common side effect, is seen during commencement of treatment. Based on some experimental findings in primates,[129] alpha-adrenergic antagonists have also been used in patients with decentralized bladders with reduced compliance. Worthwhile clinical effects in humans with similar neuropathies have not been reported. These agents are also being widely used in prostatism, and although they do not dramatically improve flow rates, they do decrease irritative symptoms, which suggest that the latter may be mediated by alpha-receptors in a bladder that is obstructed as a result of prostatic enlargement. Effective use of these for detrusor hyperreflexia with obstruction due to distal sphincter dyssynergia has not been reported.

Another use for alpha-adrenergic blocking agents is for long-term control of the efferent vascular effects of autonomic dysreflexia when all other measures have failed. In this situation, phenoxybenzamine may be the drug of choice despite its possible long-term carcinogenic effects, as it has both alpha$_1$- and alpha$_2$-blocking actions.

Alpha-adrenergic agonists have been used in the treatment of incontinence secondary to sphincter weakness in patients with myelodysplasia, the aim being to increase smooth muscle tonus.[12] Ephedrine is usually given in doses of 25 mg two or three times a day depending on the age of the patient.

The beta-blocking agent propranolol is another adrenergic agent that has been found to increase bladder storage in cats. However, it has been used without significant effect in the treatment of patients with neurogenic bladder dysfunction.[64]

CALCIUM CHANNEL BLOCKERS. Calcium channel blocking agents, including nifedipine, terodiline, and verapamil, have been employed to improve urinary bladder function.[10] At present, only terodiline, which possesses additional antimuscarinic properties, holds promise.[78] However, this agent is not available in the United States, and it has been withdrawn from use in Europe because it was associated with cardiac arrhythmias.

MUSCLE RELAXANTS. Muscle relaxants such as diazepam, dantrolene, and baclofen have been reported to be effective in the treatment of detrusor-sphincter dyssynergia, although sphincterotomy seems to be a more effective treatment for this problem. Baclofen has been used intrathecally by continuous infusion from an implanted pump for the treatment of severe lower limb spasticity,[166] and it was found that detrusor reflex and pelvic floor spasticity were both reduced. This might be useful clinically in patients with detrusor hyperreflexia and incontinence who rely on intermittent self-catheterization. However, as patients with severe spasticity may be quadriplegic and unable to perform self-catheterization, the effect of intrathecal baclofen on the lower urinary tract may make emptying worse for those using condom catheter drainage with or without having undergone prior sphincterotomy. The method is still under trial, and although there have been no reports of cases of intrathecal side effects from the catheter or the drug, the method must be regarded as experimental.

ESTROGEN. Estrogen is another drug that has been employed in patients with urinary bladder problems; it is used for the treatment of stress incontinence in women.[132, 155] It may be helpful when sphincter weakness is present in women with pelvic floor denervation and activity-related incontinence.

Surgical Treatment of the Detrusor: Failure to Store

Causes for failure of the bladder to act as a reservoir, or *failure to store*, include detrusor hyperreflexia that is uncontrolled by pharmacotherapy and poor bladder compliance with high-end filling pressure at low capacity. Several approaches have been tried, but the present standard management consists of augmentation of the bladder using a detubularized segment of bowel.[120, 121, 133, 161] Other methods, which involve surgical denervation[148–150] or intrathecal administration of baclofen to pharmacologically inhibit the detrusor reflex, are considered experimental.

AUGMENTATION CYSTOPLASTY

This operation consists of partially dividing the bladder into two parts and sewing in a patch of bowel that has been reconstructed in such a way that its tubular configuration and peristaltic functions have been destroyed (Fig. 13–6). Almost any segment of the gastrointestinal tract can be used, but small bowel is preferred over large bowel. Stomach is being tried because its low pH and reduced amount of mucus may lessen the incidence of bacteriuria.[1] Patients considering augmentation cystoplasty must be committed to performing a self-catheterization program indefinitely and must be prepared to undergo major surgery that carries a small risk of immediate bowel complications, such as obstruction or anastomotic leak with peritonitis or fistula formation. Long-term alteration in bowel function, usually lessened constipation, may occur, but diarrhea is sometimes a long-term problem. This procedure produces an excellent low-pressure reservoir with a capacity of 600 mL or more. Bacteriuria and symptomatic urinary tract infection can still occur and presence of mucus is often a prob-

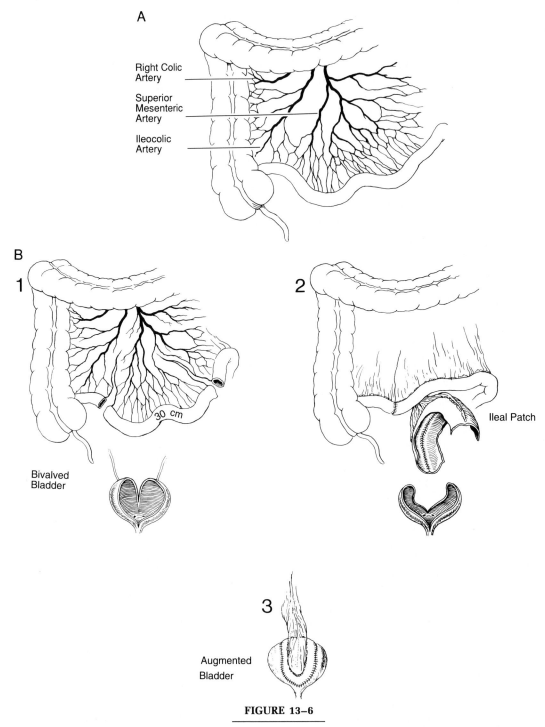

FIGURE 13-6

A, Terminal ileum, cecum, and ascending and right transverse colon with blood supply. This segment is most commonly used for reconstructive procedures. *B*, Bladder augmentation. *1*, The bladder is bivalved from near the anterior bladder neck to near the trigone posteriorly and a 30-cm segment of terminal ileum is taken. *2*, This segment is opened and reconstructed as a U-shaped patch. *3*, The patch is sewn into the bivalved bladder.

lem, especially with bladder infections. If an adequate amount of small bowel is used, anticholinergic or other similar drugs are rarely needed. However, bladders augmented with large bowel and stomach have more activity at least initially, and may require the use of these agents. A follow-up of more than 10 years is not yet available, but because carcinoma may develop in augmented bladders, all patients should have yearly cystoscopy beginning 10 or 15 years after an augmentation.

To avoid the use of bowel, an autoaugmentation procedure has been tried in children with myelodysplasia.[56] In this procedure, the thickened detrusor muscle is dissected off the mucosa, which then is allowed to bulge freely and without resistance. Results have been mixed, and this procedure is still experimental.

DENERVATION PROCEDURES FOR CONTROL OF DETRUSOR HYPERREFLEXIA

Operative approaches for denervation to control detrusor hyperreflexia include sectioning of sacral nerve roots, which is carried out by a neurosurgeon,[148–150] and sectioning of peripheral innervation of the urinary detrusor, which is performed by a urologist.[105, 136] When these procedures are performed on patients with detrusor hyperreflexia whose neurologic reflex control is already impaired, the postoperative goal is to increase detrusor reflex threshold at the expense of voluntary control of bladder emptying.

RHIZOTOMY. The original rhizotomies used by neurosurgeons in the treatment of patients with spinal cord injury were extensive procedures that reduced adductor muscle spasticity and increased bladder capacity.[131] This procedure converted a suprasacral injury into a cauda equina injury. The same result was subsequently obtained by instillation of absolute alcohol into the lumbosacral subarachnoid space.

To delimit the scope of the original rhizotomies and to reduce their complications, a limited rhizotomy was developed that focused specifically on improving bladder function.

By sectioning the sacral innervation of the urinary detrusor, the detrusor reflex threshold is raised and some central neural innervation is preserved. The procedure involves initial cystometric determination of detrusor reflex threshold followed by measurement of the response after sacral nerve root blocks. Following percutaneous blockade of the sacral nerve roots using local anesthetic, results can be assessed by cystometry. At this point, detrusor hyperreflexia can be managed either by application of phenol to a specific sacral nerve root or by a percutaneous radiofrequency-induced coagulative lesion of the root.[135]

Patients with spinal cord injuries are also candidates for limited selective differential sacral rhizotomy,[148–150] in which an operating microscope is used to select individual nerve fascicles in the nerve roots that have been defined during the preoperative evaluation. To verify the preoperative predictions, a topical anesthetic is applied to the nerve root and cystometry is carried out. If the results are satisfactory, the appropriate fascicles are sectioned. Postoperative results have been moderately good in this population of patients, but there is a tendency over time for the detrusor reflex to be rerouted through intact nerve roots. To avoid this, bilateral S2, 3, and 4 rhizotomies may be necessary; these, however, are likely to cause problems with sexual and bowel function.[76]

OTHER DENERVATION PROCEDURES

Other denervation procedures for the treatment of detrusor hyperreflexia include supratrigonal transection of the detrusor muscle, ganglionectomy, and bladder hyperdistension.

Supratrigonal transection of the detrusor muscle involves surgical interruption of motor and sensory innervation of the urinary detrusor above the trigone. A circumferential incision is made at this site with subsequent resuturing of bladder tissue.[136]

Ganglionectomy involves a surgical approach through the vagina with removal of ganglia in the area of the bladder neck.[105]

For bladder hyperdistension, the bladder

is allowed to overfill for several hours while the patient is under spinal anesthesia[181] so that consequent rupture of nerve endings in the bladder occurs. This novel approach to the creation of a docile reservoir was discovered in men with complete spinal cord lesions, in whom the bladder was intentionally allowed to overdistend during the initial phase of spinal shock. One year from injury, the prevalence of detrusor areflexia had increased from the expected 15% to 63%.[86] No longer-term results or other series using this method have been reported.

Surgical Treatment of the Detrusor: Failure to Empty

This is usually due to detrusor areflexia or hypocontractility with poor detrusor contraction, so the rise in bladder pressure is low or poorly sustained.

ELECTRICAL STIMULATION

For the past four decades, electrical stimulation of the detrusor muscle[43, 45] and the external urinary sphincter[52] has been under investigation, both in experimental animal models and in humans. The procedure aims to bring about voluntary control of detrusor muscle contraction, but results have been frequently discouraging.

Various sites employed for stimulation include: (1) the detrusor muscle itself,[43, 45] (2) pelvic nerves, (3) selected areas in the conus medullaris,[138] and (4) sacral anterior roots.[47, 48, 170] The latter may be approached at either an intraspinal extradural or an intradural location.

Stimulation at any of these four locations is accomplished by means of an implanted receiver of amplitude-modulated radiofrequency pulses, which are generated by an external transmitter. Stimulation at the first three sites has been reported in patients with spinal cord injuries. At present, only the fourth site is being actively investigated in patients with injuries above the conus.

Implantation with electrical stimulation of the sacral anterior roots in selected patients frequently results in consistent rises in intravesical pressure and adequate voiding.[47, 48, 102] However, postoperative problems include pain on voiding, autonomic dysreflexia, damage to the sacral anterior roots, cerebrospinal fluid leaks, and device failures. Dorsal rhizotomies can be performed to alleviate the first two of these complications. Pelvic floor contraction during anterior root stimulation obstructs voiding even after bilateral dorsal rhizotomies at S2, 3, and 4. At some centers, selective pudendal neurectomies[170] or selective division of the ventral roots is performed,[102] whereas at others, intermittent stimulation to produce poststimulus voiding is performed, which is said to empty the bladder at acceptable intravesical pressures.[48] In male patients with bilateral complete rhizotomies, reflex erections are abolished in all cases and usable electrically induced erections occur in fewer than 30%. Many patients find, however, that bowel evacuation is easier with this stimulation.[47] One can only wonder what quality of life would be attained in these patients if they were treated by more traditional methods. Electrical stimulation may offer promise in the future, but it can only be considered experimental at present.

Surgical Treatment of the Sphincters: Failure to Store

Failure of sphincter mechanisms resulting in clinically significant activity-related incontinence occurs with myelodysplasia in either sex and with infrasacral lesions mostly in women. In men with infrasacral lesions, enough passive resistance is often produced by elastic tissue and smooth muscle in the urethra to ensure that continence is maintained during moderate activity. More active men may have significant problems with incontinence and will be candidates for treatment. Alpha-adrenergic agonists may help minor incontinence; for more severe cases, options consist of some form of surgical procedure to produce compression at the urethra or bladder neck region. Injections with Teflon paste and collagen are still, to some degree, experimental.[122] Standard management consists of placing a fascial sling around the bladder neck (after which the patient performs intermittent self-catheterization) or implantation of an artificial sphincter.

ARTIFICIAL SPHINCTER

An artificial urinary sphincter device has been in use since 1973 for the control of urinary incontinence in patients with neurologic bladder dysfunction.[156, 157] This method, introduced by Scott and progressively improved by his colleagues, is used for the treatment of patients with myelodysplasia and infrasacral spinal cord injury.

The device consists of an inflatable cuff, reservoir, pump, and control assembly (Fig. 13–7). The prosthesis is coated with Silastic and implanted near the bladder, with the cuff placed around the bladder neck. The pump is located in the labia or scrotum, which makes it accessible for external manual manipulation. By squeezing the pump, fluid is expelled from the cuff into the balloon reservoir, which permits voiding. Fluid from the reservoir is then automatically and gradually transferred back to the cuff over an interval of several minutes, with voiding occurring during the interval.

Postoperative complications include urethral erosion[73, 90] and upper urinary tract deterioration.[23] Preoperative evaluation must reveal a docile bladder with adequate capacity (greater than 300 mL) and low pressure. Compliance should be greater than 10 mL/cm H_2O with detrusor hyperreflexia controllable by pharmacotherapy. If the bladder is inadequate as a reservoir, augmentation cystoplasty can be combined with implantation of the artificial sphincter.[83] Despite careful preoperative selection, about 10% of patients with myelodysplasia develop hyperreflexia with activation of the device, probably as a result of stimulation of hitherto dormant urethrovesical reflexes.[154] Careful observation of the urinary tract in the first year after implantation is essential; if bladder function

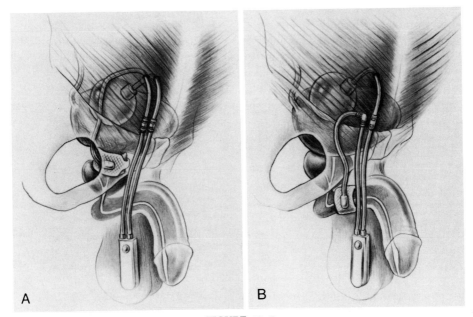

FIGURE 13–7

A, Bladder neck placement of an artificial urinary sphincter. The cuff is placed around a space that has been developed at the bladder neck, just at the top of the prostate, and the tubing is brought alongside the tubing from the pressure-regulating balloon (reservoir) and through the deep fascia to be connected to the tubing from the pump. The pump is placed within the scrotum and is activated externally by the patient. *B*, Bulbourethral placement. In this illustration the cuff is more superficial and the exit tubing lies outside the pelvis. Again, the pressure-regulating balloon (reservoir) is placed in the retropubic space and exit tubing comes through the deep fascia before connecting to the pump in the scrotum.

changes and does not respond to pharmaco-therapy, augmentation can be done as a secondary procedure.

Surgical Treatment of the Sphincters: Failure to Empty

SPHINCTEROTOMY

In male patients who are unable or unwilling to do intermittent catheterizations, sphincterotomy is frequently used to convert the lower urinary tract into a low-pressure system that empties reflexly at a lower capacity with lower residual volumes.[99, 152, 153] Most patients have suprasacral lesions with detrusor–external sphincter dyssynergia and an open bladder neck. However, it is not uncommon to find that the bladder neck does not open well at low detrusor pressures and is also potentially obstructive. It is important to select patients who have adequate bladder contractions, because a hypocontractile detrusor may account for most of the early failures.[128] These hypocontractile or areflexic bladders may be the result of occult lumbosacral dysfunction.[20]

In this procedure, the distal sphincter is usually incised anteriorly so as to avoid the termination of the pudendal artery, at which point it runs lateral to the distal sphincter and enters the corpus cavernosum to form the deep cavernosal artery.[111] In this way, risk of erectile dysfunction is minimized. The bladder neck can also be incised as indicated, and this is usually performed posterolaterally.

The operation has relatively high perioperative morbidity from bleeding, clot retention, infection, and dysreflexia. Long-term failure as a result of restricturing is also common. An implantable stainless steel stent, which may lead to more permanent results, is currently under trial (Fig. 13–8).[130] This stent becomes incorporated into the urethral wall as the epithelium grows through the spaces in the mesh, and in 3 to 6 months the wires are usually completely covered. Apart from a more permanent result, the advantage of this procedure compared with the standard sphincterotomy is that no incision is required and, therefore, no resultant bleeding or erectile dysfunction occurs.

OTHER METHODS TO REDUCE OUTLET RESISTANCE

Intrathecal baclofen administration has been discussed as a method of decreasing re-

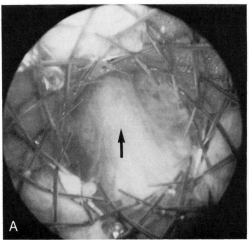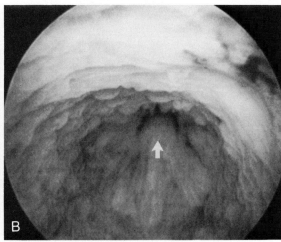

FIGURE 13–8

A, View through the cystoscope of the placement of an intraurethral stent instead of sphincterotomy. The proximal end of the stent mesh can be seen just distal to the verumontanum (*arrow*). B, Similar view 6 months later shows the cobblestone appearance of epithelium that now covers the stent; the verumontanum again is seen at the center of the image (*arrow*).

flex detrusor activity; it also decreases pelvic floor activity by its action on somatic reflexes.[75, 166] The overall effect of this therapy is to increase storage rather than to increase emptying, and its use is still experimental.

Injection of botulinum toxin into the sphincter has also been used experimentally, but its effects last only a few months.[67]

Finally, prostatic hypertrophy may occur in older men with neurogenic bladder disease. However, even if the patient has a lesion that is incomplete enough to allow spontaneous voiding, results after a prostatectomy are often unsatisfactory. Before resorting to prostatectomy, every nonsurgical method of treatment (e.g., administration of 5-alpha-reductase inhibitors[84] and alpha-adrenergic blocking agents[58, 98, 118]) should be given a fair trial.

Urinary Diversion

In some patients, either because of changes in the urethra and penile skin (e.g., fistulae, strictures, and skin ulceration) or because of intractable incontinence and perineal decubitus ulcers, some form of diversion of urine away from the perineum is necessary. The simplest means of accomplishing this is to close the bladder neck and insert a suprapubic catheter.[57] If the bladder has to be diverted or removed because of severe structural-functional changes or ureteral reflux, the options lie between a standard refluxing (or preferably a non-refluxing) bowel conduit (Fig. 13–9) or a continent diversion[18] (Fig. 13–10). In the latter, an internal reservoir is formed from a segment of bowel and a valved efferent loop is constructed with its opening on the anterior abdominal wall through which the patient performs self-catheterization every 4 to 6 hours. Naturally, a patient must be committed to an intermittent self-catheterization program. However, as severe bladder, urethral, and penile changes in structure result from an individual's failure to care for himself or herself, such a patient is usually not a good candidate for continent diversion. However, a place exists for the more elective construction of a continent system with a self-catheterizable abdominal stoma in paraplegic women in whom urethral catheterization is technically

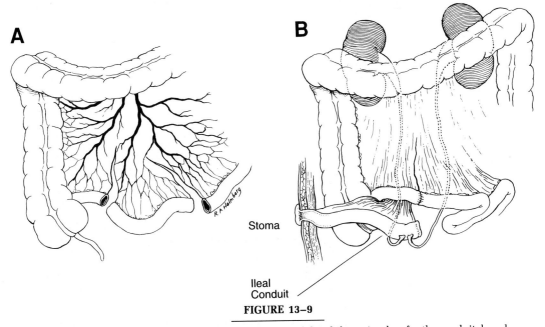

A

B

Stoma

Ileal
Conduit

FIGURE 13–9

Ileal conduit construction. *A*, Approximately 10 cm of distal ileum is taken for the conduit, based on the terminal branches of the superior mesenteric artery. *B*, Urine is conducted to the skin from the retroperitoneum, where the ureters are anastomosed.

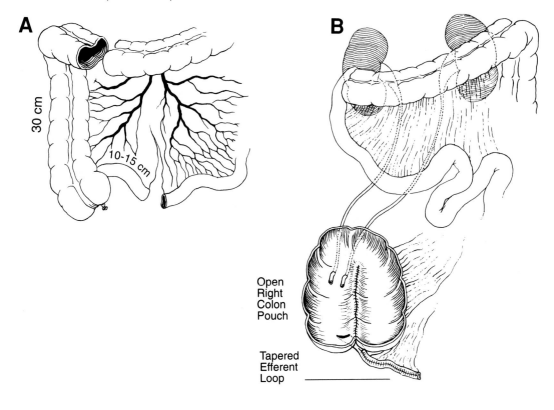

A

30 cm

10–15 cm

B

Open
Right
Colon
Pouch

Tapered
Efferent
Loop

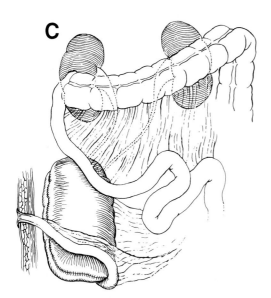

C

FIGURE 13–10

Continent diversion using only right colon for the pouch.
A, Segment consisting of terminal ileum, cecum, and ascending and beginning of right transverse colon is used based on the ileocecal and right colic arteries. *B,* The pouch is constructed in a U-shaped configuration. The efferent loop relies on the ileocecal valve for continence and is tapered to make catheterization easier with a 16F catheter; the tapering may also contribute to continence. *C,* The pouch is placed on the right side of the abdomen with the stomal opening in the right ileal fossa.

difficult. If the upper tracts are normal and reflux is not present, the bladder neck can be closed and the body of the bladder bivalved as during an augmentation procedure (Fig. 13–11).[57] The length of bowel that is used can be shorter because the patient's own bladder is being incorporated into the reservoir;

perhaps the procedure should be called a *continent augmentation.* The most difficult aspect of the continent diversion is the creation of a continence mechanism. Generally, the modified terminal ileum and ileocecal valve is the most reliable segment, and all or part of the right colon, with or without an

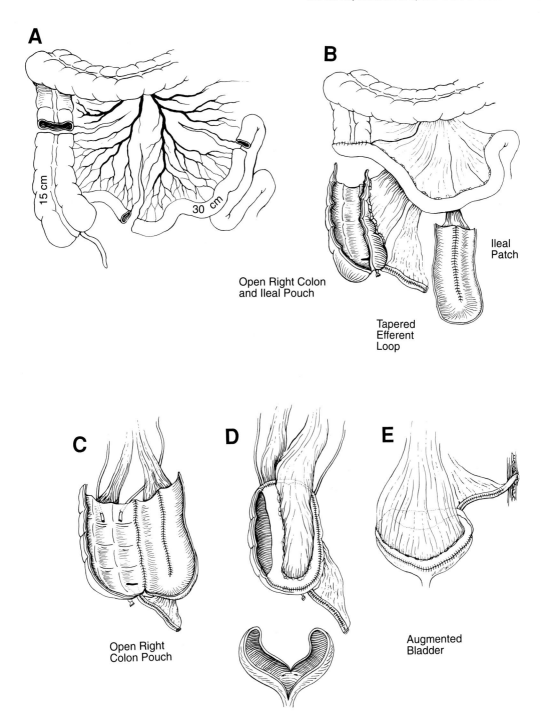

A

15 cm

30 cm

B

Open Right Colon
and Ileal Pouch

Ileal
Patch

Tapered
Efferent
Loop

C

Open Right
Colon Pouch

D

E

Augmented
Bladder

FIGURE 13–11

Continent augmentation employing the bladder and a composite bowel pouch. *A,* A 15-cm segment of cecum and part of the ascending colon with the terminal 40 cm of ileum are used. *B,* The cecum and ascending colon and 30 cm of small bowel (except the terminal 10 cm) are opened. The ileum is reconfigured as a U-shaped patch, and the terminal 10 cm of ileum is tapered to form the efferent loop. *C,* The U-shaped patch is incorporated into the opened cecum and ascending colon. *D,* The pouch is partly closed and the bladder is bivalved. *E,* The pouch is sewn into the bladder and the efferent loop is brought out to the skin at a convenient site, which is often in the left iliac fossa. The bladder neck may be left alone if it is competent, but if not it can be closed or made competent with a fascial sling or artificial sphincter.

additional small bowel patch, forms the reservoir. Problems with diarrhea resulting from malabsorption of bile salts may be less common when the ileocecal valve remains. However, the other continent mechanisms are less reliable and excess bile salts can be eliminated from the colon by oral administration of cholestyramine.

Management of Complications of Neurogenic Bladder Dysfunction

BACTERIURIA

Urinary tract infection, often combined with increased pressure and obstruction, is the final common pathway to renal damage in patients with spinal cord neurogenic bladder disease. Clearly, it is as important to treat the underlying obstruction, stones, ureteral reflux, and high bladder pressures as it is to give antibiotics. The management of asymptomatic bacteriuria is more controversial.[70, 167] Patients with indwelling catheters should not be given prophylactic antibiotics because production of resistant organisms is inevitable. High-volume fluid intake with excellent catheter care and hygiene are essential. Symptomatic bacteriuria must be treated, but short courses of antibiotics should be given unless severe pyelonephritis is present. In patients performing clean intermittent catheterization, many studies have shown no overall benefit from suppressive antibiotics.[8, 134] Treatment for symptoms that include increased spasms as well as the more obvious signs (fever; cloudy, foul-smelling urine; urinary frequency; and incontinence) gives patients and their physicians a certain amount of latitude in managing this common problem. In patients using condom catheters or no collecting devices, justification may exist for expecting suppressive antibiotics to be effective against bacteriuria. However, patients with badly managed condom catheters are at a considerably increased risk of recurrent urinary tract infection, and the bacteria are likely to become resistant to multiple antibiotics.[141]

AUTONOMIC DYSREFLEXIA

Autonomic dysreflexia with paroxysmal hypertension induced by bladder filling in the patient with a suprasacral spinal cord injury is managed with preventive techniques, such as the avoidance of bladder distension.[162] Its occurrence is rare in patients with lesions below T6 and its severity is greater as the level and completeness of the lesion increases. Calcium channel blocking agents such as nifedipine are also prescribed for these patients.[59, 119] They can be given either on a regular basis, orally, or for management of an acute episode, sublingually. Phenoxybenzamine (10 to 30 mg/day) is useful in the prevention of autonomic dysreflexia when all other causes have been eliminated. It is particularly helpful after surgery, such as a sphincterotomy, when increased afferent stimulation from the lower tract is present for 6 weeks or so, until reepithelialization of the incised area has occurred.

HYPERCALCIURIA AND STONES

Hypercalciuria (greater than 200 mg every 24 hours) occurs 4 weeks after spinal cord injury in all patients; it reaches a maximum at about 16 weeks, and may persist for as long as 12 to 18 months.[172] The incidence of renal stone formation after spinal cord injury is 1.0% to 1.5% over the first 6 to 9 months and 8% over the next 10 years. The former is probably metabolic and the latter is probably infectious in origin. Bladder stones in the first 6 to 9 months are more common in patients with an indwelling catheter (8.8%) than in patients performing clean intermittent catheterization (2.3%); this is the result of presence of bacteriuria, a foreign body, and hypercalciuria. Despite the benefits of increased fluids in patients with a Foley catheter, the incidence of upper tract stones in the first 6 to 9 months is not lower than in patients performing intermittent catheterization.[61] Other metabolic factors have been described as affecting the long-term risk of stone formation after spinal cord injury,[50, 51, 158] but the majority of stones that occur more than 2 years after injury are struvite (infective) in origin (Fig. 13–12).[14, 175]

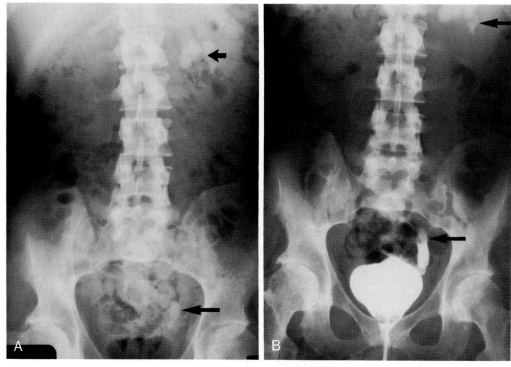

FIGURE 13–12

A, Plain film of the abdomen in a 26-year-old with C6 quadriplegia shows an incomplete staghorn calculus (*short arrow*) and opacities lying along the course of his left lower ureter (*long arrow*). *B,* A cystogram shows left reflux, which confirms filling defects in the lower ureter resulting from presence of the stones. The bladder neck and prostatic urethra are open secondary to sphincterotomies. Renal and ureteral calculi are seen (*arrows*).

Bladder stones are most effectively and safely treated by using an electrohydraulic probe after treatment of bacteriuria. For removal of fine particles after lithotripsy, daily intravesical instillation (via a catheter) of 30 mL of citric acid, glucono-deltalactone, and magnesium carbonate (Renacidin), which is held in the bladder for 10 to 30 minutes, should be continued for about a week. In some patients, Renacidin has been used on a regular basis for prevention of bladder stones.

Calyceal calculi that are asymptomatic or small (less than 1 cm in diameter) should be followed up without treatment. However, chances of calyceal calculi becoming symptomatic over 5 years are about 50%, and 50% of these patients will need an invasive procedure for complications such as obstruction.[80] Therefore, calculi that are growing or that are in the renal pelvis, and therefore more likely to cause obstruction, should be considered for treatment. As extracorporeal shockwave lithotripsy (ESWL) is performed with less morbidity, using "tubless" machines that do not require anesthesia, indications for treatment of asymptomatic calculi may change. For symptomatic renal calculi, ESWL is appropriate for stones with a combined diameter of less than 3 cm. For larger stones and in patients with deformed collecting systems, a percutaneous approach is preferable. As a majority of stones are infective in origin, patients should be given antibiotics before treatment. Although struvite (infective) stones break well with ESWL, clearance of the fragments is often impaired in immobile patients,[142] and recurrence is likely unless the stones or infections are cleared from the kidney. Ureteral stones can be treated by the usual techniques, but urgent drainage procedures are often required as obstruction combined with infection is common in this population and may present silently, with fever as the only symptom.

URETERAL REFLUX AND URETERAL DILATION

Dilated upper tracts as a result of reflux or obstruction at the ureterovesical junction are in most cases the result of high bladder pressures (Fig. 13–13), bladder wall hypertrophy, and, sometimes, a paraureteral diverticulum. The first goal is to lower bladder pressure by use of medications and clean intermittent self-catheterization. If this fails, reimplantation of the ureter into the bladder combined

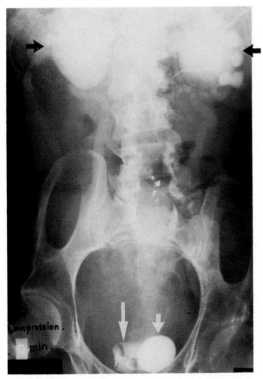

FIGURE 13–13

Excretory urogram of a 23-year-old man with myelodysplasia 6 months after implantation of an artificial sphincter. Cuff (*long white arrow*) and reservoir or pressure-regulating balloon (*short white arrow*) are seen just above the symphysis. Bilateral hydronephrosis and dilated calyces (*black arrows*) are evident with tortuous ureters to the pelvic brim. The pelvis is filled with a large bladder shadow, indicating chronic retention. The artificial sphincter in this individual rendered him continent initially. Although this proceeded to a state of chronic retention, it was successfully managed with intermittent self-catheterization.

with augmentation is the next logical step in patients with the will and the ability to do intermittent self-catheterization. The alternative is a sphincterotomy and possible treatment of any reflux with endoscopic injections of Teflon paste.[147]

Management of the Neurogenic Bladder in Common Spinal Cord Diseases

SUPRASACRAL

SPINAL CORD INJURY AND TUMORS. After the injury, a Foley catheter is kept in place until the patient's condition is stable, and fluid intake can be restricted until a urine output of 1500 to 2000 mL/day is achieved. Intermittent sterile catheterization is then begun (by a dedicated catheterization team, if possible); many patients can learn sterile self-catheterization while in the hospital.[28, 71] Bladder volumes of 500 to 600 mL should be the maximum allowed, and if larger volumes are produced after the patient is recumbent in the evenings, an extra catheterization should be ordered to avoid exceeding the upper limit. If and when reflex detrusor contractions return, and the patient begins to have episodes of incontinence, anticholinergic pharmacotherapy can be instituted.

For long-term therapy, clean intermittent self-catheterization and anticholinergic pharmacotherapy are the mainstays of management in motivated patients with spinal cord injury who have sufficient hand function. In a number of patients, drugs do not work satisfactorily and these individuals become candidates for simple bladder augmentation or, perhaps, continent augmentation. At present, these are the most successful methods of restoring the reservoir functions of the bladder so that intermittent catheterization can be continued.

In patients who are unable or unwilling to do self-catheterization, a condom catheter may allow reflex voiding at acceptable pressures. The so-called balanced bladder occurs in approximately 15% of patients with spinal cord injury.[101] Most patients, however, require sphincterotomy for adequate low pressure emptying. Surveillance of urinary tract function in the population with spinal cord injury is important because with care, many persons in this group will have a normal life span. A suggested surveillance schedule is given in Table 13–4.

MULTIPLE SCLEROSIS. Five percent of patients who are later diagnosed with multiple sclerosis have only urinary symptoms at initial presentation. Eventually, urinary manifestations develop in 90% of patients in the course of the disease.[4] Although multiple sclerosis may present with pure encephalopathic, pure myelopathic, or pure conal manifestations, most patients have combinations of two or more of these. Patients usually initially manifest urinary frequency, urgency, and urge incontinence with increased resid-

ual volumes. On urodynamic evaluation, the detrusor is hyperreflexic, but it fails to contract in a sustained fashion and the bladder fails to empty. Detrusor-sphincter dyssynergia and bladder wall and upper tract changes are unusual[82, 127] despite published reports of the high prevalence of upper tract damage.[25] Management is problematic, as treatment of hyperreflexia with anticholinergics worsens retention, but most patients are unable to manage self-catheterization because of poor upper limb strength or coordination. Many patients, especially women, require indwelling catheters at an early stage.

Patients with other neurologic conditions (e.g., degenerative myelopathies, spinal vascular disease, cervical spondylosis with acute myelopathy, and amyotrophic lateral

---

TABLE 13–4

ROUTINE URINARY TRACT SURVEILLANCE AFTER SPINAL CORD INJURY

Initial rehabilitation admission
    Urinalysis, initially and as needed
    Urine culture and sensitivity, weekly
    Intravenous pyelogram (IVP) (often done 1 to 3 mo after spinal
        cord injury)
    Renal ultrasound (baseline test)
    Postvoiding residual urine volume (PVR)
    Cystometrogram and/or urodynamic studies (usually no
        cystogram at this point)
    24-Hour urine for creatinine clearance
Yearly evaluations
    IVP at first annual evaluation and then every 3 yr (assuming all
        previous tests are normal)
    Urodynamic studies at first annual evaluation and then as
        determined on individual basis (often needed annually for
        the first few years)
    Renal ultrasound and kidney-ureters-bladder x-rays for annual
        evaluations in which no IVP or cystourethrogram (CUG) is
        obtained
    CUG at first annual evaluation, either with urodynamic studies
        or by radiologic examination, then every 3 yr with IVP (usually
        no CUG with indwelling catheters)
    24-Hour urine for creatinine clearance annually
    Urinalysis and culture and sensitivity annually
    PVR (by portable ultrasound or by catheter) annually, unless an
        indwelling catheter is present
    Other tests of renal function as needed
Cystoscopy
    Generally performed in patients after 10 yr of chronic,
        continuous indwelling catheterization (urethral or suprapubic)
        or sooner (at 5 yr) if patient is at high risk (heavy smoker, age
        > 40 yr, or history of complicated urinary tract infections) or
        in any patient with symptoms that warrant such a procedure

sclerosis) may all have varying manifestations of neurologic bladder disease, ranging from urgency resulting from mild hyperreflexia to a hypocontractile detrusor with poor emptying or to an obstructed bladder with severe detrusor-sphincter dyssynergia.

INFRASACRAL LESIONS

Conal and cauda equina damage (injury, disk disease, lumbar spondylosis, and tumors are some of the mechanical lesions that can affect this region of the spinal cord and cauda equina[72, 92, 144]) result in the bladder being insensate and hypocontractile or noncontractile and the pelvic floor flaccid. With conal lesions, bladder and pelvic floor innervations are more likely to be affected equally and completely. With cauda equina lesions, the bladder nerves are usually more easily damaged, which may lead to an areflexic detrusor with innervated pelvic floor muscles and sphincters.[34] Patients may void by using Valsalva's maneuver, but men may require relaxation of the bladder neck with alpha-adrenergic blockade or surgical resection. Women, having lower outflow resistance than men, void more easily, but tend to have development of stress incontinence. With the latter, a bladder neck sling and clean intermittent self-catheterization are indicated; occasionally, an artificial sphincter with continuation of Valsalva voiding is useful. Men with poor bladder compliance, which is more common after radical pelvic surgery than with infrasacral spinal lesions,[164] may respond both to anticholinergic agents and to alpha-adrenergic blockade; if responses are not impressive, these patients are often candidates for either bladder augmentation with continued clean intermittent self-catheterization or sphincterotomy with use of a condom catheter.

Autonomic neuropathy resulting from diabetes[32] (or, to a lesser extent, alcoholism) commonly causes a neurogenic bladder. Changes are initially confined to the visceral afferent nerves and the patient is often asymptomatic. Eventually, either because of motor involvement or because the bladder muscle becomes overstretched, the detrusor becomes hypocontractile or areflexic and a variable degree of retention develops. Management consists of timed voidings in the early stages when detrusor function is preserved; when retention develops, intermittent catheterization is recommended most frequently.

MIXED SUPRASACRAL AND INFRASACRAL LESIONS

Myelodysplasia is the most common disease producing a mixed pattern of detrusor and sphincter dysfunction.[126] Theoretically, any combination of detrusor and sphincter activity can be found, but the most common (and most debilitating) finding is a hyperreflexic and/or noncompliant bladder with dyssynergic or nonrelaxing and fixed sphincters. Patients with these lesions are at risk from bladder wall and upper tract changes and require intermittent catheterization and control of high bladder pressures with drugs or, if pharmacotherapy fails, with bladder augmentation.

Summary

No simple methods exist for evaluation or treatment of neurologic disease and urinary bladder dysfunction. This is partly a result of scarcity of data on the human physiology of voiding. In some patients, therapeutic possibilities are few and expectations must be modest. Many strategies can be pursued, and patient evaluation, including laboratory studies, can help in the selection process. However, the extent of neurologic deficit defines the extent to which normal bladder function can be reestablished.

Requirements for normal bladder function consist of: (1) the capacity to initiate voiding under appropriate circumstances; (2) no urinary leakage during the intervoiding interval; and (3) total evacuation of urine with preservation of its sterility.

Neurologic disease frequently interferes with one or all of the elements of normal bladder function. Most medical and surgical strategies for attaining effective bladder function require patient understanding and cooperation, as well as the ability to conduct simple tasks. When there is a neurologic deficit, these faculties are frequently impaired.

Hence, assessment of neurologic disease is an important factor in understanding the nature of bladder dysfunction as well as in determining the therapeutic approach. The clinical neurologist should be a more frequent participant in the care of such patients than is currently the case. To accomplish this, the neurologist must demonstrate the contribution of neurologic evaluation, including electrodiagnostic studies, to diagnosis and to the ultimate selection of therapy.

Clinical neurologists could also benefit from a training period on a urology service. Differences in terminology, which can frustrate communication in the treatment of patients, would become evident. In addition, the neurologist's ability to translate the nervous system disease process into neuroanatomic and, hence, neurophysiologic changes in bladder function would facilitate management. Productive research and improved patient care would emerge from this fusion of disciplines.

REFERENCES

1. Adams MC: Gastrocystoplasty: An alternative solution to the problem of urologic reconstruction in the severely compromised patient. J Urol 140: 1152–1156, 1988.
2. Anderson JT, Bradley WE: Postural detrusor hyperreflexia. J Urol 116:75–78, 1976.
3. Anderson JT, Bradley WE: The syndrome of detrusor-sphincter dyssynergia. J Urol 116:493–495, 1976.
4. Anderson JT, Bradley WE: Bladder and urethral innervation in multiple sclerosis. Br J Urol 48: 239–243, 1976.
5. Anderson JT, Bradley WE: The urethral closure pressure profile. Br J Urol 48:341–345, 1976.
6. Anderson JT, Bradley WE: Cystometry: Detrusor reflex activation, classification and terminology. J Urol 118:623–625, 1977.
7. Anderson JT, Bradley WE, Tim GW: The urethral electromyographic and gas pressure profile. Scand J Urol Nephrol 10:185–188, 1976.
8. Anderson RU: Prophylaxis of bacteriuria during intermittent catheterization of the acute bladder. J Urol 123:364–366, 1980.
9. Anderson RU, Hsieh-Ma ST: Association of bacteriuria and pyuria during intermittent catheterization after spinal cord injury. J Urol 130:299–301, 1983.
10. Anderson K-E, Forman A: Effects of calcium channel blockers on urinary tract smooth muscle. Acta Pharmacol Toxicol 58(suppl II):193–200, 1986.
11. Andrew J, Nathan PW: Lesions of the anterior frontal lobes and disturbances of micturition and defecation. Brain 87:233, 1964.
12. Awad SA, Downie JW, Kirulata HG: Alpha-adrenergic agents in urinary disorders of the proximal urethra: I. Sphincteric incontinence. Br J Urol 50:332–335, 1978.
13. Awad SA, Bryniak SR, Lowe PJ, et al: Urethral pressure profile in female stress incontinence. J Urol 120:475–479, 1978.
14. Barrington FJF: The relationship of the hindbrain to micturition. Brain 44:23, 1921.
15. Barrington FJF: The effect of lesions of the hind and midbrain on micturition in the cat. Q J Exp Physiol 15:181, 1925.
16. Barrington FJF: The component reflexes of micturition in the cat: I and II. Brain 54:177, 1931.
17. Barrington FJF: The component reflexes of micturition in the cat. Brain 64:239, 1941.
18. Bejany DE, Chao R, Perito PE, et al: Continent urinary diversion and diverting colostomy in the therapy of non-healing pressure sores in paraplegic patients. Paraplegia 31:242–248, 1993.
19. Benson GS, Sarshik SA, Raezer DM, et al: Bladder muscle contractility: Comparative effects and mechanisms of action of atropine, propantheline, flavoxate and imipramine. Urology 9:31–35, 1977.
20. Beric A, Light JK: Function of the conus medullaris and cauda equina in the early period following spinal cord injury and the relationship to recovery of detrusor function. J Urol 148:1845–1848, 1992.
21. Bhatia NN, Bradley WE, Haldeman S: Urodynamics: Continuous monitoring. J Urol 128:963–968, 1982.
22. Bickel A, Culkin DJ, Wheeler JS Jr: Bladder cancer in spinal cord injury patients. J Urol 146:1240–1242, 1991.
23. Bitsch M, et al: Upper urinary tract deterioration after implantation of artificial urinary sphincter. Scand J Urol Nephrol 24:31–34, 1990.
24. Blaivas JG: Videourodynamics. In Krane RJ, Siroky MB (eds): Clinical Neurourology, ed 2. Boston, Little Brown, 1992, pp 265–274.
25. Blaivas JG, Barbalias GA: Detrusor-external sphincter dyssynergia in men with multiple sclerosis: An ominous urological condition. J Urol 131:91–94, 1984.
26. Blaivas JG, Fisher DM: Combined radiographic and urodynamic monitoring: Advances in technique. J Urol 125:693–694, 1981.
27. Blaivas JG, Singha HP, Zayed AAH: Detrusor external sphincter dyssynergia: A detailed EMG study. J Urol 125:545, 1981.
28. Bors E, Comarr A: Neurological Urology: Physiology of Micturition, Its Neurological Disorders and Sequel. Baltimore, University Park Press, 1971.
29. Bradley WE: Urethral electromyography. J Urol 108:563–564, 1972.
30. Bradley WE: Electroencephalography and bladder innervation. J Urol 118:412, 1977.
31. Bradley WE: Cystometry and sphincter electromyography. Mayo Clin Proc 51:329–335, 1976.
32. Bradley WE: Diagnosis of urinary bladder dysfunction in diabetes mellitus. Ann Int Med 92:323–326, 1980.
33. Bradley WE: Aspects of diabetic autonomic neuropathy: Introduction and workshop summary. Ann Intern Med 92:289–342, 1980.
34. Bradley WE, Anderson JT: Neuromuscular dysfunction of lower urinary tract in patients with lesions of the cauda equina and conus medullaris. J Urol 116:620–621, 1976.
35. Bradley WE, Rockswold GL, Timm GW, et al: Neurology of micturition. J Urol 115:481, 1976.
36. Bradley WE, Scott FB: Physiology of the urinary bladder, In Harrison JH, et al (eds): Campbell's Urology, ed 4. Philadelphia, WB Saunders, 1978.

37. Bradley WE, Scott FB, Timm GW: Sphincter electromyography. Urol Clin North Am 1:69, 1974.
38. Bradley WE, Sundin T: The physiology and pharmacology of urinary tract dysfunction. Clin Neuropharmacol 5:131–158, 1982.
39. Bradley WE, Teague CT: Spinal cord organization of micturition reflex afferents. Exp Neurol 22:504–516, 1968.
40. Bradley WE, Teague CT: Cerebellar control of the urinary bladder. Exp Neurol 23:399, 1969.
41. Bradley WE, Timm GW: Cystometry: III. Cystometry. Urology 5:843–848, 1975.
42. Bradley WE, Timm GW: Cystometry: VI. Interpretation. Urology 7:231–235, 1976.
43. Bradley WE, Timm GW, Chou SN: A decade of experience with electronic stimulation of the micturition reflex. Urol Int 26:283–303, 1971.
44. Bradley WE, Timm GW, Rockswold GL: Detrusor and urethral electromyography. J Urol 114:891–894, 1975.
45. Bradley WE, Wittmers LE, Chou SN, et al: Use of a radio transmitter receiver unit for the treatment of neurogenic bladder. J Neurosurg 19:782–786, 1962.
46. Bradley WE, Conway CJ, McCormick S: Discriminator and integrator instrument for an on line frequency analysis of single unit discharges. Electroencephalogr Clin Neurophysiol 22:177–179, 1967.
47. Brindley GS, Rushton DN: Long-term follow-up of patients with sacral anterior root stimulator implants. Paraplegia 28:469–475, 1990.
48. Brindley GS, Polkey CT, Rushton DN, et al: Sacral anterior root stimulators for bladder control in paraplegia: The first 50 cases. J Neurol Neurosurg Psychiatry 49:1104–1114, 1986.
49. Burgio KL, Sturtzman RE, Engel BT: Behavioral training for post-prostatectomy urinary incontinence. J Urol 141:303–306, 1989.
50. Burr RG, Nuseibeh I: Biochemical studies in paraplegic renal stone patients: I. Plasma biochemistry and urinary calcium and saturation. Br J Urol 57:269–274, 1985.
51. Burr RG, Nuseibeh I, Abiaka CD: Biochemical studies in paraplegic renal stone patients. II. Urinary excretion of citrate, inorganic pyrophosphate, silicate and urate. Br J Urol 57:275–278, 1985.
52. Caldwell KPS, Flack FC, Broad AF: Urinary incontinence following spinal cord injury treated by electronic implant. Lancet 1:846–847, 1965.
53. Cardenas DD, Kelly E, Krieger JN, et al: Residual urine volumes in patients with spinal cord injury: Measurement with a portable ultrasound instrument. Arch Phys Med Rehabil 69:514–516, 1988.
54. Cardenas DD, Kelly E, Mayo ME: Manual stimulation of reflex voiding after spinal cord injury. Arch Phys Med Rehabil 66:459–462, 1985.
55. Cardenas DD, Mayo ME: Bacteriuria with fever after spinal cord injury. Arch Phys Med Rehabil 68:291–293, 1987.
56. Cartwright PC, Snow BW: Bladder autoaugmentation: Early clinical experience. J Urol 142:505–508, 1989.
57. Chao R, Mayo ME, Bejany DE, et al: Bladder neck closure with continent augmentation of suprapubic catheter in patients with neurogenic bladders. J Am Paraplegia Soc 16:18–22, 1992.
58. Chapple CR, Stott M, Abrams PH, et al: A 12 week placebo-controlled double-blind study of prazosin in the treatment of prostatic obstruction due to benign prostatic hyperplasia. Br J Urol 70:285–294, 1992.
59. Comarr AE: Autonomic dysreflexia. J Am Paraplegia Soc 7:4, 1984.
60. De Groat WC: Nervous control of the urinary bladder of the cat. Brain Res 87:201–211, 1975.
61. DeVivo MJ, Fine PR, Cutter GR, et al: The risk of renal calculi in spinal cord injury patients. J Urol 131:857–860, 1984.
62. Dick HC, Bradley WE, Scott FB, et al: Pudendal sexual reflexes. Urology 3:376–379, 1974.
63. Diokno AC, Sonda LP, Hollander JB, et al: Fate of patients started on clean intermittent self-catheterization therapy 10 years ago. J Urol 129:1120–1122, 1983.
64. Donker P, Van der Sluis C: Action of beta-adrenergic blocking agents on the urethral pressure profile. Urol Int 31:6, 1976.
65. Dow RS, Moruzzi G: The Physiology and Pathology of the Cerebellum. Minneapolis, University of Minnesota Press, 1958.
66. Drach GW, Layton TN, Binard JE: Male peak urinary flow rate: Relationships to volume voided and age. J Urol 122:210–214, 1979.
67. Dykstra DD, Sidi AA: Treatment of detrusor-sphincter dyssynergia with botulinum A toxin: A double-blind study. Arch Phys Med Rehabil 71:24–26, 1990.
68. Eardley I, Nagendran K, Kirby RS, et al: A new technique for assessing the efferent innervation of the human striated urethral sphincter. J Urol 144:948–951, 1990.
69. Ek A, Bradley WE: History of cystometry. Urology 22:335–350, 1983.
70. Erickson RP, Merritt JL, Opitz JL, et al: Bacteriuria during follow-up in patients with spinal cord injury: I. Rates of bacteriuria in various bladder-emptying methods. Arch Phys Med Rehabil 63:409–412, 1982.
71. Fam BA, Rossier AB, Blunt K, et al: Experience in the urologic management of 120 early spinal cord injury patients. J Urol 119:485–487, 1978.
72. Fanciullacci F, Sandri S, Politi P, et al: Clinical, urodynamic and neurophysiological findings in patients with neuropathic bladder due to a lumbar intervertebral disc protrusion. Paraplegia 27:354–358, 1989.
73. Fischman IJ, Shabsigh R, Scott FB: Experience with the artificial urinary sphincter model AS800 in 148 patients. J Urol 141:307–310, 1989.
74. Frewen WK: The management of urgency and frequency of micturition. Br J Urol 52:367–369, 1980.
75. Frost F, Nanninga J, Penn R, et al: Intrathecal baclofen infusion: Effect on bladder management programs in patients with myelopathy. Am J Phys Med Rehabil 142:112–115, 1989.
76. Gasparini ME, Schmidt RA, Tanagho EA: Selective sacral rhizotomy in the management of the reflex neuropathic bladder: A report on 17 patients with long-term follow-up. J Urol 148:1207–1210, 1992.
77. Gerridzen RG, Thijssen AM, Dehoux E: Risk factors for upper tract deterioration in chronic spinal cord injury patients. J Urol 147:416–418, 1992.
78. Gerstenberg TC, Klarskov P, Ramirez D, et al: Terodilene in the treatment of women with urgency and motor urge incontinence: A clinical and urodynamic double-blind crossover study. Br J Urol 58:129, 1986.
79. Gleason D, Reilly B: Gas cystometry. Urol Clin North Am 6:1, 1979.

80. Glowacki JS, Beecroft ML, Cook RJ, et al: The natural history of asymptomatic urolithiasis. J Urol 147:319–321, 1992.

81. Golji H: Complications of external condom drainage. Paraplegia 19:189–197, 1987.

82. Gonor SE, Carroll DJ, Metcalfe JB: Vesical dysfunction in multiple sclerosis. Urology 25:429–431, 1985.

83. Gonzalez R, Nguyen DH, Koleilat N, et al: Compatibility of enterocystoplasty and the artificial urinary sphincter. J Urol 142:502–504, 1989.

84. Gormley GJ, Stoner E, Bruskewitz RC, et al: The effect of finasteride in men with benign prostatic hyperplasia. N Engl J Med 327:1185–1191, 1992.

85. Gosling JA, Dixon JH, Critchley HO, et al: A comparative study of the human external sphincter and periurethral levator ani muscles. Br J Urol 53:35–41, 1981.

86. Gosling JA, Dixon JS, Humpherson JR: Functional Anatomy of the Urinary Tract: An Integrated Text and Color Atlas. Baltimore, University Park Press, 1982.

87. Gosling JA, Dixon JS, Lendon RG: The autonomic innervation of the human male female bladder neck and proximal urethra. J Urol 118:302–305, 1977.

88. Griffiths DJ: Urodynamic assessment of bladder function. Br J Urol 49:29–36, 1977.

89. Griffiths CJ, Assi MS, Styles RA, et al: Ambulatory monitoring of bladder and detrusor pressure during natural filling. J Urol 142:780–784, 1989.

90. Gundian JC, Barrett DM, Parulkar BG: Mayo Clinic experience with use of AMS 800 artificial urinary sphincter for urinary incontinence following radical prostatectomy. J Urol 142:1459–1461, 1989.

91. Hackler RH, Hall MK, Zampieri TA: Bladder hypocompliance in the spinal cord injury population. J Urol 141:1390–1393, 1989.

92. Hald T, Bradley WE: The Urinary Bladder: Neurology and Dynamics. Baltimore, Williams & Wilkins, 1982.

93. Haldeman S, Bradley WE, Bhatia NN: Evoked responses from pudendal nerve. J Urol 128:974, 1982.

94. Haldeman S, Bradley WE, Bhatia NN, et al: Pudendal somatosensory evoked potentials. Arch Neurol 39:280, 1982.

95. Haldeman S, Glick M, Bhatia NN, et al: Colonometry, cystometry and evoked potentials in multiple sclerosis. Arch Neurol 39:698–701, 1982.

96. Haldeman S, Bradley WE, Bhatia NN, et al: Pudendal evoked responses. Arch Neurol 39:280–283, 1982.

97. Hansen MV, Ertekin C, Larsson L-E: Cerebral evoked potentials after stimulation of the posterior urethra in man. Electroencephalogr Clin Neurophysiol 77:52–58, 1990.

98. Hedlund H, Andersson K-E: Effects of prazosin in men with symptoms of bladder neck obstruction and a nonhyperplastic prostate. Scand J Urol Nephrol 23:251–254, 1989.

99. Herr HW, Engelman ER, Martin DC: External sphincterotomy in traumatic and nontraumatic neurogenic bladder dysfunction. J Urol 113:32–34, 1975.

100. Hodgkinson CP: Direct urethrocystometry. Am J Obstet Gynecol 79:648–664, 1960.

101. Hoffberg HJ, Cardenas DD: Bladder trabeculation in spinal cord injury. Arch Phys Med Rehabil 67:750–753, 1986.

102. Hohenfellner M, Paick JS, Trigo-Rocha F, et al: Site of deafferentation and electrode placement for bladder stimulation: Clinical implications. J Urol 147:1665–1670, 1992.

103. Hublet D, Kaechkenbeck B, Baker DE: Etude comparative entre la cystometrie a l'eau et au gaz. Acta Urol Belg 48:4, 1980.

104. Hunt GM, Whitaker RH: A new device for self-catheterization in wheelchair bound women. Br J Urol 66:162–163, 1990.

105. Ingelman-Sundberg A: Denervation of the bladder. In Stanton SL, Tanagho EA (eds): Surgery of Female Incontinence. New York, Springer-Verlag, 1980, pp 93–97.

106. Iwatsubo E, Komine S, Yamashita H, et al: Overdistension therapy of the bladder in paraplegic patients using self-catheterization: A preliminary study. Paraplegia 22:210–215, 1984.

107. Jacobs SC, Kaufman JM: Complications of permanent bladder catheter drainage in spinal cord injury patients. J Urol 119:740–741, 1978.

108. Johnson ET: The condom catheter: Urinary tract infection and other complications. South Med J 76:579–582, 1983.

109. Kaneko S, Bradley WE: Penile electrodiagnosis. J Urol 137:933–935, 1987.

110. Kaufman JM, Fam B, Jacobs SC, et al: Bladder cancer and squamous metaplasia in spinal cord injury patients. J Urol 118:967, 1977.

111. Kiviat MD: Transurethral sphincterotomy: Relationship of site of incision to postoperative potency and delayed hemorrhage. J Urol 114:399–401, 1975.

112. Kiviat MD, Zimmerman TA, Donovan WH: Sphincter stretch: A new technique resulting in continence and complete voiding in paraplegics. J Urol 114:895–897, 1975.

113. Krane RJ, Olsson CA: Phenoxybenzamine in neurogenic bladder dysfunction: II. Clinical considerations. J Urol 110:653–656, 1973.

114. Krieger JN, Rudd TG, Mayo ME: Infection stones in patients with myelomeningocele and ileal conduit urinary tract diversion. Arch Phys Med Rehabil 66:360–362, 1985.

115. Lapides J, Diokno AC, Silber SJ, et al: Clean intermittent self-catheterization in the treatment of urinary tract disease. J Urol 107:458–461, 1972.

116. Leach GE, Farsaii A, Kark P, et al: Urodynamic manifestations of cerebellar ataxia. J Urol 128:348–350, 1982.

117. Learmonth JA: A contribution to the neurophysiology of the urinary bladder in man. Brain 54:147, 1931.

118. Lepor H, Meretyk S, Knapp-Moloney G: The safety, efficacy and compliance of terazosin therapy for benign prostatic hyperplasia. J Urol 147:1554–1557, 1992.

119. Lindan R, Leffler EJ, Kedia KR: A comparison of the efficacy of an $alpha_1$-adrenergic blocker as the slow calcium channel blocker in the control of autonomic dysreflexia. Paraplegia 23:34–38, 1985.

120. Linder A, Leach GE, Raz S: Augmentation cystoplasty in the treatment of neurogenic bladder dysfunction. J Urol 129:491, 1983.

121. Lockhart JL, Bejany DE, Politano VA: Augmentation cystoplasty in the management of neurogenic bladder disease and urinary incontinence. J Urol 135:969, 1986.

122. Lockhart JL, Walker JD, Vorstman B, et al: Periurethral polytetrafluoroethylene injection following urethral reconstruction in female patients with urinary incontinence. J Urol 140:51–52, 1988.

123. Madersbacher H, Jilg G: Control of detrusor hyperreflexia by the intravesical instillation of oxybutynine hydrochloride. Paraplegia 29:84–90, 1991.
124. Mayo ME: The value of sphincter electromyography in urodynamics. J Urol 122:357–360, 1979.
125. Mayo ME, Ansell JS: Urodynamic assessment of incontinence after prostatectomy. J Urol 122:60–61, 1979.
126. Mayo ME, Chapman WH, Shurtleff DB: Bladder function in children with meningomyelocele: Comparison of the cine-fluoroscopy and urodynamics. J Urol 121:458–461, 1979.
127. Mayo ME, Chetner MP: Lower urinary tract dysfunction in multiple sclerosis. Urology 34:67–70, 1992.
128. Mayo ME, Kiviat MD: Increased residual urine in patients with bladder neuropathy secondary to suprasacral spinal cord lesions. J Urol 123:726–728, 1980.
129. McGuire EJ, Savastano JA: Effect of alpha-adrenergic blockade and anticholinergic agents on the decentralized primate bladder. Neurourol Urodyn 4:139–142, 1985.
130. McInerney PD, Vanner TF, Harris SAB, et al: Permanent urethral stents for detrusor sphincter dyssynergia. Br J Urol 61:291–294, 1991.
131. Meirowsky AM, Scheibert CD, Hinchey TR: Studies on the sacral reflex arc in paraplegia: I. Response of the bladder to surgical elimination of sacral nerve impulses by rhizotomy. J Neurosurg 7:33–38, 1950.
132. Miodrag A, Castleden CM, Vallance TR: Sex hormones and the female urinary tract. Drugs 36:491–504, 1988.
133. Mitchell ME, Piser J: Intestinocystoplasty and total bladder replacement in children and young adults: Followup in 129 cases. J Urol 138:579, 1987.
134. Mohler JL, Cowen DL, Flanigan RC: Suppression and treatment of urinary tract infection in patients with an intermittently catheterized neurogenic bladder. J Urol 138:336–340, 1987.
135. Mulcahy JJ, Young AB: Percutaneous radiofrequency sacral rhizotomy in treatment of the hyperreflexic bladder. J Urol 120:557–558, 1978.
136. Mundy AR: Bladder transection for urge incontinence associated with detrusor instability. Br J Urol 52:480, 1980.
137. Murnaghan GF: Neurogenic disorders of the bladder in parkinsonism. Br J Urol 33:403–409, 1961.
138. Nashold BS, Friedman H, Grimes J: Electrical stimulation of the conus medullaris to control bladder emptying in paraplegia: A 10 year review. Appl Neurophysiol. 45:40–43, 1982.
139. Nathan PW, Smith MC: The centripetal pathway from the bladder and urethra within the spinal cord. J Neurol Neurosurg Psychiatry 14:262–280, 1951.
140. Nathan PW, Smith MC: The centrifugal pathway for micturition in the spinal cord. J Neurol Neurosurg Psychiatry 21:177–189, 1958.
141. Newman E, Price M: External catheters: Hazards and benefits of their use by men with spinal cord lesions. Arch Phys Med Rehabil 66:310–313, 1985.
142. Niefrach WL, Davis RS, Tometi FW, et al: Extracorporeal shock-wave lithotripsy in patients with spinal cord dysfunction. Urology 38:152–156, 1991.
143. Perkash I, Friedland GW: Transrectal ultrasonography of the lower urinary tract: Evaluation of bladder neck problems. Neurourol Urodyn 5:299, 1986.
144. O'Flynn KJ, Murphy R, Thomas DG: Neurogenic bladder dysfunction in lumbar intravesical disc prolapse. Br J Urol 69:38–40, 1992.
145. O'Grady F, Cattell W: Kinetics of urinary tract infection: II. The bladder. Br J Urol 38:156–162, 1966.
146. Onuf (Onufrowicz) B: On the arrangement and function of the neuron groups of the sacral cord in man. Arch Neurol Psychopathol 3:387–411, 1900.
147. Puri P, Guiney EJ: Endoscopic correction of vesicoureteric reflux secondary to neuropathic bladder. Br J Urol 58:504–506, 1986.
148. Rockswold GL, Bradley WE, Chou SN: Differential sacral rhizotomy in the treatment of neurogenic bladder dysfunction. J Neurosurg 38:748–754, 1973.
149. Rockswold GL, Bradley WE, Chou SN: Effect of sacral nerve blocks on the function of the urinary bladder in humans. J Neurosurg 40:83–89, 1974.
150. Rockswold GL, Chou SN, Bradley WE: Reevaluation of differential sacral rhizotomy for neurological bladder disease. J Neurosurg 48:773–778, 1978.
151. Rockswold GL, Bradley WE, Timm GW, et al: Electrophysiological technique for evaluating lesions of the conus medullaris and cauda equina. J Neurosurg 45:321–326, 1976.
152. Ross JC, Gibbon NOK, Damanski M: Division of the external sphincter in the treatment of the neurogenic bladder: A 10 year review. Br J Surg 54:627–628, 1967.
153. Ross JC, Gibbon NOK, Sham Sunder G: Division of the external urethral sphincter in the neuropathic bladder: A 20 year's review. Br J Urol 48:649–656, 1976.
154. Roth DR, Vyas PR, Kroovand RL, et al: Urinary tract deterioration associated with the artificial urinary sphincter. J Urol 135:528–530, 1986.
155. Rud T: The effect of estrogens and progestogens on the urethral pressure profile in urinary continence and stress incontinent women. Acta Obstet Gynecol Scand 59:265–270, 1980.
156. Scott FC, Bradley WE, Timm GW: Treatment of urinary incontinence by implantable prosthetic sphincter. Urology 1:252–259, 1973.
157. Scott FC, Bradley WE, Timm GW: Treatment of urinary incontinence by an implantable prosthetic urinary sphincter. J Urol 112:75–80, 1974.
158. Sharma S, Vaidyanathan S, Thrind SK, et al: The effect of dicolfenac sodium on urinary concentration of calcium, uric acid and glycosaminoglycans in traumatic paraplegics. Br J Urol 68:240–242, 1991.
159. Shaw J: Urethral pressure profile. In Krane RJ, Siroky MB (eds): Clinical Neurourology, ed 2. Boston, Little Brown, 1991, pp 185–199.
160. Shoukry I, Susset JG, Elhilali MM, et al: Role of uroflowmetry in the assessment of lower urinary tract obstruction in adult males. Br J Urol 47:559–566, 1975.
161. Sidi AA, Becher EF, Reddy PK, et al: Augmentation enterocystoplasty for the management of voiding dysfunction in spinal cord injury patients. J Urol 143:83–85, 1990.
162. Sires Trop C, Bennett CJ: Automatic dysreflexia and its urological implications: A review. J Urol 146:1461–1469, 1991.
163. Siroky MB, Olsson CA, Krane RJ: The flow rate nomogram: II. Clinical correlation. J Urol 123:208–210, 1980.

164. Sislow JG, Mayo ME: Reduction in human bladder wall compliance following decentralization. J Urol 144:945–947, 1990.
165. Staskin DR: Hydronephrosis after spinal cord injury: Effects of lower urinary tract dysfunction on upper tract anatomy. Urol Clin North Am 18:309–316, 1991.
166. Steers WD, Meythaler JM, Haworth C, et al: Effects of acute bolus and chronic continuous intrathecal baclofen on genitourinary dysfunction due to spinal cord pathology. J Urol 148:1849–1855, 1992.
167. Stickler DJ, Chawla JC: An appraisal of antibiotic policies for urinary tract infections in patients with spinal cord injuries undergoing long-term intermittent catheterisation. Paraplegia 26:215–225, 1988.
168. Sung JH: Autonomic neurons affected by lipid storage in the spinal cord in Fabry's disease: Distribution of autonomic neurons in the sacral cord. J Neuropathol Exp Neurol 38:87–98, 1979.
169. Sussett JG, Galea G, Read L: Biofeedback therapy for female incontinence due to low urethral resistance. J Urol 143:1205–1208, 1990.
170. Tanagho EA, Schmidt RA, Orvis BR: Neural stimulation for control of voiding dysfunction: A preliminary report in 22 patients with serious neuropathic voiding disorders. J Urol 142:340–345, 1989.
171. Taylor MC, Bradley WE, Bhatia N, et al: The conus demyelination syndrome in multiple sclerosis. Acta Neurol Scand 69:80–89, 1984.
172. Tori JA, Kewalramani LS: Urolithiasis in children with spinal cord injury. Paraplegia 16:357–365, 1979.
173. Thyberg M, Gedda S, Johansen PB, et al: Continuous monitoring of detrusor pressure in patients with a reflex urinary bladder after spinal cord injury. Scand J Rehabil Med 21:115–121, 1989.
174. Von Garrelts B: Analysis of micturition: A new method of recording the voiding of the bladder. Acta Chir Scand 112:326–340, 1956.
175. Wan J, Fleenor S, Kielczewski P, et al: Urinary tract status of patients with neurogenic dysfunction presenting with upper tract stone disease. J Urol 148:1126–1128, 1992.
176. Wear JB Jr, Wear RB, Cleeland C: Biofeedback in urology using urodynamics: Preliminary observations. J Urol 121:464–468, 1979.
177. Webb RJ, Styles RA, Griffiths CJ, et al: Ambulatory monitoring of bladder pressure in low compliance neurogenic bladder dysfunction. J Urol 148:1477–1488, 1992.
178. Wein AJ, Hanno PM, Dixon DO, et al: The reproducibility and interpretation of carbon dioxide cystometry. J Urol 120:205–206, 1978.
179. Wein AJ, Malloy TR, Shofer F, et al: The effects of bethanechol chloride on urodynamic parameters in normal women and women with significant residual urine volumes. J Urol 124:397–399, 1980.
180. Wein AJ: Classification of neurogenic bladder dysfunction. J Urol 125:606, 1981.
181. Whitfield HN, Mayo M: Prolonged bladder distension in the treatment of the unstable bladder. Br J Urol 47:635, 1975.
182. Wyndaele JJ: Is impaired perception of bladder filling during cystometry a sign of neuropathy? Br J Urol 270–273, 1993.

CHAPTER 14

Disturbed Sexual Function in Patients with Spinal Cord Disease

John J. Mulcahy, M.D., Ph.D., F.A.C.S.

Loss of sexual function can be devastating to a man with spinal cord disease. Younger men, in particular, assume that the ability to achieve an erection is as natural a part of life as is eating, breathing, or sleeping. Any distortion of this function is a cause for great concern and when erectile ability is lost, deep depression often ensues. When loss of erectile ability is combined with malfunction of other body parts, as often occurs in spinal cord disease, a man's total body image is severely altered. If the progression of loss of erectile abilities with aging is examined, patient attitudes may correlate with age-specific expectations about sexual performance. In the teen years, through the 20s, and into the mid-30s, erections are automatic and can usually be achieved even under adverse circumstances. In this age group it may be said that the problem is avoiding, not achieving, an erection. In the late 30s and into the 40s, more direct stimulation by a partner is needed and distraction by fatigue, anxiety, or obsessive-compulsive behavior may affect the ability to achieve an erection. During the late 50s and beyond, the incidence of impotence or inability to achieve a sufficient erection increases. By their late 50s, perhaps 25% of men are not functioning well sexually because of physical impairment of blood flow. By the late 60s, this number probably increases to 50%. With decreased sexual prowess, a concomitant decrease in libido or sexual drive occurs. Although sexual drive may be present well into older age, the drive tends to be less strong and the ability to become interested in other things when sexual stimulation is not available is easier. In view of this, the attitude of a man suddenly faced with spinal cord disease that affects his erectile ability varies with age.

MECHANISM OF ERECTION

Since 1970, knowledge of the anatomy and physiology of the erectile mechanism has greatly increased. Before that time, interest in studying this area was considered inappropriate by many, and monies for research were not forthcoming. The advent of penile prostheses in the early 1970s represented an effective treatment for organic impotence. This treatment was fairly aggressive, and many patients were unwilling to undergo a surgical procedure to restore erectile function. This gave impetus to the study of anatomy and pathophysiology in an attempt to uncover new and less aggressive ways of managing the problem. As a result of these gains, it is known that the erectile bodies are covered by an elastic membrane, the tunica albuginea. As the erectile bodies fill with blood, this membrane stretches and the penis becomes three times larger. At the point at which the membrane can stretch no further, arterial pressure pushing against the taut membrane gives rigidity to the penis (Fig. 14–1). It was once thought that the interstices of the erectile body were sponge-filled cavities that pas-

sively accepted the flow of blood. It is now known that these are endothelium-lined lacunar spaces surrounded by smooth muscle.[34] These spaces enlarge in response to smooth muscle relaxation caused by specific neurotransmitters. Enlargement of the lacunar spaces allows the erectile bodies to be filled more completely and also results in compression of the venules that course between lacunar spaces, providing a valve-like mechanism that traps the blood in the erectile bodies. One of these transmitter substances, nitric oxide, has recently been identified.[28] If an impulse or stimulus to generate an erection occurs in one portion of the penis, it is rapidly transmitted throughout both corporal bodies through gap junctions.[17] These are specialized junctional complexes between cells that allow free movement of relatively large molecules, thus avoiding the problems of membrane permeability, suboptimal dissociation constants, and other impediments to particle movement and rapid impulse transmission (Fig. 14–2).

In the flaccid state, arteriolar flow into the erectile bodies is low and the smooth muscles are contracted. Whatever blood enters the erectile bodies exits easily through open venules. In the erect state, under the influence of neurotransmitters, arteriolar flow increases, smooth muscle relaxation occurs, and the lacunar spaces expand. As these fill with blood, the membrane covering the erectile bodies is stretched maximally and rigidity occurs. Trapping of blood by the compression of venules between expanding lacunar spaces is essential for maintaining blood within the erec-

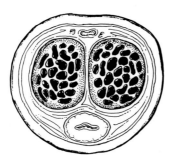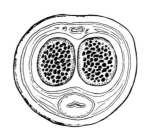

FIGURE 14–1

Cross-section of penis in erect (*left*) and flaccid (*right*) states. Blood enters erectile bodies to stretch elastic covering membrane to its limits, resulting in rigidity.

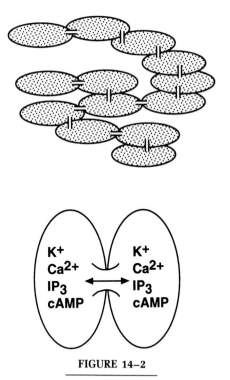

FIGURE 14–2

Propagation of an impulse producing relaxation among smooth muscle cells throughout the penis via gap junctions. K^+ = potassium; Ca^{2+} = calcium; IP_3 = inositol phosphate; cAMP = cyclic adenosine monophosphate.

tile bodies. Without such compression, blood would seep out through the venules and an incomplete or short-lived erection would occur, a condition known as *venous leak impotence*.[40]

TYPES OF IMPOTENCE

It had been estimated that 10 million men in the United States, about 10% of the population, were incapable of achieving erection suitable for intercourse. Recent epidemiologic studies have shown that this figure far underestimates the true incidence. The real figure may be as high as 20% to 30%.[23] Certainly the vast majority of these patients are older than 50 years. When Kinsey chronicled the sexual habits of the American male in 1948, he estimated that about 90% of erectile troubles were psychological.[29] Today our opinion is the reverse of his, i.e., it is thought that the vast majority of erectile difficulties have a physical basis.

Psychological Impotence

In psychological impotence, a situation or an emotion interferes with proper sexual performance. In subsequent sexual encounters, failure occurs due to persistence of the distraction. After a number of failures, when a sexual encounter occurs, the recollection of previous failures generates anxiety that interferes with concentration and results in another failure. A vicious cycle of performance anxiety has been created. Failure leads to more anxiety about subsequent sexual encounters; more anxiety leads to failure. To break this vicious cycle, sex therapists have prescribed exercises that allow foreplay but prohibit intercourse. This is intended to eliminate the anxiety of having to perform, but has only been modestly successful.[3]

Vascular Impotence

Three mechanisms may inhibit erections on a physical basis: hormonal, neurologic, and vascular. As the incidence of hormonal and neurologic disease causing impotence is relatively low, it can be concluded that the majority of causes of erectile dysfunction are vascular in nature. As men age, "hardening" of the arteries takes a toll, and the smaller helicine arteries in the corpora cavernosa seem to be an early target of occlusive vascular disease. The entire picture of impotence in the aging male is not completely clear. A transmitter substance, as yet undiscovered, may diminish in concentration in the penis with age. My experience with the impotence of aging, however, supports a vascular etiology. Men with diseases that tend to predispose to premature atherosclerosis, such as hypertension, hypercholesterolemia, heavy cigarette smoking, and diabetes mellitus, tend to manifest impotence at a relatively early age. Men who exercise regularly, stay fit and trim, avoid smoking, maintain normal blood pressure, and are otherwise generally healthy tend to maintain erectile abilities well into advanced age.

Hormonal Impotence

Two hormones tend to affect erectile function adversely when their concentrations are abnormal: prolactin and testosterone. If prolactin levels are high, lack of interest in sexual matters and erectile dysfunction are usually present. Pituitary evaluation should be undertaken in this group, as more than 50% of men with elevated prolactin levels will have an adenoma. Prompt restoration of sexual drive and erectile abilities as well as regression of the adenoma, is usually seen on institution of bromocriptine therapy.[24] Signs of testosterone deficiency are not quite as dramatic. Normal sex drive, normal erectile abilities, low sex drive, poor erectile abilities, or any combination of these may be present. A serum testosterone level is diagnostic. If sexual drive decreases or a minor impairment of erectile abilities occurs, replacing testosterone by an intramuscular injection may restore each of these to normal function. Empiric use of bromocriptine or testosterone to restore sexual abilities when the levels of prolactin and testosterone are normal has not been successful. If testosterone levels are kept above the normal limits, polycythemia and depression of high-density lipoprotein (HDL) cholesterol levels may be seen. Testosterone should be replaced with caution in the older population as it tends to stimulate the growth of prostate cancer.

Neurologic Impotence

A number of neurologic diseases and injuries have been associated with the development of erectile difficulties, namely, temporal lobe lesions, spinal cord injuries, multiple sclerosis, Parkinson's disease, and tabes dorsalis. There appears to be an "erection center" in the brain, although its location has not been identified. In addition, one or more erection centers are present in the spinal cord. The presence of cerebral connections with the spinal erection mechanism is not essential, even for volitional erections, as some paraplegics have been noted to continue to have erections following their injuries. Bors and Comar[11] studied neuroanatomy and sexual function in spinal cord injury extensively. Ninety percent of patients with complete transection of the cord above the sacral area could have erections, but only in response to tactile stimuli (reflex erections). An intact pudendal nerve was required for this phenomenon. In patients with cauda equina injuries, no reflex erections were possible, but about 25% of such patients were able to have psychogenic erections. This suggests that thoracolumbar spinal outflow from the T12–L1 level can produce psychogenic erections even when complete destruction of the sacral cord has occurred. Hence, for physical impotence to occur following spinal cord trauma, both the thoracolumbar and sacral erection centers must be affected.

IMPOTENCE EVALUATION

The most important element in differentiating psychological from organic impotence is the patient history. An experienced interviewer who is well-versed in types of sexual dysfunction can usually determine which disorder is predominant. It should also be appreciated, however, that any man who has lost his erectile abilities, whether from a psychological or physical cause, will manifest a certain amount of depression, which in itself will pose a psychological impediment to proper erectile performance. When a true determination must be made between psychogenic and organic sources of impotence, the gold standard is nocturnal penile tumescence monitoring. All men have erections during rapid eye movement (REM) sleep (about 20% of sleep time) if they are capable of achieving erections. The expansion of the penis and the rigidity developed under these circumstances can be measured. The most common method of measurement is the snap gauge test, in which a band is placed around the penis and secured with a Velcro connection.[21] The band has three bridges made of breakable plastic that snap apart at varying increments of penile expansion and rigidity. A more sophisticated and expensive nocturnal penile tumescence monitoring device is the Rigiscan[2] (Fig. 14–3). This computerized monitor measures the expansion of the penis and the rigidity, at both the base and the tip, continuously, over a period up to 10 hours during sleep (Fig. 14–4). The duration of each rigidity episode and the degree of rigidity can be quantified over this period. The test may be done in a sleep laboratory in association with electroencephalographic (EEG) monitoring or, for convenience, it may be done at home for 2 to 3 successive nights. Results of nocturnal penile tumescence monitoring should be interpreted with caution in the patient with spinal cord disease. A patient with reflex erections may show an apparently normal tracing.

Biothesiometry of the penis has been suggested as a useful test for patients suspected of having a neurogenic source of impotence.[38] Vibratory sensitivity in the glans and shaft of the penis are tested and compared with vibratory sensitivity in the index finger (Fig. 14–5). A positive result, i.e., poor appreciation of vibratory sensitivity in the penis, only reveals a sensory deficit and only suggests, but does not prove, that a compromise of the motor input to the erectile mechanism may be present as well. If biothesiometry results are abnormal, somatosensory evoked potentials following stimulation of the dorsal nerve of the penis have been recommended[31] (Fig. 14–6). These may localize a lesion to the nervous system but not conclusively prove that the deficit in erectile function is neurogenic; they add little in the way of directing appropriate therapy. Evoked potentials are rarely used in the clinical evaluation of impotence. Other tests have been advocated for the evaluation of erectile dysfunction, such as duplex sonography, which outlines the arterial input to the erectile bodies[33]; cavernosometry, which measures the intracorporeal pressures in response to infusion of solutions designed to raise intracorporeal pressure; cavernosography, which detects aberrant venous drainage channels from the erectile bodies[9]; and pelvic arteriography, which detects blockage of the arteries entering the erectile bodies.[10]

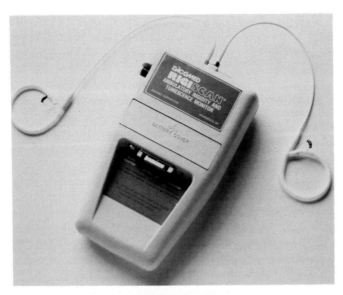

FIGURE 14–3

The Rigiscan nocturnal penile tumescence monitoring device is placed in a holster that is strapped to the thigh during sleep. Cloth-covered stainless steel loops are placed at the base and the tip of the penis during sleep to measure changes for up to 10 hours in penile circumference and degree of rigidity. (Courtesy of Dacomed Corp., Minneapolis.)

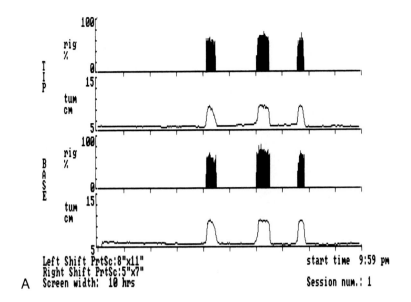

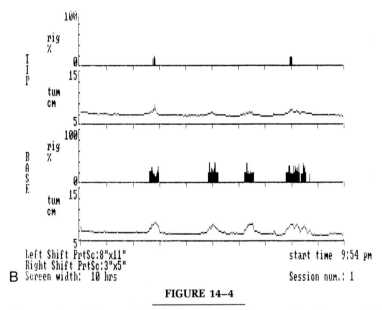

FIGURE 14–4

A, Normal tracing from Rigiscan nocturnal penile tumescence monitor: three episodes of good rigidity at base and tip are seen. Expansion of the penis from 6 to 10 cm at base and tip occurred during erection. B, Abnormal tracing from Rigiscan nocturnal penile tumescence monitor: very little expansion or rigidity of the penis was noted during sleep.

These tests have special, limited applications and should be used in patients who would be considered candidates for vascular procedures to restore function of the erectile mechanism; this is a very small group of patients.

MEDICAL TREATMENT

In consideration of the physiology of erections, it would seem that agents that increase blood flow and relax smooth muscle would

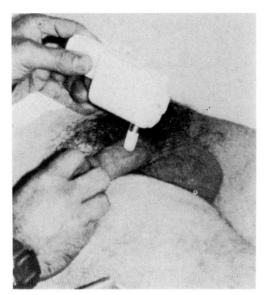

FIGURE 14–5

Biothesiometry vibrator applied to penis. Frequency of vibrations is fixed but amplitude of vibrations is variable. Response is noted from stimulation at different sites on the glans and the shaft of the penis. (From Padma-Nathan H, Goldstein I: Neurologic assessment of the impotent patient. In Montague DK (ed): Disorders of Male Sexual Function. Chicago, Year Book Medical Publishers, 1988, pp 86–94, with permission.)

have the best effect on the generation of an erection. Smooth muscle relaxant medications are available in three forms: oral, transdermal, and intracorporeal. The oral forms of these medications have relatively mild effects in treating erectile disability.[36] The medications will improve an erection that is 67% firm to the point at which it reaches 80% of optimal rigidity. They work in select cases and seem to have a more beneficial effect on idiopathic impotence of aging and hypertension-related erection difficulties, both of which are forms of vascular disease. Studies are being performed to test the effects of transdermal and intraurethral topical applications of these compounds. Preliminary results indicate that the creams and pastes are mildly helpful but no dramatic effects have occurred. Smooth muscle relaxants administered by intracorporeal injection are most effective. Three agents are in common use today but none has yet been approved by the FDA for use in improving the quality of erections, although these medications have been approved for other uses. The safety and efficacy of these agents have been well documented in the literature.[18, 19] Papaverine acts by relaxing smooth muscle and has been available for many years. Cardiologists have used it to attempt to improve cardiac blood flow in cases of angina and it has also been used by neurologists in an attempt to increase the blood flow to the spinal cord in multiple sclerosis. Its most common use, other than for penile injection, is in angiography to increase the blood flow to a particular vascular bed for radiographic study. The maximum dosage used for intracorporeal injections is in the range of 60 mg/day. This is far less than the toxic doses used by cardiologists who were giving 90 to 120 mg every 4 hours in an attempt to relieve angina. Prostaglandin E_1 (Prostin) is the most powerful smooth muscle relaxant among the prostaglandins. It is used to relax the smooth muscles of the patent ductus arteriosus in newborns who are awaiting corrective cardiac surgery. It is almost completely metabolized in the penis when injected intracorporeally, and what little medication enters the sytemic circulation is metabolized within one passage through the lungs. Phentolamine (Regitine) is an alpha-blocking agent, and when used alone it has been ineffective in improving erections. It acts on the alpha-receptors of blood vessels to increase blood flow, but it has no effect on the smooth muscle of the corporeal sinusoids. Improving the blood flow to the penis alone is ineffective in the absence of sinusoidal expansion, which occurs with smooth muscle relaxation. Phentolamine has been used in association with papaverine and with prostaglandin E_1 to augment the effects of these two smooth muscle relaxants. The maximum dose used for intracorporeal injection is 2 mg/day. During a phentolamine test for pheochromocytoma, 5 mg of the drug is given intravenously. If a 20 mm Hg or greater drop in blood pressure is noted, the result is considered positive for pheochromocytoma. When given in toxic doses, papaverine and phentolamine inhibit atrioventricular node conduction and result in aberrant intraventricular conduction. Because of its rapid metabolism, prostaglandin E_1 has not caused toxic cardiovascular effects.

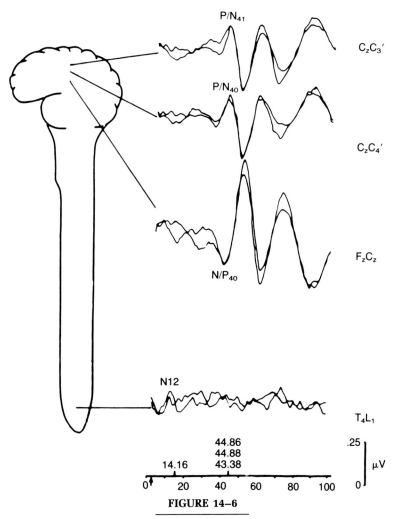

FIGURE 14–6

Cerebral (P/N$_{41}$, P/N$_{40}$, N/P$_{40}$) and sacral (N$_{12}$) wave forms during a dorsal nerve somatosensory evoked potential test. (From Padma-Nathan H, Goldstein I: Neurologic assessment of the impotent patient. In Montague DK (ed): Disorders of Male Sexual Function. Chicago, Year Book Medical Publishers, 1988, pp 86–94, with permission.)

Various protocols have been proposed for use of these agents to improve erections.[4, 45] Prostaglandin and papaverine have been used alone or in combination with phentolamine. Some protocols encourage the use of a mixture of all three agents. Drawbacks of papaverine include the fact that it has been associated with scar tissue formation with prolonged use in animals.[1] The pH of this agent is in the range of 3, and it cannot be buffered to physiologic pH. Prostaglandin E$_1$ injections are painful in about 30% of patients; because of this, some patients have avoided its use. The response in generating erections with each of these agents or a com-

bination of agents is dose-dependent. If the patient has a minor problem of vascular inflow or if deficit of neural input to the erectile mechanism is present, a relatively low dose is needed to create a very good erection. If relatively poor blood flow is present, high doses are needed to achieve a beneficial effect. If a high dose is given to a patient with a relatively minor inflow problem, priapism or prolonged painful erection can result. This can easily be reversed by using sympathomimetic amines, such as phenylephrine or epinephrine, in very dilute doses injected directly intracorporeally.[27] These agents cause vasoconstriction and reduction of the erectile state. With experience, an estimate of the effective therapeutic range of these agents can be made on the basis of the history. If a physician is unfamiliar with these agents, it is safer to start with a low dose (in the range of 15 mg of papaverine or 5 μg or less of prostaglandin E_1). In young patients with neurogenic impotence (e.g., paraplegics), erectile dysfunction results from an almost purely neural deficit. The penile vascular inflow in such cases is uncompromised and a low dose of these medications gives a very good result. A test dose resulting in an erection of 75% optimal rigidity lasting 45 minutes in the office is ideal. The injected medication is designed to support or complement a patient's partial erection. Except in cases of complete impotence due to a neurologic injury, in which the erection must be totally restored, this complementary effect has been adequate and beneficial. The appealing feature of supporting a partial erection, rather than replacing it, has made this the most popular method of restoring erectile abilities when the deficit is the result of a physical injury. In many cases, psychogenic impotence is treated with a pharmacologic erection program as well. Since the metabolism of prostaglandin E_1 is

so rapid and occurs almost completely in the penis, there is less likelihood of priapism occurring with this agent than with papaverine or phentolamine. A 30-gauge $^1/_2$ in. needle applied to either a tuberculin syringe or a 3-cc syringe is ideal for administration of these agents. They are delivered to the upper outer portion of either erectile body, and injection in one site results in improved blood flow and rigidity in the entire corpus cavernosum on each side (Fig. 14–7). The response takes about 10 to 15 minutes as impulses, analogous to a domino effect, are propagated via gap junctions. Using this injection program in patients receiving anticoagulants has posed no problem. The patient merely compresses the bleeding site for an additional period of time. Obese patients with a very large panniculus who have difficulty seeing their penis may need the help of a partner to retract the panniculus and to inject the medication. In patients with cardiac intraventricular conduction problems, prostaglandin E_1 may be a better choice as papaverine and phentolamine may precipitate heart block if higher doses are used in patients with marginal cardiac conduction. When in doubt, consult with the patient's cardiologist. De-

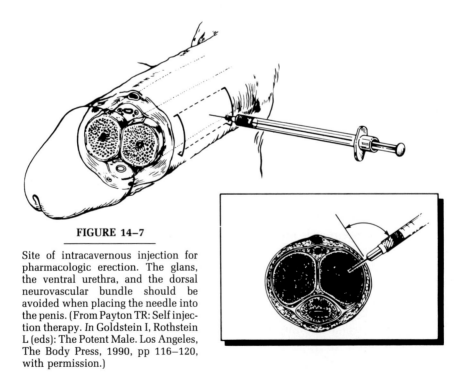

FIGURE 14–7

Site of intracavernous injection for pharmacologic erection. The glans, the ventral urethra, and the dorsal neurovascular bundle should be avoided when placing the needle into the penis. (From Payton TR: Self injection therapy. *In* Goldstein I, Rothstein L (eds): The Potent Male. Los Angeles, The Body Press, 1990, pp 116–120, with permission.)

spite good results in restoring erections in most patients, the dropout rate from pharmacologic erection programs is greater than 50% within the first 6 months. The effectiveness of these agents in patients with spinal cord disease has been noted in a number of series.[8, 46]

VACUUM ERECTION DEVICES

Vacuum erection devices have grown in popularity in recent years due to their relatively low cost and lack of invasiveness. To use these devices, a large plastic cylinder is placed over the penis. A seal is created at the base, where the penis joins the body, and negative pressure is created within the cylinder, usually by a hand pump attached to the opposite end. The negative pressure created by this vacuum draws blood into the penis. Pressures in the range of 200 cm H_2O have been achieved with these devices, which is certainly adequate to create good penile turgidity. When the penis becomes sufficiently rigid to allow intercourse, a heavy rubber band is quickly slipped off of the proximal end of the cylinder onto the penis, thus trapping blood in the erectile bodies (Fig. 14–8). This results in a hinged erection that can be directed toward the vagina and used for approximately a half hour, at which point the rubber band is removed. These devices have been relatively safe. If the patient falls asleep with the constricting band in place, necrosis of the penis does not occur, as blood flow continues in and out of the penis at a much slower than normal rate. This device should be used with caution or not at all by patients receiving major anticoagulants such as warfarin (Coumadin). In such patients, hematomas have developed. Scar tissue has been reported over the long term in some patients using vacuum devices because of repeated minor trauma from the tightly constricting rubber band. The key to success with these devices is persistence on the part of the physician or his or her associate in working with and instructing the patient to achieve a successful outcome. There is a long learning curve associated with the successful use of these devices. A number of series

have reported good results with the use of these devices in patients with spinal cord disease.[32, 47]

PENILE PROSTHESES

The third option for treating patients with spinal cord disease who have developed physical erectile difficulties is the use of a penile prosthesis. These devices were introduced in the early 1970s. When properly placed, they give a predictable and reliable result. When the patient is informed of the function and limitations of these devices, gratification is the norm. The satisfaction rate in patients with these devices is in the range of 80%, and that of their partners is about 70% in most series.[22] This is by far the highest satisfaction rate of any of the three modalities used for treating physical erectile difficulties. The most common reason for dissatisfaction with an implant is penile size. A patient can expect to lose between 0.5 and 1 in. in penile length following implantation of one of these devices when the length of the erection is compared with the patient's original, natural erection. With an exceptionally large penis, even more loss of length can be expected. Two types of prostheses are available, semirigid rods and inflatables. Mechanical problems plagued the original inflatable prostheses, but the manufacturers attended to those problems and modified, reinforced, or eliminated areas that tended to wear or malfunction (Fig. 14–9). During the first 5 years, 5% to 10% of patients' inflatable devices will need repair. Semirigid rods have had fewer mechanical problems but have been less desirable because they are firm all the time (Fig. 14–10). The patient chooses the type of prosthesis with some guidance by the physician, who can elucidate the features, functions, and limitations of each of the two types. Patients with diminished manual or mental dexterity are encouraged to choose the semirigid rod type, as these require little skill in their operation. Inflatable prostheses have resulted in fewer problems with distal erosion, as they are relatively soft the majority of the time. Patients with spinal cord disease who have impaired sensation in the penis or who

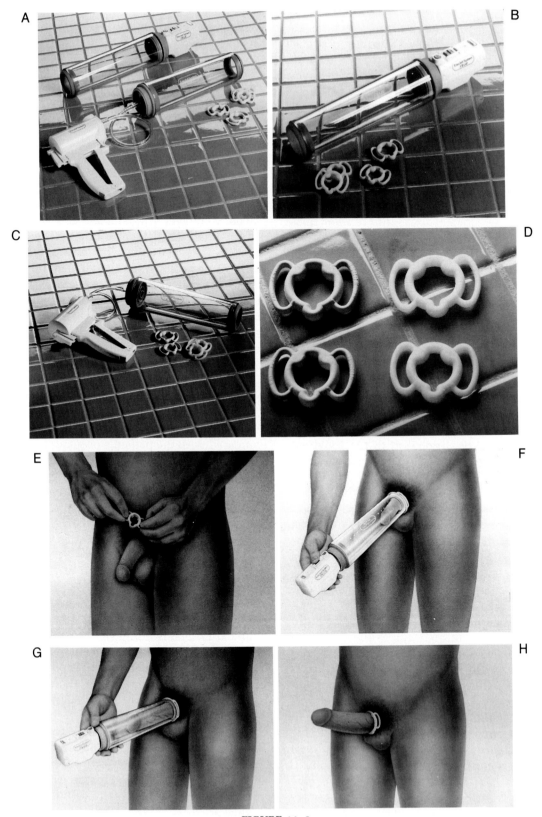

FIGURE 14–8

Vacuum erection device: Erecaid system. *A–D*, Components include a pump, plastic cylinder, lubricating jelly, and constriction rings. *E*, Constriction ring is applied and the cylinder is placed over the flaccid penis. *F* and *G*, A vacuum, created by pumping air out of the cylinder, draws blood into the penis. *H*, A hinged erection is maintained. (Courtesy of Osbon Corp., Augusta, Ga.)

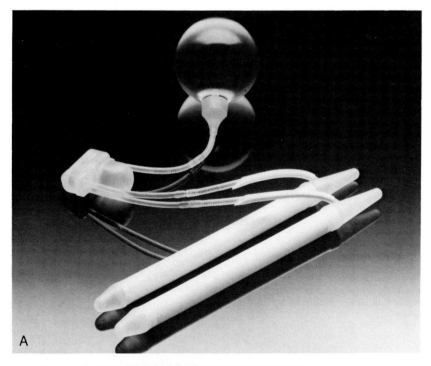

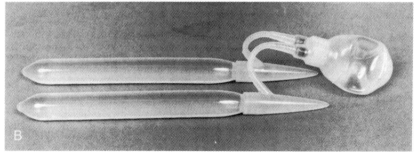

FIGURE 14-9

Two types of inflatable penile prostheses. *A*, Three-piece inflatable penile prosthesis. Via a scrotal pump, fluid is pumped from an abdominally located reservoir into the two longitudinal cylinders, one of which is located in each erectile body. (Courtesy of American Medical Systems, Minnetonka, Minn.) *B*, Two-piece inflatable penile implant. Fluid passes between a combined reservoir pump located in the scrotum and two longitudinal penile cylinders for alternating penile rigidity and flaccidity. (Courtesy of Mentor Corp., Goletta, Calif.)

are using intermittent or indwelling catheters have greater problems with erosion of these implants through the skin. Patients who are using indwelling or intermittent catheterization in association with a penile prosthesis have been advised to have a perineal urethrostomy created to facilitate catheterization through this orifice. A greater than 50% erosion rate has been seen when catheters are used through the urethra adjacent to penile prosthesis cylinders.[42] Either an inflatable or a semirigid prosthesis may be helpful for holding on a condom-type catheter. Before

considering a penile prosthesis, patients are encouraged to try a pharmacologic erection program or vacuum erection device. Both of these modalities are reversible, with virtually no damage to the penis, if they are unacceptable to the patient or are ineffective in restoring adequate erections. Once the patient has a penile implant placed, the other two modalities are not likely to be successful in restoring satisfactory erections if, for some reason, the implant must be removed.

With advances made since the mid-1970s in the treatment of erectile difficulties, it is

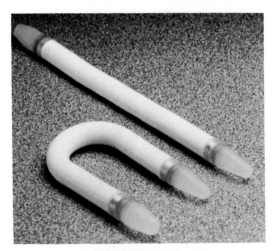

FIGURE 14–10

Mechanical semirigid rod implant. Paired, permanently firm, but bendable, cylinders are placed in each erectile body. (Courtesy of Dacomed Corp., Minneapolis.)

virtually unnecessary for any man to suffer from this affliction. Despite the high percentage of patients with this problem, a very low percentage seek treatment. Motivation for treatment is related to many factors, the two most influential of which are (1) age-dependent sex drive and (2) attitude and availability of a partner. Basic scientific research in the area of erectile dysfunction is actively looking for even simpler ways of restoring erectile ability. Compliance with treatments would be greater if such goals were to be achieved, as indicated by the remark heard from numerous patients: "Don't you just have a pill that will do the job?"

MECHANISM OF EJACULATION

Ejaculation occurs when a complex interaction of psychic and tactile stimuli result in a neuromuscular response. Ejaculation is considered in two phases: emission and ejaculation. The emission phase includes bladder neck closure and pulsatile bulbar contraction with seminal expulsion.[43] In the emission phase, the vas deferens, seminal vesicles, and prostate contract, which results in the deposition of sperm-rich seminal fluid in the prostatic urethra. Closure of the bladder neck prevents retrograde flow of the emission fluid

into the bladder.[30] The phenomena of emission occur under the influence of the sympathetic outflow from the thoracolumbar area of the cord through the hypogastric nerve. Subsequently, rhythmic contraction of the bulbocavernosus and ischiocavernosus muscles results in the forceful, pulsatile ejaculation of the emission fluid through the anterior urethra. These phenomena are under neural control with origins in the S2–4 segment of the spinal cord and efferent and afferent limbs coursing through the pudendal nerve (Fig. 14–11). Thus, both emission and ejaculation are the result of complementary sympathetic and somatic innervations. It is postulated that two centers are present in the nervous system for the regulation of the ejaculation mechanism. Supraspinal centers are present in the cerebral areas, but the location of these has not been identified. A reflex ejaculation center located between T12 and L2 in the spinal cord is believed to coordinate emission and ejaculatory events in concert with the higher cerebral centers.[6]

Aberrations of Ejaculation and Fertility

Ejaculatory failure is common in patients with spinal cord injury. In persons with complete upper motor neuron lesions, absence of ejaculation is seen almost universally.[5] Up to 30% of patients with incomplete upper motor neuron lesions can experience ejaculation, whereas 17% of patients with complete lower motor neuron lesions and 60% of patients with incomplete lower motor neuron lesions exhibit weak emission with dribbling semen expulsion. Fertility rates among men with spinal cord injury are poor, in the range of less than 10%.[12] Problems of ejaculation are compounded by suboptimal testicular function. The presence of elevated temperature in the groin due to chronic sedentary habitus; loss of the thermoregulatory mechanism of the pampiniform plexus; recurrent urinary tract infections, prostatitis, and epididymoorchitis; and the use of medications that may suppress spermatogenesis all contribute to the low rate of spontaneous fatherhood in these patients. Testicular biopsy in patients

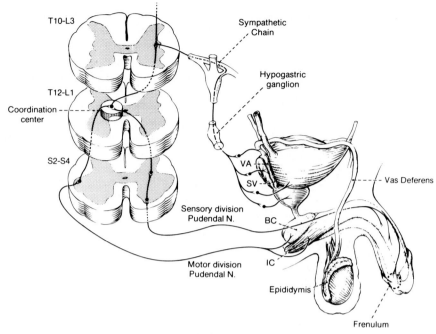

FIGURE 14-11

Neuroanatomic mechanism of ejaculation. Sensory afferent fibers arrive at the sacral cord via the sensory division of the pudendal nerve, while efferent motor fibers to the periurethral and the perineal musculature exit from the sacral cord and travel within the motor division of the pudendal nerve. Sympathetic axons leave the lower thoracolumbar cord to innervate the vasal ampulla (VA), seminal vesicles (SV), and bladder neck. The reflex center that coordinates the sequence of ejaculatory events is located somewhere around T12. BC = bulbocavernosus muscle; IC = ischiocavernosus muscle.

with spinal cord injury has shown a spectrum of pathologic findings including arrest of maturation, tubular atrophy, interstitial fibrosis, Leydig's cell hyperplasia, and hypospermatogenesis.[39] Efforts to cool and aerate the groin and to provide heat dissipation with applications of ice packs have proved helpful in certain instances.[37]

In an effort to induce ejaculation, a number of treatments have been tried in patients with spinal cord injury. Intrathecal neostigmine has been used with guarded success.[25] This compound, when injected into the cerebrospinal fluid, causes direct stimulation of the ejaculatory centers located between T12 and L2. Severe hypertension secondary to autonomic dysreflexia has occurred with such treatments, and thus this type of treatment has fallen out of popularity. Vibrator stimulation of the frenular surface of the glans, promulgated by Brindley, has seen modest success.[13] Vibration acts by stimulating the

ejaculatory coordination center in the spinal cord. It is ineffective with lesions below T12, which would eliminate reflex stimulation of this center. Semen retrieval was seen in up to 60% of patients subjected to this treatment. Autonomic dysreflexia with hypertension may also occur with this type of treatment and should be watched for.

Rectal probe electroejaculation has recently seen a gain in popularity in men with spinal cord injury as well as in patients who are experiencing ejaculation problems following retroperitoneal lymph node dissection for testis cancer.[41, 20] This was first reported to be successful in men with spinal cord injury by Horne and colleagues[26] in 1948, having arisen from successful use of this type of treatment in veterinary medicine. Electrical currents from the probe produce direct local stimulation of the ejaculatory nerves, which run near the posterior surface of the prostate (Fig. 14-12). A 90% success

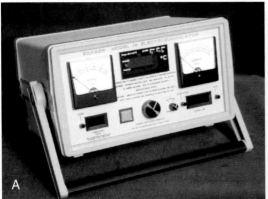
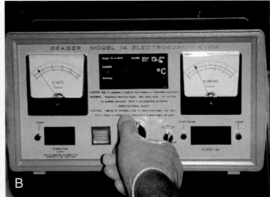
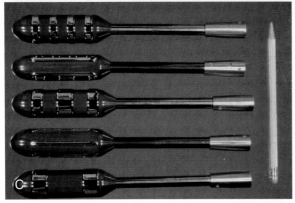

FIGURE 14–12

New design of electrostimulation equipment for fertility purposes in spinal cord–injured and other neurologically impaired men: model 14 with wide electroprobes as shown. (For further information please contact Dr. S. Seager, National Rehabilitation Hospital, 102 Irving St. N.W., Washington, D.C., 20010–2949.)

rate has been achieved using this technique for the retrieval of semen.[15] As with vibratory stimulation of the glans, autonomic dysreflexia is a well-recognized entity accompanying this treatment, and pretreatment with sublingual nifedipine can help avoid the hypertension that frequently accompanies it.[44] Sperm that are harvested by vibration or electroejaculation may be processed and instilled in utero by a husband insemination technique. Coordination with the wife's fertility cycle and techniques of reproductive endocrinology to assist impregnation, such as outlined here, are used with this technique.[14] Frequently, low sperm counts with low motility are found, and techniques of assisted reproduction (e.g., in vitro fertilization) have also proved successful. If retrograde ejaculation occurs, harvesting of semen from urine may be achieved. The urine is alkalinized prior to ejaculatory inducement and the

semen-rich urine is retrieved by catheterization. The sperm is then concentrated, separated, and energized by the addition of nutritive media.

SEXUAL DYSFUNCTION IN FEMALES WITH SPINAL CORD INJURY

Sexual dysfunction and fertility in females with spinal cord injury have received less attention than have male problems in this area. This may be due to the fact that fewer than 20% of patients with spinal cord injury are female and their responses to sexual excitement are less obvious and less readily measurable. Vaginal lubrication, clitoral engorgement, and labial swelling can certainly be significantly impaired with spinal cord injury.[7] Various levels of cord injury involve absence or presence of psychogenic or reflex stimulation of these events. In addition, bowel and bladder soiling and pelvic muscle spasticity, which may accompany sexual activity, may prove embarrassing and discourage women with spinal cord injuries from seeking sexual contact. Advice regarding elimination of body wastes prior to such activity and premedication with muscle relaxants may help allay some of the apprehension and avoid embarrassing accidents. Following a spinal cord injury, amenorrhea is usually seen during the period of spinal shock, which lasts about 3 to 9 months. Otherwise, hormonal aberrations are uncommon and pregnancy may readily occur.[35] Hypertension can be dangerous to the fetus, and recurrent urinary tract infections may increase the risk of toxemia. Childbirth can occur as usual, although women with lesions above the T6 level should be premedicated to avoid autonomic dysreflexia. In spinal cord–impaired women with higher-level lesions, abdominal contractions are not effective and it may be necessary to use forceps to aid in delivery.[16]

SUMMARY

Individuals with spinal cord injury have major obstacles to overcome in attempting to restore normality to their daily lives. A compromised body image compounded by erectile or ejaculatory failure (for men) or embarrassing accidents and pelvic spasticity during sexual activity (for women) certainly add to the patients' problems. With knowledge of the pathophysiology of these problems and the effective treatment regimens that are available, many of these obstacles can be overcome, restoring some functional ability to patients with these serious handicaps.

REFERENCES

1. Abozied M, Junemann, KP, Luo JA, et al: Chronic papaverine treatment: The effect of repeated injections on the simian erectile response and penile tissue. J Urol 138:1263, 1987.
2. Allen RP, Smolev JK, Engel RM, et al: Comparison of Rigiscan and formal nocturnal penile tumescence testing in the evaluation of erectile rigidity. J Urol 149:1265, 1993.
3. Barlow DH: Causes of sexual dysfunction: The role of anxiety and cognitive interference. J Consult Clin Psychol 54:140, 1986.
4. Bennett AH, Carpenter AJ, Barada JH: An improved vasoactive drug combination for a pharmacological erection program. J Urol 146:1564, 1991.
5. Bennett CJ, Segar SW, Vasher EA, et al: Sexual dysfunction and electroejaculation in men with spinal cord injury: Review. J Urol 139:453, 1988.
6. Benson GS, McConnell J: Erection, emission and ejaculation: Physiologic mechanisms. In Lipschultz LI, Howards SS (eds): Infertility in the Male, ed 2. St. Louis, Mosby–Year Book, 1991, pp 155–176.
7. Berard EJJ: The sexuality of spinal cord injured women: Physiology and pathophysiology: A review. Paraplegia 27:99, 1989.
8. Bodner DR, Leffler B, Frost F: The role of intracavernous injection of vasoactive medications for the restoration of erection in spinal cord injured males: A 3 year follow-up. Paraplegia 30:118, 1992.
9. Bookstein JJ, Valji K, Parsons L, et al: Penile pharmacocavernosography and cavernosometry in the evaluation of impotence. J Urol 137:772, 1987.
10. Bookstein JJ, Valji K, Parsons L, et al: Pharmacoarteriography in the evaluation of impotence. J Urol 137:333, 1987.
11. Bors E, Comar AE: Neurological disturbances of sexual function. Urol Surv 10:191, 1960.
12. Brindley GS: The fertility of men with spinal injuries. Paraplegia 22:337, 1984.
13. Brindley GS: Reflex ejaculation under vibratory stimulation in paraplegia men. Paraplegia 19:229, 1981.
14. Brody S, Gibbons WE, Lamb DJ: Assisted reproductive techniques in the treatment of male infertility. In Lipshultz LI, Howards SS, (eds): Infertility in the Male, ed 2. St Louis, Mosby–Year Book, 1991, pp 427–447.
15. Buch JP, Zorn BH: Evaluation and treatment of infertility in spinal cord injured men through rectal probe electroejaculation. J Urol 149:1350, 1993.
16. Charlifue SW, Gerhart KA, Menter RR, et al: Sexual issues of women with spinal cord injuries. Paraplegia 30:192, 1992.
17. Christ GJ, Moreno AP, Melman A, et al: Gap junction mediated intercellular diffusion of Ca^{++} in cultured human corporeal smooth muscle cells. Am J Physiol 263:C373, 1992.
18. Diagnostic and therapeutic technology assessment (DATTA): Vasoactive intracavernous pharmacotherapy for impotence: Intracavernous injections of prostaglandin E_1. JAMA 265:3321, 1991.
19. Diagnostic and therapeutic technology assessment (DATTA): Vasoactive intracavernous pharmacotherapy for impotence: papaverine and phentolamine. JAMA 264:752, 1990.
20. Donohue JP, Foster RS, Rowland RG, et al: Nerve sparing retroperitoneal lymphadenectomy with preservation of ejaculation. J Urol 144:287, 1990.
21. Ek A, Bradley WE, Krane RJ: Nocturnal penile rigidity measured by the snap gauge band. J Urol 129:964, 1983.
22. Fallon B, Ghanem H: Sexual performance and satisfaction with penile prostheses in impotence of various etiologies. Int J Impotence Res 2:35, 1990.
23. Feldman H, Goldstein I, Hatzichristou DG, et al: Impotence and its medical and psychological correlates: Results of the Massachusetts Male

Aging Study. Int J Impotence Res 4(suppl 2):A17, 1992.

24. Foster RS, Mulcahy JJ, Callahagn JT, et al: Role of serum prolactin determination in evaluation of the impotent patient. Urology 36:499, 1990.

25. Guttman L, Walsh, JJ: Prostigmin assessment test of fertility in spinal man. Paraplegia 9:39, 1970.

26. Horne HW, Paull DP, Munro D: Fertility studies in the human male with traumatic injuries of the spinal cord and cauda equina. N Engl J Med 239:959, 1948.

27. Junemann KP, Alken P: Pharmacotherapy of erectile dysfunction: A review. Int J Impotence Res 1:71, 1989.

28. Kim N, Azadzoi KM, Goldstein I, et al: A nitric oxide-like factor mediates nonadrenergic-noncholinergic neurogenic relaxation of penile corpus cavernosum smooth muscle. J Clin Invest 88:112, 1991.

29. Kinsey AC, Pomeroy WB, Martin CE: Sexual Behavior in the Human Male. Philadelphia, WB Saunders, 1948.

30. Koraitim M, Schafer W, Melchior H, et al: Dynamic activity of bladder necks and external sphincter in ejaculation. Urology 10:130, 1977.

31. Krane RJ, Siroky MB: Studies on sacral evoked potentials. J Urol 124:872, 1980.

32. Lloyd EE, Toth LL, Perkash I: Vacuum tumescence: An option for spinal cord injured males with erectile dysfunction. SCI Nursing 6:25, 1989.

33. Lue TF, Mueller SC, Jow YR, et al: Functional evaluation of penile arteries with duplex ultrasound in vasodilator-induced erection. Urol Clin North Am 16:799, 1989.

34. Lue TF, Tanagho EA: Physiology of erection and pharmacologic management of impotence. J Urol 137:829, 1987.

35. McCluer S: Reproductive aspects of spinal cord injury in females. In Leyson, JFJ (ed): Sexual Rehabilitation of the Spinal Cord Injured Patient. Clifton, NJ, Humana Press, 1991, pp 181–206.

36. Morales A, Surridge DH, Marshall PG, et al: Nonhormonal pharmacological treatment of organic impotence. J Urol 128:45, 1982.

37. Mulcahy JJ: Scrotal hypothermia and the infertile man. J Urol 132:469, 1984.

38. Padma-Nathan H, Goldstein I: Neurological assessment of the impotent patient. In Montague DK (ed): Disorders of Male Sexual Function. Chicago, Year Book Medical Publishers, 1988, p 86.

39. Perkash I, Martin DE, Warner H, et al: Reproductive biology of paraplegics: Results of semen collection, testicular biopsy, and serum hormone evaluation. J Urol 134:284, 1985.

40. Rajfer J, Rosciszewski A, Mehringer M: Prevalence of corporeal venous leakage in impotent men. J Urol 140:69, 1988.

41. Sarkarati M, Rossier A, Fam BA: Experience in vibratory and electro-ejaculation techniques in spinal cord injury patients: A preliminary report. J Urol 138:59, 1987.

42. Steidle CP, Mulcahy JJ: Erosion of penile prostheses: A complication of urethral catheterization. J Urol 142:736, 1989.

43. Thomas AJ: Ejaculatory dysfunction. Fertil Steril 39:445, 1983.

44. VerVoort SM, Donovan WH, Dykstra DD, et al: Increased current delivery and sperm collection using nifedipine during electro-ejaculation in men with high spinal cord injury. Arch Phys Med Rehabil 69:595, 1988.

45. Waldhauser M, Schramek P: Efficacy and side effects of prostaglandin E$_1$ in the treatment of erectile dysfunction. J Urol 140:525, 1988.

46. Wyndaele JJ, deMeyer JM, deSy WA, et al: Intracavernous injection of vasoactive drugs: One alternative for treating impotence in spinal cord injury patients. Paraplegia 24:271, 1986.

47. Zasler ND, Katz PG: Synergist erection system in the management of impotence secondary to spinal cord injury. Arch Phys Med Rehabil 70:712, 1989.

CHAPTER 15

Rehabilitation in Patients with Spinal Cord Disorders

Marca L. Sipski, M.D.
Ronald Tolchin, D.O.
Donna Ferrara, M.D.

The rehabilitation of an individual with spinal cord disorder (SCD) or spinal cord injury (SCI) encompasses a wide range of issues. To effectively rehabilitate the individual with SCD or SCI, collaboration of a multifaceted team of professionals is necessary to tackle the multiple problems that may occur as a result of the disorder. The SCD results not only in neurologic impairment but also in changes in numerous organ systems. Therefore, an important part of the rehabilitation process is educating the individual about these changes and how to adapt to altered bodily functions. Paralysis and loss of sensation often result in an inability to perform such daily functions as dressing, bathing, grooming, and walking, and the individual must relearn such activities during rehabilitation. Moreover, these changes may cause persons to lose the capability to participate in their usual home life and educational, vocational, and recreational activities.

The goal of SCD rehabilitation is to maximize the physical, medical, emotional, educational/vocational, and social functioning of the individual. The extent to which this is possible is dependent on the age of the individual, preexisting medical conditions, the neurologic impairment, the available personal and financial resources, and the degree of motivation. This chapter provides an overview of this process and the expected results.

Spinal cord disorders generally result in multisystem impairment and an array of functional problems. As such, the rehabilitation of individuals with SCD primarily occurs on an inpatient basis. Through inpatient rehabilitation, individuals with SCD are trained to become as independent as possible in self-care and mobility. Basic equipment is also prescribed, such as wheelchairs and commodes, and education is provided in management of bladder, bowel, skin, and respiratory changes resulting from the SCD. Rehabilitation is continued on an outpatient basis, and may even be of greater importance as vocational, adjustment, and community integration issues are emphasized. Moreover, advanced mobility training, fine motor skills training, and fitness issues are also commonly addressed during the outpatient phase.

When an individual with SCD arrives at the rehabilitation center, he or she is evaluated by an interdisciplinary team of professionals. These generally include a physiatrist, psychologist, physical therapist, occupational therapist, social worker, speech therapist, vocational counselor, therapeutic recreation specialist, and rehabilitation nurse. Other team members may include case managers, rehabilitation counselors, peer counselors, and pastoral care specialists. Based on evaluations performed by the team members and with the patient's input, an individualized list of the patient's problems is developed (Table 15–1). This problem list, along with the patient's age, medical status, support systems, and insurance coverage, are all considered in the development of short-term and long-term goals for the inpatient rehabilitation phase. For individuals with SCD who have a diminished life expectancy, such as patients with acquired immunodeficiency syndrome (AIDS) or metastatic cancer, goals will obviously be more limited and more functionally oriented than for an otherwise young and healthy individual with a long life expectancy.

Regardless of the etiology of the impairment, to ensure maximum cohesiveness of the team and participation of the patient and family, it is important that both the patient and the family members understand and agree with the goals for rehabilitation. In addition, they must realize their responsibilities as part of the interdisciplinary team. The

TABLE 15–1

SAMPLE PROBLEM LIST

Medical concerns secondary to
  Paraplegia
  Spinal cord injury
  Neurogenic bladder
  Neurogenic bowel
Dependent for activities of daily living including
  Dressing
  Bathing
  Feeding
  Grooming
  Homemaking
Dependent for mobility including
  Transfers
  Bed mobility
  Wheelchair management and mobility
  Elevations
Adjustment to disability
Lack of knowledge in patient and family regarding
  disability
Discharge planning
  Lack of accessible environment
  Appropriate equipment
  Lack of appropriate homecare
Educational/vocational
  Need for vocational retraining
  Need for further education
Community integration
  Need to develop new leisure skills
  Dependent on others for mobility in the community
  Dependent on others for driving

importance of the family's learning about the SCD and its effects cannot be overemphasized. Adequate preparation for confronting such situations as a blocked catheter or autonomic dysreflexia can help avoid unnecessary morbidity and mortality. Although family members may have difficulty accepting the fact that the patient will need to be discharged at a wheelchair level of functioning, it is in the family's best interest to begin to approach and plan for the realities of discharge early in the rehabilitation process.

Determination of the level of injury is most accurately done utilizing criteria described in the recently developed International Standards for Neurologic Classification of Spinal Cord Injury (American Spinal Injury Association [ASIA], 1992). Quantitative and qualitative degrees of injury are assigned on the basis of a comprehensive neurologic examination assessing motor, sensory, and reflex function and level of injury. Functional classification is also performed. First a motor examination is conducted (Fig. 15–1). Activity of key muscles is tested and assigned a grade of 0 to 5 based on strength. Sensory examination using pinprick and light touch is also performed in each of 32 dermatomes on both the right and left sides of the body. Sensation to pinprick is tested with a disposable safety pin, whereas light touch is tested with a cotton wisp. Sensation in each of the dermatomes is ascribed a numeric grade based on a scale of 0 to 2 (0 signifies that no sensation is present; 1, sensation is present but it is altered or diminished; and 2, normal sensation is present). Dermatomes that cannot be accurately tested are graded NT. Rectal examination is also performed to determine the presence or absence of voluntary rectal contraction and the presence or absence of the ability to perceive the examiner's finger. Finally, reflex testing and determination of position sense and vibration sense are recommended.[1]

Based on the neurologic examination, various levels can be assigned to the impairment. The motor level is described as the most caudal normal motor level for each side of the body. Because the key joint movements test the innervation from two neurologic segments, motor function may be considered fully intact at a given level provided all cephalic motor groups are graded at 5, and that level is assigned a value of 3. The sensory level is defined separately for both the right and left sides as the most caudal level at which normal or grade 2 sensation is preserved. The neurologic level takes into account both the motor and sensory levels to specify the most caudal normal level of neurologic functioning, both motor and sensory, and the skeletal level describes the level of the spinal column at which the most bony damage is located.[1]

Whether an injury is complete is determined by the presence or absence of voluntary contraction of the rectal sphincter and the ability of the individual to perceive sensation in the perianal area. When an injury is considered complete, it is also appropriate to assign a zone of partial preservation if there is an area caudal to the level of injury at which

incomplete preservation of neurologic function is noted. Additionally, based on the pattern of neurologic function below the level of injury, the patient is assigned a score on the ASIA impairment scale (see Fig. 15–1). Moreover, the motor grades for each of the ten levels are tabulated to arrive at an ASIA motor score and the individual sensory grades are added to develop a numeric sensory score.[1] Finally, utilizing the functional independence measure, the functional status of the individual for a variety of activities is described.[2]

Once the level and degree of injury are ascertained, functional potential can be predicted. Although many charts are available to predict functional potential based on the level of injury, they cannot be used in isolation. Functional potential is dependent on level of injury; however, it is also dependent on age, preexisting medical history, current medical problems, support systems, and motivation. In addition, although charts that describe functional potential are based on complete loss of function below the level of injury, most individuals do not fit into this neurologic pattern and the potential for a higher level of functioning must be considered (Table 15–2).

To provide the reader with a more complete understanding of functional potential, the functional potential of individuals with various levels of injury is described. Those individuals with complete levels of injury at or above C3 generally require some means of artificial ventilation as they usually do not have adequate vital capacity to breathe independently. They also require total assistance in all activities of daily living including dressing, feeding, and grooming. These persons are totally dependent for bladder and bowel care. It is necessary for them, however, to be able to tell others how to do these activities for them. This provides individuals with the independence to spend their time with whom they choose. They are dependent for transfers but should be able to instruct others in assisting them. To achieve independence in mobility, they require the use of an electric wheelchair with an electric reclining function. These should be activated via mouth, chin, or voice control. Finally, these individ-

STANDARD NEUROLOGICAL CLASSIFICATION OF SPINAL CORD INJURY

MOTOR

KEY MUSCLES

		R	L	
C2				
C3				
C4				
C5	Elbow flexors			
C6	Wrist extensors			
C7	Elbow extensors			
C8	Finger flexors (distal phalanx of middle finger)			
T1	Finger abductors (little finger)			

0 = total paralysis
1 = palpable or visible contraction
2 = active movement, gravity eliminated
3 = active movement, against gravity
4 = active movement, against some resistance
5 = active movement, against full resistance
NT = not testable

L2	Hip flexors
L3	Knee extensors
L4	Ankle dorsiflexors
L5	Long toe extensors
S1	Ankle plantar flexors

Voluntary anal contraction (Yes/No)

TOTALS [ ] + [ ] = [ ] MOTOR SCORE
(MAXIMUM) (50) (50) (100)

SENSORY

KEY SENSORY POINTS

• Key Sensory Points

	LIGHT TOUCH		PIN PRICK	
	R	L	R	L
C2				
C3				
C4				
C5				
C6				
C7				
C8				
T1				
T2				
T3				
T4				
T5				
T6				
T7				
T8				
T9				
T10				
T11				
T12				
L1				
L2				
L3				
L4				
L5				
S1				
S2				
S3				
S4-5				

0 = absent
1 = impaired
2 = normal
NT = not testable

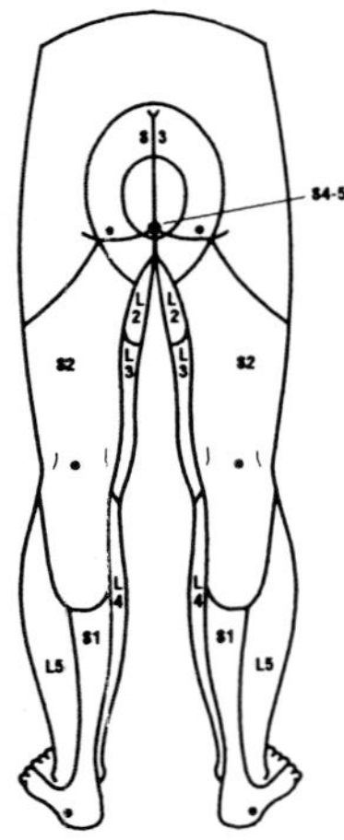

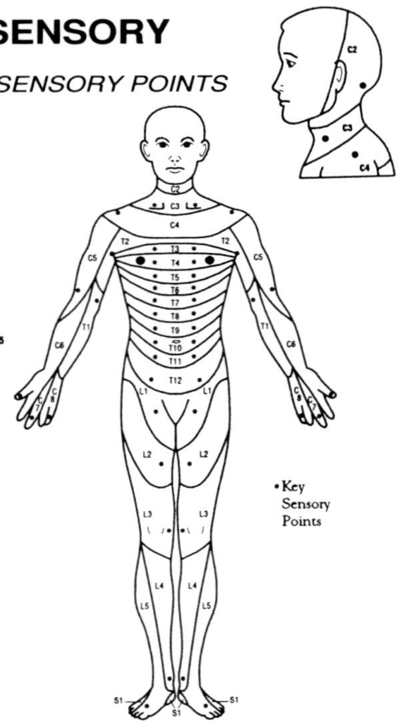

Any anal sensation (Yes/No)

TOTALS [ ] + [ ] = [ ] PIN PRICK SCORE (max: 112)
(56) (56)

[ ] + [ ] = [ ] LIGHT TOUCH SCORE (max: 112)
(56) (56)

(MAXIMUM)

NEUROLOGICAL LEVEL
The most caudal segment with normal function

	R	L
SENSORY		
MOTOR		

COMPLETE OR INCOMPLETE?
Incomplete = presence of any sensory or motor function in lowest sacral segment

[ ]

ZONE OF PARTIAL PRESERVATION
Partially innervated segments

	R	L
SENSORY		
MOTOR		

Version 4d
GHC 1992

This form may be copied freely but should not be altered without permission from the American Spinal Injury Association

FIGURE 15-1

Sample chart for indicating neurologic classification of spinal cord injury. (Courtesy of the American Spinal Injury Association, Atlanta.)

Functional Independence Measure (FIM)

LEVELS		
	7 Complete Independence (Timely, Safely) 6 Modified Independence (Device)	No Helper
	Modified Dependence 5 Supervision 4 Minimal Assist (Subject = 75%+) 3 Moderate Assist (Subject = 50%+) **Complete Dependence** 2 Maximal Assist (Subject = 25%+) 1 Total Assist (Subject = 0%+)	Helper

	ADMIT	DISCH
Self Care		
A. Eating	☐	☐
B. Grooming	☐	☐
C. Bathing	☐	☐
D. Dressing-Upper Body	☐	☐
E. Dressing-Lower Body	☐	☐
F. Toileting	☐	☐
Sphincter Control		
G. Bladder Management	☐	☐
H. Bowel Management	☐	☐
Mobility		
Transfer:		
I. Bed, Chair, Wheelchair	☐	☐
J. Toilet	☐	☐
K. Tub, Shower	☐	☐
Locomotion	W☐ C☐	W☐ C☐
L. Walk/wheelChair	☐	☐
M. Stairs	☐	☐
Communication	A☐ V☐ V☐ N☐	A☐ V☐ V☐ N☐
N. Comprehension	☐	☐
O. Expression	☐	☐
Social Cognition		
P. Social Interaction	☐	☐
Q. Problem Solving	☐	☐
R. Memory	☐	☐
Total FIM	☐	☐

NOTE: Leave no blanks; enter 1 if patient not testable due to risk.

COPY FREELY - DO NOT CHANGE
RESEARCH FOUNDATION OF THE STATE UNIVERSITY OF NEW YORK

ASIA IMPAIRMENT SCALE

☐ **A = Complete:** No motor or sensory function is preserved in the sacral segments S4-S5.

☐ **B = Incomplete:** Sensory but not motor function is preserved below the neurological level and extends through the sacral segments S4-S5.

☐ **C = Incomplete:** Motor function is preserved below the neurological level, and the majority of key muscles below the neurological level have a muscle grade less than 3.

☐ **D = Incomplete:** Motor function is preserved below the neurological level, and the majority of key muscles below the neurological level have a muscle grade greater than or equal to 3.

☐ **E = Normal:** Motor and sensory function is normal.

CLINICAL SYNDROMES

☐ Central Cord
☐ Brown-Sequard
☐ Anterior Cord
☐ Conus Medullaris
☐ Cauda Equina

FIGURE 15–1 *Continued*

uals may be able to write, type, draw, or perform other activities by using a mouthstick.

Individuals with complete injuries at C4 without biceps function are generally able to breathe on their own. They are, however, dependent on others for the same activities as those with injuries at C3 or above and must learn to be independent in instructing others to perform these activities for them. Moreover, they will need to use an electric wheelchair with mouth, chin, or voice control. If individuals have biceps function, they may be able to utilize a balanced forearm orthosis (Fig. 15–2) to perform activities such as eating, writing, or brushing their teeth by employing limited arm strength. This may also allow propulsion of the wheelchair using a joystick rather than mouth, chin, or voice control.

Persons with complete injuries at C5 have, by definition, normal strength and sensation at C4 in addition to elbow flexion strength of 3/5 or greater bilaterally. They are able to use an electric wheelchair with a joystick and can usually propel a manual wheelchair with lugs for short distances. They are generally able to eat, write, and groom themselves independently with assistive devices after setup

TABLE 15–2

LEVEL OF INJURY AND MAXIMAL FUNCTIONAL POTENTIAL FOR TETRAPLEGICS*

LEVEL OF INJURY	GROOMING	FEEDING	DRESSING	BLADDER AND BOWEL CARE	TRANSFERS	WHEELCHAIR MANAGEMENT AND MOBILITY
C1–3†	Dependent‡	Dependent‡	Dependent‡	Dependent‡	Dependent‡	Independent with electric reclining wheelchair with voice control, chin control, or sip-and-puff control
C4	Dependent	Dependent	Dependent‡	Dependent‡	Dependent‡	Independent with same chair as C1–3 patient
C4 with some elbow flexor function (up to grade 2+)	May be able to perform independently with balanced forearm orthosis (BFO) adaptive devices and setup	May be able to perform independently with BFO adaptive devices and setup	Dependent‡	Dependent‡	Dependent‡	Independent with electric wheelchair; may be able to use joystick and BFO
C5	Independent with assistive devices and setup	Independent with assistive devices and setup	Requires minimal to moderate assistance with setup for upper body but dependent for lower body	Dependent‡	Requires moderate assistance with transfer board	Independent in electric wheelchair with joystick; may be able to propel a lightweight manual wheelchair with lugs for short distance

270

Injury level						
C5 with some wrist extensor function (up to grade 2+)	Independent with assistive devices and setup	Independent with assistive devices and setup	Requires minimal assistance for upper body with setup; dependent for lower body	Dependent‡	Requires minimal to moderate assistance with transfer board	Independent in electric wheelchair with joystick; able to propel manual lightweight wheelchair with lugs for longer distances
C6	Independent with assistive devices and setup	Independent with assistive devices and setup	Independent with upper body dressing; moderate assistance needed for lower body dressing	May be able to perform catheterization with assistive device; dependent for bowel care‡	Requires minimal assistance with transfer board	Independent in lightweight manual wheelchair propulsion; needs electric wheelchair for community distances
C6 with some elbow extensor function (up to grade 2+)	Independent	Independent	Independent with upper body dressing; requires minimal assistance with lower body dressing	Requires minimal assistance or independent with adaptive equipment	Requires minimal assistance with transfer board; may do some level surface transfers independently	Independent in lightweight manual wheelchair propulsion
C7	Independent	Independent	Independent	Independent with adaptive equipment	Independent on all surfaces	Independent in lightweight manual wheelchair propulsion

*Assuming individual is in good physical condition and has symmetrical injury with 0 total motor score below designated injury level.
†Will be dependent on external means of ventilatory support.
‡Potential for independence in instructing others.

and to put on a loose top after setup. They are able to assist with transfers; however, they probably need moderate assistance (or 50% assistance) from another individual to perform them. In addition, they need a sliding or transfer board to perform transfers. Individuals with an injury at the C5 level need maximal assistance for lower body dressing and bed mobility. In addition to the strength in their elbow flexors, some individuals with C5 level injuries have preservation of wrist extensor strength (up to grade 2) bilaterally, which may enable such individuals to propel a manual wheelchair without lugs and to perform activities of daily living and transfer activities at a greater level of independence than the others.

Individuals with a C6 injury level have normal strength in elbow flexion bilaterally in addition to a minimum of grade 3 wrist extensor strength bilaterally. They are able to perform transfers with minimal assistance using a board, are generally able to do upper body dressing independently after setup, and should need only minimal to moderate assistance with lower body dressing. They are generally able to propel a manual wheelchair without lugs, but may need to use an electric wheelchair for traveling long distances. They are often able to drive an adapted van. Some individuals with C6 level injuries may have preservation of partial elbow extension. If this is the case, these individuals may be able to perform certain activities such as bed mobility, lower body dressing, or transfers nearly independently.

Individuals with C7 level complete injuries have normal strength in elbow flexion and wrist extension in addition to a minimum of 3/5 strength bilaterally in elbow extension. These individuals are fortunate in that they have the capability to be fully independent in dressing, bathing, grooming, writing, bed mobility, transfers, and wheelchair mobility. They are generally capable of performing range-of-motion independently and living independently in a wheelchair-accessible environment. Moreover, they are often able to drive a car with hand controls as opposed to requiring an adapted van.

With more caudal levels of injury, an individual's potential to achieve independence becomes greater and greater. For instance an elderly, obese male with L1 paraplegia will certainly have a greater chance of achieving independence at a wheelchair level than he would if he suffered from C7 tetraplegia. In sum, to determine an individual's functional potential, information based on the "optimal potential" is useful; however, the overall status and functioning of each individual must be taken into account.

MEDICAL CONCERNS

The importance of proper management of the medical consequences of SCD cannot be overestimated. The impairment affects all organ systems so aggressive preventive management of potential complications is necessary. For instance, the importance of proper control of the neurologic bowel via a routine bowel program cannot be overemphasized. Similar concerns can be brought up for other systems such as genitourinary and respiratory. These issues are extremely important in the rehabilitation process; however, as they are discussed in great detail throughout this text, they are not described here.

ACTIVITIES OF DAILY LIVING

Activities of daily living (ADLs) consist of the tasks a person needs to perform in everyday life. In rehabilitation of the individual with SCD, it is the team's responsibility to define these and facilitate their performance. Most commonly, ADLs are centered around self-maintenance activities, such as feeding, dressing, and grooming. However, more complex skills may also be included, such as cooking a meal or making a bed.

ADLs are not as simple or basic as they may appear at first glance. ADLs are the result of integrating a number of subskills into patterns of routine performance. Spinal cord disorders may cause a reduction in the ability to perform the subskills or patterns necessary to perform routine ADLs. Depending on the patient's degree of impairment, varying degrees of independence can be achieved.

For the person with tetraplegia, assistive

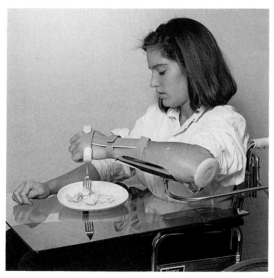

FIGURE 15–2

Balanced forearm orthosis. (From DeLisa J: Rehabilitation Medicine: Principles and Practice, ed 2. Philadelphia, JB Lippincott, 1993.)

equipment may be useful to maximize independence in ADLs. This may include electronic assistive equipment, hand splints, and devices such as built-up handles, attachments to faucet handles, reachers, overhead rings, or mats to anchor plates and tableware. Upper extremity orthoses may also be useful to allow individuals with SCI to achieve maximal independence in ADLs. In persons with C4 tetraplegia, mobile arm supports or a balanced forearm orthosis can be used to aid weak shoulder musculature and allow greater functional use of the arm. In individuals with weakened pinch, a manually operated ratchet wrist or powered prehension orthosis may provide finer dexterity.[3]

MOBILITY

Optimal mobility is accomplished through a coordinated program of training in functional activities. Neurologically intact musculature must be strengthened, with particular attention to the trapezius, deltoid, triceps, latissimus dorsi, and wrist extensor muscles, since these are key muscles for crutch walking and for independent transfers to and from a bed or wheelchair.[3]

Mobilization of the patient with SCD begins with the placement of the patient in a reclining wheelchair, followed by a progressive increase in the angle of elevation. As the upright position is better tolerated, a more vigorous therapy program is pursued. Mat activities concentrate on improving balance, strength, and endurance, which are essential to facilitate subsequent independence in bed mobility, wheelchair transfers, and dressing. The importance of being able to move around in bed should not be underestimated. Patients in wheelchairs must also learn to transfer themselves to and from a bed, commode, shower or tub, car, and floor. Those individuals who live in a home with stairs may also need to learn to "bump" up and down stairs. Skills for independence in the community, such as ramp and curb negotiations and the ability to perform "wheelies" and to ride escalators, are developed as well. Finally, the wheelchair user should also be taught proper maintenance, handling, and storage of the wheelchair and the simple repairs needed to prevent mechanical breakdowns and to extend the useful life of the wheelchair.[4]

One of the first questions asked by the newly injured individual is, "Will I walk again?" This is also a primary concern for the family. Recent reports have revealed that younger age[5] and the preservation of pinprick sensation in the lower extremities [6] are positive predictors of the ability to walk in persons with incomplete SCI. Within other patterns of injury, one study noted that patients who were able to walk (1) had pelvic control; (2) had fair or better function of hip flexors; (3) had fair or better function of the quadriceps in at least one leg; (4) required either no braces or a maximum of one short leg brace and one long leg brace; and (5) had no fixed joint deformity or significant spasticity.[7] More recently the ambulatory motor index (AMI), which is derived from the manual muscle grades of both lower extremities, was developed as an indicator of the degree of paralysis and was noted to be useful in predicting the ability to ambulate.[8]

STANDING AND AMBULATION

Many devices are available to the person with spinal cord disorders for assistance with standing and walking, and the use of these devices depends on the patient's level of injury. For tetraplegic individuals, assisted standing may be considered as a means of achieving an upright posture. Several options exist to allow standing. These include mechanical or power stand-up wheelchairs and power, manual, or hydraulic standing frames.[9]

Options for braces include metal, plastic, air-filled, and electric devices. The Craig-Scott orthosis differs from conventional long leg braces (knee-ankle-foot orthoses, or KAFOs) in reducing unnecessary hardware. A minimum number of straps and bands are featured, with the primary knee stabilizing force provided by a rigid anterior closure below the knee.[10] The reciprocal gait orthosis (RGO) provides support to the hip joints in addition to the knees and ankles. The uprights extending from the hip joints to the midthoracic region provide additional support to the trunk muscles. A cable system in this orthosis allows reciprocal flexion at the hips. This is usually initiated by the patient's lifting his or her pelvis. The reciprocal gait orthosis has also been combined with electrical stimulation to allow improved ambulation.[11] The Vannini-Rizzoli stabilizing orthosis (boot) permits standing and ambulation in paraplegics by immobilizing the ankle and foot in 15 degrees of plantar flexion, which stabilizes the knee in an upright position.[12]

The level and degree of SCD determine what type of orthotic device will be needed. The RGO can allow individuals with SCD at levels as high as C7–8 to ambulate. This ambulation, however, is primarily for exercise purposes because of the high energy expenditure that is required. Individuals with SCD to a level of about T11–L2 can often ambulate indoors with bilateral knee-ankle-foot, Craig-Scott, or Vannini-Rizzoli orthoses and crutches. For lower-level paraplegia, such as at L3–S3 levels, full ambulation is expected. These individuals are generally able to ambulate indoors and outdoors with braces stabilizing the knees and ankles, as appropriate, combined with crutches, canes, or whatever assistive device provides the best gait.

As mentioned earlier, orthoses and assistive devices allow some persons with low-level tetraplegia and many with paraplegia to ambulate (ranging from standing to therapeutic indoor/functional, or community ambulation). A wheelchair, however, continues to be the preferred means of mobility for the majority of these patients. Reasons include decreased energy expenditure, convenience, efficiency, safety, and decreased likelihood of mechanical failure.[13]

STRENGTHENING EXERCISES AND RANGE OF MOTION

Early rehabilitation helps to prevent complications of imposed immobility and disuse. During this time, goals for maximizing functional independence are set. One of the universal goals of rehabilitation of the SCD patient necessary to achieve maximal functional independence is working to optimize function in weakened and intact muscles both above and below the level of injury.

To maximize strength, optimal range of motion must be present in all muscle groups. To maintain range of motion, patients with SCD should be put through full passive range of motion in all extremity joints at least twice daily; this will prevent contractures and decrease spasticity. Both the patient and a family member should also be taught to perform these range-of-motion exercises independently. An exception to this is in persons with C5 and C6 tetraplegia, in whom finger flexors should be permitted to tighten to help form a natural tenodesis (Fig. 15–3) to aid in grasp. This process is called *selective stretch*.

When joint range of motion becomes restricted, it is imperative to try to increase it to a point at which the extremity can function. Increases in range of motion can be achieved through passive exercise, serial casting, or the use of dynamic or passive splints. Proper positioning between exercises will also assist in maintaining gains in range of motion.

Muscle strengthening and endurance training are accomplished through a program of

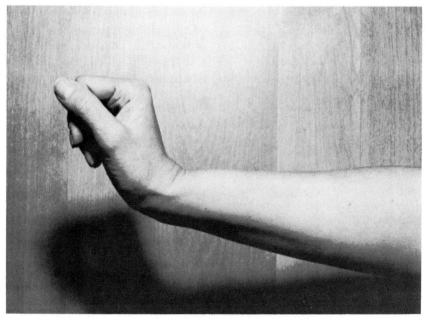

FIGURE 15–3

Wrist extension tenodesis. (From Sipski ML, Hendler S, DeLisa JA: Rehabilitation of patients with spinal cord disease. *Neurol Clin* 9:705–725, 1991.)

active assistive, active, and progressive resistive exercises for the innervated muscles. Different exercise equipment such as power boards, Velcro weights, dumbbells, rickshaws, latissimus bars, and pulley systems with weights may be utilized to increase strength. Upper extremity ergometers are often used to improve endurance. Biofeedback has also recently been used for severely weakened muscles, grade 1 or less, that may initially fail to be strengthened by traditional means.

ADJUSTMENT

Learning to live with a disability is a lifelong process. The sudden onset of a disabling condition such as an SCD often necessitates a major shift in roles, activities, and life goals for the patient and family. Furthermore, these changes lead to a process of continual "adjusting" rather than a finite end point of "adjustment."[13]

Although each person responds according to his or her unique personality and life process, some common issues confront all individuals during the early period following injury. Numerous earlier theories hypothesize stages of adjustment that indicate the need for patients to "work through" the following substages: shock, fear and anxiety, grief and mourning, aggression or rebellion. It has been further hypothesized that without progression through these stages the individual can not adjust properly.

In contrast, more recent research has supported the notion that individuals with SCD adjust in their own way and time and that there is not one correct means of adjusting. Taylor's theory of successful adaptation addressed three areas: *meaning, mastery,* and *self-enhancement.* In the meaning stage, Taylor[14] described that all patients in the study asked themselves the same question, "Why did this happen to me?" Those who adjusted well were able to move beyond this issue. By mastery, Taylor found that those individuals who were socially integrated felt an increased sense of control in their lives. Sometimes this control was realistic, although at other times it was overoptimistic and unrealistic. In either event, a perceived sense of control, realistic or unrealistic, seemed to aid in adjustment. Self-enhancement has to do with the longer-term process of adjustment. Those individuals who adjusted well came to view their illnesses or disabilities in a less negative manner. In fact, these individuals believed that they were better or stronger people for having experienced their catastrophic situation.[14]

Perhaps one of the earliest, most significant adjustment issues after SCI or SCD relates to loss of control and feelings of helplessness. Fear, grief, and anger may also prevent the rehabilitation process from being effective unless each of these feelings is properly dealt with. Only then will the individual be able to reach maximal functional potential. By 1 year after SCI, most affected persons do not demonstrate appreciably more distress than able-bodied persons. Most persons with SCI maintain emotional stability over time and are not substantially more hostile or depressed than their able-bodied peers, nor do they necessarily experience diminished self-esteem or increased dissatisfaction with life.[13] Despite an increased understanding of the adjustment process, there remains a lack of consensus as to the critical elements necessary for good adjustment. Factors that may predict good adjustment include supportive interpersonal relationships with family and friends; young age; female gender; preinjury personality characteristics that include high ego strength, ability to delay gratification, and conscientiousness; and development of coping mechanisms.[15]

PATIENT/FAMILY TEACHING

As part of an effective rehabilitation program for individuals with SCD, the importance of patient/family teaching cannot be overemphasized. The myriad of changes in physical function must be understood by the patient and family. Unless this is the case, individuals with SCD may inadvertently find themselves receiving unnecessary care in an emergency room for problems that are more appropriately solved in the home setting. For instance, individuals with poikilothermia must be forewarned not to spend excessive time outdoors to avoid development of hypo-

thermia or hyperthermia. Furthermore, if such a problem occurs, they must know the proper methods of treatment. Education can also be helpful for the caregivers. For instance, learning the proper way to assist in a transfer can prevent back strain and pain in the caregiver.

DISCHARGE PLANNING

Discharge planning must be emphasized from the first day of the patient's rehabilitation. The patient must be made aware of the need to ascertain that the home environment is as accessible as possible. The occupational therapist should review the floor plan of the patient's living environment and make specific suggestions for improvement in accessibility. For those individuals who must go home to an inaccessible environment, proper safety measures should be considered, such as obtaining a cordless phone, instituting a lifeline system, or notifying the police and fire departments of their living situation.

Prescribing and obtaining appropriate equipment are also an integral part of discharge planning. Depending on the situation, the individual with SCD may need to purchase or rent an electric or manual wheelchair. The wheelchair should be customized and a detailed prescription provided by the rehabilitation center to allow safe and effective use. Moreover, the patient should be provided with a customized wheelchair cushion to allow proper positioning and assist in prevention of pressure sores. Other pieces of equipment that may be appropriate include assistive devices such as canes, crutches, walkers, shower/commode chairs, tub benches, and lifting devices.

To complete the discharge planning process, appropriate home health assistance must be arranged. Unfortunately, although many patients may need home health care, obtaining such care is often dependent on whether or not a patient has insurance coverage. When this is not the case, the family must choose whether they will provide attendant care on their own, which often requires giving up jobs in the process, or pay for attendant care with their own funds. Furthermore, follow-up services must be decided on prior to discharge from inpatient rehabilitation, including decisions about who will function as the individual's primary care physician and whether the individual needs continuing physical or occupational therapy or psychotherapy after discharge.

POSTDISCHARGE/COMMUNITY INTEGRATION

Perhaps the greatest challenge for the individual with SCD is the return to living in the community for the remainder of his or her life. Full success with this task is difficult to measure because what may be deemed successful for one person may be intolerable for another. Three areas of adaptiveness are thought to be the most important: (1) maintaining health and avoiding the preventable complications of the SCD; (2) leading an active and productive life; and (3) achieving an appropriate degree of life satisfaction.[16]

In attempts to achieve community integration, the first problem individuals with SCD may face on discharge is lack of structure. During the rehabilitation stay, almost each hour of the day was accounted for. After discharge, because there is no set schedule, it is often difficult to fill the day with activities. Because of this, the individual may not want to get up early in the morning. This in turn may place a burden on the family or caretaker. Most individuals do not return immediately to work on leaving the rehabilitation center.

Another problem that may be encountered is internal architectural barriers in the home. The change from the rehabilitation environment to the home environment may present new obstacles and may limit the individual's ability to perform certain activities independently. For example, it may be significantly more difficult for the individual to propel a wheelchair on thick pile carpeting than on linoleum or tile. Although the individual may have gone out on weekend passes to the home environment and felt these architectural barriers were not problems, they oftentimes become more significant once the individual is home on a permanent basis.

Several basic movements need to be negotiated by the individual with SCD on entering into the home environment. Individuals must learn how to negotiate their transfers into and out of bed, onto and off the toilet, and onto and off various surfaces such as couches. They must be able to dress in the bed and propel the wheelchair throughout the home in and out of various doorways. Negotiating architectural barriers may also mean finding new ways to prepare meals or perform chores around the house. Home modifications may have to be made.

Other stress factors on the family or care provider are present once the individual is in the home environment. For example, the free time that the spouse or family member had while the patient was in the rehabilitation setting is no longer available. The spouse or family member may have to assume all of the responsibilities that the nursing staff had in the rehabilitation setting. Moreover, physicians are not available "around the clock" to take care of medical questions as they are in the rehabilitation setting. These responsibilites may create feelings of anger in the caregiver and dependency in the individual with SCD.

For individuals with SCD, lack of transportation can become a barrier against going out into the community. For individuals who are able to learn to drive, it may be appropriate to modify a current vehicle with hand controls. For other individuals, a van with modifications may need to be purchased or another individual may need to be hired to do the transporting. Public transportation may also be appropriate to allow the individual to get around. Regardless of the method, if the individual does not master transportation issues, he or she may be confined to the house and may never reintegrate into the community.

Assuming the individual with SCD can make his or her way out of the house and into the community, new sets of barriers present themselves. These include narrow doors, hallways, parking spaces, stairs, escalators, and bathrooms. In addition, in order to travel long distances, other barriers must be overcome. For example, if the individual is using air travel, then the issue of accessibility becomes paramount. Hotel accessibility and special needs during overseas travel must also be considered. Solutions to these problems are often not clear. Creativity and good problem-solving skills are often necessary.

Although the transition into the community is laden with significant physical and psychological barriers, these are surmountable. Recently, the Americans with Disability Act has attempted to break down many of the physical barriers that individuals with SCD face in the community. Regardless of specific barriers, once an individual with SCD successfully reintegrates into the community, his or her life is generally more rewarding.[16–18]

FITNESS

Fitness is an increasing concern among individuals with SCD who strive toward wellness. Weight gain is one of the sequelae of decreased basal metabolism after SCI or SCD and general fitness provides a means of counteracting it. This becomes a concern, as weight gain can ultimately restrict mobility and increase the risk of complications. In addition, fitness has such added benefits as improved strength and endurance, maintenance of normal blood pressure, reduction in serum cholesterol level, and improvement in pulmonary function.[19]

Endurance training is directed at the cardiorespiratory system and intact peripheral musculature. The goal of endurance training is to increase the amount of work that an individual can achieve before reaching the level of fatigue. This involves the use of the aerobic and anaerobic energy systems, which improve oxygen transport and the efficiency of oxygen extraction from the blood. Endurance training in SCD is primarily aimed at the use of the intact upper extremity musculature and diaphragm. Training is either continuous (aerobic) or interval (anaerobic). Interval training is preferred for the high-level paraplegic or tetraplegic individual, as it better meets the needs of the smaller muscle groups of the upper extremities and simulates the short-duration functional activities of the individual. Interval training over time also improves vital capacity and forced expiratory volume in 1 second (FEV_1).[20]

An alternative approach to the fitness and conditioning of an individual with SCI or SCD is through the use of functional electrical stimulation (FES), which can be used to provide a cardiovascular conditioning/fitness program. FES is the application of electrical current to neural tissue to control lost motor function or to perform a functional task. It can be applied to a variety of systems including phrenic nerve stimulation, upper extremity function, or lower extremity function for standing/ambulating, or as computerized lower extremity cycle ergometry. The bicycle ergometers, REGYS (designed for institutional use) and ERGYS (their counterpart for home use), have been shown to produce muscle hypertrophy, strengthening, and increased endurance.[21, 22] Unfortunately, benefits can only be maintained through regular use of the ergometers and in one study only 19 of 28 patients who owned ERGYS units were regular users.[23]

Overall, fitness not only improves cardiovascular performance and endurance but also has an impact on psychosocial issues. These may include improved alertness, emotional stability, and self-esteem and reduction in stress and anxiety. Fitness can be achieved through a variety of wheelchair sports, functional electrical stimulation, or participation in recreational activities.

MEDICAL MAINTENANCE

Medical maintenance initially begins in the rehabilitation setting and continues thereafter. The patient must know the details of his or her condition as well as the medical constraints. Once discharged, the patient should be well aware of what medications he or she is receiving and the reasons for each, as well as the possible complications and side effects. If other mechanical devices are needed for medical maintenance, such as respiratory or ventilatory equipment, the patient and the family should know how to troubleshoot related issues appropriately.

Follow-up medical care must be available after discharge to ensure prevention of known complications. Local medical care should be arranged in addition to routine follow-up pertinent to SCD issues. Patients should have copies of their medical records or discharge summaries to present in emergencies. Visiting nurse arrangements also need to be made prior to discharge.

Various medical problems arise from time to time in the spinal cord–impaired individual. This individual and his or her representative caretaker should have the confidence and security of working closely with a team of persons qualified to address issues pertinent to SCD. They should also be able to reach the staff in the event that acute medical issues arise. In addition, during off hours, the emergency medical system should be easily accessible to the individual or family. There should be regular follow-ups for immunizations, vaccines, and screening measures for malignancy and cardiovascular disease. These should become an integral part of SCD follow-up care.[24–27]

MARITAL AND FAMILY CONCERNS

Individuals with SCDs must make extremely difficult adjustments in their lives. One of the major effects of SCD is alteration in sexual function. This may be manifested by altered lubrication, impotence, and problems with ejaculation and orgasm. Moreover, infertility may result in males and difficulty with pregnancy may result in females. Although these issues are paramount, as they are discussed elsewhere in the text (see Chapter 16), they are not reviewed here. The reader is referred elsewhere for a more complete discussion of this topic.[28] As a result of altered body functioning, one of the most difficult adjustments that must be made pertains to the marriage relationship. Postdisability marital stability is of great concern because rehabilitation outcome is related, in part, to the strength and quality of patients' marital relationships.[29]

Although results of reseach assessing the impact of SCD on marriage are mixed, certain conclusions seem evident. SCD forces a slower pace of life and leads to decreased social opportunities. Often, the partner must serve a dual role as lover and caretaker, which creates deleterious situations and conflicts. Friends and even family members who have difficulty adjusting to the disability may distance themselves. Monetary costs involved with SCD place a tremendous burden on the marriage and family. If a man with SCD cannot return to work, a role reversal may be necessary, with the wife working and the husband remaining in the home.[28] This situation and others can create frustration within the marriage. This has led some researchers to believe that marriages that occur after SCD, in which the spouse accepts the burdens associated with SCD from the start, are more likely to succeed. Crewe and Krause[30] found that those married after injury reported greater satisfaction with their sex lives, living arrangements, social lives, health, emotional adjustment, and sense of control over their lives, and they indicated that loneliness was less of a problem. They were also far more likely to be working and to be socially active outside their homes.[30]

One study evaluated the impact of SCI on marriage and divorce rates of individuals 3 years after injury. Observed and expected marriage and divorce rates were compared. The study concluded that individuals with SCI experience more divorces and fewer marriages than their noninjured counterparts.[29] In a similar study, it was concluded that SCI significantly affects marriage and divorce rates, particularly for women with SCD.[31]

Possible interpretations of these findings include the likelihood that those in preinjury marriages are burdened with the losses due to the SCD and are resentful of the resultant change in their lifestyles. They also might have lost confidence in their ability to control their future decisions and actions. Disability was something that neither of the partners had bargained for as part of their marriage agreement, and it often seems to cause resentment. Frequently, partners need to adjust to a reversal of roles or to learn new ways of communicating feelings and needs. Spouses in postinjury marriages may have unusual qualities or values that contribute to the success of these unions. They may have the independence and maturity necessary to look beyond society's stereotypes and to pursue intimate involvement with someone with a disability. They may also possess better-than-average communication skills that help them to overcome initial barriers in nonverbal communication and spontaneous action imposed by the SCI.[32]

Marital therapy procedures developed with able-bodied couples are quite applicable to SCD couples. Therapy might focus on increasing positive interaction between spouses, decreasing the frequency of negative behavior between spouses, reducing the reactivity of each spouse to negative events in the relationship, and enhancing communication. During rehabilitation, strong emphasis should be placed on assisting the couple in developing activities that can be done together. Mutually enjoyable activities can enhance the marital relationship and thus have a favorable impact on long-term outcome for the person with injury.

PARENTING

Individuals with SCI who have or plan to have families often express concerns about the impact of their disability on their children. To date, however, few empirical studies have been conducted to assess the impact of disability on childrearing.[28]

Buck and Hohmann[33] compared adult children reared by fathers with SCI with a group of children who had able-bodied fathers. Children of fathers with SCI were noted to be well adjusted. Fathers with SCI tended to express physical and verbal affection toward their children significantly more often than did able-bodied fathers, and their children responded more quickly and willingly to their father's requests and commands than did children of able-bodied fathers. Children of disabled parents held more positive attitudes toward their fathers than did children of able-bodied fathers and, perhaps not surprisingly, they also felt more protective of their parents.[33–35]

Although there are no empiric data, it is postulated that the effect of having a mother with SCI will similarly affect the child. Certainly many mothers with SCI are successful parents; however, this is an area in which further research is necessary to address the impact of SCI.

DRIVING

Driving is particularly important in areas where access to public transportation is difficult or other methods of transportation are unavailable. This can mean the difference between dependence and independence in the community. Driving can also provide a way of obtaining vocational and community reintegration. The Commission for Accreditation of Rehabilitation Facilities now requires a center for rehabilitation to provide driver rehabilitation services, usually under the auspices of occupational therapy providers. Various medical and legal issues must be taken into account prior to the initiation of driving by a disabled person.[36]

Medically, the individual's physical, visual, perceptual, and cognitive functions need to be considered. An assessment of the physical strength, range of motion, and coordination of the individual must be performed. In addition, the individual must have knowledge of the rules of the road as well as of the mechanics of driving. The rules and mechanics of driving are learned through driver's training. This may include a predriving evaluation, simulator training, and behind-the-wheel training. Once the individual is deemed ready to attempt a state road examination, the test can be set up between the local division of motor vehicles and the driver rehabilitation instructor. If additional equipment is needed, the individual will have a change in his or her license.

Considerations of what type of vehicle an individual should drive take into account the individual's ability to perform car transfers and to lift his or her wheelchair into and out of the car. For those who are able to transfer and lift the wheelchair into and out of a car, it is relatively obvious that they should drive a car. For those who are unable to lift their wheelchair, options exist to provide assistance in lifting a folding wheelchair. These include a "car topper," which will load the wheelchair into a car-top luggage holder; having someone else load the wheelchair into the car; and using two wheelchairs, one that is left at home and the other that is left at a regular destination (for example, at work).

A van is necessary for individuals who use power wheelchairs. This should be equipped with an elevator lift as well as a system to anchor the chair into the driver's position, or the capacity to transfer into a driver's seat. Options that may be necessary inside an adapted vehicle may include a chest strap to stabilize the individual in the vehicle; modified steering, acceleration, and braking systems (Fig. 15–4); air conditioning; and automated door-opening systems.[37, 38]

VOCATIONAL REHABILITATION

The purpose of vocational rehabilitation is to evaluate, remediate, educate, explore career opportunities, provide job training and job site analysis, develop job-seeking skills, provide job development and specialized placement, and provide follow-up services.

To provide these services the vocational counselor may work with the individual as both an inpatient and an outpatient. Through vocational rehabilitation, individuals are encouraged to identify their needs and goals and are taught problem-solving skills. The vocational counselor initiates and maintains contact with the patient's previous employer if there is a desire to return to the previous job. Later, the counselor and the patient can make a job site visit and address various concerns by all parties about the patient's returning to work. These should include any potential architectural barriers. In addition, the vocational counselor refers the patient to the Office of Vocational Rehabilitation (OVR) for the state and maintains communication with that agency. The capabilities of OVR vary from state to state, but this agency may be a source of financing for therapy, education, training, job placement, equipment supplies, and architectural modifications necessary for the individual to return to work.[39]

Vocational rehabilitation is important after SCD because of the large impact that SCD

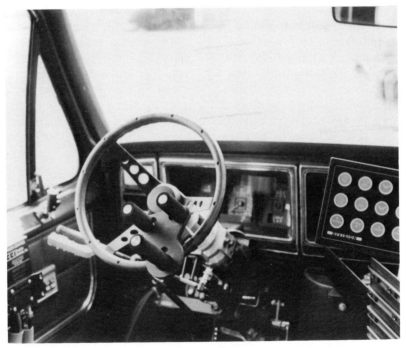

FIGURE 15–4

Steering system on adapted van.

may have on vocational skills. Vocational adjustment is paramount in importance, particularly when it is closely correlated with survival. Therefore, one of the most important goals of rehabilitation may be to return to work. Goldberg and Freed followed a group of persons with SCI and found 13% to 48% to be employed.[40, 41] This is a significant decrease from the 60% who were employed prior to injury.

It is difficult to predict who will be successful at returning to work. The effect of level of injury on employment status is uncertain.[42–44] Time since injury, however, may be a significant factor in employment rates. In a longitudinal study by Krause,[42] 48% of the participants were working at the time of the study. At some point after injury, almost 75% of the participants had worked. This approximates the preinjury rate for the study population of 85%.[42] Employment rates were found to improve dramatically with increasing time since injury. Krause noted that education was the most important factor for returning to work. In addition, the younger the person at the time of injury, the more likely the individual is to return to employment. Preinjury vocational interests and attributes, concomitant medical concerns, duration of disability, and male gender have also been noted to be important in vocational rehabilitation.[42]

Other requirements for successful vocational rehabilitation include elimination of financial disincentives, such as a loss of benefits that may occur with return to work, availability of attendant care, and environmental accessibility.[44–46] Barriers preventing persons with SCD from working need to be identified and ultimately overcome. Overall, only a small number of individuals return to the same job they had before injury. To maximize vocational rehabilitation for SCD individuals, issues may need to continue to be addressed long after the illness. Furthermore, continued training and education may be warranted. Education, preinjury vocational interests and attributes, severity of impairment, medical problems associated with disability, age, duration of disability, financial disincentives to work, and gender-linked factors must all be taken into account when an individual plans to return to work.

RECREATION

Recreation and leisure activities can help restore independence to an individual with SCD, and improve the quality of life. Recreation can also ease the traumatic adjustment process. The overall goal is to encourage each person to reach his or her fullest potential. It is important to allow individuals to perform, whenever possible, the same activities they enjoyed prior to injury. This may be done with appropriate modifications. Benefits may include self-acceptance, confidence, feelings of enjoyment, and fun.

Adaptive equipment needs and resources are important considerations in therapeutic recreation. It is important to plan equipment needs ahead of time so that cost can be reduced and proper customization of equipment can be achieved. Specialized equipment for recreational activity (e.g., skiing) is often needed but should not be recommended until proper investigation of the limitations and practicality of participation in the activity has been made. Environmental issues, such as whether an individual can tolerate the weather in which a sport is played, must also be considered prior to embarking on any recreational pursuit.[47]

For the individual with high-level tetraplegia, activities include those that are accessed via head, mouth, or chin control. These may include sip-and-puff tool operation (e.g., paint brushes), ham radio operation, and playing table games with magnetic pieces that are moved with a mouth stick. In addition, electronic video games and card games can be operated by adaptive equipment. For those interested in outdoor activities such as fishing, adaptive fishing reel equipment can be operated electrically by a drive belt on the electric sip-and-puff–controlled wheelchair. Moreover, radio-controlled sailing or the operation of model sailboats by radio control is available. Other aquatic activities include rafting and boating, utilizing the proper safety considerations and personnel. Camping is also an option for individuals with SCD.

Imaginative applications are almost limitless in adapting activities for the individual with SCD. These include kite flying, hot air ballooning, and hunting. Photography is also an avenue in which creativity and self-expression can be achieved. Many adaptations can be made to cameras and darkroom equipment, should the individual desire to develop his or her own pictures.

For the able-bodied, competitive sports have been classified according to weight, age, sex, or other physical characteristics to equalize the competition. In individuals with disabilities, the categories have been based on severity of impairment to equalize the competition. In competitive sports for the SCD individual, it is often necessary to amend the rules, modify the playing area, or alter the distances. The rules of many sports have been modified to take into account the presence of wheelchairs. Modifications are minimized to ensure as much of a full experience as possible in the sport. These activities teach the concepts of team work, cooperation, and accepting victory and defeat. Competitive team sports that are available to persons in wheelchairs include football, soccer, softball, volleyball (Fig. 15–5), quad rugby, goalball, and beep baseball.

For persons who wish to participate in individual (nonteam) sports, mountain climbing, wheelchair racing, white water rapid rafting, archery, bowling, golf, wheelchair dancing, and many other activities are available. The martial arts are also available, including judo, tae kwon do, and karate, which teach concentration, practice, and discipline. Wheelchair tennis, snowmobiling, and mountain climbing are other possibilities. In summary, despite the occurrence of SCD, leisure and recreational activities remain an important part of life that should be encouraged to the fullest extent possible.[48, 49]

INDEPENDENT LIVING CENTERS

The movement for independent living centers began in the 1970s in Berkeley, California, and was initiated by a group of disabled individuals who had a strong desire to live independently and avoid institutional living. Further, they wished to avoid being confined to the home environment. In 1977 the ILRU (Independent Living Research Utilization Program) was established as a national database of independent living center programs.[50]

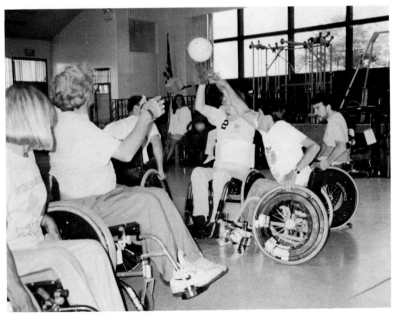

FIGURE 15–5

Wheelchair volleyball.

Independent living is defined as the ability of a disabled individual to actively and genuinely share in the joys and responsibilities of community life.[50] The basic premise behind this is that every individual has the potential to live more independently in society. There are three concepts of independent living. The first is physical modification, which consists of the modification of the physical environment to make activities of daily living more feasible. The second concept is that of independent living rehabilitation. In this realm, vocational rehabilitation services are available to disabled individuals when vocational objectives are feasible. The third, consumer rights, focuses on the attitudes and rights of individuals with disabilities: individuals with disabilities have the right to services that enable them to be equal and independent members in the community. Independent living centers encourage consumers and professionals to advocate change in the general attitudes and provision of services that are necessary for individuals with disabilities to take part in community life.

Other services offered by an independent living center include permanent residential facilities, transitional living programs, attendant referral, attendant management training, peer counseling, financial counseling, family counseling, newsletters, public relations activities, promotion of consumer involvement, and civic activities and community affairs. In addition, there are programs to increase public awareness of disabilities and projects to reduce community barriers.

The majority of consumers using an independent living center come from the immediate community surrounding it. A minority come from rural areas and other cities and states. The contribution made by individuals with disabilities to the community is largely a result of the independent living movement. A large array of networks of independent living programs exists across the country. In fact, more than 300 independent living centers in the United States today can be located or accessed through the state office of vocational rehabilitation or protection and advocacy offices, or under Social Services in the telephone directory.[51–55]

AGING

Aging with an SCD has only recently been addressed[56]; in the past, individuals with SCD did not live for extended periods. Now that improved methods of medical management are available, the individual with SCD has a greater life expectancy, and more research is being done into the aging process. Current efforts are focusing on how the aging process in SCD is similar to that in able-bodied population and on how the unique requirements of living with an SCD result in acceleration of specific aspects of the aging process (e.g., individuals with SCD who must rely extensively on use of the upper extremities to bear weight have more rapidly occurring degenerative changes in the shoulders). To consider the effects of aging on a person with SCD, any underlying disease process and the age of the individual at the time he or she contracts the disease and develops spinal cord dysfunction must be taken into account. For some individuals, such as those with transverse myelitis, which develops at an early age, the effects of aging are probably similar to those of the individual who suffers SCI at an early age. In contrast, the individual with SCD due to metastatic cancer or AIDS oftentimes dies early as a result of the disease process.

Acknowledgment

Grateful acknowledgment is made to Susan M. Gilbert for her support in preparation of this chapter. Work for this chapter was supported in part by funds from the National Institute on Disability and by Rehabilitation Research grant H133N00022.

REFERENCES

1. American Spinal Injury Association (ASIA): Standards of Neurological and Functional Classification of Spinal Cord Injury. Chicago, ASIA, 1992.
2. Hamilton BB, Laughlin JA, Granger CV, et al: Interrater agreement of the seven level functional independence measure (FIM). *Arch Phys Med Rehabil* 72:790, 1991.
3. Sipski ML, Hendler S, DeLisa JA: Rehabilitation of patients with spinal cord disease. *Neurol Clin* 9:705–725, 1991.
4. Staas WE, Ditunno JF: Traumatic spinal cord injury. *Phys Med Rehabil Clin* 3:863–864, 1992.
5. Penrod LE, Hegde SK, Ditunno JR: Age effect on prognosis for functional recovery in acute, traumatic central cord syndrome. *Arch Phys Med Rehabil* 71:963–968, 1990.

6. Crozier KS, Graziana V, Ditunno JF, et al: Spinal cord injury: Prognosis for ambulation based on sensory examination in patients who are initially motor complete. Arch Phys Med Rehabil 72:119–121, 1991.

7. Hussey RW, Stauffer ES: Spinal cord injury: Requirements for ambulation. Arch Phys Med Rehabil 54:544–547, 1973.

8. Waters RL, Yakura JS, Adkins R, et al: Determinants of gait performance following spinal cord injury. Arch Phys Med Rehabil 70:811–818, 1989.

9. Jaeger RJ, Yarkony GM, Roth EJ: Rehabilitation technology for standing and walking after spinal cord injury. Am Phys Med Rehabil 68:128–133, 1989.

10. Lehmann JF, Warren CG, Hertling D, et al: Craig Scott orthosis: A biomechanical and functional evaluation. Arch Phys Med Rehabil 57:438–442, 1976.

11. Hirokawa, Grimm M, Le T, et al: Energy consumption in paraplegic ambulation using the reciprocating gait orthosis and electric stimulation of the thigh muscles. Arch Phys Med Rehabil 71:687–694, 1990.

12. Kent HO: Vannini-Rizzoli stabilizing orthosis (boot): Preliminary report on a new ambulatory aid for spinal cord injury. Arch Phys Med Rehabil 73:302–307, 1992.

13. Richards JS: Psychological adjustment to spinal cord injury during first post discharge year. Arch Phys Med Rehabil 67:362–365, 1986.

14. Taylor SE: Adjustment to threatening events: A theory of cognitive adaptation. Am Psychol 38:1161–1173, 1983.

15. Judd FK, Webber JE, Brown DJ, et al: Psychological adjustment following traumatic spinal cord injury: A study using the psychosocial adjustment to illness scale. Paraplegia 29:173–179, 1991.

16. Woodbury B, Redd C: Psychosocial issues and approaches. In Buchanan LE, Nawoczensik DA (eds): Spinal Cord Injury: Concepts and Management Approaches. Baltimore, Williams & Wilkins, 1987, pp 187–217.

17. Tunks E, Bahry N, Basbaum M: The resocialization process after spinal cord injury. In Block RE, Basbaum M (eds): Management of Spinal Cord Injuries. Baltimore, Williams & Wilkins, 1986, pp 387–409.

18. Trieschman RB: Spinal Cord Injuries: Psychological, Social, and Vocational Rehabilitation, ed 2. New York, Demos Publications, 1988, pp 147–236.

19. Staas WE, Ditunno JF: A system of spinal cord injury care. Phys Med Rehabil Clin 3:901, 1992.

20. Decker M, Hall A: Physical therapy in spinal cord injury. In Bloch RE, Basbaum M (eds): Management of Spinal Cord Injuries. Baltimore, Williams & Wilkins, 1986, pp 320–347.

21. Weber RJ: Functional neuromuscular stimulation. In DeLisa JA (ed): Rehabilitation Medicine: Principles and Practice, ed 2. Philadelphia, JB Lippincott, 1993, pp 463–476.

22. Phillips CA, Petrofsky JS, Hendershot DM, et al: Functional electrical exercise: A comprehensive approach for physical conditioning of the spinal cord injured patient. Orthopedics 7:112–123, 1984.

23. Sipski ML, Alexander CJ, Harris M: Long-term use of computerized bicycle ergometry for spinal cord injured subjects. Arch Phys Med Rehabil 74:238–241, 1993.

24. Carter RE: The lifetime care process. In Whiteneck G, et al (eds): The Management of High Quadriplegia. New York, Demos Publishing, 1989, pp 291–296.

25. Cioschi H, Staas WE: Follow-up care. In Buchanan LE, Nawoczewski DA (eds): Spinal Cord Injury: Concepts and Management Approaches. Baltimore, Williams & Wilkins, 1987, pp 221–234.

26. Menter R: Aging with a spinal cord injury. Phys Med Rehabil Clin 3:879–892, 1992.

27. Short DJ: Clinical issues involving multiple organ systems. In Whiteneck GG, et al (eds): Aging with Spinal Cord Injury. New York, Demos Publications, 1993, pp 183–190.

28. Sipski ML, Alexander CJ: Sexual function and dysfunction after spinal cord injury. Phys Med Rehabil Clin North Am 3:822–823, 1992.

29. DeVivo MJ, Fine PR: Spinal cord injury: Its short-term impact on marital status. Arch Phys Med Rehabil 66:501–504, 1985.

30. Crewe NM, Krause JS: Marital relationships and spinal cord injury. Arch Phys Med Rehabil 69:435–438, 1988.

31. Brown JS, Giesy B: Marital status of persons with spinal cord injury. Soc Sci Med 23:313–322, 1986.

32. Crewe NM, Athelstan GT, Krumberger J: Spinal cord injury: A comparison of pre-injury and post-injury marriages. Arch Phys Med Rehabil 60:252–256, 1979.

33. Buck FM, Hohmann GW: Personality, behavior, values and family relations of children of fathers with spinal cord injury. Arch Phys Med Rehabil 62:432–438, 1981.

34. Buck FM, Hohmann GW: Child adjustment as related to severity of paternal disability. Arch Phys Med Rehabil 63:249–253, 1982.

35. Buck FM, Hohmann GW: Child adjustment as related to financial security and employment status of fathers with spinal cord injuries. Arch Phys Med Rehabil 65:327–333, 1984.

36. Pierce S: Legal considerations for a driver rehabilitation program. Physical Disabilities 16: 1–4, 1993.

37. Nawoczenski DA, Rinehart ME, Duncanson P, et al: Physical management. In Buchanan LE, Nawoczenski DA (eds): Spinal Cord Injury: Concepts and Management Approaches. Baltimore, Williams & Wilkins, 1987, pp 176–182.

38. Ford J, Duckworth B. Physical Management for the Quadriplegic Patient. Philadelphia, FA Davis, 1987, pp 439–470.

39. Ragnarsson KT, Gordon WA: Rehabilitation after spinal cord injury: The team approach. Phys Med Rehabil Clin 3:866–868, 1992.

40. Goldberg R, Freed M: Vocational adjustment, interests, work values, and career plans of persons with spinal cord injuries. Scand J Rehabil Med 5:3–11, 1973.

41. Goldberg RT, Freed MM: Vocational development of spinal cord injury patients: An 8-year follow-up. Arch Phys Med Rehabil 63:207–210, 1982.

42. Krause JS: The relationship of productivity to adjustment following spinal cord injury. Rehabil Counseling Bull 33:188–199, 1990.

43. DeVivo MJ, Rutt RD, Stover SL, et al: Employment after spinal cord injury. Arch Phys Med Rehabil 68:494–498, 1987.

44. Crisp R: Return to work after spinal cord injury. J Rehabil 56:28–34, 1990.

45. DeJong G, Branch LG, Corcoran PJ: Independent living outcomes in spinal cord injury: Multiple analyses. Arch Phys Med Rehabil 65:66–73, 1984.

45. Weidman CD, Freehafer AA: Vocational outcome in patients with spinal cord injury. J Rehabil 47:63–65, 1981.

47. Andrews S, Kelly C: Leisure options for the high

quadriplegic patient. *In* Whiteneck G, et al (eds): The Management of High Quadriplegia. New York, Demos Publishing, 1989, pp 281–290.

48. Ford J, Duckworth B: Physical Management for the Quadriplegic Patient. Philadelphia, FA Davis, 1987, pp 485–515.

49. Kelley JD, Frieden L: Go For It: A Book on Sport and Recreation for Persons with Disabilities. Orlando, Harcourt Brace Jovanovich, 1989.

50. Stoddard S: Independent living. *Annu Rev Rehabil* 1:231–278, 1980.

51. Trieschman RB: Spinal Cord Injuries: Psychological, Social and Vocational Rehabilitation, ed 2. New York, Demos Publications, 1988, pp 142–145, 221–235.

52. Zola IK: Social and cultural disincentives to independent living. *Arch Phys Med Rehabil* 63:394–397, 1982.

53. DeJong G, Hughes A: Independent living: Methodology for measuring longterm outcomes. *Arch Phys Med Rehabil* 63:68–73, 1982.

54. Fuhrer MJ, Rossi LD, Gerken L, et al: Relationships between independent living centers and medical rehabilitation programs. *Arch Phys Med Rehabil* 71:519–522, 1990.

55. Corbet B: What price independence? *In* Whiteneck GG, et al (eds): Aging With Spinal Cord Injury. New York, Demos Publications, 1992, pp 183–190.

56. Whiteneck GG, et al (eds): Aging with Spinal Cord Injury. New York, Demos Publications, 1992.

CHAPTER 16

Cause, Prevention, and Treatment of Pressure Sores

Robert M. Woolsey, M.D.
John D. McGarry, M.D.

The most common preventable medical complication of myelopathy is the development of pressure sores. Pressure sores develop in 20%[28] to 40%[29] of all patients with acute quadriplegia and paraplegia during the initial hospital stay, and they are severe (grade III or IV) in approximately 6%.[28] In a large group of quadriplegic and paraplegic patients observed over a 5-year period, pressure sores developed in approximately 30% of patients each year.[29] Six percent of these patients had severe sores resulting in an average hospital stay of 2 months.[29] One major rehabilitation hospital reported that the average cost of treating a severe pressure sore in 1988 was $58,000.[1]

TERMINOLOGY

The pressure sore was called a *bedsore* in the English literature and a *decubitus* in the European literature of the nineteenth century. Decubitus is a Latin noun meaning "the reclining position." (Incidentally, the plural of decubitus is *decubitus*, not *decubiti*.[3]) This early terminology reflected the fact that patients with conditions conducive to pressure sores rarely survived long enough to be out of bed. Eighty percent of American and British soldiers in World War I with spinal cord injuries died within a few weeks after injury.[6]

Physicians of the nineteenth century understood pressure sores remarkably well. Consider the following excerpts from the

"Clinical Lecture on Bed-Sores,"[25] published by Sir James Paget in 1873:

Bed sores may be defined as the sloughing and mortification or death of a part produced by pressure. When we press on any part of our bodies for a moment, on the removal of the pressure the part is quite white, owing to the blood having been pressed out. The colour immediately returns, however. In bed-sores, the pressure is continual, the blood is driven away, nourishment ceases, and death of the part takes place.

Bed-sores occur in those who are absolutely at rest. If there is the slightest movement from one side to the other bed-sores may be averted. In the case of those whose lower limbs are paralysed, there can be no motion whatever, and so they are liable to bed-sores.

Now let us look at the means of preventing bed-sores, as nine-tenths of your care must be devoted to this; for if once they appear it is very difficult to get rid of them. We have to prevent pressure on those parts where bed-sores are likely to occur. These are the middle line of the sacrum, the posterior superior spine of the ilium, then the trochanters of the femur. The chief thing is frequent change of posture.

A patient can lie on his back, each side and his face. When patients lie on their backs they may be saved for a time by dividing a mattress and leaving a space of six inches between the halves. You may thus save the sacrum which will have no pressure on it.

Paget then proceeds to describe the use of a water bed and other techniques for treating a bedsore, including debridement and packing.

Charcot[7] described the clinical features of "decubitus acutus" in detail and emphasized the rapidity with which they developed, hours or days after the onset of paralysis (Fig. 16–1). However, he stated that "we must relegate to a secondary position the influence of pressure," believing instead that a decubitus resulted from a disturbance of the "trophic" relationship existing between the central nervous system and the skin, subcutaneous tissue, muscles, and joints. He called the decubitus "a most inauspicious sign. We might, in fact, call it decubitus ominous" (because patients with them rarely survive their acute illness).[7] According to Parish and colleagues,[26] Charcot caused "an era of therapeutic nihilism" that lasted 40 years.

During and following World War II, due to the pioneering work of Sir Ludwig Guttmann and Donald Munro in the management of spinal cord injury and the control of urosepsis, the survival rate improved dramatically. It became apparent that ischial sores occurred frequently in patients using wheelchairs. Because these sores had no correlation with be-

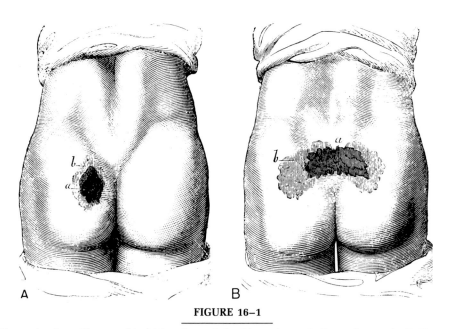

FIGURE 16–1

Illustration from Charcot of ischial and sacral decubitus ulcers. A, Zone of necrosis. B, Zone of erythema. (From Charcot JM: Lectures on Diseases on the Nervous System [translated by Seigerson G]. London, The New Sydenham Society, 1877, p 78.)

ing in bed or lying down, they could not reasonably be called bedsores or decubitus ulcers. Guttmann[15] forcefully advocated for use of the term *pressure sore* because "where there is no pressure there is no sore." Pressure sore or *pressure ulcer* is now generally accepted terminology.

PATHOGENESIS

As proposed by Paget, ischemia is generally accepted as the most important factor in the production of pressure sores. Soft tissue is squeezed between two hard surfaces—a bed or chair on the outside of the body and a bone on the inside—creating a tissue pressure that exceeds the vascular perfusion pressure.

Various experimental data have been used to try to determine in a more quantitative way what these pressures might be. The work of Landis[18] and Fronek and Zweifach[13] (Fig. 16–2) suggests that the capillary perfusion pressure is in the range of 20 to 30 mm Hg.

Animal models of pressure sore induction have all utilized an external "impounder" against a bony prominence.[9,10,17] Such external pressure over a bone exerts two effects on the intervening tissue: compression and distortion. The tissue is flattened and displaced sideways (Fig. 16–3). Compressive force has usually been measured at the external surface,[9,10,17] but it is actually greater internally at the bone surface.[19] Tissue displacement produces shearing force that is difficult to measure, but, according to Bennett and Lee,[4] it may be as significant as compressive force. Virtually all animal models have demonstrated an inverse relationship between pressure and time (Fig. 16–4).[9,10,17] High pressure causes tissue damage quickly, whereas lower pressure can be tolerated for more extended periods.

The various components of soft tissue are not equally sensitive to the effects of ischemia. Daniel and colleagues[9] and Nola and Vistens[24] have shown that muscle is damaged first, probably due to its higher metabolic requirements.

The human body has a contoured shape, an irregular skeleton, and different soft tissue consistencies and thicknesses. Several investigators have studied the distribution of pressure in supine and seated normal human subjects. The data reported by Lindan and co-workers[20] are an example (Figs. 16–5 and 16–6). It is apparent from these diagrams that the highest pressures exist over the sacrum, ischial tuberosities, heels, and knees. When the patient lies on one side, pressure exerted over the trochanteric area is even higher than

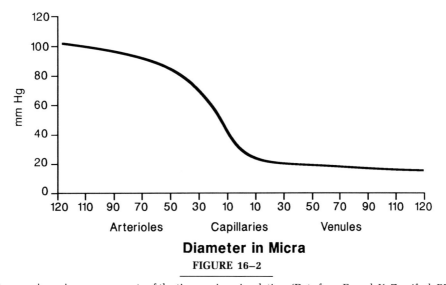

Diameter in Micra

FIGURE 16–2

Pressure in various components of the tissue microcirculation. (Data from Fronek K, Zweifach BW: Microvascular pressure distribution in skeletal muscle and the effects of vasodilation. Am J Physiol 228:791, 1975.)

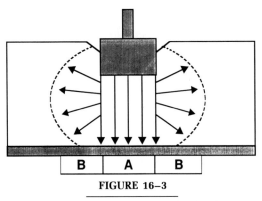

FIGURE 16–3

Pressure exerted on tissue resting on a hard surface exerts compressive force (*A*) and shearing force (*B*).

- Stage I: Nonblanchable erythema of the intact skin. This is a red or violaceous area that does not blanch when pressed on with the finger, indicating that blood has escaped from capillaries into the interstitial tissue.
- Stage II: Partial-thickness skin loss. The skin surface is broken, resulting in an abrasion or shallow crater.
- Stage III: Full-thickness skin loss and extension into subcutaneous fat.
- Stage IV: Extension into muscle and bone.

that exerted over the sacrum when the patient lies supine.[16]

As might be predicted from these data in normal human subjects, certain positions are particularly hazardous in paralyzed patients. These include lying supine (sacrum and heels), lying on one side (trochanteric area), and being seated (ischial area). Elevation of a patient's head and upper trunk to a 30- to 45-degree angle generates even more stress over the sacral area than does lying supine.

PRESSURE SORE PATHOLOGY

Because muscle is the soft tissue component most sensitive to ischemia, sores that develop in areas where a great deal of muscle intervenes between skin and bone, such as the ischial area, tend to be in a "flask" shape. Where there is little muscle, such as in the sacrum and trochanteric area, they tend to be "dish" shaped (Fig. 16–7).

Pressure sores are conventionally described in terms of stages (I–IV). Staging is useful to indicate the severity of a pressure sore; however, stages do not imply an evolutionary process in their development; that is, a stage III sore is not necessarily preceded by stages I and II.

Several pressure sore staging systems have been proposed that differ slightly from one another. All are based on the depth of the sore. The staging system recommended by the National Pressure Ulcer Advisory Panel[23] is as follows (see Fig. 16–7):

PRESSURE SORE PREVENTION

Paraplegic and quadriplegic patients are at extremely high risk for pressure sore development. Paget's advice that "nine-tenths of your care must be devoted . . . to preventing pressure sores" is indeed well taken.

Animal models have demonstrated two main variables in pressure sore production: (1) time and (2) compressive force (see Fig. 16–4). Pressure sore prevention involves control of these two factors.

Control of compressive force involves the use of pressure-reductive devices. Such de-

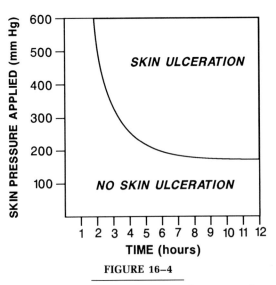

FIGURE 16–4

The relationship between pressure and time in production of skin ulcers. (Data from Kosiak M: Etiology of decubitus ulcers. Arch Phys Med Rehabil 42:19, 1961.)

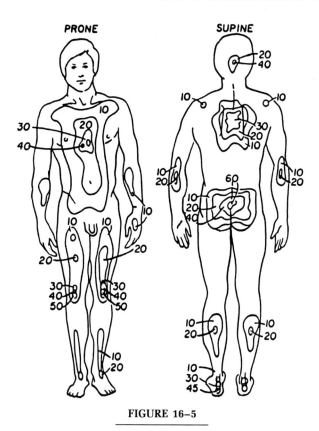

FIGURE 16–5

Skin pressures (mm Hg) measured in normal human subjects lying prone and supine. (From Constantine MB: Pressure Ulcer Principles and Techniques of Management. Boston, Little, Brown, 1980, p 17; with permission.)

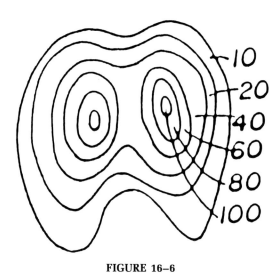

FIGURE 16–6

Skin pressures (mm Hg) measured in normal human subjects seated in a standard wheelchair. (From Constantine WB: Pressure Ulcer Principles and Techniques of Management. Boston, Little, Brown, 1980, p 18; with permission.)

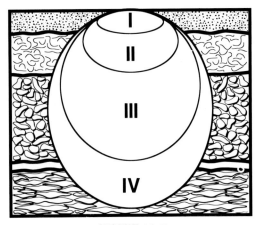

FIGURE 16–7

Pressure sore stages: I, Nonblanchable erythema—lesion is confined to skin that is not broken. II, Partial-thickness skin loss resulting in an abrasion or shallow crater. III, Full-thickness skin loss with extension to or into subcutaneous fat. IV, Extension to or into muscle or bone.

vices are available in the form of mattresses, mattress overlays, and wheelchair cushions. These are generally composed of high-density foam, gels, water, or air-filled sacks. When an individual sits or lies on such a surface, areas of higher pressure under bony prominences sink into the supporting surface, diffusing the pressure to surrounding areas (Fig. 16–8). The supporting surface must be sufficiently buoyant to avoid "bottoming out" (see Fig. 16–8), that is, yielding so much that the patient essentially sinks through the supporting surface to sit or lie on the underlying hard surface. Thus, sheepskin and "egg crate" mattresses are not very effective. The various commercially available pressure-reductive mattresses, mattress overlays, and cushions are all useful, although various studies indicate that some are better than others.[8,16]

It should be noted that some published investigations of the comparative effectiveness of various mattresses and cushions are flawed by significant methodologic problems (R.H. Graebe, personal communication, 1990).

Control of pressure exposure time is achieved by turning patients in bed from the back to one side, to the back again, and to the other side. When lying on a regular mattress, patients should be repositioned at least every 2 hours. Paraplegic patients in wheelchairs should use their arms and the armrests of their wheelchairs to lift their buttocks off the seat every 15 to 30 minutes for 5 to 10 seconds. Quadriplegics can relieve buttocks pressure by leaning forward or to one side followed by the other.

MANAGEMENT OF A PRESSURE SORE

With proper care, grade I and II pressure sores usually heal within 1 or 2 weeks.[2] However, grade III and IV pressure sores require an average of 2 months of treatment.[29] As a rule, grade III and IV sores of more than 2 cm diameter are best treated surgically.[5]

The two absolute requisites for healing a pressure sore are keeping it pressure-free and clean. Patients with a single sore can ordinarily be positioned in such a way that the sore is always pressure-free. For example, a patient with a sacral sore can lie on his or her left side, right side, and prone. Because this reduces possible weight-bearing surfaces from four to three, the risk of generating another sore is increased. A repositioning schedule should be rigidly adhered to. The prone position can be tolerated for a longer period of time. A pressure-reductive mattress or mattress overlay should be used.

Not infrequently, patients have more than one pressure sore. This further reduces possible weight-bearing surfaces to two or one. Under these circumstances, some type of turning frame or special bed is necessary.

Turning frames, such as the Stryker (Stryker Corporation, Kalamazoo, Mich.) frame and the Circ-O-lectric (Stryker Corpo-

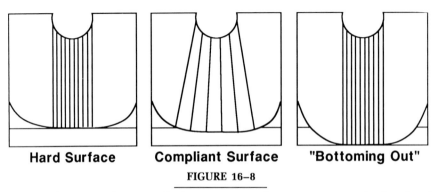

Hard Surface   **Compliant Surface**   **"Bottoming Out"**

FIGURE 16–8

Compressive force exerted on tissue by bone in a person lying or sitting on a hard surface (*left*), an effective compliant pressure-reductive device (*center*), and an ineffective pressure-reductive device that "bottoms out" (*right*).

ration, Kalamazoo, Mich.) bed, although effective, are uncomfortable for the patient and require two staff members to execute turns. At this time, turning frames are rarely used.

Specialized beds, which afford maximal pressure redistribution, are available in two varieties: the *air-fluidized bed* and the *low air-loss bed*. The air-fluidized bed consists of a container filled with tiny ceramic beads resembling fine sand through which air is continually forced by a blower, causing the beads to assume a fluidlike character (Fig. 16–9). The low air-loss bed consists of a series of 18 to 20 air-filled sacks (Fig. 16–10), each of which can be individually pressurized so that weight can be shifted from one body part to another, thereby relieving, for example, sacral pressure by shifting it to the posterior thighs and lumbar area of the back.

Both of these types of beds are expensive to rent or buy, and it is inappropriate to use them for routine pressure sore prevention for which much simpler mattress overlays will suffice.

Pressure sores must be cleaned because necrotic tissue and infection prevent healing. Exposed necrotic tissue is invariably colonized by environmental bacteria, provoking an inflammatory response in the juxtaposed viable tissue. Usually, removal of necrotic tissue is all that is needed to control the infectious component of a pressure sore.

Necrotic tissue can be removed from a pressure sore surgically, mechanically, or chemically. Usually, a combination of the three is used. Surgical debridement is mandatory if the sore is covered by a hard black eschar, which can shield the wound from any other

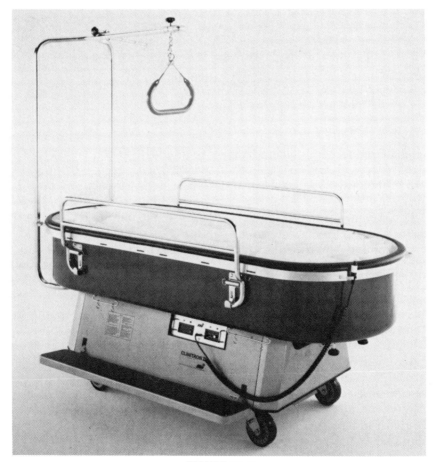

FIGURE 16–9

An air-fluidized bed. (Courtesy of Support Systems International Inc., Charleston, S.C.)

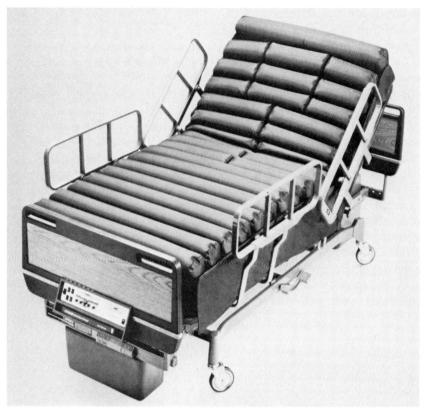

FIGURE 16–10

A low air-loss bed. (Courtesy of Support Systems International Inc., Charleston, S.C.)

type of treatment. Surgical debridement with scalpel, scissors, or both should be conservative, and only obviously necrotic tissue should be removed.

Mechanical debridement consists of packing the sore with saline-soaked gauze, which is allowed to dry for 6 to 8 hours and is then removed. Necrotic tissue will adhere to the gauze and be extracted with it. Whirlpool is also a very useful modality for mechanical debridement. Necrotic tissue is softened, agitated loose, and washed from the sore.

Chemical debridement using various enzyme preparations believed to digest necrotic tissue seems to be effective. Some of the more widely used commercial products are Travase, Elase, Santyl, Granulex, and Panafil. Because these agents can damage viable tissue, their use should be discontinued as soon as the wound is clean.[2]

Topical antiseptics and antibiotics can be useful during the cleaning process,[12] but should be discontinued as soon as they have served their purpose, because some evidence suggests that they also slow wound healing and promote the growth of resistant bacteria.

Systemic antibiotics are not useful in the treatment of pressure sores unless the patient has osteomyelitis or severe wound infection unresponsive to the usual modalities of local care. Fulminating sepsis with a 50% mortality rate has been reported in patients with pressure sores;[14] however, this must be a rare occurrence, because during a 20-year period of treating patients with pressure sores on a daily basis, we have never seen such a situation.

When the ulcer is clean, healing can be accelerated by the creation of a *tissue growth environment*. Epithelial cells, fibroblasts, endothelial cells, bloodborne cells (macrophages, lymphocytes, neutrophils, and platelets), collagen, and glycosaminoglycans all participate in healing. The signals that begin healing, the signals that end the process, and the methods by which all of the events are coordinated have only recently begun to be understood. Macrophages appear to have a predominant role in removing necrotic tissue and in attracting and stimulating other healing cells.[11] Multiple stimulant and growth factors have been recognized, and some of these may be of value in the future for hastening wound repair.[22, 27]

Wound dressings designed to maintain an optimal microenvironment for healing processes and high wound humidity are replacing sterile gauze, which has long been the standard dressing.[12] Some of the occlusive materials include hydrocolloid (DuoDerm) and semipermeable film (Op-Site, Tegaderm, Bio-occlusive, Polyskin) dressings. These dressings are mainly useful in the management of ulcers with a large open surface.

Ulcers with a small surface outlet and a large underlying cavity, such as in most ischial ulcers, should be packed with saline-soaked gauze to cause the sore to heal from the bottom up. If the surface outlet is permitted to close first, the cavity can become an abscess.

A potpourri of topical agents have been advocated as useful in the treatment of pressure sores. Parish and others[26] list 50 such agents. Reports of the effectiveness of these treatments are largely anecdotal, and some may actually be harmful. The frustration occasioned by the large number of these unproved remedies provoked one clinician to exclaim, "You can put anything you like on a pressure sore, except the patient!"[15]

SURGICAL TREATMENT

Grade III and IV ulcers heal faster and generate less scar tissue when treated surgically. Surgical treatment involves total excision of the ulcer and filling the tissue void created by its removal with some type of flap secured from adjacent tissue.[5, 21] Usually, only ischial, trochanteric, or sacral sores require flaps. The myocutaneous flap is used most commonly (Fig. 16–11).

SUMMARY

Pressure sores are a common, expensive, and preventable complication of paralysis. They are the result of ischemia produced when tissue is compressed and distorted by pressure exerted between a bone and an external hard surface for an extended period of

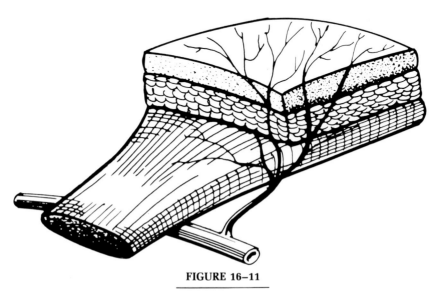

FIGURE 16–11

A myocutaneous flap. Muscle and overlying skin receive their blood supply from vessels of the muscle body. (From Black JM, Black SB: Surgical management of pressure ulcers. Nurs Clin North Am 22:433, 1987; with permission.)

time. Prevention involves control of the two variables of pressure and time. Pressure can be minimized by using various pressure-reductive devices in the form of mattresses and cushions. Control of time involves scheduled position changes. If pressure sores occur, treatment consists of keeping the sore completely pressure-free and clean. Grade I and II sores usually need no further treatment. Grade III and IV sores heal faster and more effectively when treated surgically.

REFERENCES

1. Adkins RH, Waters RL, Kendall K: The cost of pressure sores in the treatment of acute spinal injury. Presented at the American Spinal Injury Association Annual Meeting, San Diego, 1988.
2. Allman RM: Pressure ulcers among the elderly. N Engl J Med 320:850, 1989.
3. Arnold HL: Decubitus: The word. In Parish LC, Witkowski JA, Crissey JT: The Decubitus Ulcer. New York, Masson Publishing, 1983, p 1.
4. Bennett L, Lee BY: Vertical shear existence in animal pressure threshold experiments. Decubitus 1:18, 1988.
5. Black JM, Black SB: Surgical management of pressure ulcers. Nurs Clin North Am 22:429, 1987.
6. Carroll DG: History of treatment of spinal cord injuries. Md Med J 19:109, 1970.
7. Charcot JM: Lectures on Diseases on the Nervous System [translated by Seigerson G]. London, The New Sydenham Society, 1877, p 78.
8. Cochran GVB, Palmieri V: Development of test methods for evaluation of wheelchair cushions. Bull Prosthet Res 17:9, 1980.
9. Daniel RK, Priest DL, Wheatley DC: Etiologic factors in pressure sores: An experimental model. Arch Phys Med Rehabil 62:492, 1981.
10. Dinsdale SM: Decubitus ulcers: Role of pressure and friction in causation. Arch Phys Med Rehabil 55:147, 1974.
11. Eaglstein WH: Wound healing. In Thiers BH, Dobson RL (eds): Pathogenesis of Skin Diseases. New York, Churchill Livingstone, 1986, p 617.
12. Feedar JA, Kloth LC: Conservative management of chronic wounds. In Kloth LC, McCulloch JB, Feedar JA (eds): Wound Healing: Alternatives in Management. Philadelphia, FA Davis, 1990, pp 145–149, 150–161.
13. Fronek K, Zweifach BW: Microvascular pressure distribution in skeletal muscle and the effects of vasodilation. Am J Physiol 228:791, 1975.
14. Galpin JE, Chow AW, Bayer AS, et al: Sepsis associated with decubitus ulcers. Am J Med 61:346, 1976.
15. Guttmann L: Spinal Cord Injuries: Comprehensive Management and Research. Oxford, Blackwell Scientific Publications, 1973, pp 486, 506.
16. Jester J, Weaver V: A report of clinical investigations of various tissue support surfaces used for the prevention, early intervention and management of pressure ulcers. Ostomy/Wound Manage 19:39, 1990.
17. Kosiak M: Etiology of decubitus ulcers. Arch Phys Med Rehabil 42:19, 1961.
18. Landis EM: Microinjection studies of capillary blood pressure in human skin. Heart 15:209, 1930.
19. Le KM, Madsen BL, Barth PW, et al: An in-depth look at pressure sores using monolithic silicon pressure sensors. Plast Reconstr Surg 74:745, 1984.
20. Lindan O, Girbenway RM, Piazza JM: Pressure distribution on the human body: I. Evaluation of lying and sitting positions using a "bed of springs and nails." Arch Phys Med Rehabil 45:378, 1965.
21. Linder RM, Morris D: The surgical management of pressure ulcers: A systematic approach based on staging. Decubitus 3:32, 1990.
22. Mustoe TA, Pierce GF, Thomason A, et al: Accelerated healing of incisional wounds in rats induced by transforming growth factor-beta. Science 237 (4820):1333, 1987.
23. National Pressure Ulcer Advisory Panel: Pressure ulcers prevalence, cost and risk assessment: Consensus development conference statement. Decubitus 2:24, 1989.
24. Nola GT, Vistens LM: Differential response of skin and muscle in the experimental production of pressure sores. Plast Reconstr Surg 66:728, 1980.
25. Paget J: Clinical lecture on bed-sores. Student J Hosp Gaz I: 144, 1873.
26. Parish LC, Witkowski JA, Crissey JT: The Decubitus Ulcer. New York, Masson Publishing, 1983, pp 8, 39.
27. Pierce GF, Mustoe TA, Lingelbach J, et al: Platelet-derived growth factor and transforming growth factor-beta enhanced tissue repair activities by unique mechanisms. J Cell Biol 109:429, 1989.
28. Woolsey RM: Rehabilitation outcome following spinal cord injury. Arch Neurol 42:116, 1985.
29. Young JS, Burns PE, Bowen AM, et al: Spinal Cord Injury Statistics: Experience of the Regional Spinal Cord Injury Systems. Phoenix, Good Samaritan Medical Center, 1982, pp 99, 100, 108, 112.

CHAPTER 17

Medical Complications of Spinal Cord Disease

James Schmitt, M.D.
Meena Midha, M.D.
Norma McKenzie, M.D.

Spinal cord disease, especially injury to the cervical portion of the cord, can affect virtually every body system by impairing voluntary motor and autonomic nervous system functions. Impairment of voluntary motor function results in immobility (contributing to the development of decubitus ulcers) and can impair cough (contributing to pneumonia). Damage to the autonomic nervous system can affect respiration, heart rate, insulin secretion, and temperature regulation.

The diagnosis of medical conditions may be more difficult in patients with spinal cord disease as a result of impairment in sensation. The presence of spinal cord disease can obscure clinical signs, such as pain. Other signs, such as fever, can be difficult to interpret.

Advances in medical technology, including broad-spectrum antibiotics and dialysis, have significantly prolonged the life spans of patients with spinal cord injury. Such patients may therefore challenge the skills of internists and primary care physicians for many years.

PULMONARY DISORDERS

Spinal cord disease has a profound effect on pulmonary function. A complete high cervical cord lesion results in immediate life-threatening respiratory compromise. Furthermore, impaired cough and decreased lung volumes predispose the patient to the development of atelectasis and pneumonia, further impairing pulmonary function. Pulmonary complications are the major cause of death in acute spinal cord disease.[5, 36] The age of the patient, level of cord injury, and presence of preexisting medical problems, such as cardiopulmonary disease, contribute to mortality from pulmonary disorders.[50]

Pulmonary Function

The major muscles of inspiration and expiration and their segmental innervation are shown in Tables 17–1 and 17–2.[50] During inspiration, the diaphragm contracts, forcing the abdominal contents downward, and the intercostal muscles contract to expand the rib cage. Sixty-five percent of the inspiratory increase in lung volume is due to motion of the diaphragm. Passive expiration is due to the elastic recoil of the rib cage. Forced expiration, such as in cough, enlists the abdominal and intercostal muscles. The effects of spinal cord injury on pulmonary function depend on the level of the lesion (see Tables 17–1 and 17–2). Lesions of the lumbar area have little or no effect on ventilation or cough. Lesions of the thoracic cord can impair cough but have little effect on normal breathing. Lesions of the cervical cord are associated with increased effects on breathing. Lesions at C5 or higher can affect diaphragmatic function, with complete lesions at C3 or higher producing bilateral diaphragmatic paralysis, which is incompatible with

TABLE 17–2

MAJOR MUSCLES OF EXPIRATION AND THEIR SEGMENTAL INNERVATION

MUSCLE	INNERVATION
Primary	
Rectus abdominus	T6–12
Transversus abdominus	T2–L1
Internal and external obliques	T6–L1
Accessory	
Diaphragm	C3–5
Internal intercostals	T1–11

Data from Polatty RC, McElaney MA, Marcelino V: Pulmonary complications in the spinal cord injury patient. Phys Med Rehabil 1:353, 1987.

survival without artificial ventilation. The standard lung volumes and capacities are shown in Figure 17–1. McMichan and co-workers[36] found that acute traumatic quadriplegia produced decreased vital capacity and decreased maximum inspiratory and expiratory pressures. By 18 weeks after injury, these values improved. However, pulmonary function tests remained abnormal, with decreased total lung capacity, vital capacity,

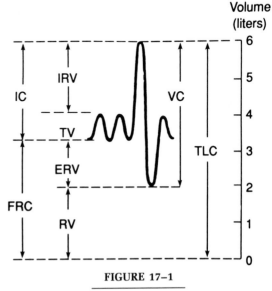

FIGURE 17–1

Normal lung volumes and capacities. TLC = total lung capacity; VC = vital capacity; IC = inspiratory capacity; FRC = functional residual capacity; IRV = inspiratory reserve volume; ERV = expiratory reserve volume; RV = residual volume; TV = tidal volume.

TABLE 17–1

MAJOR MUSCLES OF INSPIRATION AND THEIR SEGMENTAL INNERVATION

MUSCLE	INNERVATION
Primary	
Diaphragm	C3–5
External intercostals	T1–11
Accessory	
Sternocleidomastoids	C1–3
Trapezius	C1–4 and cranial nerve XI
Scalenes	C4–8 and cranial nerve XI

Data from Polatty RC, McElaney MA, Marcelino V: Pulmonary complications in the spinal cord injury patient. Phys Med Rehabil 1:353, 1987.

functional residual capacity, expiratory reserve volume, peak inspiratory and expiratory pressures, and increased residual volume. Maximal voluntary ventilation was also decreased to 43% of predicted levels. Improvement in pulmonary function after the acute injury is attributable to spasm of the intercostal and abdominal muscles, which prevents paradoxical motion of the rib cage and permits improved diaphragmatic function. Conditioning may also play a role. Unless frank respiratory failure occurs (see following section), arterial blood gas levels in quadriplegic patients are normal.

Respiratory Failure

Patients with spinal cord disease are at high risk for respiratory failure (an inability to adequately oxygenate and remove carbon dioxide from the blood). Bergofsky[6] found that in quadriplegic patients, the diaphragm contributed more that 90% of the tidal volume. High cervical cord lesions (above C3–5), which paralyze the diaphragm, can therefore result in respiratory failure and death. Such patients can survive only with life-long mechanical ventilation or phrenic nerve pacing.

Impaired cough, renal failure, and infection predispose the patient with spinal cord disease to a variety of pulmonary problems that can precipitate respiratory failure.[15] Evidence also indicates that interruption of sympathetic bronchial innervation predisposes to reversible airway obstruction in quadriplegic individuals.[57] Fishburn and others[16] found that in 50% of patients with spinal cord disease, atelectasis or pneumonia developed during the first 30 days after injury. As might be expected, the incidence of these complications was highest in high-level quadriplegia (C3–5) and lowest in paraplegic patients. The left lung was involved by these processes four times more frequently than the right lung. Fishburn and colleagues theorized that the angle between the left main stem bronchus and the trachea, which is more acute than that between the right mid-stem bronchus and the trachea, makes suctioning more difficult, thereby resulting in a predisposition to atelectasis and pneumonia.

TREATMENT OF RESPIRATORY FAILURE

In the treatment of respiratory failure,[47, 49, 50] oxygen is delivered via nasal prongs, Venturi masks (which deliver a constant oxygen concentration that can range from 24% to 50%, depending on the mask), and via partial rebreathing masks that can deliver an oxygen concentration up to 60%. Tight-fitting non-rebreathing masks deliver an oxygen concentration as high as 90% to 95%. Quadriplegic patients who use these masks should be observed closely because if the mask disconnects from the oxygen source, the patient may be unable to remove it and could suffocate.

Nebulized beta-agonists (such as metaproterenol), 0.3 mL via intermittent positive-pressure breathing (IPPB) every 4 to 6 hours, effect reversal of bronchospasm and enhance ciliary action. Theophylline relieves bronchospasm and increases the strength of diaphragmatic contraction. In an emergency situation, aminophylline (which is converted to theophylline) is given in a loading dose of 6 mg/kg intravenously. Patients already taking theophylline need a lower dose. In adults younger than 40 years with no heart or liver problems, a maintenance dose of 0.6 mg/kg/hour is given. Higher doses are needed in smokers because smoking increases the hepatic metabolism of theophylline. Lower maintenance doses are needed in older patients or in patients with hepatic or cardiac problems. Blood levels must be measured and side effects of nausea, vomiting, or arrhythmias monitored. In the patient with spinal cord injury, abdominal pain, which is also a manifestation of theophylline toxicity, can be masked. Anticholinergic agents, such as ipratropium bromide delivered by IPPB, two puffs four times a day, also relieve bronchospasm. N-Acetylcysteine (Mucomyst), 1 to 2 mL of a 10% to 20% solution diluted with 5 to 10 mL of saline given via IPPB or endotracheal tube, may be useful in removing mucus plugs. Because N-acetylcysteine can cause bronchospasm, it should be given only after an inhaled bronchodilator. When mucus plugs are refractory to these measures and to vigorous pulmonary toilet, including chest percussion, fiberoptic bronchoscopy may be necessary.

Intubation and Mechanical Ventilation

Intubation[48, 50] is performed to provide a closed system for mechanical ventilation and to provide pulmonary toilet and prevent aspiration when cough is impaired. Intubation also may be performed when the patient appears to be tiring or when his or her condition is unstable. The following clinical parameters are indications for intubation:

- PO_2 less than 60 mm Hg with oxygen therapy
- PCO_2 greater than 45 mm Hg with a pH less than 7.35
- Respiratory rate greater than 35 breaths per minute
- Maximum expiratory pressure less than 20 cm H_2O
- Maximum inspiratory pressure less than 25 cm H_2O
- Vital capacity less than 15 mL/kg or less than twice the tidal volume

These are only guidelines and need not always be followed. For example, acute respiratory failure secondary to bronchospasm might rapidly be reversed by bronchodilators, and intubation might be avoided.

A volume-cycled ventilator is preferable to a pressure-cycled ventilator. The initial ventilator settings[50] are as follows:

- Respiratory rate of 10 to 12 breaths per minute
- Tidal volume of 10 to 15 mL/kg
- Flow rate of 50 L/minute
- Pressure limit of 60 cm H_2O
- Inspired oxygen concentration less than 60% unless a higher concentration is needed

A positive end-expiratory pressure of 5 cm H_2O can improve oxygenation and prevent atelectasis. Arterial blood analyses should be repeated within 30 minutes after mechanical ventilation is instituted, and the ventilator settings changed accordingly. With prolonged intubation, a tracheostomy should be performed and a cuffed tracheostomy tube placed.

WEANING FROM THE VENTILATOR

Intubation of the patient with spinal cord injury is usually performed at the time of acute injury. Factors contributing to ventilatory failure at this time include atelectasis, pneumonia, and anesthesia for laminectomy.[33] Reversal of anesthesia, treatment of pneumonia, and strengthening of respiratory muscles can help reverse respiratory failure and permit extubation. Although criteria for weaning from ventilators vary somewhat, the following suggested by Lamid and co-workers[33] are reasonable:

- Vital capacity greater than 10 mL/kg of body weight
- Tidal volume more than 5 mL/kg of body weight
- Peak inspiratory pressure greater than 20 cm H_2O
- Respiratory rate less than 30 breaths per minute

Weaning from the ventilator can be accomplished by withdrawing mechanical ventilation and allowing the patient to breathe on a T-piece for increasing periods of time or by increasing the frequency of intermittent mandatory ventilation. Lamid and others[33] concluded that successful weaning of patients with spinal cord injury from ventilation depends on several factors, including prevention of pneumonia and urinary tract infection, relief of depression and anxiety, communication between staff and patients, and motivation of the patient by family members.

Phrenic Nerve Pacing

Phrenic nerve pacing[50] employs electrical stimulation of intact phrenic nerve fibers below the level of spinal cord injury. Contraction of the ipsilateral diaphragm during stimulation as assessed by ultrasonography or fluoroscopy confirms the efficacy of this procedure, which can free patients with paralysis of the diaphragm from the ventilator. Muscles of expiration are not affected by a phrenic nerve pacemaker. The tracheostomy is therefore left in place for suctioning and as a precaution in case of pacemaker failure.

PREVENTION OF PULMONARY COMPLICATIONS

With care, some of the pulmonary complications of spinal cord injury can be prevented. Pneumococcal vaccine and yearly influenza vaccination can prevent life-threatening lung infections. Whether pneumococcal vaccination should be repeated after the initial immunization is controversial. Certain maneuvers can improve ventilatory function. In quadriplegic individuals who have intact diaphragmatic function, vital capacity, tidal volume, and oxygenation are improved in the supine position,[50] because the diaphragm is pushed up by abdominal contents into the configuration of maximal muscle efficiency.

However, McCool and colleagues[35] found that reflex neural compensation was adequate to maintain ventilation when the quadriplegic patient was tilted from the supine to the upright position. Inspiratory muscle training has been shown to improve the strength and endurance of these muscles.[23] Glossopharyngeal breathing, which entails the use of the tongue and pharyngeal muscles to force air into the airway, improves vital capacity and cough. The patient's wearing of a corset while in the upright position further elevates the diaphragm and improves function. Patients who have function of their upper extremities can improve their ability to cough by pushing downward and upward on the abdominal contents in a manner similar to the Heimlich maneuver ("quad cough").[50] McMichan and co-workers[36] found that vigorous pulmonary toilet, including frequent change of position, incentive spirometry, IPPB every 4 hours with aerosolized isoetharine, and chest percussion, increased survival and decreased the incidence of pulmonary complications in acute quadriplegia. These principles are illustrated by the following case report:

CASE REPORT: CASE 1

A 40-year-old man with complete quadriplegia at C6 and a history of 40 pack-years of smoking presented after 3 days of progressive dyspnea. Physical examination revealed a very anxious man with a temperature of 38°C; blood pressure, 150/70 mm Hg; and respiration rate, 35 breaths per minute. Chest examination disclosed diffuse wheezes. Arterial blood gases were PO_2, 45 mm Hg; PCO_2, 62 mm Hg; and pH, 7.26. Nasotracheal intubation was performed, and ventilation with a volume-cycled ventilator was initiated. A chest radiograph showed right middle lobe pneumonia. The patient's condition improved when intravenous aminophylline and antibiotics were given. After 3 days, extubation was undertaken. Subsequent pulmonary function tests showed an FEV_1/ FVC of only 50% of predicted value.

This case illustrates the effect of chronic obstructive pulmonary disease superimposed on cervical cord injury. The elevated PCO_2 and decreased pH indicated acute ventilatory failure. Intubation and artificial ventilation were therefore needed. Antibiotics and bronchodilators rapidly reversed the ventilatory failure, and extubation was accomplished.

PERIPHERAL VASCULAR DISORDERS

Venous Thrombosis and Pulmonary Embolism

Pulmonary embolism is a major cause of death in patients with acute spinal cord injury.[10, 54] Most pulmonary emboli originate from thrombi in the deep veins of the lower extremities. The early diagnosis and treatment of thromboembolic disease is therefore of great importance in the patient with spinal cord disease.

Virchow's classic triad of risk factors for deep vein thrombosis are hypercoagulability, decreased blood flow, and injury to the vessels. The first two are clearly present in the patient with spinal cord disease.

The formation of a clot is a complex process involving the coagulation cascade and platelets.[12] Abnormalities in coagulation factors that increase the risk of thrombosis have been found in spinal cord disease. Myllynen and others[43] found that factor VIII antigen (which reflects endothelial damage) and factor VIII procoagulant activity increase during the 10 to 12 days of immobilization in acute spinal cord disease. These investigators also found that a ratio of factor VIII antigen to procoagulant activity of greater than 2 : 1 accurately predicted the development of deep vein thrombosis. Petäjä and colleagues[44] found fibrinolytic activity to be decreased during the first 24 hours after spinal trauma. Patients with spinal cord disease who have end-stage renal disease appear to be especially predisposed to thrombotic complications. Vaziri and co-workers[66] found that antithrombin III levels were lower in patients with spinal cord disease who had end-stage renal disease than in ambulatory patients with end-stage renal disease. Factor XII and VIII activities were found to be higher in patients with spinal cord disease who had renal failure when compared with controls.[67] In addition, tissue damage at the time of injury increases platelet number and adherence to surfaces.

Myllynen and others[42] used radiolabeled fibrinogen and venography to compare the incidence of deep vein thrombosis in patients who had acute spinal cord disease with that in nonparalyzed patients with spinal fractures. Whereas 64% of patients with spinal cord disease had documented deep vein thrombosis, none of the nonparalyzed patients had deep vein thrombosis. These data dramatically illustrate the importance of immobilization in the genesis of deep vein thrombosis in patients with spinal cord disease.

DIAGNOSIS OF DEEP VEIN THROMBOSIS

The lack of awareness of physical signs of deep vein thrombosis in patients with spinal cord disease makes the use of diagnostic studies even more important. Calf pain is usually not present. Leg swelling may not be present or may be attributed to other causes. Unexplained fever in a patient with spinal cord injury should raise the suspicion of deep vein thrombosis.[69] The possibility that untreated deep vein thrombosis may result in pulmonary embolism and death necessitates use of a sensitive diagnostic procedure (one with few false-negatives results). Conversely, anticoagulant therapy can produce hemorrhage and even death. Therefore, when physicians commit patients to long-term anticoagulation on the basis of positive test results, they should ensure that the diagnostic procedure has a high degree of specificity (few false-positive results).

The venogram provides the gold standard for the diagnosis of deep vein thrombosis. This procedure can be performed in any radiology department, has few complications, has a high sensitivity and specificity, and can be performed as the initial diagnostic procedure in suspected deep vein thrombosis. However, venography is an invasive procedure associated with some morbidity. Less invasive procedures are available for the diagnosis of deep vein thrombosis.[10, 26, 40, 72]

Impedance plethysmography can be performed at the bedside. Thrombosis results in reduced venous blood flow, which decreases an electrical signal. Impedance plethysmography detects proximal venous obstruction with a sensitivity as high as 93% to 98% but is unreliable in the detection of calf thrombi. Venous Doppler ultrasound detects thrombi in the calf with 50% or greater accuracy. The reliability of a combination of positive impedance plethysmography and venous Doppler findings in detecting deep vein thrombosis of the lower extremity approaches that of venography.

The radiolabeled fibrinogen technique is expensive and is used primarily as a research tool. However, this method can detect a very small thrombus because radiolabeled fibrinogen is taken up into the forming thrombus.

More recently, real-time ultrasonography[72] and color Doppler ultrasonography[17] have been found to be extremely sensitive techniques for the diagnosis of lower extremity deep vein thrombosis. Duplex imaging, which combines ultrasonic imaging and

Doppler information, is now supplanting former techniques.[72] The duplex scan diagnoses symptomatic above-knee thrombosis with as high as 100% sensitivity and 98% specificity. For thrombosis below the knee, sensitivity and specificity are as great as 91% and 96%, respectively.

DIAGNOSIS OF PULMONARY EMBOLISM IN SPINAL CORD DISEASE

Unexplained symptoms of dyspnea, cough, hemoptysis, or apprehension should raise the suspicion of pulmonary embolism. Signs such as hemoptysis, cyanosis, hypotension, pleural friction rub, fever, or loud S2, S3, or S4 gallop also may indicate that a pulmonary embolism has occurred. Hypoxemia is usually present.[61] As in many other disorders, these findings can be obscured or difficult to interpret in patients with spinal cord injury. For example, the quadriplegic individual may not be able to sense chest pain or may be dyspneic from some other cause. There-fore, the physician must be vigilant, especially in the period immediately following acute spinal cord injury. When pulmonary embolism is suspected, a ventilation/perfusion scan should be performed immediately. Areas that are ventilated but not perfused are likely sites of pulmonary embolism. A high probability scan shows normal ventilation of areas that on perfusion scan are characterized by multiple defects that are wedge-shaped or segmental or that occur as concave defects on the lateral edges of the lung or on a pleural surface (Figs. 17–2 and 17–3). A high-probability scan is usually sufficient to make the diagnosis of pulmonary embolism. A totally negative perfusion scan excludes pulmonary embolism. In the patient with spinal cord injury, mucus plugs can cause dyspnea and hypoxemia and abnormal perfusion scans.[13] However, in the patient with mucus plugs, decreased ventilation of the affected area is also present, which differentiates the mucus plug from pulmonary embolism. Pulmonary angiography should be considered

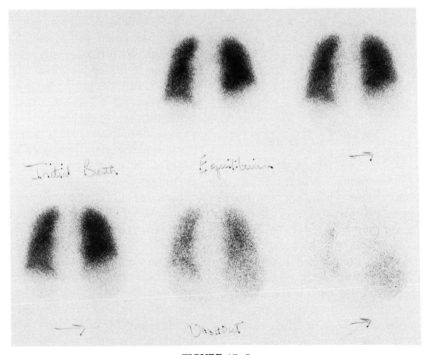

FIGURE 17–2

Normal xenon ventilation scan showing even distribution of ^{133}Xe in the lungs. (Courtesy of the Department of Nuclear Medicine, Hunter Holmes McGuire Veterans Administration Medical Center, Richmond, Va.)

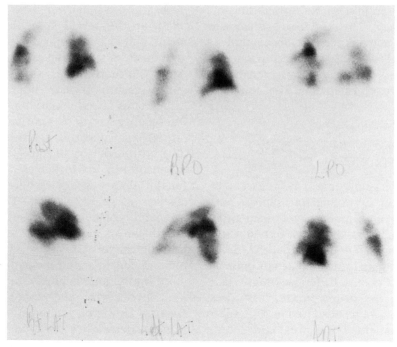

FIGURE 17-3

Abnormal technetium 99 m macroaggregated albumin lung scan showing multiple segmental perfusion defects. (Courtesy of the Department of Nuclear Medicine, Hunter Holmes McGuire Veterans Administration Medical Center, Richmond, Va.)

when the ventilation/perfusion scan is of intermediate or low probability, when there is increased risk of bleeding from anticoagulants, or if the use of thrombolytic therapy or surgical treatment (such as embolectomy) is contemplated.

TREATMENT OF DEEP VEIN THROMBOSIS AND PULMONARY EMBOLISM

Most pulmonary emboli arise from clots in the lower extremities. Therefore, the treatment of these two conditions is similar. The goal of anticoagulant therapy is to prevent further clot formation. Within 1 to 3 weeks, the clot will endothelialize and attach to the vessel wall, and the threat of dislodgment will be minimized.[40] Heparin activates antithrombin III, which inhibits the clotting cascade at several points.[12] A loading dose of 5000 to 7000 units is given intravenously.[37,61] A continuous infusion of heparin at a rate sufficient to maintain the activated partial thromboplastin time (PTT) at a level of 1.5 to 2.5 times the control is started. Although

there is a wide dosage range, the most common dose is on the average of 1000 units per hour. Within a day after starting heparin, administration of warfarin can begin. Heparin is continued until the prothrombin time on warfarin is 1.5 to 2 times that of the control, and then is discontinued.

Subcutaneous heparin given at an initial dose of 250 units/kg every 12 hours has been found to be as effective as intravenous heparin in preventing pulmonary emboli. Algorithms for adjustment of heparin dose are available.[37] Loading doses of warfarin are not required. Ten milligrams is administered daily for 2 to 4 days and then adjusted to maintain a therapeutic prothrombin time. Warfarin inhibits synthesis of vitamin K–dependent factors II, VII, IX, and X and also reduces levels of protein C (a naturally occurring antithrombic protein). Because protein C has a short half-life, warfarin could initially induce a temporary hypercoagulable state before the synthesis of cofactors with a longer half-life is inhibited. This is another reason why heparin is needed during the first

24 hours of treatment. Clinical studies[40] suggest that the rate of recurrence of venous thromboembolism after 4 weeks of anticoagulation is no greater than that after 6 months. However, 3 months of warfarin therapy is the standard recommendation. During this period the muscles of the patient with spinal cord injury become spastic, thereby increasing venous tone, and the hypercoagulable state of acute tissue injury abates. Recurrence of thrombosis is an indication for a longer duration of warfarin therapy.[40]

Occasionally, anticoagulation is contraindicated in patients with spinal cord disease or such patients have recurrent pulmonary embolism despite adequate anticoagulation. In these instances, the vena cava can be interrupted to prevent clots from passing from the venous system to the lungs. Placement of the Greenfield filter, which is inserted into the vena cava via the right internal jugular vein or common femoral vein, is the most common method of interrupting the vena cava[28] (Fig. 14–4). Patients with spinal cord disease are at increased risk for complications from Greenfield filter placement. Balshi and colleagues[2] found that in 13 instances in which a Greenfield filter was placed in quadriplegics, five cases of abnormality in the filter were seen (distal migration, deformity, occlusion). Laparotomy for bowel perforation was required in two of these patients. The occurrence of these complications correlated with the use of quad cough physical therapy. In patients with pulmonary compromise who require vigorous pulmonary toilet, vena caval interruption by some other means should be considered.

PREVENTION OF DEEP VEIN THROMBOSIS IN SPINAL CORD INJURY

The high incidence of deep vein thrombosis and pulmonary embolism during the first 3 months after spinal cord injury makes prophylaxis of deep vein thrombosis desirable. This need becomes more pressing in view of the fact that that pulmonary embolism can occur within 24 hours of a negative iodine 125–labeled fibrinogen scan and impedence plethysmography of the lower extremities.[18] Several methods of prophylaxis have been

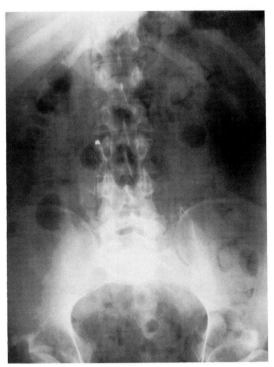

FIGURE 17–4

Greenfield filter in the inferior vena cava of a patient with spinal cord injury. (Courtesy of the Department of Radiology, Hunter Holmes McGuire Veterans Administration Medical Center, Richmond, Va.)

effective. Low-dose heparin (5000 units two to three times daily or three times a day subcutaneously) prevents thrombosis with little or no increase in the risk of bleeding in ambulatory patients.[61] However, this dose of heparin may be ineffective in preventing thrombosis in patients with acute spinal cord injury.[22] Green and others[20] found that adjusting the heparin dose upward to prolong the activated partial thromboplastin time to 1.5 times the control level was superior to low-dose therapy in preventing deep vein thrombosis, but the larger dose of heparin increased the risk of hemorrhagic complications. Low molecular weight heparin given once daily has been shown to be superior to standard heparin therapy in preventing thromboembolic disease and in decreasing hemorrhagic complications.[21] External pneumatic calf compression and electrical stimulation of the calf can disperse the high concentrations of clotting factors associated with venous stasis and may thereby prevent deep vein thrombosis.[22]

Combining administration of aspirin and dipyridamole with external pneumatic calf compression may result in fewer thrombotic events than occur with calf compression alone.[22] Dihydroergotamine prevents deep vein thrombosis in patients without spinal cord injury[41] and has an additive effect when given in combination with heparin. However, we are unaware of any controlled studies of the use of dihydroergotamine in patients with spinal cord injury.

Arterial Disease in Spinal Cord Injury

Patients with spinal cord disease are susceptible to the same vascular problems as the general population; however, neurologic deficits can obscure their diagnosis. An abdominal aortic aneurysm can present as abdominal and back pain, symptoms that may not be present in the patient with spinal cord injury.[61] Aneurysms of the thoracic aorta can cause neurologic deficits,[34] which can be masked in patients with cervical cord lesions. The only sign of an aortic aneurysm may be a decreased pulse amplitude and a mass on palpation of the abdomen. Likewise, intermittent claudication of the calf, an important symptom of peripheral vascular disease, may not be evident in the patient with spinal cord disease, nor are paralysis, poikilothermy, or paresthesias. Pallor and decreased pulses may be the only signs[61] of arterial disease in the lower extremities of the patient with spinal cord injury.

Arterial disease is occasionally a cause of spinal cord disease. Acute aortic thrombosis[60] and dissecting aneurysm[74] can present as painless paraplegia. Paraplegia can result from surgical trauma to the aorta, intercostal artery ligation, and emboli to the spinal cord[8] or after cardiac arrest.[29] The following case report demonstrates a vascular etiology of paraplegia:

CASE REPORT: CASE 2

A 41-year-old man sustained a back injury after being blown out of a gun truck in Vietnam. He subsequently experienced right lower extremity weakness with foot drop. Workup revealed a T11 spinal arteriovenous malformation. This was resected with improvement of symptoms. However, after 3 years, symptoms recurred, and a recurrence of the arteriovenous malformation was found. It was again resected, but symptoms failed to improve. This unusual case represents a potentially correctable cause of paraplegia due to a vascular abnormality.

RENAL DISORDERS

Renal failure commonly complicates spinal cord disease. Tribe and Silver[62] reported that 50% of all patients in an autopsy series of spinal cord–injured patients between 1945 and 1967 died of renal failure.

Barton and colleagues[3] reported renal pathologic findings revealed from the review of autopsy material from 21 patients with spinal cord injury who had been treated with hemodialysis and compared this data with autopsy findings in 43 patients who had undergone ambulatory dialysis. The most common pathologic diagnosis in patients with spinal cord disease was chronic pyelonephritis, which was found in 100% of kidneys (Fig. 17–5). Less common findings were amyloidosis (81%) (Fig. 17–6), calculous disease (57%), obstructive uropathy (57%), acute pyelonephritis (29%), nephrosclerosis (29%), and abscess (24%). These findings were in contrast to those in ambulatory patients with end-stage renal disease in whom nephrosclerosis and interstitial nephritis were the most common causes of renal failure. Sepsis was the most common cause of death in patients with spinal cord disease who had end-stage renal disease (62%); there was a 12% incidence of sepsis in ambulatory patients with end-stage renal disease.

Assessment of Renal Function in Spinal Cord Disease

The glomerular filtration rate must decrease 30% before the serum creatinine level

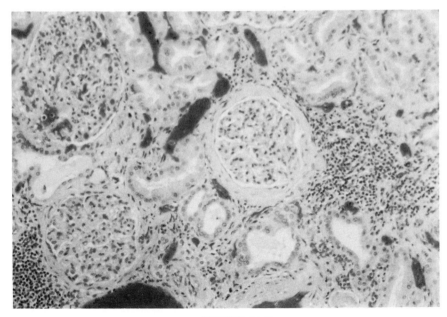

FIGURE 17–5

Chronic pyelonephritis in a quadriplegic man: autopsy specimen shows interstitial infiltration of inflammatory cells (magnification ×400). (Courtesy of B. Kipreos, M.D. Department of Pathology, Hunter Holmes McGuire Veterans Administration Medical Center, Richmond, Va.)

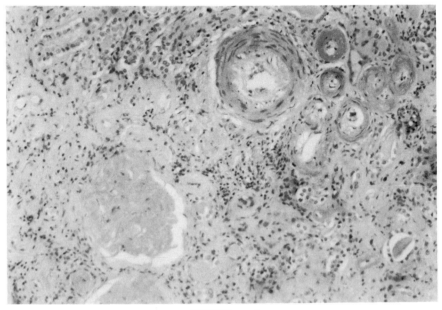

FIGURE 17–6

Amyloidosis of the kidney of a quadriplegic man; autopsy specimen shows deposition of amyloid in the interstitium and vessel walls (magnification ×400). (Courtesy of B. Kipreos, M.D., Department of Pathology, Hunter Holmes McGuire Veterans Administration Medical Center, Richmond, Va.)

rises. The serum creatinine level is therefore a poor indicator of early impairment of renal function. The formula reported by Cockroft and Gault[11] permits determination of creatinine clearance based on the level of serum creatinine and factors that affect creatinine production (age, body weight, and gender). This formula (for a male) is as follows:

Creatinine clearance

$$= \frac{(140 - \text{age}) \times \text{body weight (kg)}}{72 \times \text{serum creatinine (mg/dL)}}$$

In females, the calculated value of creatinine clearance is multiplied by a correction factor of 0.85. Because of decreased muscle mass, this formula overestimates the creatinine clearance in patients with spinal cord disease, especially quadriplegic patients in whom muscle atrophy is most extreme. Nomograms are available by which creatinine clearance can be estimated from serum creatinine levels in patients with spinal cord injury.[39]

Biochemical Features of End-Stage Renal Disease

The biochemical features of end-stage renal disease in patients with spinal cord disease are somewhat different from those in ambulatory patients with renal failure. Vaziri and co-workers[64] found that the mean serum creatinine level in patients with spinal cord disease who had end-stage renal disease was 8.2 mg/dL as compared with 11.3 mg/dL in ambulatory patients with renal failure. Patients with spinal cord disease had higher daily urine outputs of lower specific gravity and higher glucose and protein excretion than did control subjects, presumably due to the effects of chronic pyelonephritis, obstructive uropathy, and amyloidosis on the renal tubules. Patients with spinal cord injury also had higher urine pH and higher fractional potassium excretion than did control subjects. The increased urine pH is due in part to infection with urease-producing bacteria.

PREVENTION OF RENAL FAILURE

High bladder pressures, which cause vesicoureteral reflux and pyelonephritis, can be reduced by maintaining a postvoiding residual volume of less than 10% of bladder capacity. Guttman and Ranakel[24] have described a method of intermittent catheterization that permits maintenance of sterile urine. If the patient cannot catheterize himself or herself, urethral sphincterotomy with placement of a Texas catheter may be indicated. Hall and colleagues[25] found that refluxing renal units were associated with a higher risk of formation of renal stones than were nonrefluxing units, and that Foley catheter drainage increased the risk for development of kidney and bladder stones. The foreign body is presumably a nidus for stone formation. Attention to sterile techniques during instrumentation of the bladder and aggressive treatment of infection can prevent deterioration of renal function. Extra care must be taken in the use of nephrotoxic drugs in patients with spinal cord injury.[30] The Cockroft-Gault equation overestimates the glomerular filtration rate in patients with spinal cord disease and therefore cannot be relied on for the determination of doses of nephrotoxic drugs. If possible, a drug that does not affect renal function should be substituted for a nephrotoxic drug.

Hemodialysis in Spinal Cord Disease

Renal failure can initially be treated with diet and medication. However, dialysis is usually indicated eventually. Stacy and others[58] found that the average time from the onset of spinal cord injury to the development of end-stage renal disease was 21 years. Major indications for dialysis are hyperkalemia, volume overload, and uremic syndrome.

Hemodialysis has been shown in several studies to improve survival in spinal cord patients with renal failure.[38, 58] Access to the bloodstream is created by surgical placement of an arteriovenous shunt when the creatinine clearance falls below 10 mL/minute. The most common vascular procedure performed in patients with spinal cord disease at the Hunter Holmes McGuire Veterans Administration Medical Center (Richmond, Va.) is the creation of vascular access for dialysis.[56] Patients usually undergo dialysis three times per week for periods of 4 to 6 hours. Stacy and co-workers[58] reported on 15 patients in whom end-stage renal disease was treated with hemodialysis. The 1-year survival rate was 57%, which is similar to that reported by Mirahmadi and others,[38] and less than the 80% 1-year survival rate for ambulatory patients with end-stage renal disease.

Hemodialysis presents special problems in patients with spinal cord injury. Intradialysis hypotension has been reported to occur more frequently in patients with spinal cord injury when the dialyzers needed large volumes of blood for priming.[59] Newer dialyzers that do not need large priming volumes have ameliorated this problem. Vaziri[63] noted painful muscle spasms in dialysis patients. This condition could have been provoked by dialysis and other causes and was believed to be due to uninhibited spinal reflexes. Diazepam and baclofen occasionally relieved the symptoms. Headaches, nausea, and vomiting are common in patients with spinal cord disease who undergo hemodialysis.

Peritoneal Dialysis

Peritoneal dialysis presents an attractive alternative to hemodialysis in the patient with spinal cord injury[55, 65] because it can be performed in the patient's home and does not necessitate heparinization. Speculation that peritoneal dialysis in patients with spinal cord disease would produce an unacceptable risk of complications, such as peritonitis, basal atelectasis, and hypoalbuminemia, seems to be unfounded. The incidence of peritonitis, 0.7 to 3.2 episodes per patient, is similar to that reported in patients without spinal cord injury.

Renal Transplantation

Renal transplantation has until recently been unavailable to patients with spinal cord disease. Hussey and Ha[27] reported the following case:

CASE REPORT: CASE 3

A 40-year-old man with T4 paraplegia developed chronic renal failure secondary to amyloidosis and chronic pyelonephritis. After 10 months of hemodialysis, he underwent renal transplantation. Two years after transplantation the patient had renal function that was sufficient to obviate the need for dialysis. This classic example of renal failure in a patient with spinal cord injury was managed with dialysis and renal transplantation.

It is likely that the use of renal transplantation will increase in patients with spinal cord disease in whom chronic renal failure develops.

Cardiovascular Complications of Spinal Cord Disease

With increased survival from infection and renal failure, spinal cord injury patients often live to an age at which coronary disease is clinically important. A man who becomes paraplegic at age 20 years has a life expectancy of 33 additional years.[14] Even a 20-year-old man with complete quadriplegia has a life expectancy of 22 more years. The leading cause of death for persons with neurologically incomplete paraplegia is ischemic heart disease. Overall, ischemic heart disease is the seventh most commonly reported cause of death in patients with spinal cord injury.

The aging of the population with spinal cord injuries, their need for potentially life-threatening surgical procedures, and the problem of silent myocardial ischemia make coronary artery disease in this group an increasingly important subject.

CARDIOVASCULAR EFFECTS OF SPINAL CORD INJURY

The heart and blood vessels above the diaphragm receive sympathetic innervation from the first through seventh thoracic cord segments.[1] Vasculature below the diaphragm receives sympathetic innervation from the fifth thoracic cord segments and below. Therefore, injury to the spinal cord above the T1 level may interrupt transmission of information from the brain to sympathetic neurons controlling cardiovascular function. Activation of sympathetic neurons results in cardioacceleration, increased myocardial contractility, and vasoconstriction, thereby increasing blood pressure and pulse. The parasympathetic nervous system, which slows the heart, is spared by spinal cord injury. As a result of these factors, patients with acute cervical cord injury are prone to hypotension, bradycardia, and even asystole during procedures that augment vagal tone, such as tracheal suctioning.[1, 46] Administration of atropine 10 to 15 minutes before tracheal suctioning or induction of hyperventilation immediately before suctioning prevents hypoxemia and activation of the parasympathetic nervous system.

Hypotension and bradycardia are most pronounced in the first few weeks after injury to the cervical spine. After several months these effects diminish, although orthostatic hypotension often persists in the quadriplegic individual.

Garner and colleagues[19] compared the effects of the vagotonic maneuvers of facial immersion and apnea on patients with chronic quadriplegia (mean duration of quadriplegia, 9.4 months) with response in ambulatory patients. As compared with ambulatory control subjects, who experienced a significant decrease in heart rate with each of these maneuvers, patients with quadriplegia experienced no decrease in heart rate (Fig. 17–7). This is apparently an adaptive response to unopposed parasympathetic activity in quadriplegia, and this finding may have clinical significance. Vagotonic maneuvers that are used to slow the heart and "break" supraventricular tachyarrhythmias might be ineffective in the quadriplegic patient.

In quadriplegic patients, cutaneous stimulation below the level of the lesion activates spinal reflexes that are not inhibited by the normal descending sympathetic pathways. This results in elevation of blood pressure, tachycardia, hyperhydrosis above the level

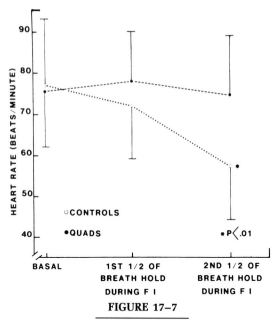

FIGURE 17–7

Heart rate (mean ± SD) in basal state and during facial immersion in normal control subjects and in quadriplegic subjects. (From Garner SH, Bloch R, Sutton JR: Heart rate response to facial immersion and apnea in quadriplegics. Arch Phys Med Rehabil 66:763, 1985.)

of the cord lesion, and various other signs, including penile erection, mydriasis, conjunctival congestion, facial flushing, nasal congestion, and paresthesia.[1] Autonomic dysreflexia is treated by reducing afferent nerve activity (e.g., by relieving bladder distension and fecal impaction). Hypertension may be controlled by alpha-adrenergic blockers (e.g., phenoxybenzamine or prazosin), direct-acting vasodilators (e.g., hydralazine, nitroprusside, or intravenous nitroglycerin), and calcium channel blockers. Use of ganglionic blockers is much less common now than in the past.

RISK FACTORS FOR CORONARY DISEASE IN PATIENTS WITH SPINAL CORD INJURY

The major risk factors for the development of coronary artery disease are smoking, hypertension, diabetes mellitus, and lipid abnormalities.

Many physicians who work with patients with spinal cord injury think that cigarette smoking is more prevalent in these patients than in the general population. However,

Krum and colleagues[31] found that the percentage of patients with spinal cord injury in Australia who smoked (31%) was not significantly different than that of ambulatory patients (28%).

Type II diabetes mellitus is found more commonly in patients with spinal cord injury than in ambulatory patients.[52] A major reason for this increased prevalence is insulin resistance, which may also contribute to the development of hypertension.

Characteristics of spinal cord injury both protect from and promote hypertension. Interruption of spinal efferent pathways prevents reflex tachycardia and vasoconstriction, which maintain blood pressure with upright posture.[1] Postural hypotension is therefore common in persons with acute quadriplegia. With rehabilitation, symptoms of hypotension decrease. However, upright hypotension is common in long-standing quadriplega. Quadriplegic patients are therefore somewhat protected from the development of hypertension.[32] However, in paraplegic individuals in whom the sympathetic control of blood pressure is relatively normal, the incidence of hypertension seems to be increased. Yekutiel and others[73] found that 34% of patients with spinal cord injury had hypertension as compared with 18.6% of ambulatory control subjects. This increase may be due, in part, to obesity and renal failure.

A decreased high-density lipoprotein (HDL) cholesterol level is a major risk factor for the development of coronary artery disease. A decreased level of the HDL_2 subfraction is an especially powerful predictor of cardiovascular risk. Brenes and colleagues[9] found that mean HDL and HDL_2 cholesterol levels in sedentary patients with spinal cord injury were extremely low. With increased physical activity, HDL cholesterol levels increased toward the normal range (Fig. 17–8).

DIAGNOSIS OF CORONARY ARTERY DISEASE IN PATIENTS WITH SPINAL CORD INJURY

Cardiac pain fibers accompany sympathetic cardiac nerves and enter the central nervous system through the dorsal and ventral roots of the first four thoracic segments

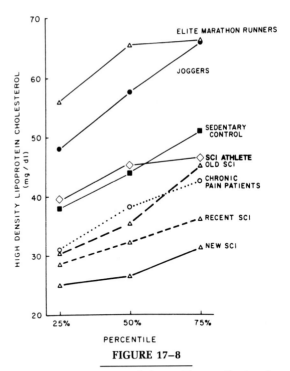

FIGURE 17–8

High density lipoprotein cholesterol by quartiles in subjects who perform various levels of physical activity. (From Brenes G, Dearwarter MS, Shapera R, et al: High density lipoprotein cholesterol concentrations in physically active and sedentary spinal cord injured patients. Arch Phys Med Rehabil 67:445, 1986.)

of the spinal cord.[1] Therefore, injury to the cervical cord might prevent transmission of pain signals to higher centers. As a result, patients with cervical spine lesions may not be able to sense cardiac pain. Quadriplegic patients may therefore develop complications of myocardial infarction, such as congestive heart failure or even sudden cardiac death, without experiencing chest pain.[68]

The diagnosis of myocardial ischemia in these patients is difficult. The resting electrocardiogram is not a sensitive indicator of ischemia, and some form of stress testing is usually required. In ambulatory patients, arm crank ergometry is as sensitive as leg exercise in detecting myocardial ischemia.[68] However, quadriplegic patients have a reduced ability to perform arm crank ergometry (or may be unable to perform it at all). Therefore, alternate methods of diagnosing myocardial ischemia are necessary.

Dipyridamole induces coronary artery vasodilation.[45] Injection of the radioisotope thallium 201 during infusion of dipyrida-mole allows detection of ischemic or "cold" areas of myocardium. Initially cold areas that take up the isotope after 2 to 4 hours indicate reversible ischemia as opposed to infarction, in which failure to take up the isotope is un-changing. We and others[51] have safely uti-lized dipyridamole-thallium scans in diag-nosing myocardial ischemia in patients with spinal cord injury. Alternatively, dobuta-mine, which increases myocardial work and oxygen demand, can be used in conjunction with thallium 201 in diagnosing myocardial disease.

In a 1992 report, both dipyridamole and dobutamine infusions were combined with echocardiography in diagnosing ischemia.[45] Myocardial ischemia produces decreased systolic wall motion or paradoxical systolic wall motion. Stress echocardiography using these pharmacologic agents is a sensitive method of diagnosing coronary disease.

Angiography remains the gold standard for the diagnosis of coronary artery disease. However, in the patient with spinal cord in-jury, technical concerns must be taken into account. Large volumes of contrast material might decrease renal function, and impaired pulmonary function makes it difficult for some quadriplegic patients to lie flat during the procedure.

TREATMENT OF ISCHEMIC HEART DISEASE IN PATIENTS WITH SPINAL CORD INJURY

MEDICAL TREATMENT OF CORONARY ARTERY DISEASE.[53] Nitrates relieve anginal symptoms, primarily by reduction of preload, which re-duces myocardial work and improves suben-docardial perfusion. These agents also im-prove coronary blood flow and reduce afterload. Sublingual nitroglycerin relieves angina within 2 minutes, and relief continues for 15 to 30 minutes. If pain fails to abate by the third dose, medical attention should be obtained because of the possibility of myocar-dial infarction.

Long-acting oral nitrates (e.g., isosorbide 5 to 20 mg sublingually every 3 to 4 hours or up to 40 mg orally, three times daily) and topical nitrates (e.g., 2% nitroglycerin oint-ment applied to skin, 1 to 2 in. every 4 to 6

hours) reduce frequency of anginal episodes. By withholding nitrates at night, nitrate toler-ance can be prevented. Because nitrates pro-duce hypotension they should be used cau-tiously in quadriplegic persons who are already predisposed to postural hypotension.

Beta-blockers exert their antianginal effects by decreasing myocardial contractility and slowing heart rate. Propranolol (20 to 60 mg four times daily) acts on beta$_1$- and beta$_2$-receptors. Selective beta$_1$-receptor blockers (such as metoprolol, 50 to 100 mg twice daily) are less likely to produce bronchospasm or exacerbate peripheral vascular disease. Be-cause quadriplegic patients are usually sed-entary and may have decreased sympathetic activity, the benefits of treatment with beta-blockers is uncertain.

Side effects of beta-blockers that are espe-cially important in the patient with spinal cord injury are postural hypotension, bron-chospasm, and salt retention. Adrenergic symptoms of hypoglycemia may be de-creased in insulin-treated quadriplegic pa-tients and it is likely that the use of beta-blockers in these patients would further impair the recognition of symptoms of hypo-glycemia. In addition, beta-blockers decrease HDL cholesterol levels, which are already de-creased in patients with spinal cord injury.

Calcium channel antagonists are periph-eral and coronary vasodilators and have vary-ing effects on myocardial contractility and conduction. Nifedipine (10 to 30 mg three or four times daily) has no effect on atrioventric-ular conduction. Its negative inotropic effects are offset by its vasodilating properties. Dilti-azem (30 to 90 mg four times daily) prolongs atrioventricular conduction and exerts a modest degree of negative inotropism. Ver-apamil (40 to 120 mg three times daily) has the greatest effect on atrioventricular conduc-tion and myocardial contractility of the cal-cium channel blockers and therefore should be avoided in patients with significant left ventricular dysfunction or heart block. Ver-apamil also may cause constipation, which may be especially troubling in the patient with spinal cord injury.

Aspirin decreases platelet adhesiveness and may prevent coronary thrombosis. If there is no contraindication (such as gastrointestinal bleeding), aspirin (80 to 325 mg/day) should probably be used in all patients with known coronary disease.

INVASIVE THERAPY OF CORONARY ARTERY DISEASE. Invasive therapy of coronary artery disease is indicated in patients with angina that is resistant to medical management. However, because of the absence of chest pain in some patients with spinal cord injury, it may be unclear when a patient's condition is refractory to medical therapy. Percutaneous transluminal coronary angioplasty and coronary artery bypass grafts prolong life in ambulatory patients with left main coronary artery disease and in patients with triple-vessel disease, especially when left ventricular dysfunction is present. However, the effect of these procedures on the longevity of patients with spinal cord injury has not been established.

PREVENTION OF CORONARY ARTERY DISEASE IN PATIENTS WITH SPINAL CORD INJURY

Early modification of cardiovascular risk factors may prevent later cardiovascular morbidity and mortality.[7,71] Cessation of smoking is of primary importance and may be facilitated by use of nicotine gum or transdermal patches.

Diets for spinal cord injury patients should take into account their decreased daily energy expenditures. Hypercholesterolemia is treated with reduction in daily cholesterol and fat intake.

When diet fails to do so, drugs may be used to control lipid levels. Bile acid binders produce a modest reduction in serum cholesterol level. However, these drugs cause constipation and may increase serum triglyceride levels. Hydroxymethylglutaryl–coenzyme A (HMG-CoA) reductase inhibitors are the most potent agents used for lowering serum cholesterol levels. Nicotinic acid and gemfibrosil lower serum cholesterol levels and also increase HDL levels, especially in patients with hypertriglyceridemia. However, nicotinic acid produces such effects as flushing, carbohydrate intolerance, and hyperuricemia.

Therapeutic guidelines for control of blood

pressure in patients with spinal cord injury have not been established. Secondary causes, such as autonomic dysreflexia, should be ruled out. It seems prudent to maintain an upright blood pressure of 140/85–90 mm Hg or below. Antihypertensive agents must be used with caution. Diuretics may aggravate postural hypotension and beta-blockers may exacerbate bradycardia. Peripheral alpha-blockers, such as prazosin, may have the advantage of reducing urethral sphincter tone but may also produce postural hypotension. Loss of sympathetic reflexes results in increased reliance of the renin-angiotensin system for maintenance of blood pressure, especially when hypovolemia has been induced by diuretics.[1] Therefore, angiotensin-converting enzyme inhibitors should be used cautiously in patients with spinal cord injury. If these agents are to be used, a small test dose with a short-acting agent such as captopril should be given first, with careful monitoring of blood pressure. Use of calcium channel blockers for the control of blood pressure has the potential advantage of protecting the patient from myocardial ischemia, which may be silent.

Exercise reduces cardiovascular risk by increasing HDL levels and promotes cardiovascular fitness in other ways. Recently, Bauman and colleagues[4] have found that functional electrical stimulation–induced lower extremity exercise training produced an average 6 mg/dL increase in serum HDL cholesterol levels in patients with quadriplegia.

Some of the principles in the preceding discussion are illustrated by the following case report.

CASE REPORT: CASE 4

A 47-year-old man with T4–5 incomplete paraplegia and a history of insulin-treated diabetes mellitus and hypercholesterolemia noted onset of substernal tightness occurring two or three times per day. This was initially felt to be due to a hiatus hernia. However, because of strong family history of coronary disease, a dipyridamole-thallium scan was performed. Multiple reversible defects, consistent with myocardial ischemia, were found. Cardiac catheterization demonstrated 95% stenosis of the right coronary artery, 50% stenosis of the left anterior descending artery, and total occlusion of both obtuse marginal arteries.

PTCA was performed with reduction of the right coronary occlusion.

The patient was placed on a regimen of one enteric-coated aspirin per day; diltiazem, 90 mg every 6 hours; and nitroglycerin as needed; he experienced reduction of frequency of chest pain.

As compared with quadriplegic patients, who may not sense chest pain, this paraplegic man developed typical anginal symptoms. Because of his inability to walk on a treadmill, dipyridamole-thallium testing was performed, which demonstrated reversible ischemia; the condition responded to PTCA and medication.

SUMMARY

Spinal cord injury increases the risk of many life-threatening medical problems, including respiratory failure, pulmonary embolism, renal failure, and ischemic heart disease. Respiratory failure results from paralysis of muscles of inspiration and of expiration. Respiratory failure in patients with spinal cord injury can be prevented by proper positioning of the patient, training of ventilatory muscles, pulmonary toilet, and aggressive use of antibiotics and bronchodilators. When respiratory failure occurs, it can be managed by administration of oxygen, intubation, and mechanical ventilation, and, in instances of paralysis of the diaphragm, diaphragmatic pacing.

The risk of deep vein thrombosis and pulmonary embolism in acute spinal cord disease is increased by the immobilization of the patient and abnormalities in clotting factors. Thrombotic disease in spinal cord disease can be prevented by intermittent calf compression and heparinization. If pulmonary embolism develops, acute heparinization should be undertaken, followed by a regimen of warfarin for at least 3 months. If anticoagulation is contraindicated, a Greenfield filter

can be placed. However, concurrent use of quad cough places the patient at increased risk for complications from the Greenfield filter.

Chronic pyelonephritis and systemic amyloidosis are the most common causes of renal failure in the patient with spinal cord disease. Renal failure can be prevented by maintenance of a low postvoiding residual volume, avoidance of indwelling catheters, use of medications that are not nephrotoxic, and rapid treatment of infection. Hemodialysis and peritoneal dialysis can extend the life of the patient with spinal cord disease in whom renal failure develops, and successful use of renal transplantation has been reported.

The aging of the population with spinal cord injury has resulted in increased emphasis on ischemic heart disease. Cigarette smoking and decreased HDL levels are major coronary risk factors found in patients with spinal cord disease. Quadriplegic patients with coronary disease may not sense chest pain. Infusions of dobutamine and dipyridamole mimic the effects of exercise on myocardial blood flow, and, when used in conjunction with thallium 201 labeling or echocardiograms, accurately diagnose myocardial ischemia in patients with spinal cord injury.

REFERENCES

1. Arrowwood JA, Mohanty PK, Thomas MD: Cardiovascular problems in the spinal cord injury patient. Phys Med Rehabil 1:443, 1987.
2. Balshi DD, Contelmo NDL, Monzoian JO: Complications of caval interruption by Greenfield filter for deep venous thrombosis in quadriplegics. J Vasc Surg 9:558, 1989.
3. Barton CH, Vaziri ND, Gordon S, et al: Renal pathology in end-stage renal disease associated with paraplegia. Paraplegia 22:31, 1984.
4. Bauman WA, Spungen AM, Petry C, et al: The effects of functional electrical stimulation-induced lower extremity exercise training on total and regional lean tissue mass and on high density lipoprotein cholesterol, In Proceedings of the 38th Annual Meeting of the American Paraplegia Society. Las Vegas, 1992.
5. Bellamy R, Pitts FW, Stauffer ES: Respiratory complications in traumatic quadriplegia. J Neurosurg 39:596, 1973.
6. Bergofsky EE: Mechanism for respiratory insufficiency after cervical cord injury: A source of alveolar hypoventilation. Ann Intern Med 61:435, 1964.
7. Bierman EL: Atherosclerosis and other forms of arteriosclerosis, In Wilson JD, Braunwald E, Isselbacher KJ, et al (eds): Harrison's Principles of Internal Medicine, ed 12. McGraw-Hill, 1991, pp 992–1001.

8. Bockenek WL, Bach JR: Fibrocartilagenous emboli to the spinal cord. J Am Paraplegia Soc 13:18, 1990.

9. Brenes G, Dearwarter MS, Shapera, R, et al: High density lipoprotein cholesterol concentrations in physically active and sedentary spinal cord injured patients. Arch Phys Med Rehabil 67:445, 1986.

10. Chu DA, Ahln MD, Ragnarsson KT: Deep venous thrombosis: Diagnosis in spinal cord injured patients. Arch Phys Med Rehabil 66:365, 1985.

11. Cockcroft DW, Gault MH: Prediction of creatinine clearance from serum creatinine. Nephron 16:31, 1976.

12. Davey FD: Blood vessels and hemostasis, In Henry JB (ed): Clinical Diagnosis and Management by Laboratory Methods. Philadelphia, WB Saunders, 1979, pp 1109–1170.

13. Dee PM, Surratt PM, Bray ST, et al: Mucous plugging simulating pulmonary embolism in patients with quadriplegia. Chest 85:363, 1984.

14. Devivo MJ: Life Expectancy and Causes of Deaths in Persons with Spinal Cord Injuries. Birmingham, Research Update Medical Rehabilitation Research and Training Center, University of Alabama, 1990.

15. Fairsthter RD, Vaziri ND, Gordon S: Frequency and spectrum of pulmonary diseases in patients with chronic renal failure associated with spinal cord injury. Respiration 44:58, 1983.

16. Fishburn MJ, Marino RJ, Ditunno JF: Atelectasis and pneumonia in acute spinal cord injury. Arch Phys Med Rehabil 71:197, 1990.

17. Foley WD, Middleton WD, Lawson TL: Color-doppler ultrasound imaging of lower extremity venous disease. AJR 152:371, 1989.

18. Frisbie JH, Sarkarati M, Sharma GVRK, et al: Venous thrombosis and pulmonary embolism occurring at close intervals in spinal cord injury patients. Paraplegia 21:270, 1983.

19. Garner SH, Bloch R, Sutton JR: Heart rate response to facial immersion and apnea in quadriplegics. Arch Phys Med Rehabil 66:763, 1985.

20. Green D, Lee MY, Ito VY, et al: Fixed- vs adjusted-dose heparin in the prophylaxis of thromboembolism in spinal cord injury. JAMA 260:1255, 1988.

21. Green D, Lee MY, Lim AC, et al: Prevention of thromboembolism after spinal cord injury with low molecular weight heparin. Ann Intern Med 113:571, 1990.

22. Green D: Prophylaxis of thromboembolism in spinal cord injured patients. Chest 102:649S, 1992.

23. Gross D, Ladd HW, Riley EJ: The effect of training on strength and endurance of the diaphragm in quadriplegia. Am J Med 68:27, 1980.

24. Guttman L, Ranakel H: The value of intermittent catheterization in the early management of traumatic paraplegia and tetraplegia. Paraplegia 4:63, 1966.

25. Hall MA, Hackler RF, Zampieri TA, et al: Renal calculi in spinal cord injured patients: Association with reflux, bladder stones and Foley catheter drainage. Urology 34:126, 1989.

26. Hume M: Acute venous thrombosis, In Spittel JA (ed): Clinical Vascular Disease. Philadelphia, FA Davis, 1983, pp 121–131.

27. Hussey RW, Ha CYL: Renal transplantation in a patient with spinal cord injury (abstract). J Am Paraplegia Soc 13:93, 1990.

28. Jarrell BE, Posuniak E, Roberts J, et al: A new method of management using the Kim-Ray Greenfield filter for deep venous thrombosis and pulmonary embolism in spinal cord injury. Surg Gynecol Obstet 15:316, 1983.

29. Kim SW, Kim RC, Choi BH, et al: Non-traumatic ischemic myelopathy: A review of 25 cases. Paraplegia 26:262, 1988.

30. Kolb K: Pharmacokinetic and pharmacodynamic alterations in drug therapy caused by spinal cord injury. Phys Med Rehabil 1:375, 1987.

31. Krum H, Howes LG, Brown DJ, et al: Risk factors for cardiovascular disease in chronic spinal cord injury patients. Paraplegia 30:381, 1992.

32. Kunin CM: Blood pressure in patients with spinal cord injury. Arch Intern Med 127:285, 1971.

33. Lamid S, Ragalie GF, Welton K: Respirator-dependent quadriplegia: Problems during weaning period. Am J Paraplegia 8:33, 1985.

34. Lindsay J: Aortic dissection, In Spittel JA (ed): Clinical Vascular Disease. Philadelphia, FA Davis, 1983, p 108.

35. McCool FD, Brown R, Mayewski R, et al: Effects of posture on stimulated ventilation in quadriplegia. Am Rev Respir Dis 138:101, 1988.

36. McMichan JC, Michel L, Westbrook PR: Pulmonary function following traumatic quadriplegia. JAMA 243:528, 1980.

37. Merli GM: Management of deep vein thrombosis in spinal cord injury. Chest 102:652S, 1992.

38. Mirahmadi MK, Vaziri ND, Ghobadi M, et al: Survival on maintenance hemodialysis in patients with chronic renal failure. Paraplegia 20:43, 1982.

39. Mohler JL, Barton SD, Blouin RA, et al: The evaluation of creatinine clearance in spinal cord injury patients. J Urol 136:366, 1986.

40. Mohr DN, Ryu JH, Litin SC: Recent advances in the management of venous thromboembolism. Mayo Clin Proc 63:281, 1988.

41. Multicenter Trial Committee: Dihydroergotamine-heparin prophylaxis of postoperative deep vein thrombosis. JAMA 251:2960, 1984.

42. Myllynen P, Kammonen M, Rokkanen P, et al: Deep vein thrombosis and pulmonary embolism in patients with spinal cord injury: A comparison with nonparalyzed patients immobilized due to spinal fractures. J Trauma 25:541, 1985.

43. Myllynen P, Kammonen M, Rokkanen P, et al: The blood FVIIIag:FVIIIc ratio as an early indicator of deep vein thrombosis during post-traumatic immobilization. J Trauma 27:287, 1987.

44. Petäjä J, Myllynen P, Rokkanen MD, et al: Fibrinolysis and spinal cord injury. Acta Chir Scand 155:241, 1989.

45. Picano E: Stress echocardiography. Circulation 85:1604, 1992.

46. Piepmeier JM, Lehmann KB, Lane JG: Cardiovascular instability following acute cervical spinal cord trauma. J Neurotrauma 2:153, 1985.

47. Pierson DJ: Drugs used to improve pulmonary function, In Luce JM, Pierson DJ (eds): Critical Care Medicine. Philadelphia, WB Saunders, 1988, pp 247–255.

48. Pierson DJ: Endotracheal intubation, In Luce JM, Pierson DJ (eds): Critical Care Medicine. Philadelphia, WB Saunders, 1988, pp 204–210.

49. Pierson DJ: Supplemental oxygen therapy, In Luce JM, Pierson DJ (eds): Critical Care Medicine. Philadelphia, WB Saunders, 1988, pp 211–217.

50. Polatty RC, McElaney MA, Marcelino V: Pulmonary complications in the spinal cord injury patient. Phys Med Rehabil 1:353, 1987.

51. Raza M, Spungen AM, Zhang R: Thallium-201 myocardial imaging after dipyridamole infusion in subjects with quadriplegia (abstract). J Am Paraplegia Soc 16:51, 1993.

52. Schmitt JK, Adler RA: Endocrine metabolic consequences of spinal cord injury. Phys Med Rehabil 1:425, 1987.

53. Selwyn AP, Braunwald E: Ischemic heart disease, In Wilson JD, Braunwald E, Isselbacher KJ, et al (eds): Harrison's Principles of Internal Medicine, ed 12. McGraw-Hill, 1991, pp 964–971.

54. Simon RJ: Thrombosis of the inferior vena cava in a patient with spinal cord injury. Arch Phys Med Rehabil 68:178, 1987.

55. Smith B, Sica DA, Stacy W: Peritoneal dialysis in spinal cord injury. Nephron 44:245, 1980.

56. Sobel M, McNeil P, Hussey R, et al: Vascular surgery in the spinal cord injured patient (abstract 55), In Proceedings of the 36th Annual Meeting of the American Paraplegia Society. Las Vegas, 1990, p 32.

57. Spungen AM, Dicpinigaitis PV, Almenoff PL, et al: Pulmonary obstruction in individuals with cervical spinal cord lesions unmasked by bronchodilator administration. Paraplegia 31:404, 1993.

58. Stacy WK, Falls WF, Hussey RW: Chronic hemodialysis of spinal cord injury patients. J Am Paraplegia Soc 6:7, 1983.

59. Stacy WK, Midha M: The kidney in the spinal cord injury patient. Phys Med Rehabil 1:415, 1987.

60. Sumpio BE, Gusberg RJ: Aortic thrombosis with paraplegia: An unusual consequence of blunt abdominal trauma. J Vasc Surg 6:412, 1987.

61. Tikoff G, Marcelino M: Peripheral vascular disease in spinal cord injury patients. Phys Med Rehabil 1:457, 1987.

62. Tribe C, Silver JR: Renal Failure in Paraplegia (monograph). London, Pitman Medical, 1969, pp 54–90.

63. Vaziri ND: Long-term hemodialysis in end-stage renal disease associated with paraplegia. Int J Artif Organs 7:111, 1984.

64. Vaziri ND, Bruno A, Mirahmadi MK, et al: Features of residual renal function in end-stage renal failure associated with spinal cord injury. Int J Artif Organs 7:319, 1984.

65. Vaziri ND, Lopez G, Nikakhtar B, et al: Peritoneal dialysis in renal failure associated with spinal cord injury. J Am Paraplegia Soc 7:63, 1989.

66. Vaziri ND, Winer RL, Alikhani S, et al: Antithrombin deficiency in end-stage renal disease associated with paraplegia: Effect of hemodialysis. Arch Phys Med Rehabil 66:307, 1985.

67. Vaziri ND, Winer RL, Tohey J, et al: Intrinsic coagulation pathway in end-stage renal disease associated with spinal cord injury treated with hemodialysis. Int J Artif Organs 9:155, 1985.

68. Walker WC, Khokhar MS: Silent cardiac ischemic in cervical spinal cord injury: Case study. Arch Phys Med Rehabil 73:91, 1992.

69. Weingarden SI, Weingarden DS, Balen MD: Fever and thromboembolic disease in acute spinal cord injury. Paraplegia 26:35, 1988.

70. White RH, McGahan JP, Daschbach MM: Diagnosis of deep vein thrombosis using duplex ultrasound. Ann Intern Med 111:297, 1989.

71. Williams H: Hypertensive vascular disease, In Wilson JD, Braunwald E, Isselbacher KJ, et al (eds): Harrison's Principles of Internal Medicine, ed 12. McGraw-Hill, 1991, pp 1001–1015.

72. Yao JT: Deep vein thrombosis in spinal cord injured patients: Evaluation and assessment. Chest 102:645S, 1992.

73. Yekutiel M, Brooks ME, Ohry A, et al: The prevalence of hypertension, ischemic heart disease and diabetes in traumatic spinal cord injured patients and amputees. Paraplegia 27:58, 1989.

74. Zull D, Cydulka R: Acute paraplegia: A manifestation of aortic dissection. Am J Med 84:765, 1988.

CHAPTER 18

Spinal Cord Compression

Stephen G. Waxman, M.D., Ph.D.
Thomas N. Byrne, M.D.

Because spinal cord compression, if left untreated, can lead to paraplegia or quadriplegia, prompt diagnosis is mandatory. However, diagnosis can be difficult. This may be due in part to the fact that numerous etiologies exist, both neoplastic and nonneoplastic, for spinal cord compression. Table 18–1 lists some of these. The diagnosis of spinal cord compression can be further confounded by similarities between its clinical presentation and those of noncompressive myelopathies. For example, cervical spondylotic myelopathy, the most common cause of spinal cord compression, is usually characterized by a prolonged clinical history, frequently with remissions and exacerbations, and can be confused with neurodegenerative or demyelinating diseases. Alternatively, acute and subacute transverse myelitis, the prototype of intramedullary spinal cord disease, has a clinical presentation that frequently cannot be distinguished from that of neoplastic cord compression. Thus, in a series of patients initially suspected of having transverse myelitis, nearly 50% were found to have neoplastic cord compression.[1]

This chapter reviews only the most typical clinical presentations of spinal cord compression and emphasizes three of the most common causes, which can be considered prototypical disorders: cervical spondylotic myelopathy, metastatic epidural spinal cord compression, and epidural abscess. The reader is referred elsewhere for a comprehensive review of the subject.[2]

TABLE 18-1

SOME CAUSES OF SPINAL
CORD COMPRESSION

Spondylosis
Herniated intervertebral disk
Spinal stenosis
Metastatic neoplasms (epidural, intradural-
    extramedullary, intramedullary)
Primary neoplasms (epidural, intradural-extramedullary,
    intramedullary)
Abscess
Hematoma
Congenital deformities
Syringomyelia
Ankylosing spondylitis
Rheumatoid arthritis
Sarcoidosis
Paget's disease

CLINICAL PRESENTATION OF SPINAL CORD COMPRESSION

The four cardinal signs of spinal cord compression are pain, weakness, sensory loss, and autonomic disturbances.

Pain

Pain may be local, radicular, referred, or funicular. Local pain arises from injury to the vertebral column and surrounding tissues. It is usually aggravated by activity. Although a common early symptom, it is seen so often in clinical practice that clinicians may dismiss the importance of this finding. Radicular pain, which is often aggravated by Valsalva's maneuver, is typically associated with spinal root compression. During Valsalva's maneuver, Batson's plexus becomes engorged and the compressed contents of the spinal canal are further compromised. Nonradicular referred pain may be funicular in origin or referred from visceral sites, which is termed *referred pain*. Finally, pain with recumbency can be of special diagnostic significance because it is frequently seen in cases of neoplastic spinal cord compression, whereas musculoligamentous strain and pain due to

degenerative joint disease are typically alleviated by bed rest.

Motor Disorders

Motor disorders are second only to pain as the most common presenting manifestation of spinal cord compression. Weakness can occur in a lower motor neuron or upper motor neuron pattern. The location of upper motor neuron weakness does not always correspond to the expected pattern. For example, compressive lesions on the left side of the cord might be expected to cause pyramidal signs in the left leg before causing signs in the right leg. However, because of contrecoup injuries to the opposite side of the cord and vascular factors, this pattern of weakness may not occur. McAlhany and Netsky[3] found that regions of spinal ischemia and demyelination cannot be predicted on the basis of the location of the compression in relation to the cord.

The rate of evolution of weakness is not helpful in distinguishing between intramedullary and extramedullary lesions. While slow progressive weakness may be the rule, rapid deterioration in motor function has been reported in intramedullary tumors, extramedullary-intradural tumors, and extradural tumors.[4] Rapid decline in motor function may be a result of cord ischemia, edema, or hemorrhage.[5]

Elsberg[6] noted that weakness as a result of intramedullary tumors may characteristically spread in the limbs from a proximal to a distal location because of lamination of the corticospinal tract. Intramedullary lesions in the cervical region, such as gliomas or syringomyelia, may cause unilateral or bilateral arm paresis with sparing of lower extremity strength early in the course of disease[7] (*suspended area of weakness*). With the exception of foramen magnum tumors, extramedullary cervical neoplasms infrequently give a clinical picture of bilateral arm weakness with preservation of leg strength. Neoplasms of the foramen magnum are often characterized by unilateral arm weakness before progression to leg weakness occurs.[8]

Sensory Disturbances

Sensory disturbances may begin with subjective complaints of paresthesias. Isolated sensory loss in the absence of other complaints and other signs on examination is a rare presenting manifestation of either intramedullary or extramedullary spinal tumors. The pattern and evolution of sensory loss may be helpful in distinguishing between intramedullary and extramedullary tumors. For example, dissociated sensory loss (preservation of dorsal column function with loss of spinothalamic function), is considered characteristic of intramedullary lesions; however, extramedullary tumors have also been reported to cause this sensory pattern.[6]

Extramedullary compression is often manifested by an ascending sensory level, whereas intramedullary growths may cause a suspended sensory level that is most prominent at the level of the tumor. This phenomenon is due to the lamination of the spinothalamic tracts.[9] Because the fibers conducting sensory impulses from the caudal dermatomes are most posterolateral, and those mediating sensation from rostral regions are more anteromedial, extramedullary compressive lesions may initially injure the fibers that represent the caudal locations. From a diagnostic point of view, it is important to know that the level of compression may be higher than the sensory level. In some cases it is necessary to image the entire spine rostral to the clinically affected level to rule out a compressive lesion with certainty. Conversely, intramedullary growths involve the more medial fibers initially and later invade the more laterally placed pathways. Thus, intramedullary tumors may appear to cause a descending sensory loss.

Although these patterns of sensory loss may be of great diagnostic value, the evolution of sensory loss does not always follow these patterns. For example, if an intramedullary growth is eccentric it may give rise to an ascending sensory level rather than to a suspended sensory loss. Exceptions to the pattern of ascending sensory levels are found not infrequently with epidural tumors. Moreover, benign extramedullary tumors in the region of the foramen magnum frequently cause position sense loss that is more marked in the upper extremity than in the lower extremity ipsilateral to the tumor.[10] These examples of variability may result from the presence of coup and contrecoup injuries as demonstrated in a clinicopathological study of extramedullary spinal tumors described by McAlhaney and Netsky.[3]

Autonomic Disorders

Sphincter disturbances are considered unusual early manifestations of extramedullary and intramedullary masses, except when the conus or cauda equina is the site of involvement. In the large series of intramedullary tumors reported by Sloof and associates,[11] only 3% of patients manifested sphincter disturbances as the first symptom. Most authors report that sphincter disturbance occurs after motor and sensory disturbances are already present unless the lesion is in the region of the conus or cauda equina.[4]

Other autonomic symptoms generally do not provide help in distinguishing between intramedullary and extramedullary disorders, as they are found in both instances. For example, Horner's syndrome has been found to occur with both extramedullary and intramedullary growths.[4] The superior sulcus tumor as described by Pancoast is a common cause of Horner's syndrome.

CERVICAL SPONDYLOTIC MYELOPATHY

Cervical spondylotic myelopathy has been defined by Rowland[12] as "a condition in which the spinal cord is damaged, directly by traumatic compression or indirectly by arterial deprivation, venous stasis, or other consequences of the proliferative bony changes that characterize spondylosis."

Cervical spondylosis and cervical spondylotic myelopathy are extremely common. Radiographically, cervical spondylosis without neurologic complaints has been reported in 50% of individuals over the age of 50 years and in 75% of those over age 65 years.[13] Limitation of neck movement was found in 40%

of those older than 50 years. Furthermore, 60% had some neurologic sign referable to the cervical spondylosis. Cervical spondylotic myelopathy is the most frequent cause of myelopathy in the general population.[14]

The importance of the premorbid diameter of the cervical canal in the development of cervical spondylotic myelopathy has been recognized repeatedly. In a study of the anteroposterior dimension of the cervical spines of patients with myelopathy secondary to cervical spondylosis, Payne and Spillane[15] reported that the diameter of the spinal canal at the C4–7 levels was smaller in patients with myelopathy than in those without myelopathy. As the degenerating cervical disk narrowed, the resulting apposition of the vertebral bodies caused deformity of the uncovertebral joints and narrowing of the intervertebral foraminae, with formation of an osteophytic bar along the anterior spinal canal wall that presumably produced myelopathy.

In addition to anterior compression by osteophytes and disk material, the spinal cord may be compressed posteriorly by the ligamentum flavum when the neck is hyperextended. Thus, hyperextension of the neck may result in repeated trauma. The fact that the lower cervical spine is the most common location for cervical spondylosis may be a result of the extensive mobility at that level.

Controversy has surrounded the pathogenesis of cervical spondylotic myelopathy. The most important factors appear to be spinal canal size, impairment of blood supply to the spinal cord, and mechanical factors.[16] Although pathologic studies[17, 18] have supported the hypothesis that interference with the blood supply to the cord is the probable cause of spondylotic myelopathy, the temporal profile of cervical spondylotic myelopathy is unlike that of other ischemic disorders, and anterior spinal artery thrombosis has only rarely been verified pathologically.[19] Alternatively, mechanical compression of the cord during neck movement has been proposed.[16] This mechanical hypothesis may explain the exacerbation of symptoms encountered with flexion and extension of the cervical spine and the clinical improvement that is often seen following immobilization with a cervical collar. Exacerbation of symp-

toms and signs of myelopathy may also be seen with neck flexion.[20]

Clinical Features

Clinical features of cervical spondylotic radiculopathy and myelopathy are often present in the same patient. Symptoms may begin either in upper or lower extremities.

Pain in the neck, shoulder, and/or arm is a common presenting complaint and may be dermatomal or myotomal in distribution. Paresthesias and muscle weakness in the distribution of the affected nerve roots are often encountered. Reduction in the biceps (C5 and 6), brachioradialis (C5 and 6), or triceps (C7) reflexes may be seen. The depressed tendon reflexes may be associated with hyperactive reflexes caudal to the level of spondylosis when radiculopathy and myelopathy occur simultaneously.

Symptoms and signs of myelopathy include spasticity, weakness, sensory findings, and, later, bowel and bladder complaints. Although the patient may only complain of unilateral lower extremity symptoms, the neurologic examination usually reveals signs of bilateral disturbance of long tract function. Spasticity is an especially prominent sign, and "jumping legs" may be reported. Sensory complaints in the lower extremities are often not prominent. When sensory abnormalities are found in the lower extremities, vibratory sensation usually is more impaired than is position sense, and pain and temperature are typically unimpaired unless spinal damage is advanced. Lhermitte's sign also is often reported.[21]

Diagnostic Imaging Studies

With cervical spondylosis, plain x-rays of the cervical spine most frequently show narrowing of the intervertebral disk spaces, accompanied by narrowing of the spinal canal and/or the intervertebral foramina by adjacent osteophytes, and sclerosis of the vertebral end plates. Although a good correlation does not exist between the specific findings on plain x-ray films and the clinical manifestations,[22] it has been suggested that if the anteroposterior dimension of the canal is greater than 13 mm, then cord compression from spondylotic changes alone is unlikely.[23] Alternatively, since the findings suggestive of cervical spondylosis are so common on radiologic examination, a frequent clinical pitfall lies in erroneously attributing neurologic symptoms to spondylosis seen on x-ray in cases in which these radiologic findings are incidental and asymptomatic.

Computed tomography (CT) and magnetic resonance imaging (MRI) are used most frequently to image the spinal canal. Since cervical spondylosis most frequently occurs in the low cervical spine, CT is at a disadvantage, given the artifacts created by the shoulders. This has led to the use of MRI as the imaging modality of choice in many centers.[24, 25] When CT scanning is combined with intrathecal contrast agents, soft disk herniation may be differentiated from spondylosis.[25, 26]

Natural History and Therapy

Few studies are extant of the natural history of cervical spondylotic myelopathy. Lees and Turner[27] reported their findings on the long-term follow-up of 44 patients who had cervical spondylotic myelopathy when first seen at the neurology outpatient department. Only 8 patients underwent surgical intervention. These authors concluded that in most patients, cervical spondylotic myelopathy is a chronic disorder characterized by long periods of nonprogressive disability that are interrupted by shorter periods of exacerbation of myelopathy. Furthermore, they noted that disability and myelopathy may improve with conservative management alone. In a minority of patients, the course of cervical spondylotic myelopathy was characterized by progressive deterioration.

In another study of the long-term prognosis of cervical spondylotic myelopathy, Epstein and co-workers[28] found that among 114 nonsurgical patients culled from the literature, the condition of 36% improved, that of 38% remained stable, and that of 26% deteriorated. They found that when progressive my-

elopathy does occur, it may display a pattern of stepwise worsening interrupted by long periods of stability, improvement, or slow deterioration; when intervals of stability or improvement occur, they may last for many years. In other patients, deterioration may be slow and steady without remissions or stabilization. In another review, LaRocca[29] concluded that it is not possible to predict precisely the clinical course of an individual patient. This difficulty in prognosis jeopardizes the assessment of any therapy and leads to controversy in the management of cervical spondylotic myelopathy.

Management

Contemporary management of cervical spondylotic myelopathy includes nonsurgical and surgical approaches.[24] Surprisingly, surgical and nonsurgical treatment have never been compared in a prospective, controlled clinical trial. Recommendations regarding management need to be considered within this context and should be individualized. In patients without major deficits or signs of disease progression, a conservative approach, including rest, cervical traction, and stabilization of the neck with a collar, followed by physical therapy, is often successful. However, if the patient is moderately or severely disabled from progressive spondylotic myelopathy, surgery should be considered. Furthermore, surgery should also be considered if signs of progressive myelopathy develop or progress despite conservative management.[29] However, surgical complications also need to be recognized when considering this approach. Polkey[30] reported a mortality rate of 1.8% among 169 patients undergoing laminectomy for spondylosis and a 2% frequency of permanent neurologic worsening. Furthermore, among patients undergoing anterior decompression by corpectomy, Saunders and colleagues[31] reported a perioperative complication rate of 57% with a persistent sequela rate of 7.5%. Given the lack of evidence that surgery is superior to medical management and the enormous expense of surgical treatment (estimated to be $600,000,000 annually in the United States),

Rowland[12] called for a controlled clinical trial to compare surgical and nonsurgical treatments for cervical spondylotic myelopathy.

METASTATIC EPIDURAL SPINAL CORD COMPRESSION

Spinal neoplasms can be classified according to location, i.e., epidural, intradural-extramedullary (leptomeningeal), and intramedullary (Fig. 18–1). Although the histologic features of primary spinal tumors that occur in these locations reflect the tissues found in each of these sites, metastases from any primary tumor elsewhere may grow in epidural, leptomeningeal, or intramedullary locations. This chapter emphasizes the diagnosis and management of epidural metastases, given their far greater frequency and concomitant clinical importance.

Metastatic epidural spinal cord compression (MESCC) occurs in approximately 5% of patients who die of cancer.[32] It has been estimated that among the approximately 400,000 individuals dying of cancer annually in the United States, between 60,000 and 160,000 harbor spinal metastases and MESCC develops in 20,000.[2] Left untreated, MESCC ultimately leads to paraplegia and sphincter paralysis. Alternatively, if treated before neural injury occurs, most patients retain neurologic function.

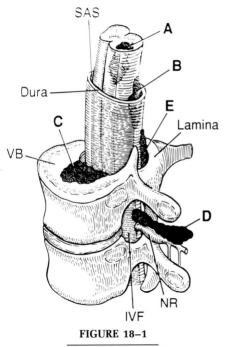

FIGURE 18–1

Anatomic locations of spine metastases. A, Intramedullary metastases are located within the spinal cord. B, Leptomeningeal metastases are located in the subarachnoid space and may be extramedullary and intradural. Epidural metastases arise from the extension of metastases located in the following adjacent structures: the vertebral column (C); the paravertebral spaces via the intervertebral foraminae (D); or, rarely, the epidural space itself (E). As epidural metastases grow they compress adjacent blood vessels, nerve roots, and spinal cord, resulting in local and referred pain, radiculopathy, and myelopathy. IVF = intervertebral foramen; NR = nerve root; SAS = subarachnoid space; VB = vertebral body. (From Byrne TN: Spinal cord compression from epidural metastases. N Engl J Med 327:614–619, 1992; with permission.)

Pathogenesis and Pathology

In approximately 85% of cases of MESCC,[33] metastasis begins in the vertebral column and extends into the epidural space to cause neural compression. Vertebral metastases have been reported to occur in 15% to 41%[2] of patients dying of malignancy. The high frequency of vertebral metastases is due both to hemodynamic factors and to the propitious environment of the bone marrow for growth of tumor cells. In the hemodynamic model, the metastatic cascade is based on the anatomy of the draining veins. Batson[34] showed in human cadavers a valveless system of veins in the epidural space that acts as a source of collateral circulation for veins draining the pelvic, abdominal, and thoracic cavities. In living primates, he demonstrated that the epidural plexus did not fill after injection of the dorsal vein of the penis unless the abdomen was compressed, mimicking a Valsalva maneuver. Batson hypothesized that in the human, this vertebral venous plexus of low intraluminal pressure could be filled by venous effluent draining from breast, intrathoracic, and intra-abdominal organs during coughing, sneezing, and straining.

Batson's hypothesis was confirmed by Coman and DeLong,[35] who injected cancer cells into the femoral veins of animals either with (experimental group) or without (control group) external abdominal pressure. Whereas in the control group only lung metastases were seen in the majority of animals, spine metastases occurred in the majority of animals in the experimental group. Alternatively, Arguello and co-workers[36] found that intracardiac injection of tumor cells in animals led to subchondral metastases in vertebral bodies, which they attributed to hematopoietic growth factors that have been shown to stimulate cancer cell growth in vitro.

MESCC arises from metastasis to one of three locations: the vertebrae (85% of cases); the paravertebral tissues (10% to 15% of cases); or, rarely, the epidural space itself. Compression of the spinal cord by tumor or, less frequently, by bone fragments occurs as tumor destroys the vertebra.

Approximately two-thirds of cases of MESCC due to lymphoma and pediatric neoplasms occur via extension into the vertebral canal through the intervertebral foramina. In such cases, plain x-ray films of the spine and radionuclide bone scan are usually negative.

Spinal cord pathologic characteristics in cases of MESCC include edema, demyelination, hemorrhage, and cystic necrosis. McAlhany and Netsky[3] undertook a clinicopathologic study of 19 tumor patients with extramedullary spinal cord compression. No correlation existed among the axial location of the neoplasm, the presenting clinical manifestations, and the pathologic findings that were present ipsilateral and/or contralateral to the mass. Hashizume and others[37] found "pencil-shaped softening" within the ventral portion of the posterior column of the cord at the level of epidural tumors that may extend over several segments of the spinal cord. This region corresponds to that involved in cases of venous infarction, but it is also considered a watershed zone for arterial circulation.[38]

MESCC is thoracic in approximately 70% of cases, cervical in 10%, and lumbar in 20%.[33] MESCC occurs at multiple noncontiguous levels in 10% to 38% of cases.[2]

Both circulatory disturbances and direct neural compression have been cited as causes of neurologic injury in MESCC. When carcinoma cells were injected into the epidural space in rats, vasogenic edema of the spinal cord was an early pathologic finding.[39] Furthermore, horseradish peroxidase, which is normally excluded from the spinal cord, entered the cord at the site of compression, which suggests a breakdown of the blood–spinal cord barrier as a cause of edema. The administration of corticosteroids caused a reduction of vasogenic edema, which paralleled improved neurologic function in the animals. Other studies have emphasized the possible role of prostaglandins in the evolution of compressive myelopathy.[40]

The most common primary tumors to cause MESCC are breast, lung, and prostate cancer, which constitute nearly 50% of all primary neoplasms. Other frequently occurring primary neoplasms include lymphoma, renal carcinoma, melanoma, multiple myeloma, and sarcoma.[33] Among children with MESCC, the most common primary tumors are sarcoma, neuroblastoma, and lymphoma[41] (Table 18–2).

Clinical Presentation

As with other causes of spinal cord compression, the major presenting clinical signs and symptoms of MESCC are pain, weakness, sensory loss, and autonomic disturbances. In approximately 95% of adults and 80% of children, progressive axial, referred, and/or radicular pain is the most common initial complaint in both vertebral metastatic disease and MESCC.[33, 41] A characteristic feature of pain resulting from MESCC is its frequent exacerbation by recumbency; this finding is highly atypical of other causes of spinal pain, such as degenerative joint disease.

Weakness is rarely the sole manifestation of MESCC. Only 2 of 130 patients in one series[33] had isolated weakness as the initial manifestation of cord compression (Table 18–3). Alternatively, at the time of diagnosis, subjective weakness was found in more than 76% and objective signs of weakness in 87% of patients.

Furthermore, sensory loss is rare as a sole presenting manifestation of MESCC (see Table 18–3). Caution is advised when attributing a sensory level to a lesion at that same level in the spine. As the somatotopically arranged spinothalamic tracts are progressively

TABLE 18–2

RELATIVE FREQUENCIES OF PRIMARY TUMORS CAUSING METASTATIC EPIDURAL SPINAL CORD COMPRESSION IN MALES AND FEMALES (%)

	STARK ET AL.[62]		BARRON ET AL.[32]	
	MALE	FEMALE	MALE	FEMALE
Lung	53	12	32	14
Breast	0	59	0	39
Prostate	8	NA*	8	NA*
Kidney	3	3	12	6
Myeloma	Excluded		8	6
Lymphoma	Excluded		20	9
Melanoma	0	1	—	—
Gastrointestinal tract	5	3	5	5
Female reproductive organs	NA*	6	NA*	6
Miscellaneous	31	16	15	15

From Byrne TN, Waxman SG: Spinal Cord Compression: Diagnosis and Principles of Treatment. Philadelphia, FA Davis, 1990.
* NA = not applicable.

compressed, an ascending sensory level may occur with MESCC. This has clinical implications, as a sensory level may mislead the examiner, and it underscores the need for radiographic examination of the entire spinal canal in patients with symptoms or signs of MESCC.

Finally, sphincter disturbances are rarely the sole presenting manifestation of MESCC unless the lesion is located at the conus medullaris or cauda equina.[33] At the time of diagnosis, however, sphincter disturbances are often present along with pain (see Table 18–3). Sphincter disturbance is a poor prognostic indicator for continued ambulation after therapy. Rare presentations of MESCC include Brown-Séquard syndrome, herpes zoster–like symptoms, and truncal ataxia.[33]

Cerebrospinal fluid (CSF) abnormalities with MESCC are nonspecific; typically, the protein content is elevated, the glucose level is normal, and, occasionally, a mild CSF pleocytosis is found.

Although not all investigators have had similar experiences, some report that lumbar puncture may result in neurologic deteriora-

tion in patients with extramedullary neoplasms. In a retrospective series, Hollis and co-workers[42] found that 14% of 50 patients had "significant neurological deterioration" after lumbar puncture. No deterioration was seen in patients undergoing myelography via a cervical (C1–2) puncture. The mechanism of neurologic deterioration in such patients is uncertain, but one hypothesis involves impaction of the spinal cord tumor, also known as "spinal coning." Despite these occasional reports, the quantitative risk is difficult to establish. For example, among several hundred patients from whom data were accumulated, no neurologic deterioration was reported after myelography in several series.[43] As there is no specific information to be gained from CSF analysis that assists in making a diagnosis of MESCC, a lumbar puncture should not be performed to "rule in or rule out" this diagnosis. If CSF analysis is indicated for diagnosis of infectious or neoplastic meningitis, close neurologic observation following lumbar puncture is mandatory and neurosurgical consultation may be necessary. Furthermore, although MRI may preclude the

TABLE 18–3

SIGNS AND SYMPTOMS OF METASTATIC
EPIDURAL COMPRESSION IN 130 PATIENTS

SIGN/SYMPTOM	FIRST SYMPTOM		SYMPTOMS AT DIAGNOSIS	
	NO.	%	NO.	%
Pain	125	96	125	96
Weakness	2	2	99	76
Autonomic dysfunction	0	0	74	57
Sensory complaints	0	0	66	51
Ataxia	2	2	4	3
Herpes zoster	0	0	3	2
Flexor spasms	0	0	2	1

From Gilbert RW, Kim JH, Posner JB: Epidural spinal cord compression from metastatic tumor: Diagnosis and treatment. Ann Neurol 3:40–51, 1978.

need for myelography in most patients, it is not readily available in many centers, and patients with pacemakers or claustrophobia are not candidates for MRI. In this setting, myelography should not be delayed or avoided if it is needed to confirm the diagnosis of MESCC and to plan therapy (see following).

Diagnostic Imaging Studies

The diagnostic imaging test of choice in evaluating patients for MESCC is MRI, performed in a timely fashion (Fig. 18–2). Carmody and co-workers[44] and Smoker and colleagues[45] have found unenhanced MRI to be equivalent to myelography in detecting MESCC and to be superior in detecting vertebral metastases and paravertebral masses. Alternatively, myelography should be performed when management is delayed by inability to schedule MRI in a timely fashion, in patients unable to undergo MRI (e.g., those with pacemakers or pain precluding recumbency) or when a technically adequate MRI cannot be obtained.

Sze and colleagues[46] have shown that contrast-enhanced MRI is superior to unenhanced studies for detecting leptomeningeal metastases and intramedullary tumors,[47] and

may provide additional information regarding epidural disease. Moreover, in cases of MESCC, regions of vertebral enhancement may correspond to areas of active tumor proliferation, and visualization may be useful for directing biopsies[47] (Fig. 18–3).

Clinical Approach to the Patient with Suspected Spinal Metastasis

Cancer patients with clinical evidence of spinal metastases fall into four groups: (1) patients with axial pain, normal neurologic examination findings, and abnormal plain radiographs; (2) patients with axial pain, normal neurologic examination findings, and normal radiographs; (3) patients with radiculopathy; and (4) patients with clinical manifestations of MESCC.

NECK/BACK PAIN, NORMAL NEUROLOGIC FINDINGS, AND POSITIVE PLAIN FILMS. The management of the cancer patient with neck or back pain, normal neurologic examination findings, and metastatic disease on conventional radiographs (which explains the pain) is controversial. While myelography or MRI to define radiotherapy ports is recommended by many authors,[48, 49] many physicians[50, 51] irradiate symptomatic vertebral metastases with-

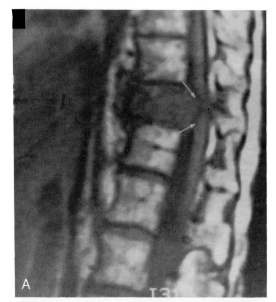

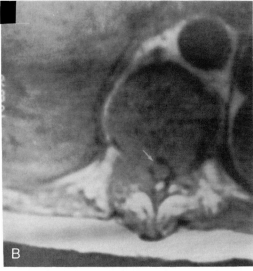

FIGURE 18–2

Nonenhanced magnetic resonance image of the thoracic spine in a patient with breast cancer, back pain, and gait difficulty. *A,* Sagittal image shows a T9 vertebral metastasis that extends into the spinal canal and compresses the spinal cord (*arrows*). *B,* Axial view through the T9 vertebral body shows tumor compressing the spinal cord (*arrow*). (From Byrne TN, Waxman SG: Spinal Cord Compression: Diagnosis and Principles of Treatment. Philadelphia, FA Davis, 1990.)

out further imaging. Arguments for and against definitive canal imaging have been discussed elsewhere.[43] Ultimately, if definitive canal imaging is not performed, a greater onus is placed on the physician, initially, to be confident of normal neurologic examina-tion findings and, subsequently, to be clini-cally vigilant to recognize early symptoms of MESCC.

PAIN, NORMAL NEUROLOGIC FINDINGS, AND NORMAL PLAIN FILMS. In cancer patients who experience unexplained axial or radicular pain, have normal neurologic examination findings, and have negative plain films, MRI of the involved region is indicated to distin-guish benign from malignant disease. If MRI is unavailable, CT and myelography should be considered.

RADICULOPATHY. The manifestations of rad-iculopathy include pain, weakness, sensory loss, and/or reflex loss in a single nerve root distribution. Since MESCC is present in a large proportion of cancer patients with radi-culopathy, MRI is indicated to identify adja-cent levels of vertebral metastases that could cause confounding referred or radicular pain and to define the extent of epidural tumor. If MRI is unavailable, CT and myelography should be considered.

CLINICAL MANIFESTATIONS OF MESCC. Cancer patients with mild, stable, or equivocal clini-cal manifestations of MESCC should undergo total spine MRI or myelography by the next day.[48] Patients with significant neurologic signs or rapidly progressive neurologic dete-rioration should be given intravenous corti-costeroids (see following) and undergo an im-mediate total spine MRI or myelography.

If the noncontrast spinal MRI is negative but clinical suspicion of a spinal tumor re-mains, contrast-enhanced MRI or myelogra-phy should be considered.

Therapy

Management of metastatic epidural com-pression usually consists of administration of corticosteroids and radiotherapy, but recent favorable results with anterior decompres-sion have renewed surgical interest.

Corticosteroids improve neurologic func-tion and alleviate pain acutely; they should be administered promptly to patients with clinical manifestations of metastatic epidural compression confirmed by diagnostic im-aging or when strong clinical suspicion exists but confirmation by diagnostic imaging is

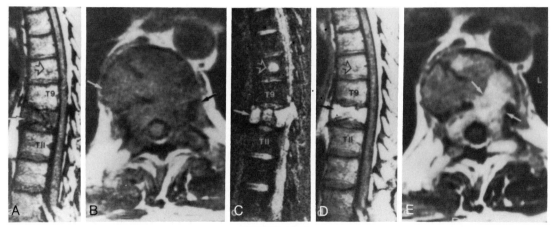

FIGURE 18–3

Thoracic spine magnetic resonance image of spine of patient with metastasis from plasmacytoma. Sagittal (A) and axial (B) images show partial collapse of T10 vertebral body and replacement of normal bone marrow with low-intensity tumor (*solid arrows*). A poorly defined hypointense focus in the T8 vertebral body is present (*open arrow*, A). C, Both lesions are seen on the T2-weighted images. After administration of gadolinium-DTPA, the T1-weighted sagittal (D) and axial (E) scans show enhancement of the T10 lesion (*solid arrows*), which extends into the spinal canal. In contrast, the T8 lesion is poorly seen due to the fact that it is isointense with the remainder of the vertebral body (*open arrow*). E, The axial scan shows more enhancement (*arrows*) on the left (L) than on the right side of the vertebral body. Although tumor may permeate the entire vertebral body, multiple biopsies on the right were negative, whereas biopsy of the enhanced region on the left revealed tumor. (From Sze G, Krol G, Zimmerman RD, et al: Gadolinium-DTPA: Malignant extradural spinal tumors. Radiology 167:217–223, 1988.)

pending.[52] The dose of dexamethasone, the corticosteroid reported to be used most often, remains controversial. While some authors recommend 4 mg four times daily,[52, 53] laboratory studies have shown a dose-related benefit with dexamethasone[39] leading to the clinical use of a loading dose of 100 mg followed by 24 mg four times daily.[48] We most often give 10 to 100 mg of dexamethasone in an immediate intravenous dose followed by 4 to 24 mg four times daily. The larger doses are reserved for patients with profound or rapidly progressive neurologic injury and the lower doses for those with mild or equivocal signs. Steroid administration is usually continued throughout radiation therapy at a tapering dose. One tapering schedule that has been useful in many patients is an approximately one-third reduction in dose every 3 to 4 days (e.g., from 16 to 12 to 8 mg). An increase in steroids followed by tapering may be attempted if initial tapering is not tolerated and neurologic deterioration occurs. The toxic effects of high-dose corticosteroids must be considered.

Several retrospective studies[33, 54] and one small prospective study[55] have failed to demonstrate a difference in neurologic outcome between radiotherapy vs. laminectomy followed by radiotherapy. Furthermore, laminectomy (removal of the posterior arch of the spinal canal) has been associated with a significant increase in morbidity, including spinal instability.[54] Thus, radiotherapy alone has become the primary definitive treatment in most cases of metastatic epidural compression.

Neurologic prognosis is primarily dependent on the level of neurologic function at the time of initiation of radiotherapy. The proportion of patients who are ambulatory following radiotherapy declines, respectively, from greater than 80%, to less than 50%, to less than 10% for patients who are ambulatory, paraparetic, and paraplegic at the initiation of treatment.[33, 54]

Since most cases of metastatic epidural compression begin as metastases to the vertebral body, it is the most common site for the initiation of cord compression. In carefully selected patients, the principle of relieving the compression of the spinal cord that results from the effects of metastatic epidural lesions by removing tumor or bone from the area of compression (rather than by just enlarging the spinal canal by laminectomy) has shown promise. This has led to the procedure of anterior decompression (vertebral body resection) and stabilization.[56, 57] Harrington[56] reported the neurologic outcome in 40 patients with major neurologic deficits preoperatively who underwent vertebral body resection followed by stabilization. Of these, 21 had complete neurologic recovery postoperatively. In addition, of 13 plegic patients, 7 had no neurologic deficit postoperatively. Harrington stressed, however, that many patients are too debilitated from underlying disease to undergo major surgery, even in the presence of vertebral collapse or instability with neurologic compromise, and he emphasized that the procedure is hazardous. Further studies comparing this procedure with radiotherapy are needed to determine the clinical and diagnostic imaging criteria that might be indications for surgery as initial therapy.

While many surgical indications still need to be defined, it has been suggested that surgery be considered in the following circumstances:[43, 48] (1) in patients without a diagnosis, (2) in patients who have previously had radiation at the affected site and whose neurologic conditions are deteriorating because of metastatic epidural compression, (3) in patients with progressive deterioration of neurologic condition during radiotherapy despite large doses of corticosteroids, and (4) in patients with symptomatic spinal instability or bone compression of neural structures. Surgery is also considered in patients with radiotherapy-resistant tumors and intractable pain.

EPIDURAL ABSCESS

Although spinal epidural abscess has been a rare condition, its frequency is increasing as the number of immunocompromised patients rises. Epidural infection occurs as a result of extension from adjacent osteomyelitis of the vertebral column or by hematogenous dissemination from a distant infection.

Early diagnosis and treatment are essential for a successful outcome in this disorder, which often responds favorably to early intervention. Patients with acute epidural abscesses often display other signs of acute infection, including tachycardia and fever. The patient with a chronic abscess, however, may appear to be generally well.

The clinical presentation of spinal epidural abscess includes local pain followed by radicular pain. Percussion tenderness over the spinal column, which is highly suggestive of epidural abscess, is not always present. Neurologic deficit ensues, leading to complete transverse myelopathy if not treated. The course often progresses through four stages: (1) local pain and tenderness; (2) radicular pain; (3) weakness and sphincter dysfunction; and (4) paraplegia or quadriplegia. The tempo of progression of clinical manifestations may be measured over several months or may evolve over days. The pathogenesis of neurologic dysfunction appears to involve cord compression, venous congestion, thrombosis, and infarction.[58]

The most common organism to be isolated is *Staphylococcus aureus*, which accounts for 44% to 71% of reported cases.[58] Identification of the causative organism requires culture of the abscess directly or isolation of the organism from blood, CSF, or a primary source elsewhere. The CSF usually shows signs of parameningeal infection, i.e., pleocytosis, elevated protein level, and normal glucose level. However, lumbar puncture is contraindicated if epidural abscess is suspected at the level of puncture, as puncture of the abscess can contaminate the CSF and lead to meningitis.

MRI usually provides excellent anatomic visualization of the vertebral body, disk space, and spinal canal. On T1-weighted images, the lesion is typically isointense or hypointense, and on T2-weighted images it is hyperintense. Following the administration of gadolinium, the lesion may enhance diffusely or at the periphery.[59, 60]

Mainstays of management of spinal epidural abscess have included surgical drainage and intravenous antibiotic therapy. With the advent of MRI, some clinicians have attempted to manage patients with few or no neurologic signs with the administration of antibiotics alone.[58, 61] This management is controversial. As discussed by Corboy and Price[58] and Wheeler and others,[61] unexpected sudden worsening in neurologic function has been reported in 19% of patients receiving intravenous antibiotics while awaiting surgical drainage. Thus, there is a risk in delaying surgical intervention. Furthermore, patients with epidural abscesses that compress the thecal sac appear to be at greatest risk for sudden unexpected deterioration of their neurologic condition. Patients in whom medical management alone has been successful are those with no or minimal neurologic dysfunction. Further studies are needed to define which cases can be managed safely with antibiotics alone.

REFERENCES

1. Ropper AH, Poskanzer DC: The prognosis of acute and subacute transverse myelopathy based on early signs and symptoms. Ann Neurol 4:51–59, 1978.
2. Byrne TN, Waxman SG: Spinal Cord Compression: Diagnosis and Principles of Treatment: Contemporary Neurology Series. Philadelphia, FA Davis, 1990.
3. McAlhany HJ, Netsky MG: Compression of the spinal cord by extramedullary neoplasms: A clinical and pathological study. J Neuropathol Exp Neurol 14:276–287, 1955.
4. Guidetti B, Fortuna A: Differential diagnosis of intramedullary and extramedullary tumors. In Vinken PJ, Bruyn GW (eds): Handbook of Clinical Neurology, vol 19. Amsterdam, Elsevier North-Holland, 1975, pp 51–75.
5. Kato A, Ushio Y, Hayakawa T, et al: Circulatory disturbance of the spinal cord with epidural neoplasm in rats. J Neurosurg 63:260–265, 1985.
6. Elsberg CA: Surgical Diseases of the Spinal Cord, Membranes and Nerve Root. New York, Hoeber, 1941.
7. Shenkin HA, Alpers BJ: Clinical and pathological features of gliomas of the spinal cord. Arch Neurol Psychiatry 52:87–105, 1944.
8. Stein B, Leeds NE, Taveras J, et al: Meningiomas of the foramen magnum. J Neurosurg 20:740–751, 1963.
9. Tilney F, Elsberg CA: Sensory disturbances in tumors of the cervical spinal cord: Arrangement of fibers in the sensory pathways. Arch Neurol Psychiatry 15:444–454, 1926.
10. Dodge HW, Love JG, Gottlieb CM: Benign tumors at the foramen magnum. J Neurosurg 13:603–617, 1956.
11. Sloof JL, Kernohan JW, MacCarty CS: Primary Intramedullary Tumors of the Spinal Cord and Filum Terminale. Philadelphia, WB Saunders, 1964.
12. Rowland L: Surgical treatment of cervical spondy-

lotic myelopathy: Time for a controlled trial. Neurology 42:5–13, 1992.
13. Pallis C, Jones AM, Spillane JD: Cervical spondylosis. Brain 77:274–289, 1954.
14. Adams RD, Victor M: Diseases of the spinal cord, peripheral nerve, and muscle. In Adams RD, Victor M (eds): Principles of Neurology, 5th ed. New York, McGraw-Hill, 1993, pp 1059–1290.
15. Payne EE, Spillane JD: Cervical spine: An anatomicopathological study of 70 specimens using a special technique with particular reference to the problem of cervical spondylosis. Brain 80:571–596, 1957.
16. Bohlman HH, Emery SE: The pathophysiology of cervical spondylosis and myelopathy. Spine 13:843–846, 1988.
17. Taylor AR: Vascular factors in the myelopathy associated with cervical spondylosis. Neurology 14:62–68, 1964.
18. Hughes JT: Pathology of the Spinal Cord. Philadelphia, WB Saunders, 1978.
19. Hughes JT, Brownell B: Cervical spondylosis complicated by anterior spinal artery thrombosis. Neurology 14:1073–1077, 1964.
20. Adams CBT, Logue V: Studies in cervical spondylotic myelopathy: II. Observations on the movement and contour of the cervical spine in relation to the neural complications of cervical spondylosis. Brain 94:569–586, 1971.
21. Vollmer T, Brass L, Waxman S: Lhermitte's sign in a patient with herpes zoster. J Neurol Sci 106:153–157, 1991.
22. Plum F, Olson ME: Myelitis and myelopathy. In Baker AB, Baker LH (eds): Clinical Neurology. Hagerstown, Md, Harper & Row, 1973, pp 1–52.
23. Brain WR, Wilkinson M: Cervical Spondylosis and Other Disorders of the Cervical Spine. London, Heinemann, 1967.
24. Saunders R, Bernini P (eds): Cervical Spondylotic Myelopathy. Boston, Blackwell Scientific Publications, 1992.
25. Kricun R, Kricun ME: Computed tomography. In Kricun ME (ed): Imaging Modalities in Spinal Disorders. Philadelphia, WB Saunders, 1988, pp 376–467.
26. Daniels DL, Grogan JP, Johansen JG, et al: Cervical radiculopathy: Computed tomography and myelography compared. Radiology 151:109–113, 1984.
27. Lees F, Turner JWA: Natural history and prognosis of cervical spondylosis. Br Med J 2:1607–1610, 1963.
28. Epstein JA, Janin Y, Carras R, et al: A comparative study of the treatment of cervical spondylotic myeloradiculopathy. Acta Neurochir 61:89–104, 1982.
29. LaRocca H: Cervical spondylotic myelopathy: Natural history. Spine 13:854–855, 1988.
30. Polkey C: Immediate effects of cervical and upper dorsal laminectomy. Proc Soc Br Neurosurg 47:106, 1984.
31. Saunders R, Bernini P, Shiffeffs T, et al: Central corpectomy for cervical spondylotic myelopathy: A consecutive series with long-term follow-up evaluation. J Neurosurg 74:163–170, 1991.
32. Barron KD, Hirano A, Araki S, et al: Experiences with metastatic neoplasms involving the spinal cord. Neurology 9:91–106, 1959.
33. Gilbert RW, Kim JH, Posner JB: Epidural spinal cord compression from metastatic tumor: Diagnosis and treatment. Ann Neurol 3:40–51, 1978.
34. Batson OV: The function of the vertebral veins and

their role in the spread of metastases. Ann Surg 112:138–148, 1940.

35. Coman DR, DeLong RP: The role of the vertebral venous system in the metastasis of cancer to the spinal column. Cancer 4:610–618, 1951.

36. Arguello F, Baggs RB, Duerst RE, et al: Pathogenesis of vertebral metastasis and epidural spinal cord compression. Cancer 65:98–106, 1990.

37. Hashizume Y, Iljima S, Kishimoto H, et al: Pencil-shaped softening of the spinal cord: Pathologic study in 12 cases. Acta Neuropathol 61:219–224, 1983.

38. Hughes JT: Venous infarction of the spinal cord. Neurology 21:794–800, 1971.

39. Ushio Y, Posner R, Posner JB, et al: Experimental spinal cord compression by epidural neoplasms. Neurology 27:422–429, 1977.

40. Siegal T, Siegal TZ, Sandbank U, et al: Experimental neoplastic spinal cord compression: Evoked potentials, edema, prostaglandins, and light and electron microscopy. Spine 12:440–448, 1987.

41. Lewis DW, Packer RJ, Raney B, et al: Incidence, presentation, and outcome of spinal cord disease in children with systemic cancer. Pediatrics 78:438–442, 1986.

42. Hollis PH, Malis LI, Zappulla RA: Neurological deterioration after lumbar puncture below complete spinal subarachnoid block. J Neurosurg 64:253–256, 1986.

43. Byrne TN: Spinal cord compression from epidural metastases. N Engl J Med 327:614–619, 1992.

44. Carmody RF, Yang PJ, Seeley GW, et al: Spinal cord compression due to metastatic disease: Diagnosis with MR imaging versus myelography. Radiology 173:225–229, 1989.

45. Smoker WRK, Godersky JC, Knutzon RK, et al: The role of MR imaging in evaluating metastatic spinal disease. AJR 149:1241–1248, 1987.

46. Sze G, Abramson A, Krol G, et al: Gadolinium-DTPA in the evaluation of intradural extramedullary spinal disease. AJNR 9:153–163, 1988.

47. Sze G, Krol G, Zimmerman D, et al: Intramedullary disease of the spine: Diagnosis using gadolinium-DTPA–enhanced MR imaging. AJNR 9:847–858, 1988.

48. Posner JB: Back pain and epidural spinal cord compression. Med Clin North Am 71:185–204, 1987.

49. Portenoy R, Lipton RB, Foley KM: Back pain in the cancer patient: An algorithm for the evaluation and management. Neurology 37:134–137, 1987.

50. Calkins AR, Olson MA, Ellis JH: Impact of myelography on the radiotherapeutic management of malignant spinal cord compression. Neurosurgery 19:614–616, 1986.

51. Rodichok LD, Ruckdeschel JC, Harper GR, et al: Early detection and treatment of spinal epidural metastases: The role of myelography. Ann Neurol 20:696–702, 1986.

52. Weissman DE: Glucocorticoid treatment for brain metastases and epidural spinal cord compression: A review. J Clin Oncol 6:543–551, 1988.

53. Vecht ChJ, Haaxma-Reiche H, Putten WLJV, et al: Initial bolus of conventional versus high-dose dexamethasone in metastatic spinal cord compression. Neurology 39:1255–1257, 1989.

54. Findlay GFG: Adverse effects of the management of malignant spinal cord compression. J Neurol Neurosurg Psychiatry 47:761–768, 1984.

55. Young RF, Post EM, King GA: Treatment of spinal epidural metastases: Randomized prospective comparison of laminectomy and radiotherapy. J Neurosurg 53:741–748, 1980.

56. Harrington KD: Anterior cord decompression and spinal stabilization for patients with metastatic lesions of the spine. J Neurosurg 61:107–117, 1984.

57. Siegal T, Siegal T: Surgical decompression of anterior and posterior malignant epidural tumors compressing the spinal cord: A prospective study. Neurosurgery 17:424–432, 1985.

58. Corboy J, Price R: Myelitis and toxic, inflammatory and infectious disorders. Curr Opin Neurol Neurosurg 6:564–570, 1993.

59. Nussbaum E, Rigamonti D, Standiford H, et al: Spinal epidural abscess: A report of 40 cases and review. Surg Neurol 38:225–231, 1992.

60. Kricun R, Shoemaker E, Chovanes G, et al: Epidural abscess of the cervical spine: MR findings in five cases. AJR 158:1145–1149, 1992.

61. Wheeler D, Keiser P, Rigamonti D, et al: Medical management of spinal epidural abscesses: Case report and review. Clin Infect Dis 15:22–27, 1992.

62. Stark RJ, Henson RA, Evans SJW: Spinal metastases: A retrospective survey from a general hospital. Brain 105:189–213, 1982.

63. Sze G, Krol G, Zimmerman RD, et al: Gadolinium-DTPA: Malignant extradural spinal tumors. Radiology 167:217–223, 1988.

CHAPTER 19

The Neurogenic Bowel

Walter E. Longo, M.D.
Anthony M. Vernava III, M.D.

The devastation of permanent injury to the spinal cord affects more than 20,000 persons each year.[1, 2] Other less common causes of acute myelopathy include multiple sclerosis, idiopathic transverse myelitis, spinal cord infarction, and extramedullary or intramedullary hemorrhage. The resulting neural impairment, whether it is quadriplegia, paraplegia, or significant paresis, results not only in a profound change in physiology, but also in lifestyle. Chronic constipation and a variety of gastrointestinal complications continue to plague individuals who have sustained any degree of spinal cord injury.[3] Fecal impaction is the most common gastrointestinal complication sustained by the patient with spinal cord injury and, along with fecal incontinence, remains a very costly and frustrating problem for both patient and physician. It is, therefore, imperative for the clinician to be familiar with bowel dysfunction in the spinal cord–impaired patient. This group of patients is often referred to the physician with regard to bowel management, or a consultation may be requested in the perioperative period when bowel dysfunction commonly occurs. Management of this problem requires an understanding of the alterations in the mechanisms regulating colorectal and anal function. It is the aim of this chapter to: (1) review the normal colorectal and anal physiology in the neurally intact human; (2) describe the altered colorectal and anal physiology in the spinal cord–injured patient; (3) discuss strategies for investigation of constipation and fecal incontinence in the spinal cord–injured patient; (4) discuss

331

therapeutic measures for constipation and fecal incontinence in the spinal cord–injured patient; and (5) review some of the commonly occurring gastrointestinal and anal diseases seen in patients with spinal cord injury.

NORMAL COLORECTAL PHYSIOLOGY

The intrinsic innervation of the large bowel consists of many nerve cell bodies and endings that lie between the circular and longitudinal muscle coats, and that have their cell body within the wall of the colon. The cell bodies of these neurons can be found in the submucosal ganglia (Meissner's plexus) and the myenteric ganglia (Auerbach's plexus).[4] Both of these groups of plexus are interconnected through interneurons and act as a single functional unit. The extrinsic innervation of the colon is accomplished by way of the autonomic nervous system; it is subdivided into sympathetic and parasympathetic divisions. The nerve supply closely follows the blood supply and pursues a different course to the right colon from that followed to the left colon and rectum.[5, 6] The sympathetic supply to the right colon originates in the lateral columns of the lower six thoracic segments of the spinal cord. These preganglionic fibers pass via white rami communicantes to the sympathetic chain and travel via thoracic splanchnic nerves to synapse at the celiac and superior mesenteric plexus. Postganglionic fibers are distributed along the superior mesenteric artery and its branches course to the small intestine and right colon. The sympathetic supply to the left colon and upper rectum commences in the lateral columns of the first three lumbar segments of the spinal cord and pass, via white rami communicantes, to the sympathetic chain. By way of the lumbar splanchnic nerves, it joins the preaortic plexus to synapse at the inferior mesenteric plexus. The postganglionic fibers travel via the inferior mesenteric artery to the left colon and upper rectum.[7, 8] The sympathetic supply to the lower rectum and anal canal originates from three roots, one from the aortic plexus and two from the lumbar splanchnic nerves. After uniting to form the hypogas-

tric plexus, the presacral nerve descends into the pelvis and bifurcates to form the two pelvic plexus. The postganglionic fibers supply the lower rectum and anal canal. Sympathetic stimulation results in a decrease in contractility and motility of the colon and in constriction of the internal anal sphincter.

The parasympathetic output to the colon and anorectum originates from the tenth cranial nerve nuclei in the medulla oblongata via the vagus nerve. The parasympathetic innervation to the right colon is carried by the posterior vagus nerve. These fibers pass through the celiac plexus to the preaortic and superior mesenteric plexus and follow the blood vessels to the small intestine and right colon to the level of the midtransverse colon. The parasympathetic innervation pathways to the left colon and anorectum arise from the sacral parasympathetic centers S2 through S5 within the spinal cord and travel along the presacral nerve to the inferior mesenteric plexus and are then distributed along the course of the inferior mesenteric artery. Parasympathetic stimulation results in increases in contractility, motility, and tone of the colon, and relaxation of the involuntary internal anal sphincter.[9]

The physiology of continence is complex, and the mechanisms involve both conscious and involuntary components.[5, 10, 11] Stool characteristics, propulsion in the distal bowel, reservoir function of the rectum, sensory mechanisms, rectosphincteric reflexes, anorectal angulation, and resistance from the anal canal must all be considered to understand the mechanisms of fecal continence and defecation.

The main functions of the rectum and anus are to preserve fecal continence; to distinguish between solids, liquids, and gas; to maintain nocturnal control; and to act as a reservoir so that defecation can be voluntarily deferred. Continence is a function of the left portion of the colon (water absorption), the rectum (reservoir), and the anus (high-pressure zone). Normally, the fecal mass does not pass beyond the rectosigmoid sphincter until the act of defecation occurs.[10] The anorectal angle, normally maintained at 80 degrees by the puborectalis sling, acts as a flap valve to occlude the anal canal. The involuntary and sphincter muscles generate a resting anal canal pressure that further occludes the anal canal. Accumulation of stool in the rectum causes distension of the rectal wall. This stretch provokes a reflex relaxation (negative inhibitory reflex) of the internal sphincter, allowing the rectal contents to descend into the anal canal. Increasing abdominal pressure assists the defecation reflex, resulting in evacuation of the rectum. Alternatively, if defecation is to be deferred continued voluntary constriction of the external sphincters is necessary until the negative inhibitory reflex subsides.[12-15] The rectum accommodates to its contents and to intrarectal pressure drops. Thus, defecation occurs by reflex evacuation of the rectum once increased rectal pressure incites the negative inhibitory reflex.

Fecal output differs markedly throughout the world because of differences in culture, diet, and psychosomatic factors.[16] Similarly, wide variations in fecal measurements and gastrointestinal transit times occur, not only between individuals but also on repeated measurements within the same individual.[17, 18] Stool consistency is probably the most important physical characteristic that influences fecal continence and is an important determinant of the ease of defecation. Stool frequency is the essential clinical parameter of stool output. Early epidemiologic surveys have shown that 95% of adult subjects pass between 3 and 21 bowel movements per week. Information concerning bowel habits obtained from more than 14,000 individuals chosen at random revealed that most persons defecate every day.[16-20]

The human large intestine has three functional regions. The cecum and ascending and transverse colon serves as a site for temporary stasis, absorption, and bacterial fermentation of contents. The distal colon has a function directed primarily to the formation, containment, and convenient evacuation of solid stools. The anorectal region acts as a site of temporary storage, programmed for convenient evacuation. Although the rectum plays a crucial role in voluntary defecation, it is not essential for continence.

The epithelium of the anal canal is profusely supplied with organized and free nerve endings that extend cranially from the anal margin to as far as the top of the columns of Morgagni. Voluntary sphincter contraction depends partly on sensory input from the anal canal; however, normal anal sensation is not essential for fecal continence. The major role of anal sensation appears to be to discriminate between flatus and feces and to indicate the necessity to begin or terminate defecation.[21]

ALTERED PHYSIOLOGY IN THE SPINAL CORD PATIENT

Spinal Shock

When the spinal cord is transected, a permanent loss of all voluntary and sensory function and a temporary loss of reflex function occurs in all segments below the lesion. The latter effect, called *spinal shock*, may last for 3 to 4 weeks. During the phase of spinal shock all motor, sensory, and reflex functions are lost. There is a loss of facilitation from above the lesion and a loss of inhibitory reflexes below the transection. In rat studies, motility of the distal colon significantly dropped after acute thoracic spinal cord transection.[22] The termination of spinal shock is heralded by an initial return to, followed by an exaggeration of, intestinal reflex activity.

Gastrocolic Reflex

In humans, eating a meal stimulates an increased level of colonic electromyographic activity. This response of the colon to food ingestion is generally called the *gastrocolic reflex*. The response of the colon is dependent on the caloric load of the meal, and fat appears to be the predominant determinant of this colonic response. The mechanism that mediates the gastrocolic reflex remains unknown; however, it seems likely that this response is non-neurally mediated and may depend on circulating humoral factors.[23-25] Connell and others[26] investigated alterations in motility of the pelvic colon in patients with clinically complete transverse spinal cord lesions. In these studies, food ingestion increased both the duration of colonic activity and the amplitude of colonic motility. This increase was similar to that observed in normal subjects. In contrast, studies by Glick and colleagues[27] failed to demonstrate any evidence of a gastrocolic reflex in nine patients with spinal cord injuries. One possible explanation for these discrepancies is that motility patterns were measured in different locations in these two studies. Connell and co-workers placed the recording tips at 15, 20, and 25 cm from the anus. Glick and colleagues placed the recording electrodes 12 and 18 cm from the anal verge. Thus, the first group was measuring largely sigmoid and rectosigmoid motility, whereas the second group was primarily measuring rectosigmoid and rectal motility. In any case, it seems likely that the gastrocolic reflex remains active in at least some patients with spinal cord injuries.

Alterations in Colorectal Compliance and Motility

Two studies have demonstrated decreased colonic compliance in patients with spinal cord injuries.[28, 29] In these studies, water at room temperature was perfused into the rectum at a constant rate. Changes in intraluminal pressure were measured. In both of these studies, intracolonic pressure in the spinal cord–injured patients increased rapidly to about 40 mm Hg with instillation of as little as 300 mL of water. In contrast, similar intracolonic pressure in normal subjects was achieved only with infusion of more than 2000 mL of water. This loss of compliance was attributed to the interruption of the inhibitory input to sigmoid motility from the central nervous system. Rectal compliance appears to be normal in spinal cord–injured patients. Frenckner[29] measured rectal compliance in eight patients with transverse lesions of the spinal cord and in eight normal subjects. Compliance was determined by inflation of a latex balloon in the rectum with graded volumes of air up to 300 mL. No difference in rectal pressures was noted between the spinal cord–injured patients and normal control subjects at any volume of inflation. These three studies indicate that rectal com-

pliance appears to be normal, but that sigmoid compliance is decreased in spinal cord patients.

In humans, the effect of spinal cord injury on the motility of the large bowel has shown that the decrease in transit time occurs mainly at the level of the left colon and rectum (hindgut). Connell and co-workers[30] studied 26 patients with a wide spectrum of spinal cord injuries. They found that the resting unstimulated motility of the sigmoid colon differed in patients with high-level spinal cord lesions when compared with both that of normal subjects and that of patients with low-level thoracolumbar spinal cord lesions. In patients with high-level cord transection with intact isolated cord below the lesion, resting colonic activity was reduced compared with that of normal subjects, whereas in patients with low-level cord lesions a significant increase in colonic motility was noted. It was postulated that an inhibitory center in the lumbar outflow exists, and that in patients with low-level spinal cord injuries this outflow is inhibited, resulting in increased sigmoid activity.

Alterations in the Anal Sphincter

Several subsequent studies have shown that resting anal pressures and the rectoanal inhibitory reflex in spinal cord patients are similar to those observed in normal subjects.[31, 32] These findings indicate that regulation of the internal sphincter is independent of cerebral nervous connections. The function of the striated component of the anal sphincter also has been studied in spinal cord–injured patients.[29] In eight patients with transverse injuries of the spinal cord, rectal distension with a balloon stimulated contraction of the striated sphincter muscles. Contractions of the striated muscles in spinal cord patients occurred less frequently and at greater volumes of inflation than in normal controls. In all of the spinal cord patients, the balloon was reflexively defecated after inflation. This did not occur in any of the normal control subjects, which indicates that spinal cord–injured patients lose the ability to delay reflex evacuation of the rectum by voluntarily increasing the activity of the striated muscles of the anal sphincter. Furthermore, this suggests that reflex contraction of the external sphincter after rectal distension is mediated by a spinal reflex arc and that cerebral centers participate in determining the magnitude of this response.

INVESTIGATION OF CONSTIPATION AND FECAL INCONTINENCE IN THE SPINAL CORD–INJURED PATIENT

Complete transection of the spinal cord is inevitably followed by constipation that is refractory to medical management.[33, 34] Several mechanisms may be involved in the pathogenesis of this constipation, including lack of sensation and of conscious urge to defecate, body immobilization, and motor paralysis of the abdominal and perineal muscles. Negligent performance of their bowel regimen or dehydration result in development of fecal impaction in many patients with spinal cord injury.

Fecal impaction should be suspected when the patient manifests unexplained constipation or diarrhea. Pain, fever, abdominal distension, nausea and vomiting, and autonomic hyperreflexia may also be present. At times, loops of fecally loaded bowel can be palpated and impacted feces are usually present in the rectum. The patient responds promptly to emergency decompression of the bowel with manual disimpaction and provocation of the defecation reflex. Once the rectum is evacuated, high colonic irrigations should be instituted. Vital signs should be monitored for autonomic hyperreflexia, which should be treated appropriately if it occurs. Stool should be checked for occult blood. The patient's standard bowel regimen should be reinstated. An oral cathartic regimen should also be instituted at that time.

If recurrent bouts of fecal impaction take place despite maximizing the patient's bowel program, the physician should be alerted to the possibility of a correctable cause of constipation other than the colonic inertia that occurs with spinal cord injury. Dietary and extracolonic causes should be sought before invasive testing is performed. In cases of refractory, continuous fecal impaction, it has been our policy to give the patient polyethylene glycol cathartic and to perform colonoscopy to eliminate the possibility of a nearly obstructing neoplasm. We combine colonoscopy with a barium enema to rule out the possibility of extrinsic compression or stricture from either diverticular disease or ischemia.

If a problem with the pelvic floor is a diagnostic possibility, anal mamometry, proctography, and electromyographic pudendal nerve latencies may be beneficial in excluding a rare, surgically correctable cause of chronic constipation related to the pelvic floor, such as internal procidentia. We subscribe to the algorithm proposed by Wexner and Jagelman for the workup of chronic constipation.[35] The ability to manipulate the pelvic floor in spinal cord–injured patients to improve the ability to evacuate is unknown. Rectal compliance appears to be normal in patients with spinal cord injury. The resting anal pressures are also similar to those observed in normal subjects. Although spinal cord–injured patients lose the ability to delay reflex evacuation as a result of denervation of the striated anal sphincter, many paraplegic patients use abdominal muscles to strain and aid in evacuation. Some of these patients may be experiencing a paradoxical action of the puborectalis, and may benefit from biofeedback.

Fecal continence depends on the resting tone of the anal sphincter and on the ability of the subject to contract the external sphincter in response to factors that threaten continence, such as increases in intra-abdominal pressure, rectal distension with feces, and rectal contraction. These responses are mediated by spinal reflexes because they are present in patients with complete spinal transection, but they appear to be greatly modulated by conscious mechanisms in normal subjects. Spinal disease or injury could result in incontinence by impairing these responses.

Anorectal pressures and sphincter responses to stimuli that would threaten fecal continence were studied in 20 patients with spinal disease, all of whom had fecal incontinence.[36] The patients were divided into subgroups according to the level of the spinal lesion. Patients with high-level spinal lesions had impaired rectal sensation and an impaired ability to consciously contract the external anal sphincter. In contrast, the external sphincter responses to rectal distension and increases in intra-abdominal pressure were present and often were much enhanced. This observation supports the contention that these responses are spinal reflexes and are heavily modulated by cortical influences. The impairments of conscious external sphincter contraction and rectal sensitivity were not as marked in patients with low-level spinal lesions. However, the external sphincter responses to increases in intra-abdominal pressure and rectal distension were either absent or altered, and most patients had anal leakage during these maneuvers. The low resting pressures in this group may be caused by reduced tonic sphincter activity. Patients with mixed lesions showed manometric features of both high- and low-level lesions; had the lowest basal, squeeze, and residual pressures; and showed an absence of external sphincter activity.

The results of this study show that patients with spinal diseases have a variety of abnormalities in anorectal function that could lead to fecal incontinence and that marked differences in function are present depending on the site of the lesion.

THERAPEUTIC MEASURES FOR SPINAL CORD–INJURED PATIENTS

Bowel Training

Immediately after injury, an adynamic ileus develops in patients with spinal cord injury. Consequently, oral intake of fluid is withheld initially, and intravenous fluids are administered. While the adynamic ileus persists, manual disimpaction of feces and enemas are required to evacuate the rectum. Once the stage of spinal shock passes and reflex activity returns, the patient is trained to evacuate the rectum by using the rectal reflexes. It is important to realize that not all patients need to have a bowel movement

every day; however, to avoid accidents, the entire sigmoid colon must be completely evacuated at regular intervals. The goal of bowel education is to establish routine defecation for the patient. By maintaining proper fecal consistency and by stimulating peristalsis at regular intervals, a conditioned reflex can be developed to ensure adequate fecal elimination for the patient at predictable times. The results of adequate bowel training are gratifying to both the patient and the physician. A well-established and controlled bowel regimen can help the patient to once again become a functional member of society.

Bowel training includes several important components. The patient should eat a well-balanced diet that includes adequate hydration and roughage. This serves to maintain a bulky, moist stool that can be evacuated more readily. A medical regimen for maintaining stool consistency with either fecal moistening agents or bulk-producing agents may be beneficial. In most patients, evacuation can be accomplished best in the morning, shortly after breakfast, because the meal induces a gastrocolic reflex. Increased colonic motor activity peaks about 30 minutes after eating. At initiation of bowel training in the spinal cord unit, a suppository is given every night for 2 weeks accompanied by digital stimulation. The suppository and digital stimulation cause reflex evacuation.

After 2 weeks the regimen is advanced to suppositories given every other day, at which time movements should be fairly regular, with no accidents occurring between administration of suppositories. According to the patient's ability to evacuate, bowel programs can often be advanced to a regimen of evacuation every third day. Digital stimulation of the anal canal serves both to manually disimpact the rectum and to relax the internal sphincter musculature by inciting a local reflex. Finally, the patient produces an increase in intra-abdominal pressure by massaging the abdomen firmly, attempting to follow the course of the large intestine with massaging motions. In some patients, additional stimulation of the rectum is required. Fleet enemas can be administered directly following breakfast. Because of the loss of voluntary control of the external sphincter, the patient with an injured spinal cord will find it difficult to retain the enema. Consequently, enemas are best instilled above the rectosigmoid junction.

It is important that the spinal cord–injured patient choose foods high in bulk and fiber, such as fruit, vegetables, and whole-grain breads. Spicy or greasy foods can cause diarrhea. In patients who have no fluid restriction, six to eight glasses of water should be drunk every day. Activity is important. Lack of activity can cause constipation. A regular pattern of evacuation avoids accidents. A bowel routine is best done on a commode chair, but can also be done on an absorbent bed pad. Meticulous skin cleansing is needed to prevent skin breakdown.

PROKINETIC AGENTS

Erythromycin

The macrolide antibiotic erythromycin has been shown to be a stimulant of gastric and small bowel motor activity.[37–41] Erythromycin mimics the effect of the gastrointestinal polypeptide motilin on gastrointestinal motility by binding to motilin receptors in the gastric antrum and proximal duodenum. The effect of erythromycin on gastric emptying was studied in 10 patients with insulin-dependent diabetes and gastroparesis. After the intravenous administration of 200 mg of erythromycin, the prolonged gastric-emptying time for both liquids and solids was shortened to normal. Motilin receptors have also been demonstrated in the colon. Erythromycin and motilin act on the same receptor, as evidenced by ^{125}I-motilin binding studies. Administration of erythromycin in healthy volunteers resulted in accelerated colonic transit and increased stool frequency. Erythromycin has been shown to improve ileus in two patients with Ogilvie's syndrome. In both patients, oral erythromycin (500 mg four times a day), resulted in the passing of flatus within 24 hours of erythromycin administration. Although reflex ileus after acute spinal cord injury has not been thought to be part of Ogilvie's syndrome, these conditions may be related in that both result from interference with normal extrinsic mechanisms that control colonic motility.

We have selectively administered oral erythromycin to spinal cord–injured patients with refractory constipation.

Cisapride

Cholinergic agents have been used in an attempt to overcome the lack of parasympathetic stimulation, but they are associated with significant side effects.[42–46] Cisapride has been described as a noncholinergic gastrointestinal motor stimulant that acts through increased release of acetylcholine in the intramural plexuses. Its prokinetic effects on gastrointestinal motility have been demonstrated in patients with motility disorders of the upper gastrointestinal tract. Its effect on fecal stasis caused by spinal cord injury have been relatively unknown. In one study, two patients with intractable constipation and an atonic bladder (due to a partial spinal cord lesion in one case and a sacral nerve lesion in the other) were treated with cisapride (10 mg, orally, four times a day). In both patients, daily spontaneous evacuation was achieved within a few days and was maitained for at least 40 months. The effect was dose-dependent. Normal bladder function was not achieved. In a similar report, treatment with cisapride (10 mg, orally, four times a day) combined with the administration of a suppository of bisacodyl in a patient with T11 paraplegia resulted in dramatic improvement in bowel evacuation. When use of the suppository was withdrawn, defecation became difficult. However, the combination of cisapride administration and bisacodyl suppositories was markedly better than the use of suppositories alone. These preliminary results justify further clinical trials of cisapride as a useful therapy of intractable constipation in patients with spinal cord injury.

OTHER MEASURES

Enema Continence Catheter

The enema continence catheter, designed by Shandling and Gilmour,[47] includes a latex catheter with balloon (used for administering barium enemas), an inflator, a length of tubing, and a plastic bag to hold the solution.[47-49] Thirty-one children with spinal cord impairment and their families were taught to administer a 20 mL/kg saline enema through this device. The children's bowel function was evaluated 18 and 20 months after the start of the program. The proportion of continent stools rose from 28% to 94%; the proportion of constipated stools dropped from 55% to 15%. The catheter was efficacious in 90% of the children in this study, which is similar to the 70% success rate seen by Walker and Webster,[49] who reported a 70% success rate with no complications. This procedure has inherent risks, such as allergic reaction to latex, electrolyte disturbances, bacteremia, and the potential for perforation of the rectum (as with any other enema). Nevertheless, the enema continence catheter may provide significant improvement in select patients, especially in the pediatric population. Randomized controlled studies of this device need to be performed.

Brindley Stimulator

The Brindley stimulator acts on the anterior roots of the sacral nerves S2, 3, and 4 and thus affects only the sacral parasympathetic outflow.[50-53] The effect of pelvic parasympathetic stimulation by the Brindley stimulator was investigated in 10 patients with severe constipation due to complete spinal cord injury; results were compared with those of 10 non–spinal cord–injured patients. In a third group of patients with spinal cord injury, a Brindley S2, 3, and 4 anterior sacral nerve root stimulator was implanted. Without the Brindley stimulator, the 10 spinal cord–injured patients had a prolonged oral–anal transit time, a diminished fecal water content, and a reduced frequency of defecation when compared with the 10 non–spinal cord–injured patients. Paraplegics with an implanted Brindley stimulator had a significant increase in frequency of defecation compared with the spinal cord–injured group that did not use the stimulator. The predominant effect of the Brindley stimulator is stimulation of left colonic motility and emptying of the distal colon. The right portion of the colon is unaf-

fected and allows for continued water absorption. This form of treatment of constipation of the spinal cord–injured patient requires the surgical implantation of this device and its inherent complications.

Colostomy

Colostomy has been advocated for treatment of chronic gastrointestinal effects of spinal cord injury such as incontinence, prolonged evacuation, megacolon, perineal ulcers, and rectal neoplasia. Stone and co-workers[54] reported the results in 20 patients who were treated with a colostomy for various complications of spinal cord injury.[54] None of the 19 living patients wished to have his or her colostomy reversed. Among patients with intractable constipation, quality of life was dramatically improved, and colostomy simplified bowel care, relieved abdominal distension, and was well tolerated. Stone and others[54] recommended that colonic transit time and anorectal manometry be performed preoperatively in these patients. Patients with normal colonic transit time and pelvic floor disorders can be treated with a sigmoid colostomy. Patients with prolonged left colon transit time are best served with a right transverse colostomy. Ileostomy is best reserved for a dilated nonfunctioning right colon.

The physician is called on to evaluate refractory constipation in the spinal cord–injured patient. Initial evaluation of these patients should be the same as that performed in able-bodied patients to uncover a potentially correctable cause of constipation, such as colorectal cancer or extracolonic pathologic lesions. Once the evaluation has been performed, a strict bowel regimen consisting of digital stimulation, suppositories, and an oral cathartic should be undertaken, with planned evacuation at a regular time each day. It is important to realize that a successful bowel regimen may be different and unique for each patient. Other measures, such as administration of prokinetic agents, use of mechanical stimulators, and creation of stomas, are reserved for patients in whom all other measures fail. It is quite rewarding to the patient and physician when bowel function no longer rules the life of the patient with spinal cord injury, who may now feel more like a functioning member of society. Refractory fecal incontinence, by and large, necessitates creation of a stoma.

GASTROINTESTINAL DISEASE

Acute Inflammatory Conditions

The thoracolumbar output of the spinal cord constitutes the motor, sensory, and autonomic nervous system for the abdomen and pelvis. The thoracic spinal cord below T6 innervates the abdominal wall and overlying skin. Pain from visceral inflammation is carried mostly by sympathetic nerve fibers to the lower half of the thoracic and upper lumbar cord.[55] The sacral parasympathetic system receives pain fibers from, and is responsible for the motility of, the left colon. The vagus nerve from the brain stem is responsible for movement in the right colon. Pain, often mild, may be experienced even by the patient with complete spinal cord transection. Many explanations for this phenomenon have been proposed. Accessory pain fibers may develop. Pain fibers may pass upward for several segments in the sympathetic ganglionic chain before entering the cord, thus bypassing the damaged level. The vagus nerve may, under certain circumstances, carry painful impulses from abdominal viscera.

Patients with neurologic impairment may appear to be chronically ill, malnourished, and febrile without any inflammatory visceral or anorectal disease. This, along with the fact that symptoms and findings may be absent when abdominal or anorectal sepsis is present, makes the diagnosis of acute inflammatory conditions of the colon and anorectum extremely difficult. Unnecessary surgery or delay in treatment resulting in death may occur from lack of understanding of how symptoms and signs of colorectal emergencies may be altered in the patient with spinal cord injury.

The manifestations of a colorectal emergency may be subtle. The patient senses that something is wrong, and he or she may detect an abnormality in the daily pattern of living. Loss of appetite and nausea, with or without vomiting, is usually present and is of recent onset. The patient may detect an increase in spasticity of the extremities or the urinary or anal sphincters, which results in urinary or fecal incontinence or autonomic dysreflexia.[56] The patient can be restless and sleepless or complain of tiredness and weakness. The pain is usually dull and deep-seated. If the pain is sharp, radicular, and bilateral, a neurologic lesion such as herpes zoster should be suspected. The pain from abdominal visceral inflammation may be sensed only at a referred site. Shoulder pain, for example, from diaphragmatic irritation may be the only symptom of an abdominal catastrophe. A spinal cord segment that supplies a viscus also innervates both the abdominal skin overlying the viscus and the distant skin areas that develop from the same embryonic segment as the viscus. The patient with a spinal cord lesion at T12 or below who has normal bowel and bladder function has intact sensation to the colon. He or she remains insensate to the anorectum.[57-60]

Temperature may be elevated in the presence of peritoneal or perineal inflammation.[61] Chronic urinary tract infection as a result of use of either indwelling urinary catheters or intermittent bladder catheterization may result in persistent low-grade fevers in the absence of visceral inflammation. A patient with an intra-abdominal emergency condition usually has a temperature of greater than 101°F. Temperatures greater than 103°F, especially of rapid onset, are usually indicative of urosepsis. The patient with poikilothermia from a cervical-level or high thoracic-level spinal injury may not ever manifest an elevated temperature.[62]

A newly recognized tachycardia may be the initial and only finding of visceral disease. An elevated heart rate accompanied by elevated blood pressure may be the signal of impending autonomic dysreflexia. Autonomic dysreflexia is characterized by bradycardia or tachycardia, hypertension, diaphoresis, and headache. It is the result of an outpouring of adrenergic activity as a result of visceral inflammation. Delay in recognizing the early signs of autonomic dysreflexia may lead to a delay in diagnosis. Diarrhea and incontinence are a result of stimulation of the reflex arc below the level of the spinal cord lesion, which results in increased visceral contraction.[63-66]

Abdominal findings are universally misleading. Abdominal distension is a normal finding in the patient with a spinal cord injury. However, the abdominal wall may be rigid in the absence of visceral inflammation or soft in the presence of peritonitis. In patients with cervical or high thoracic-level spinal cord lesions, the abdominal wall is extremely spastic and the abdominal viscera may not be able to be manually palpated. In patients with low thoracolumbar-level lesions, the abdominal wall is usually flaccid. Lumbosacral or cauda equina lesions do not affect the tone of the abdominal wall. Abdominal tenderness is not common in the patient with a spinal cord injury. If present, abdominal tenderness is abnormal, but its location cannot be reliably related to an intra-abdominal viscus. Spinal reflex sweating, in which the abdomen is drenched with sweat, may occur with visceral inflammation. Bowel sounds are usually hypoactive, even in the absence of visceral inflammation, and are often unreliable. Vomiting, although associated with either urinary, abdominal, or anorectal disease, may be an early sign of visceral inflammation.[67-69]

In addition to routine blood tests, urinalysis should be among the first group of diagnostic tests performed in the patient with suspected visceral inflammation to eliminate the possibility of urosepsis. Intravenous pyelography may be required to exclude nephrolithiasis. Retrograde cystography should be performed if a suspicion of urinary bladder rupture exists. Plain films of the abdomen often reveal dilated loops of bowel, which may represent a normal variant in many spinal cord patients. However, a thorough search for calcific densities about the urinary tract, air-fluid levels in the bowel, or free air should be undertaken. Free air is often the result of a perforated peptic ulcer. Appendicitis is the most common etiology of visceral inflammation in most series.[70-74]

Among 13 patients with colorectal disease whose cases have been reported from the West Haven Veterans Administration Medical Center,[75] the most common presenting symptoms were abdominal distension, vomiting, and constipation. Due to the nonspecific nature of the symptoms, the average delay in diagnosis of colorectal disease was 35.8 hours. An 84% morbidity and 22% mortality were observed. The study indicated that any deviation from the normal lifestyle of the spinal cord patient should alert the physician to the possibility of visceral inflammation. The authors concluded that close attention to the signs of autonomic dysreflexia or changes in spasticity, along with a thorough evaluation of the ill-appearing spinal cord–injured patient, may uncover occult colon or anorectal disease.

Intraoperatively, spinal cord–injured patients may experience a drop in blood pressure on induction of anesthesia as a result of lack of central neuroregulatory mechanisms. Abdominal wound closure should employ retention sutures to counteract the increased wound tension that occurs from abdominal spasticity. Postoperatively, the surgeon should be aware of hypertension, decreased pulmonary excursion, urinary tract infections, and prolonged ileus.

GASTROINTESTINAL HEMORRHAGE

It is not uncommon for the spinal cord–injured patient to be referred for evaluation of unexplained gastrointestinal hemorrhage, most commonly from a source in the upper gastrointestinal tract (e.g., peptic ulcer disease). The workup of these patients should be the same as for able-bodied individuals and should include the judicious use of endoscopy, upper and lower nuclear medicine scans, and, when indicated, arteriography. In the elderly patient, diverticular bleeding, angiodysplasia, and colorectal neoplasia should be sought. Because spinal cord–injured patients perform daily manipulation of the anorectum for bowel management, an anorectal source of bleeding needs to be evaluated by inspection, anoscopy, and proctoscopy. The finding of a potential anorectal source, however, should not preclude examination of the remainder of the large bowel when indicated. Clotting studies should be performed, and any coagulopathy should be corrected.

Early, definitive management of gastrointestinal hemorrhage is of paramount importance in the spinal cord–injured patient. In patients with borderline renal function owing to chronic renal infections, massive blood loss and replacement are not well tolerated; this has been borne out by results of previous studies. Furthermore, when arteriography is contemplated, special consideration must be made. Spinal cord–injured patients with gastrointestinal hemorrhage should be given treatment similar to that of able-bodied patients.

LARGE BOWEL OBSTRUCTION

Fecal Impaction

Fecal impaction is the most common gastrointestinal complication in spinal cord–injured patients, who suffer routinely from chronic constipation. Intestinal obstruction induces hyperactivity of bowel sounds, and continued distension may trigger autonomic dysreflexia. In the patient with suspected intestinal obstruction, digital examination should be performed initially to detect the possible presence of impacted stool in the rectal vault. If fecal impaction is found, manual disimpaction should be performed promptly. This is usually followed by immediate decompression of the rectosigmoid colon and relief of the obstruction. The abdomen should be inspected for surgical scars and the groin should be palpated for inguinal or femoral hernias. If fecal impaction is not detected, a plain film of the abdomen should be obtained. Volvulus of either the small or large intestine should be looked for.

Sigmoid Volvulus

Sigmoid volvulus is a common cause of intestinal obstruction in any group of patients who suffer from chronic constipation. This presumably results from the development of a long, redundant, atonic colon.[76] Six previous cases of sigmoid volvulus in paralyzed patients have been reported. Two other cases of intestinal volvulus, one involving the colon in an unspecified area and one involving the ileum and cecum, have also been reported.

Colorectal Neoplasia

Spinal cord–injured patients are at the same risk for development of colorectal neoplasia as their able-bodied counterparts. In any patient with refractory constipation, especially one older than 35 years or one at risk for the development of colorectal cancer, a screening procedure to evaluate the large bowel should be performed. Colonoscopy is not without its complications in patients with spinal cord injury, as the lack of visceral sensation and the inablity to perceive pain adequately could result in inadvertent perforation. Among four spinal cord–injured patients with a perforated viscus whose cases were reported by Charney and colleagues,[66] one experienced a rectosigmoid perforation secondary to colonoscopy. A contrast enema could prove to be an inadequate study if the patient is unable to retain the barium after instillation into the rectum. One spinal cord–injured patient reported to have a large bowel tumor presented with a perforated rectal carcinoma requiring proctectomy and multiple procedures for persistent pelvic sepsis. He had a long history of chronic constipation, and further evaluation had been neglected despite recurrent bouts of fecal impaction. Proctosigmoidoscopy and, when indicated, colonoscopy should be performed for detection of early colorectal neoplasia.

ANORECTAL DISEASE

Anorectal complaints in the spinal cord–injured patient are similar to those suffered by the remainder of the population. Prolapsing hemorrhoids are a common complaint in patients with spinal cord injury. Cosman et al[77] have speculated that hemorrhoidal bleeding occurs in 75% of persons with chronic spinal cord injury, and that hemorrhoidal bleeding occurs at or distal to the dentate line as a result of methods used to stimulate reflex defecation. In results of multiple banding procedures in 62 men with chronic spinal cord injury, 73% reported a significant reduction in bleeding postbanding, 20% reported a moderate reduction, and 3% reported increased bleeding. Although autonomic dysreflexia was seen in 14% of patients, no patients required readmission or treatment for hemorrhage, infection, or stricture. The authors concluded that multiple banding is a safe and effective treatment for hemorrhoidal bleeding in patients with chronic spinal cord injury. Absent anal sensation allows banding of external hemorrhoids, although symptoms of autonomic dysreflexia may occur.

In the spinal cord–injured patient, occult anorectal sepsis should be sought in the patient with evidence of a clinical illness but no clear etiology. Perforation of the rectum, retained foreign bodies, and anorectal abscess, with or without fistula in ano, may be the result of daily anorectal manipulation. This manipulation sometimes includes digital stimulation, placement of suppositories, or self-administration of enemas. Pelvic sepsis can result from rectal perforation secondary to fecal impaction or a perforated rectal neoplasm.

REFERENCES

1. Bedbrook GM, Sedgley GI: The management of spinal injuries—Past and present. Int Rehabil Med 2:45–61, 1980.
2. Michaels LS: Epidemiology of spinal cord injury. In Vinken PJ, Bruyn GW (eds): Handbook of Clinical Neurology. Amsterdam, Elsevier North Holland, 25:141–143, 1976.
3. Gore RM, Mintzer RA, Calenoff L: Gastrointestinal complications of spinal cord injury. Spine 6:538–544, 1980.
4. Cooke HJ: Neurobiology of the intestinal mucosa. Gastroenterology 90:1057–1081, 1986.
5. Goligher JC, Hughes ES: Sensibility of the rectum and colon: Its role in the maintenance of anal continence. Lancet 1:543–547, 1951.
6. Goligher J: Surgery of the anus, rectum and colon. London, Bailliere Tindal, 1984, pp 1–47.
7. Telford ED, Stopford JS: The autonomic nerve supply of the distal colon: An anatomical and clinical study. Br Med J 1:572–574, 1934.
8. Davis AA: The presacral nerve. Br Med J 2:1–6, 1934.
9. Longo WE, Ballantyne GH, Modlin IM: The colon, anorectum and spinal cord patient: A review of the functional alterations of the denervated hindgut. Dis Colon Rectum 32:261–267, 1989.
10. Connell AM: The motility of the pelvic colon: Motility in normals and in patients with asymptomatic duodenal ulcer. Gut 2:75–86, 1961.
11. Ballantyne GH: Rectosigmoid sphincter of O'Beirne. Dis Colon Rectum 29:525–531, 1986.
12. Parks AG: Anorectal incontinence. Proc R Soc Med 68:681–690, 1975.
13. Denny-Brown D, Robertson G: An investigation of the nervous control of defecation. Brain 58:256–310, 1935.
14. Schuster MM: The riddle of the sphincters. Gastroenterology 69:249–262, 1975.
15. Duthie HL: Dynamics of the rectum and anus. Clin Gastroenterol 4:467–471, 1975.
16. Davies GJ, Crowder M, Reid B, et al: Bowel function measurements of individuals with different eating patterns. Gut 27:164–169, 1986.
17. Everhart JE, Go VL, Johannes RS, et al: A longitudinal survey of self-reported bowel habits in the United States. Dig Dis Sci 34:1153–1162, 1989.
18. Wyman JB, Heaton KW, Manning AP, et al: Variability of colonic function in healthy subjects. Gut 19:146–150, 1978.
19. Rendtorff RC, Kashgarian M: Stool patterns of healthy adult males. Dis Colon Rectum 10:222–228, 1967.
20. Phillips SF, Devroede G: Functions of the large intestine. In Crane RK (ed): International Review of Physiology, Gastrointestinal Physiology, III. Baltimore, University Park Press, 1979, pp 263–291.
21. Devroede G: Defecation and continence. In Phillips SF, Pemberton JH, Shorter RG (eds): The Large Intestine: Physiology, Pathophysiology and Disease. New York, Raven Press, 1991.
22. Meshkinpour H, Harmon D, Thompson R, et al: Effects of thoracic spinal cord transection on colonic motor activity in rats. Paraplegia 23:272–276, 1985.
23. Holdstock DJ, Misiewicz JJ: Factors controlling colonic motility: Colonic pressures and transit after meals in patients with total gastrectomy, pernicious anaemia or duodenal ulcer. Gut 11:100–110, 1970.
24. Wright SH, Snape WJ Jr, Battle W, et al: Effect of dietary components on gastrocolonic response. Am J Physiol 238 (Gastrointest Liver Physiol):G228–G232, 1980.
25. Snape WJ Jr, Wright SH, Cohen S, et al: The gastrocolonic response: Evidence for a neural mechanism—neural versus hormonal mediation. Gastroenterology 77:1235–1240, 1979.
26. Connell AM, Jones FA, Rowlands EN: Motility of the pelvic colon: IV. Abdominal pain associated with colonic hypermotility after meals. Gut 6:105–112, 1965.
27. Glick ME, Meshkinpour H, Haldeman S, et al: Colonic dysfunction in patients with thoracic spinal cord injury. Gastroenterology 86:287–294, 1984.
28. Meshkinpour H, Nowroozi F, Glick ME: Colonic compliance in patients with spinal cord injury. Arch Phys Med Rehabil 64:111–112, 1983.
29. Freckner B: Function of the anal sphincters in spinal man. Gut 16:638–644, 1975.
30. Connell AM, Frankel H, Guttman L: The motility of the pelvic colon following complete lesions of the spinal cord. Paraplegia 1:98–115, 1963.
31. Denny-Brown D, Robertson G: An investigation of the nervous control of defecation. Brain 58:256–310, 1935.

32. Schuster MM, Hendrix TR, Mendeloff AL: The internal anal sphincter response: Manometric studies on its normal physiology, neural pathways, and alterations in bowel disorders. J Clin Invest 42:190–207, 1963.

33. Menardo G, Bausano G, Corazziari E, et al: Large bowel transit in paraplegic patients. Dis Colon Rectum 30:924–928, 1987.

34. Schuster MM, Hendrix TR, Mendeloff AI: The internal anal sphincter response: Manometric studies on its normal physiology, neural pathways, and alterations in bowel disorders. J Clin Invest 42:196–207, 1963.

35. Wexner SD, Jagelman DG: Chronic constipation. Postgrad Adv Colorectal Surg, 1:1–22, 1989.

36. Sun WM, Read NW, Donnelly TC: Anorectal function in incontinent patients with cerebrospinal disease. Gastroenterology 99:1372–1379, 1990.

37. Inatomi I, Satoh H, Maki Y, et al: An erythromycin derivative EM-523, induces motilin-like gastrointestinal motility in dogs. J Pharmacol Exp Ther 251:707–712, 1989.

38. Tomomasa T, Kuroume T, Arai H, et al: Erythromycin induces migrating motor complex in human gastrointestinal tract. Dig Dis Sci 31:157–161, 1986.

39. Janssens J, Peeters TL, Van Trappen G, et al: Improvement of gastric emptying diabetic gastroparesis by erythromycin: Preliminary studies. N Engl J Med 322:1028–1031, 1990.

40. Hasler W, Heldsinger A, Soudah H, et al: Erythromycin promotes colonic transit in humans: Mediation via motilin receptors. Gastroenterology 98:A358, 1990.

41. Armstrong DN, Ballantyne GH, Modlin IM: Erythromycin for reflex ileus in Ogilvie's syndrome. Lancet 337:378, 1991.

42. Reyntjens A, Verlinden M, Schuurkes J, et al: New approach to gastrointestinal motor dysfunction: Non-anti-dopaminergic, non-cholinergic stimulation with cisapride. Curr Ther Res 36:1029–1037, 1984.

43. Jian R, Ducrot F, Piepeloup C, et al: Measurements of gastric emptying in dyspeptic patients: Effect of a new gastrokinetic agent (cisapride). Gut 25:325–358, 1985.

44. Smout AJPM, Bogaard JW, Grade AC, et al: Effects of cisapride, a new gastrointestinal prokinetic substance, on inter-digestive and postprandial motor activity of the distal esophagus in man. Gut 26:246–259, 1985.

45. deGroot GH, dePaster GF: Effects of cisapride on constipation due to a neurological lesion. Paraplegia 26:159–161, 1988.

46. Etienne M, Verlinden M, Brassinne A: Treatment with cisapride of the gastrointestinal and urologic sequelae of spinal cord transection: Case report. Paraplegia 26:162–164, 1988.

47. Shandling B, Gilmour RF: The enema continence catheter in spina bifida: Successful bowel management. J Pediatr Surg 22:271–273, 1987.

48. Liptak GS, Revell GM: Management of bowel dysfunction in children with spinal cord disease or injury by means of the enema continence catheter. J Pediatr 120:190–194, 1992.

49. Walker J, Webster P: Successful management of fecal incontinence using the enema continence catheter. Z Kinderchir 42(suppl 1):43–45, 1987.

50. Brindley GS, Polkey CE, Rusthton DN: Sacral anterior root stimulators for bladder control in paraplegia. Paraplegia 20:365–381, 1982.

51. Brindley GS: An implant to empty the bladder or close the urethra. J Neurol Neurosurg Psychiatry 40:358–369, 1977.

52. Binnie NR, Smith AN, Creasey GH, et al: Constipation associated with chronic spinal cord injury: The effect of pelvic parasympathetic stimulation by the Brindley stimulator. Paraplegia 29:463–469, 1991.

53. Varma JS, Binnie NR, Smith AN, et al: Differential effects of sacral anterior root stimulation on anal sphincter and colorectal motility in spinally injured man. Br J Surg 73:478–482, 1986.

54. Stone JM, Wolfe VA, Nino-Murcia M, et al: Colostomy as treatment for complications of spinal cord injury. Arch Phys Med Rehabil 71:514–518, 1990.

55. Juler GL: Acute abdominal emergencies in spinal cord injured patients. J Am Paraplegia Soc 2:1–5, 1979.

56. McGuire TJ, Kumar VH: Autonomic dysreflexia in the spinal cord injured patient. Postgrad Med 80:81–89, 1986.

57. Guttman L: Spinal Cord Injuries, Comprehensive Management and Research, ed 2. Oxford, Blackwell Scientific Publications, 1976.

58. Guttman L: Clinical symptomatology of spinal cord lesions. In Vinken PJ, Bruyn GW (eds): Handbook of Clinical Neurology: vol 2. Localization in Clinical Neurology. New York, Elsevier, 1969, p 178.

59. Pollock LJ, Boshes B, Brown M, et al: Relation of recovery of sensation to intraspinal pathways in injuries of the spinal cord. Arch Neurol Psychiatry 70:137, 1953.

60. Hutchinson J: Temperature and circulation after crushing the cervical cord. Lancet 1:713, 1975.

61. Sugarman B: Fever in recently injured quadriplegic persons. Arch Phys Med Rehabil 63:639–640, 1982.

62. Sipski ML, Hendler S, Delisa JA: Rehabilitation of patients with spinal cord disease. Neurology Clin 9:705–726, 1991.

63. Inberg HO, Prust FW: The diagnosis of abdominal emergencies in patients with spinal cord lesions. Arch Phys Med Rehabil 49:343–349, 1968.

64. Greenfield J: Abdominal operations on patients with chronic paraplegia. Arch Surg 59:1077–1087, 1949.

65. Miller LS, Staas WE, Herbison GJ: Abdominal problems in patients with spinal cord injuries. Arch Phys Med Rehabil 56:405–408, 1975.

66. Charney KF, Juler GL, Comarr AE: General surgery problems in patients with spinal cord injury. Arch Surg 110:1083–1088, 1975.

67. Juler GL, Eltora IM: The acute abdomen in spinal cord patients. Paraplegia 23:118–123, 1985.

68. Sugarman B, Brown D, Musher D: Fever and infection in spinal cord patients. JAMA 248:66–70, 1982.

69. Hoen T, Cooper I: Acute abdominal emergencies in paraplegics. Am J Surg 75:19–24, 1948.

70. Fast A: Reflex sweating in patients with spinal cord injury—A review. Arch Phys Med Rehabil 58:435–437, 1977.

71. Nyquist R: Mortality in spinal cord injuries. Proceedings of the Ninth Annual Clinical Spinal Cord Injuries Conference, Oct. 18–20, 1960, pp 109–112.

72. Dietrick R, Russi S: Tabulation and review of autopsy findings in 55 paraplegics. JAMA 166:41–44, 1958.

73. Tibbs PA, Bivins BA, Young B: The problem of acute abdominal disease during spinal shock. Am Surg 45:366–368, 1979.

74. Stone JM, Murcia MN, Wolfe VA, et al: Chronic gastrointestinal problems in spinal cord injury patients: A prospective analysis. Am J Gastroenterol 85:1114–1119, 1990.

75. Longo WE, Ballantyne GH, Modlin IM: Colorectal disease in spinal cord patients: An occult diagnosis. Dis Colon Rectum 33:131–134, 1990.

76. Ballantyne GH: Sigmoid volvulus: High mortality in county hospital patients. Dis Colon Rectum 24:515–520, 1981.

77. Cosman BC, Stone JM, Perlcash I: Gastrointestinal complications of chronic spinal cord injury. J Am Paraplegia Soc 14:175–181, 1991.

CHAPTER 20

Orthopedic Complications of Spinal Cord Disease

Roy Ashford, M.D.

Because of altered bone physiology and unusual stresses placed on joints and ligaments, paraplegic and quadriplegic patients commonly experience orthopedic complications. In this chapter, three such orthopedic disorders are discussed: heterotopic bone formation, osteoporosis and associated pathologic fractures, and overuse syndromes. This chapter represents a cumulative summary of relevant publications from the Spinal Cord Injury Unit of Rancho Los Amigos Hospital, Los Angeles.

HETEROTOPIC BONE FORMATION

Pathologic bone formation or heterotopic ossification is most commonly a consequence of traumatic brain injury, spinal cord injury, blunt trauma, or surgical exposure. Each form of heterotopic ossification has differences that need to be recognized for treatment and prognosis. This chapter focuses on heterotopic ossification in the spinal cord–injured patient. Heterotopic ossification is rarely seen in patients with nontraumatic paraplegia or quadriplegia. For more complete information, Garland[3] has written a comprehensive description of the other forms of heterotopic ossification.

The incidence of clinically significant heterotopic ossification, i.e., that which limits joint motion (as opposed to that which is merely a roentgenographic observation), is similar when studies from similar institutions and using similar methods are compared, regardless of the etiology of heterotopic ossification. Only 10% to 20% of heterotopic ossification is clinically significant. Joint ankylosis occurs in fewer than 10% of lesions, typically in about 3%.[3] The most common locations are the hip (60% to 70%) and the knee (20% to 30%); the upper extremity (less than 10%) and other areas (less than 1%) are involved less commonly.

Three conditions can influence the incidence and location of heterotopic ossification: spasticity, local trauma, and pressure sores. Heterotopic ossification from spinal cord injury is associated with spasticity. Patients with limb spasticity have a greater risk of development of heterotopic ossification, and patients with massive amounts of bone formation usually have severe spasticity. Recurrence of heterotopic ossification after surgical resection is more typical in patients with spasticity than in any other group.

Trauma to a specific bone or joint also increases the risk of heterotopic ossification. Finally, pressure sores adjacent to proximal joints (i.e., the hip) further increase the likelihood of heterotopic ossification.

Heterotopic ossification most commonly forms near the proximal limb joints. The hip is the most common site at which heterotopic ossification occurs anteriorly and medially; it generally forms within a plane from the anterior superior iliac spine toward the lesser trochanter (Fig. 20–1). It may form proximally above the joint, distally about the lesser trochanter, or between the two. Neurogenic heterotopic ossification is para-articular; other forms may be para-articular or peri-articular. The pattern of spasticity greatly affects the site of heterotopic ossification. Patients with spinal cord injury usually have hip flexor and adductor spasticity, which increases the likelihood that heterotopic ossification will occur in those loca-

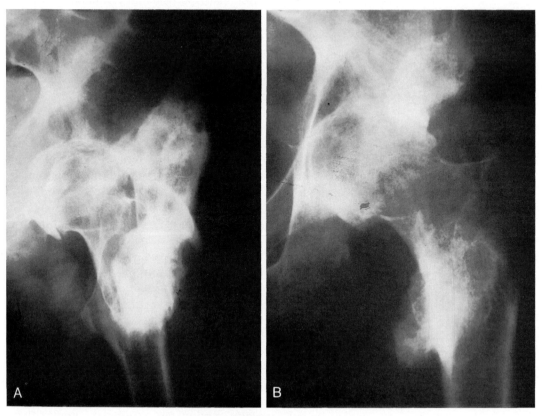

FIGURE 20–1

A, Heterotopic ossification within thigh musculature anterior to the hip joint. *B*, Successful surgical removal of bone mass pictured in *A*.

tions. If a pressure sore is present about the greater trochanter, heterotopic ossification may form in this vicinity. Although the location is uncommon, heterotopic ossification may also arise in the abductor region or at a posterior site. Shoulder and elbow are uncommon sites.

The natural history of heterotopic ossification shows that it usually begins within 3 months after the initial injury. The peak occurrence is at 2 months, but it may be as early as at 4 weeks. The natural history of the disease is shown in Figure 20–2. Garland[6] groups the majority of patients into a subset, type I, in which the evolution of heterotopic ossification occurs over a 6-month period. A small proportion of patients (10% to 20%) have a prolonged and unremitting course (type II); these patients tend to have a worse prognosis. Patients with type II disease commonly show progression to ankylosis, with years of increased radionuclide bone imaging activity.

On clinical examination, limited range of motion is the most common physical finding of heterotopic ossification, often occurring about 2 months after injury. The physical therapist is often the first to detect its presence. Localized swelling is the second most common sign. This may mimic either a septic process or phlebitis.

Chemical assays usually show an increase in serum alkaline phosphatase levels early, during active ossification. Serum alkaline phosphatase levels begin to rise, while remaining in the normal range, within 2 weeks after injury. Elevated levels occur after 3 weeks and continue to be elevated for an average of 5 months (Fig. 20–3). Most patients in whom clinically significant heterotopic ossification develops have an elevated serum alkaline phosphatase level. This level does not correlate with inactivity, peak activity, or the number of heterotopic ossification lesions.

Triple-phase bone scans are a common confirmatory tool. The first two phases are most sensitive for early detection of heterotopic ossification and can be abnormal within 2 to 4 weeks after the initial injury, even though the osseous tissue uptake, phase III, may be normal (see Fig. 20–3). The period between a positive phase I and II scan with a negative phase III scan may vary from 2 to 4 weeks before roentgenographic appearance of heterotopic ossification.[3]

Radiographs are the ultimate confirmatory test. Unfortunately, they become abnormal from 3 weeks to 2 months after the process has already begun. The site of heterotopic ossification can be determined by roentgenograms, which are an easy, inexpensive, and reliable method for following the progress of

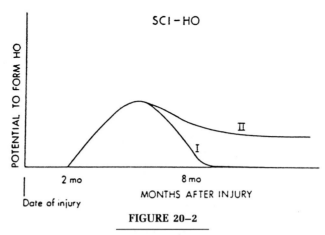

FIGURE 20–2

Two possible evolutionary patterns of heterotopic ossification. Type I shows an elevated serum alkaline phosphatase level and radiographic progression for 6 months, following which the disease becomes quiescent and the bone scan returns to normal. In type II heterotopic ossification, elevated serum alkaline phosphatase levels, radiographic progression, and the potential to form heterotopic bone persist for an extended period. (From Garland DE: Clinical observations on fractures and heterotopic ossification in spinal cord injury and traumatic brain injury patients. Clin Orthop 233:86–100, 1988, with permission.)

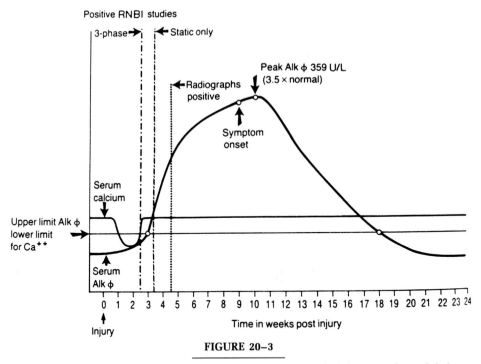

FIGURE 20–3

The developmental sequence of abnormalities of serum alkaline phosphatase, radionuclide bone images, and radiographs in relation to clinical symptoms of heterotopic ossification. (From Orzel JA, Rudd TG: Heterotopic bone formation: Clinical, laboratory and imaging correlation. J Nucl Med 26:125–132, 1985, with permission.)

heterotopic ossification and for evaluating the effect of treatment.

The treatment of heterotopic ossification depends on its clinical severity. Patients with minimal lesions may require no treatment. Others may need physical therapy, medication, controlled manipulation, surgical excision, or a combination of these treatments. The majority of patients with heterotopic ossification maintain functional joint motion with standard physical therapy and medication. Forceful manipulations are generally not performed in the patient with spinal cord injury owing to the potential for pathologic fracture. Only a small number of patients require surgery, and some surgically treated patients experience a recurrence of lesions.

Radiation therapy is used in two general situations: (1) to prevent or limit the amount of heterotopic bone formation after the primary injury and (2) to prevent recurrence of bone formation following surgical resection. As the location of heterotopic bone formation in the patient with neurologic injury cannot be predicted, and as radiation is relatively

ineffective once the lesions are detected, its use in preventing initial heterotopic ossification is limited in patients with spinal cord injury.

Diphosphonates continue to be the primary medical therapy for heterotopic ossification: they inhibit the precipitation of calcium phosphate from clear solutions, delay the aggregation of apatite crystals into layer clusters, and block the transformation of amorphous calcium phosphate into hydroxyapatite.[3] Garland[6] studied 9 spinal cord–injured patients with 14 established cases of heterotopic ossification about the hip. Etidronate disodium therapy at a dosage of 20 mg/kg/day was started at the time of diagnosis and given for 2 weeks, then decreased to 10 mg/kg/day for 2 years. This treatment did not prevent radiologic progression of lesions, even when started early in the course of disease. No joints showed ankylosis and, functionally, all hips maintained 90 degrees of motion. Although three unaffected hips in the study patients did show subsequent development of heterotopic ossification, Garland's overall clinical impression was that treatment was potentially beneficial. He recommends a 6-month treatment at an increased dose of 20 mg/kg/day, owing to the natural history of radiographic progression. Follow-up studies, although not published, have proved this to be an effective treatment regimen.

A study tested intravenous dosages of etidronate disodium, 300 mg/day for 3 to 5 days.[1] In 20 patients with documented heterotopic ossification and no deep venous thrombosis, a rapid decrease in swelling took place within 1 or 2 days. No side effects were noted. The remainder of the protocol was similar to that advocated by Garland. This seems to be the most effective treatment to date.

Indomethacin has proven effective in preventing the formation of heterotopic bone in patients who have undergone total hip arthroplasty. Indomethacin blocks the metabolic process of ossification, in contrast to the inhibition of calcification of osteoid that occurs with diphosphonates. Indomethacin is usually given orally, 25 mg three times daily, for 6 weeks following total hip arthroplasty. This treatment shows promise with spinal cord–injured patients but has not been used at Rancho Los Amigos Hospital.

Surgery is indicated for joint mobility or limp positioning. Surgery should be delayed until heterotopic ossification is in a quiescent state as indicated by a normal serum alkaline phosphatase level, mature roentgenographic appearance, and a baseline radionuclide bone imaging study. Garland recommends waiting for 1 year after the onset of heterotopic ossification before undertaking surgery. Patients with type I disease definitely should not have surgery prior to 6 months after onset. No joint pain or swelling should be present. Roentgenographic progression should have stabilized, although some involution of heterotopic bone formation may be evident. The serum alkaline phosphatase level should have returned to baseline and evidence of disease on radionuclide bone scan should have decreased or not increased from baseline. If the laboratory examinations remain abnormal, i.e., if type II disease is present, or if the patient has had ineffective prophylactic

treatment, a further delay of up to 6 months may be warranted.

Medicinal prophylaxis after surgery is desirable. Indomethacin and radiation are helpful. Etidronate disodium, if used, should be given at a dose of 20 g/kg/day for a minimum of 3 months. If any clinical or laboratory parameters are abnormal at that time, treatment should continue for 3 additional months.

To summarize the treatment of heterotopic bone formation, the practitioner must be aware that decreased motion and pain are commonly the first evidence of heterotopic ossification. This should alert the examiner that clinically significant disease may be imminent. Early confirmation of heterotopic ossification is best established by triple-phase bone scanning. Site-specific location, grading, and response to treatment are accomplished with standard roentgenograms. When the diagnosis is made, a regimen of etidronate disodium or indomethacin should be started. The protocol at Rancho Los Amigos Hospital begins with 3 days of intravenous etidronate disodium followed by 6 months of oral treatment at 20 mg/kg/day. If the disease is very active and aggressive, 6 weeks of indomethacin administration is included with the etidronate disodium therapy. For type I heterotopic ossification, after 1 year, when all tests show inactivity, surgery may be considered if incomplete range of motion or joint ankylosis is present. For type II heterotopic ossification, surgery is recommended at 1.5 years, even if the laboratory examinations are abnormal, to prevent joint ankylosis and potential pathologic fractures. Prophylactic medicinal therapy is recommended after surgical resection.

OSTEOPOROSIS AND PATHOLOGIC FRACTURES

The simplest definition of osteoporosis is a decrease in bone density to what is less-than-expected for a given individual. Osteoporosis commonly occurs in spinal cord–injured patients.[7,8] It is important because of the high rate of associated pathologic fractures (1.4% to 6%). Actually, when all pathologic fractures are considered (i.e., nondisplaced or neglected fractures), this number is likely to be higher, possibly closer to 20% to 30%. Studies at Rancho Los Amigos Hospital have noted an increased incidence of fractures 10 years after spinal cord injury.[8]

Garland and colleagues[8] have noted that bone loss in the lower extremities following a complete lesion of the spinal cord is rapid. In the first 3 months after injury, the bone is depleted by approximately 22%; an additional 5% is lost between the third and fourth months after injury, and at 14 months after injury, approximately 32% of bone has been lost. Bone depletion at 16 months after injury is essentially the same as that observed 10 years after injury, or approximately 37%. Paraplegic and quadriplegic patients have significantly different depletion patterns in the arms and trunk, but patterns are highly similar in the pelvis and lower extremities. Both groups showed significant depletion throughout the axial skeleton (except for the head) when compared with normal age-matched control patients.

Further investigation by Garland and coworkers[7] evaluated 18 spinal cord–injured patients with pathologic fractures and compared them with age-matched controls who had a similar distribution of spinal cord trauma. The average age was similar, 35 and 32 years, and in both groups approximately 10 years had elapsed from injury. They observed a significant decrease in bone mineral density in the patients with fractures as compared with that of the control group, 0.5502 g/cm^2 vs. 0.6735 g/cm^2, respectively. Both of these numbers are well below the established spine fracture threshold of 1.0 g/cm^2. Based on these numbers, Garland believes the fracture threshold about the knee is closer to 0.6 g/cm^2, or approximately 50% bone loss. This group falls below the expected steady-state loss of 33% for spinal cord–injured patients.

Treatment of osteoporosis consists of the standard modalities: vitamin D, calcium supplements, and activity. But osteoporosis with spinal cord injury is more complex. Garland (personal communication) thinks that this type of osteoporosis is attributable to more than simple disuse. The distribution of bone loss is greater in different areas of the body (e.g., the lower extremities) when compared with that in senile or postmenopausal osteoporosis. He thinks that a neurogenic contribution to bone loss, and possibly other undetermined factors, exists in patients with spinal cord injury that make standard treatments, such as sitting exercises or standing frames, ineffective for bone gain. Early treatment may best be directed at blocking the osteoclastic activity that accounts for the rapid early bone loss.[8]

Once the bone has fractured, treatment is a matter of personal preference. Outcome studies of nonoperative and operative treatment fail to demonstrate a consistent superiority of one therapeutic mode in all fracture types. Garland's preference is to treat most diaphyseal fractures with intramedullary fixation when technically possible, while most metaphyseal fractures do better with nonoperative treatment. Freedom from external support facilitates self-care, transfer training, and nursing care.[4]

In paraplegic and quadriplegic patients, fractures usually occur in the lower extremities, most commonly about the knee. Femur and tibial fractures are treated similarly. Nondisplaced metaphyseal fractures are treated nonoperatively. At Rancho Los Amigos Hospital, it was found that nonoperative treatment of displaced fractures yielded a nonunion rate of 31% in the femur and a delayed or malunion rate of up to 50% in the tibia.[4] Garland prefers treatment of long bone fractures with intramedullary fixation when appropriate, as osteoporotic bone does not hold screws well enough for plate osteosynthesis. For intracapsular hip fractures, intramedullary rod and hip screw fixation are preferred. Once fractures are stabilized, the therapist may restart early range-of-motion exercises and mobilization to prevent further deterioration.

Fracture response above the level of a spinal cord lesion is rarely modified. Traumatic heterotopic ossification, excessive callus, and angular deformities are uncommon, even in quadriplegic patients. Indications for open reduction and internal fixation of specific fracture sites in the upper extremities are similar to those in the general population.

OVERUSE SYNDROMES

Both paraplegic and quadriplegic patients rely on their upper extremities for activities of daily living, locomotion, and transfers. Such abnormal stresses lead to dysfunction and pain in the upper extremities. At Rancho Los Amigos Hospital, Gellman and others[10] reported on 84 paraplegics more than 1 year after injury. Fifty-seven (67.8%) of all patients interviewed complained of pain in one or more areas of the upper extremity. The shoulder and carpal tunnel were most commonly implicated. Sie and co-workers[12] found that about half of all quadriplegic patients complained of shoulder pain (Table 20–1). Painful elbows, forearms, and hands were also reported, but only in 5% to 8% of patients.[10]

Pain syndromes were very common initially, within the first 6 months after injury, while the patient is adapting to new body demands and functions.[10, 12] The lowest incidence was found 2 to 4 years after injury but began to increase over time beyond 5 years. During the first 5 years, 52% of patients complained of pain. This increased to 62% by 10 years, to 72% by 15 years, and after 20 years, all patients had upper extremity pain and (or) paresthesia.

Unrestricted motion of the shoulder is important for activities of daily living and for transfers. Pathologic disorders of the shoulder in spinal cord–injured patients include biceps tendinitis, rotator cuff tendinitis (impingement syndromes), adhesive capsulitis, various restrictive contractures of the capsule, subscapularis tendonitis, brachial neuritis, reflex sympathetic dystrophy, referred cervical pain, and heterotopic bone formation. Most authors agree that the two main sources of shoulder pain are bicipital tendinitis and rotator cuff pathologic disorders associated with impingement. Bayley and others[2] found a 30% incidence of shoulder pain in paraplegic patients. Half of these patients were found to have a rotator cuff tear diagnosed by arthrography; these patients were older and had chronic disease. At Rancho Los Amigos Hospital, Silfverskiold and Waters[13] found that in patients younger than 40 years, the diagnosis was almost exclusively of bicipital tendinitis.

During the first 6 months following injury, 78% of quadriplegics have shoulder pain, whereas only 35% of paraplegics are symptomatic. Both decrease to about 33% at 6 to 18 months' follow-up. On long-term follow-up, shoulder pain increases to 100% of all patients more than 20 years after injury.[9] In the quadriplegic patient, active or passive exercise in the presence of rotator cuff imbalance likely results in abnormal glenohumeral

TABLE 20–1

PREVALENCE OF UPPER EXTREMITY PAIN IN PATIENTS WITH QUADRIPLEGIA

TIME SINCE INJURY (yr)	NO.	PREVALENCE BY REGION								TOTAL PREVALENCE	
		SHOULDER		ELBOW		WRIST		HAND			
		%	(n)	%	(n)	%	(n)	%	(n)	%	(n)
<5	19	53	(10)	26	(5)	16	(3)	26	(5)	68	(13)
5–9	39	44	(17)	18	(7)	18	(7)	13	(5)	54	(21)
10–14	31	39	(12)	3	(1)	6	(2)	6	(2)	45	(14)
15–19	22	45	(10)	9	(2)	9	(2)	18	(4)	50	(11)
20+	25	52	(13)	24	(6)	24	(6)	20	(5)	64	(16)
Total	136	46		15		15		15		55	(75)

From Sie IH, Waters RL, Adkins RH, et al: Upper extremity pain in the post-rehabilitation spinal cord injured patient. Arch Phys Med Rehabil 73:44–48, 1992.

motion, subluxation, and stress, leading to synovial and capsular inflammation and rotator cuff or bicipital tendinitis. Inflammation causes pain that increases spasticity, thus creating a vicious cycle.

Patients with shoulder pain respond well to conservative therapy: range-of-motion exercises to tolerance, muscle strengthening, splinting of contractures, nonsteroidal anti-inflammatory analgesic regimens, ultrasound, and passage of time are usually sufficient in the majority of cases. Spasmolytic agents are used if evidence of increased muscle tone is present. Trigger point injections of cortisone are utilized early for localized pain, and iontophoresis with cortisone has been successful for areas of more diffuse tenderness. Operative intervention should be reserved for those cases that are refractory to conservative modalities. In patients older than 40 years, referral of rotator cuff tears to an orthopedist would be advisable.

Carpal tunnel complaints are common in paraplegics, mainly because of the stress that is imparted at extremes of motion at the wrist. Gellman and colleagues[9] found a 49% incidence of carpal tunnel syndrome in 77 outpatients at Rancho Los Amigos Hospital. The incidence increases with time from injury and was found to be as high as 89% 15 years after injury.

Carpal tunnel syndrome in paraplegic patients has clinical features that are similar to those noted in other patients: numbness, tingling, and pain in the radial three digits, abnormal sensation in the median nerve distribution, thenar muscle weakness and atrophy, and positive results of provocative tests (e.g., Tinel's and Phalen's tests).

Gellman and co-workers[9] measured carpal tunnel pressures in different wrist positions (Table 20–2). Paraplegic patients had pressures near normal in flexion and intermediate at neutral, but they were very high in extension and up to 220 mm Hg during a wheelchair-RAISE (Relief of Anatomical Ischial Skin Embarrassment) maneuver with the extended wrists supporting the body weight. The authors postulated that the etiology of carpal tunnel syndrome in paraplegic patients may be a combination of repetitive trauma from the use of a wheelchair and of

TABLE 20–2

PRESSURES IN THE CARPAL TUNNEL (IN mm Hg) IN PARAPLEGIC PATIENTS

POSITION OF THE WRIST	CARPAL TUNNEL SYNDROME (N = 8)	NO CARPAL TUNNEL SYNDROME (N = 10)
Neutral	12 (32)	8 (3)
Flexion	95 (94)	42 (31)
Extension	160 (110)	200 (30)
RAISE maneuver	220	180

From Gellman H, Chandler DR, Petrasek J, et al: Carpal tunnel syndrome in paraplegic patients. J Bone Joint Surg Am 70:517–519, 1988.

ischemia that results from repetitive transient increases in pressure.

Because of the differences in etiology and symptoms between classic carpal tunnel syndrome and the syndrome in paraplegics, Sie and colleagues[11] proposed that "repetitive contract neuropathy" may be a more appropriate term. They grouped median and ulnar nerve pathology into one subset and identified three specific "at-risk" activities. The first is performing RAISEs, in which all of the body weight is placed on a maximally extended wrist, which affects both the carpal tunnel and Guyon's canal. The second is lying prone with pressure on the flexed elbows, which compromises the integrity of the ulnar nerve. The third is resting the elbows on the wheelchair armrest for prolonged periods, which compresses the ulnar nerve.

Gellman and colleagues[9] found that the most common abnormal finding in paraplegics with carpal tunnel syndrome was decreased monofilament sensibility; next was a positive Phalen's test. A positive Tinel's sign was less frequent. Because carpal tunnel syndrome in paraplegic patients is secondary to repetitive trauma, Sie and others[12] suggested padded gloves or elbow pads to protect the nerve from repeated percussion. Carpal tunnel release in a nonpainful injury might actually render the nerve more exposed and vulnerable to repetitive trauma.[11] Carpal tunnel release is reserved for patients with pain that does not respond to padding or protection or for those with progressive neurologic deterioration.

Overuse syndromes of other parts of the upper extremity are rarely found; painful elbows, forearms, and hands were found in only 5% to 8% of the long-term study population of Gellman and colleagues.[10] The authors did note that the incidence of hand pain after 25 years rose to 40%. Because other sites of pain are seldom seen in spinal cord injury, specific treatment has not been discussed in the literature. Basic physiotherapy modalities, anti-inflammatory analgesics, trigger point injection, ice, and range-of-motion exercises have proven to be effective.

To summarize, a number of overuse syndromes occur in spinal cord–injured patients, but only two are seen commonly. In quadriplegic patients, shoulder pain is the most frequent complaint. In patients younger than 40 years, bicipital tendinitis is the usual cause, whereas rotator cuff pathology is more frequent in older patients. Both of these disorders respond to conservative modalities such as range-of-motion, stretching and strengthening exercises, nonsteroidal anti-inflammatory analgesics, steroid injection, and avoidance of aggravating activities; they seldom require operative intervention. Paraplegic patients most often complain of carpal tunnel symptoms. This overuse syndrome is also best treated conservatively with protection of the nerve by padded gloves or the temporary use of a power wheelchair to alleviate symptoms. Surgery for carpal tunnel syndrome is not recommended unless unremitting pain or neurologic deterioration is present despite conservative treatment.[11]

The studies at Rancho Los Amigos Hospital were done by retrospective questionnaires and interviews. Although the prevalence of painful symptoms is quite high, clinic visits are not as frequent as would be anticipated. Of the hundreds of outpatient clinic visits for spinal cord injuries, only two or three patients per week are seen for overuse syndromes. The key to treatment of overuse syndromes is to recognize "at-risk" activities and minimize patient exposure to them. Once an overuse syndrome is recognized, it should be treated aggressively with anti-inflammatory medications, both oral and injectable, and with physiotherapy. Patients should be educated about the frequency of such problems, instructed to avoid "repetitive trauma," and encouraged to seek early treatment before pain becomes chronic.

REFERENCES

1. Banovac K, Gonzalez F, Wade N, et al: Intravenous disodium etidronate therapy in spinal cord injury patients with heterotopic bone. Paraplegia 31:660–666, 1993.
2. Bayley JC, Cochran TP, Sledge CB: The weight bearing shoulder: The impingement syndrome in paraplegics. J Bone Joint Surg Am 69:676–678, 1986.
3. Garland DE: A clinical perspective on common forms of acquired heterotopic ossification. Clin Orthop 263:13–29, 1991.
4. Garland DE: Clinical observations on fractures and heterotopic ossification in the spinal cord and traumatic brain injured populations. Clin Orthop 233:86–100, 1988.
5. Garland DE, Orwin JF: Resection of heterotopic ossification in patients with spinal cord injuries. Clin Orthop 242:169–176, 1988.
6. Garland DE, Alday B, Venos KG, et al: Diphosphonate treatment for heterotopic ossification in spinal cord injury patients. Clin Orthop 176:197–200, 1983.
7. Garland DE, Maric Z, Adkins RH, et al: Bone mineral density about the knee in spinal cord injured patients with pathologic fractures. Contemp Orthop 26:375–379, 1993.
8. Garland DE, Stewart CA, Adkins RH, et al: Osteoporosis after spinal cord injury. J Orthop Res 10:371–378, 1992.
9. Gellman H, Chandler DR, Petrasek J, et al: Carpal tunnel syndrome in paraplegic patients. J Bone Joint Surg Am 70:517–519, 1988.
10. Gellman H, Sie IH, Waters RL: Late complications of the weight-bearing upper extremity in the paraplegic patient. Clin Orthop 233:132–135, 1988.
11. Sie IH, Waters RL, Adkins RH: Upper extremity disability due to lower extremity paralysis in paraplegia. In Current Orthopedics Mini-Symposium: Paralytic Disorders. 1991, pp 88–91.
12. Sie IH, Waters RL, Adkins RH, et al: Upper extremity pain in the post rehabilitation spinal cord injured patient. Arch Phys Med Rehabil 73:44–48, 1992.
13. Silfverskiold J, Waters RL: Shoulder pain and functional disability in spinal cord injury patients. Clin Orthop 272:141–145, 1991.
14. Waters RL, Sie IH, Adkins RH: The musculoskeletal system. In Whitneck GG (ed): Aging with Spinal Cord Injury. New York, Demos, 1993, pp 53–71.

CHAPTER 21

Pain in Spinal Cord Disorders

Robert M. Woolsey, M.D.

Pain is a prominent feature in some acute and chronic disorders of the spinal cord and cauda equina. Pain may arise from spinal bones and ligaments, spinal meninges, the cauda equina, or the spinal cord itself.[1] Since spinal trauma, the most common cause of spinal cord dysfunction, involves all of these potential sources of pain simultaneously, it is not surprising that pain is frequently a major, life-long management issue in patients with traumatic myelopathy.

To quantify the problem, the author interviewed 100 randomly selected patients who had sustained a spinal cord or cauda equina injury at least 1 year prior to entry into the study. Patients with complete lesions (no sensory or motor function below the level of injury) or incomplete lesions (some sensory or motor function below the level of injury) were included. Pain was classified according to severity and type.[2]

Two-thirds of all patients stated that they experienced chronic or recurrent pain. One-fifth of all patients rated the pain as severe, which in this study was defined as pain from which the patient was unable to divert his or her attention or pain that prevented the patient from pursuing daily activities when it was present and from which he or she felt the need to seek immediate relief.

The patients described pain that was mainly of three types. The most common pain consisted of a burning or aching sensation below the level of injury in the area of impaired or absent sensation (diffuse pain), which occurred in 38/100 patients. The next most common type of pain occurred over the site of spinal fracture (local pain); it occurred in 24/100 patients. Pain radiating into the distribution of one or several nerve roots unilaterally or bilaterally at the level of spinal cord injury (radiating pain) was the least common pain variety and occurred in 12/100 patients.

THE PAIN PATHWAY

Excellent, detailed, fully referenced accounts of the anatomy and physiology of the pain pathways are available.[3, 4] The information in this chapter, which has been abstracted from these sources unless otherwise indicated, is essential to the understanding and management of the various pain entities seen in patients with spinal cord disorders.

Pain receptors (nociceptors) are the distal terminals of small myelinated (A delta) and unmyelinated (C) fibers. Painful stimuli activate these receptors by the dual mechanism of receptor deformation and the production of "algesic substances," which result from tissue damage (Fig. 21–1). Possible "algesic

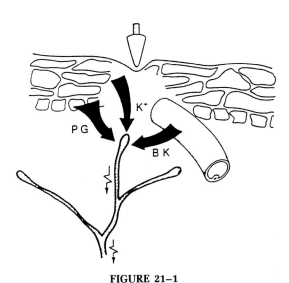

FIGURE 21–1

Pain receptor activation. A mechanical stimulus directly activates a pain receptor and damages adjacent tissue. Cell damage releases "algesic substances," which continue receptor activation after removal of the stimulus. "Algesic substances" include potassium (K^+), prostaglandin (PG), and bradykinin (BK). (From Fields HL: Pain. New York, McGraw-Hill, 1987; with permission.)

substances" include potassium, serotonin, bradykinin, histamine, prostaglandin, leukotrienes, and substance P.

Following receptor activation, pain is transmitted through peripheral nerves by two sizes of nerve fibers. The A delta fibers are thinly myelinated and conduct at a rate of 15 m/second. The C fibers are unmyelinated and conduct at a rate of 1 m/second. As these fibers approach the dorsal root entry zone, they segregate themselves from larger-diameter myelinated fibers and occupy the lateral portion of the dorsal root. On entering the spinal cord they bifurcate into an ascending process and a descending process, which traverse several cord segments in the zone of Lissauer, from which they enter the dorsal horn gray matter to terminate mainly (though not exclusively) in laminae I, II, and V.

The dorsal horn is a complex sensory information processing center consisting of connections from peripheral sensory receptors, connections to and from the brain, connections to and from other levels of the spinal cord, and local segmental excitatory and inhibitory neurons.

Centrally directed nociceptive axons arise mainly from neurons in laminae I and V. These axons cross to the contralateral anterolateral quadrant of the spinal cord where they ascend as a compact bundle, the lateral spinothalamic tract (Fig. 21–2).

On reaching the brain, the lateral spinothalamic tract bifurcates into a lateral division, which continues on to the ventral posterolateral thalamic nucleus (the neospinothalamic tract), and a medial division, which feeds into the brain stem reticular formation at all levels, where it relays to fibers destined for the medial and intralaminar thalamic nuclei (the paleospinothalamic system).

About 50% of all cells in the ventral posterolateral thalamic nucleus respond to noxious stimuli and about 15% respond only to noxious stimuli. This nucleus projects to the postcentral gyrus, mainly to Brodmann's areas 3b and 1. The medial and intralaminar thalamic nuclei project widely to the cerebral cortex, including the postcentral gyrus.

The central pain transmission system is modulated, mainly at the spinal dorsal horn

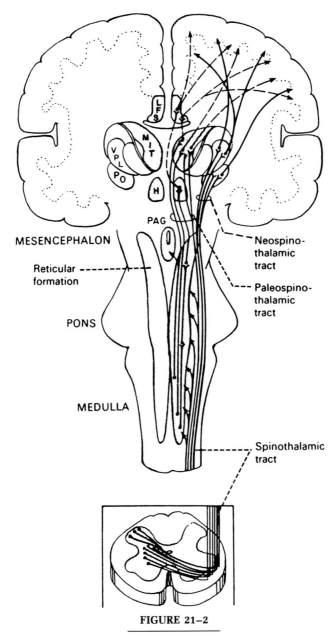

FIGURE 21–2

The central pain pathways. The axons of nociceptive projection neurons in the dorsal horn cross in the spinal cord and ascend in the white matter of the anterolateral quadrant. Some axons pass directly to the ventroposterolateral (*VPL*) and posterior (*PO*) thalamic nuclei (neospinothalamic tract), which project mainly to the postcentral gyrus. Other ascending axons enter the brain stem reticular formation, from where they relay to neurons that project to the medial/intralaminar (*MIT*) thalamic nuclei, which project widely to the cerebral cortex. (From Bonica JJ: The Management of Pain, vol I, ed 2. Philadelphia, Lea & Febiger, 1990; with permission.)

level, by descending pathways from the brain. Though the detailed anatomy of this system is still incompletely investigated, important pain-blocking areas include the periaqueductal gray, the dorsolateral pontine re-

ticular formation, and the medullary reticular formation (Fig. 21–3). The periaqueductal gray matter appears to act through the medullary reticular formation, which projects to the spinal cord by pathways located in the dorsal

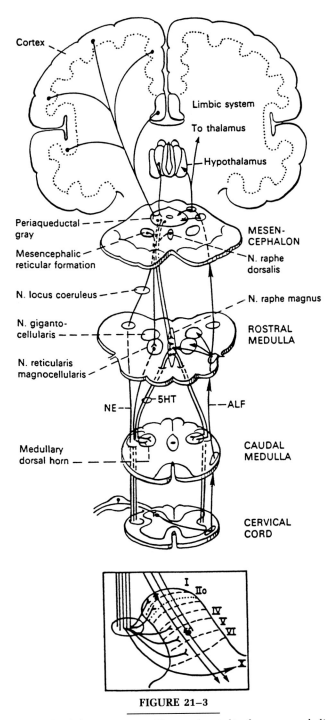

FIGURE 21-3

Descending pain control (inhibitory) systems. Neurons located in the mesencephalic periaqueductal gray matter, dorsolateral pontine reticular formation, and medullary reticular formation project axons located in the dorsal part of the lateral fasciculus of the spinal cord. These axons contact nociceptive projection neurons in the dorsal horn and release inhibitory neurotransmitters such as serotonin (5-HT) and norepinephrine (NE). (From Bonica JJ: The Management of Pain, vol I, ed 2. Philadelphia, Lea & Febiger, 1990; with permission.)

half of the lateral fasciculus. Neurotransmitters of this descending system at the spinal level include serotonin and norepinephrine, which seem to be important inhibitory agents.

PAIN PHARMACOLOGY

Peripherally acting analgesics, such as aspirin and the many other compounds classified as nonsteroidal anti-inflammatory analgesics, appear to prevent the formation of "algesic substances." The best known such mechanism, though not necessarily the most important, is the prevention of prostaglandin formation from arachidonic acid by blocking the enzyme cyclo-oxygenase[3] (Fig. 21–4).

Tricyclic antidepressant medications, especially amitriptyline, inhibit serotonin and norepinephrine reuptake by neurons, thus prolonging their inhibitory activity, which may explain the usefulness of these agents in pain management.[4]

Neurons of the periaqueductal gray mat-

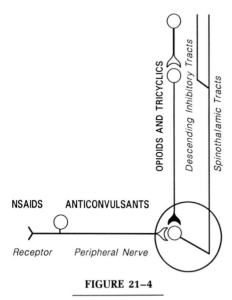

FIGURE 21–4

Presumed site of action of drugs useful in pain control. Aspirin and other nonsteroidal anti-inflammatory drugs (NSAIDs) block the formation of algesic substances. Anticonvulsants stabilize neuronal membranes to prevent ectopic impulse generation in damaged peripheral nerve. Opioid drugs and tricyclic antidepressant drugs act directly on spinal nociceptive projection neurons or by activation of descending inhibitory pathways from the brain stem.

ter, medullary reticular formation, and spinal cord dorsal horn have high concentrations of receptors for both endogenous and exogenous opioids. Centrally acting analgesics are thought to produce their effect through this pain-modulating system. At the dorsal horn level, morphine, for example, acts on the central processes of primary nociceptive afferents to inhibit neurotransmitter release and also produces postsynaptic inhibition of output neurons of the spinothalamic tract. In addition, profound analgesia is produced by injection of morphine into the periaqueductal gray matter and into the medullary reticular formation.[5] Spinal and brain-stem pain-blocking systems thus appear to function synergistically.

TYPES AND MANAGEMENT OF SPINAL CORD PAIN

Pain may be broadly classified as nociceptive or neuropathic. Nociceptive pain is "normal" pain, in which a noxious stimulus activates a pain receptor that generates impulses conducted to the spinal cord dorsal horn, from where they pass by way of the spinothalamic tract to the thalamus and sensory cortex.

Neuropathic pain arises as a result of damage to the pain transmission system. No noxious stimulus is present. The damage may have occurred to either the peripheral or the central portions of the transmission system, causing, respectively, peripheral neuropathic pain or central neuropathic pain. Both types of neuropathic pain have similar clinical features, the most fundamental of which is "anesthesia dolorosa," or pain in an area of decreased or absent sensation.

The three types of pain associated with spinal cord disorders (local pain, radiating pain, and diffuse pain) probably involve five different pain mechanisms (Fig. 21–5).

Local Pain at the Level of Spinal Disease

Spine pain is a common feature of fractures, spondylosis, acute epidural lesions, tu-

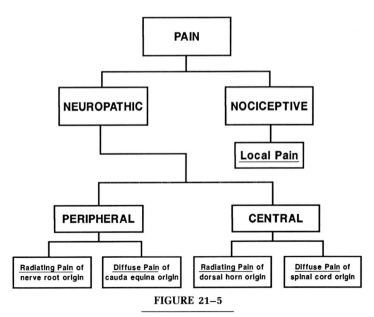

FIGURE 21–5

Possible mechanisms of pain syndromes associated with spinal cord disorders. Local pain is nociceptive. Other pain varieties are neuropathic. Radiating and diffuse pain may be of the peripheral or central neuropathic type depending on whether nerve roots or the spinal cord is involved.

mors, and intramedullary lesions, which cause enlargement of the spinal cord.[6] Pain is maximal over the spine but may extend into the paravertebral areas; with cervical or lumbar involvement it may extend into the shoulders or hips.[7,8] Local pain is nociceptive in nature owing to involvement of pain receptors in the spinal periosteum, ligaments, and meninges (see Chapter 4).

Based on their mechanism of action, it would be expected that peripherally or centrally acting analgesics or amitriptyline would control local pain. Frequently, a combination of analgesics with different sites of action on the pain pathways is more effective than a high dose of a single analgesic[9] (Fig. 21–6).

Many of the aforementioned causes of local pain are obviously amenable to surgical treatment, including those that cause chronic local pain. Bohlman and colleagues[10] reported pain relief following anterior decompression in 41/45 patients with pain following spinal fractures which had been present for an average of 4.5 years.[10]

Radiating Pain at the Level of Spinal Disease

Pain extending from the site of spinal disease into the distribution of one or several adjacent dermatomes unilaterally or bilaterally is mainly neuropathic, arising from the dorsal horn gray matter (segmental pain) or from the dorsal roots themselves (radicular pain).

Segmental pain involving several adjacent dermatomes, usually bilaterally, is most commonly seen in patients with spinal cord injury though it may also be seen in other types of intrinsic spinal cord disease. This pain is strikingly similar to that seen in patients with brachial plexus injury when one or more spinal roots are actually pulled out of the spinal cord. Severe persistent pain in a radicular distribution is seen in 90% of such patients.[11] Nashold[12] believed that this pain was caused by hyperactivity of nociceptive cells in the damaged dorsal horn; he developed the dorsal root entry zone operation, wherein most of the remaining dorsal horn is destroyed.

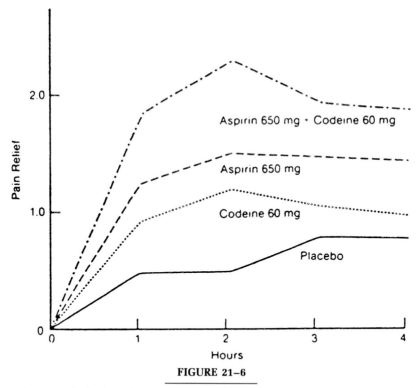

FIGURE 21–6

Nociceptive pain relief achieved using a peripherally acting analgesic (aspirin), a centrally acting analgesic (codeine), and a combination of both. (From Beaver WT: Combination analgesics. Am J Med 77:42, 1984; with permission.)

This procedure was effective in most patients. Nashold subsequently tried a dorsal root entry zone operation in patients with segmental pain secondary to spinal cord injury. Pain was relieved in 80% of patients.[12]

Radicular pain is usually unilateral and extends mainly into the distribution of a single dermatome. Radicular pain is commonly seen in patients with lumbar or cervical disk disease. It is also seen in patients with extramedullary spinal cord tumors or herpes zoster.

Pathologic evidence from patients with herpes zoster[13] and experimental evidence suggests that involvement of the dorsal root ganglion is the essential element in radicular pain.[14, 15]

Experimental acute compression of normal spinal roots alone in humans produces paresthesias, weakness, and reflex loss, but not pain.[16, 17]

Though both segmental and radicular pain are neuropathic, the site of neural involvement makes the response to analgesic medication different. Peripherally acting analgesics may be helpful in radicular pain, particularly if an inflammatory element is present. Centrally acting analgesics and amitriptyline, which act on the dorsal horn pain transmission apparatus, are usually helpful. In segmental pain the dorsal horn is disrupted, and none of these medications is effective.

Diffuse Pain Below the Level of Spinal Disease

Diffuse, usually burning or aching pain is the most common type of pain in patients with spinal cord injury. Though trauma is the most common etiology, it is seen in a variety of other spinal cord disorders.[18] This type of pain may result from injury of the cauda equina or of the spinal cord itself.

Pain arising from cauda equina involvement is of the peripheral neuropathic variety and is also seen in patients with mononeuropathies (e.g., lateral femoral cutaneous neuralgia) or polyneuropathies (e.g., diabetic polyneuropathy).[19] The possible mechanisms of peripheral neuropathic pain include: (1) deafferentation hyperactivity of dorsal horn pain transmission neurons; (2) C fiber disinhibition resulting from loss of myelinated peripheral nerve fibers, which exercise an inhibitory influence on C fibers; or (3) ectopic impulse generation in peripheral afferents in areas of damage or demyelination.

As there is no noxious stimulus, peripherally acting analgesics are not very effective against peripheral neuropathic pain, including that arising from the cauda equina. Centrally acting analgesics are effective; however, many consider the long-term use of opioids to be problematic. Tricyclic antidepressants are usually effective. Carbamazepine is frequently helpful in neuropathies that have a lancinating component (e.g., trigeminal neuralgia or tabes dorsalis).[20, 21]

Central neuropathic pain was first clearly described by Dejerine and Roussy[22, 23] in 1906 in patients with thalamic infarction. The clinical syndrome consisted of hemisensory loss and spontaneous pain in the affected area. The pain was continuous, with paroxysmal exacerbations, and could be provoked by any type of stimulus applied to the area of sensory loss. The authors presented three pathologic specimens from patients with "the thalamic syndrome," all of which showed infarction involving the ventral posterolateral thalamic nucleus.

In 1919, Holmes[24] described a series of patients who had sustained spinal cord injuries in World War I. Some patients had unilateral or bilateral pain in the distribution of one or several adjacent nerve roots at the level of the spinal cord injury (radicular or segmental pain). Other patients had diffuse pain below the level of injury. Holmes identified this syndrome as "central pain," similar to that described by Dejerine and Roussy.

The pathophysiology of central pain remains largely unknown 88 years after it was first described. Kendall,[25] in 1939, proposed that the neospinothalamic tract exercises an inhibitory influence over the paleothalamic tract. When the neospinothalamic tract is damaged or destroyed, the unregulated paleospinothalamic tract produces spontaneous pain.[26] An alternate possibility is deafferentation producing hyperexcitability of neurons at various sites in the pain transmission system. Experimental evidence from animals and humans supports this concept.[27, 28]

Either of these mechanisms of central pain should offer the possibility of treatment by surgical destruction of the malfunctioning neural systems. However, such treatments have been disappointing with less than one-third of patients relieved of pain.[18]

Available data on the effectiveness of electrical stimulation of peripheral nerves, the spinal cord, or brain in central pain management are inconclusive.[28] Peripheral nerve or dorsal spinal cord stimulation is usually not helpful. Deep brain stimulation produces pain relief in 42% of patients.[18]

Pharmacologic treatment of central pain is difficult. Because the pain mechanism is uncertain, it is impossible to formulate a coherent pharmacologic strategy. The literature consists mainly of anecdotal case reports that are confusing and contradictory. The few prospective controlled studies mostly concern pain after stroke. Peripherally acting analgesics, as would be expected, are not useful. Opioids and other centrally acting drugs have been reported to be ineffective in some studies[30, 31] but effective in others.[32, 33] In the author's experience, high doses of methadone or codeine frequently reduce the central pain of spinal cord origin to a tolerable level. Serotonin reuptake blockers have been reported to be useful in pain after stroke (amitriptyline)[34] but not in the central pain of spinal cord disease (trazodone).[35]

REFERENCES

1. Heller JG: The syndromes of degenerative cervical disease. Orthop Clin North Am 23:381–394, 1992.
2. Woolsey RM: Chronic pain following spinal cord injury. J Am Paraplegia Soc 9:39–41, 1986.
3. Bonica JJ: Anatomic and physiologic basis of nociception and pain. In Bonica JJ (ed): The Management of Pain, vol I, ed 2. Philadelphia, Lea & Febiger, 1990, pp 28–94.
4. Fields HL: Pain. New York, McGraw-Hill, 1987.
5. Jaffe JH, Martin WR: Opioid analgesics and antagonists. In Gilman AG, Rall TW, Nies AS, et al (eds): The Pharmacological Basis of Therapeutics, ed 8. New York, Pergamon Press, 1990, pp 485–521.

6. Woolsey RM, Young RR: The clinical diagnosis of disorders of the spinal cord. Neurol Clin 9:573–583, 1991.

7. McCall IW, Park WM, O'Brien JP: Induced pain referral from posterior lumbar elements in normal subjects. Spine 4:441–446, 1979.

8. O'Brien JP: Mechanisms of spinal pain. In Wall PD, Melzack R (eds): Textbook of Pain. Edinburgh, Churchill Livingstone, 1984, p 242.

9. Beaver WT: Nonsteroidal antiinflammatory analgesics and their combination with opioids. In Aronoff GM (ed): Evaluation and Treatment of Chronic Pain, ed 2. Baltimore, Williams & Wilkins, 1992, pp 369–383.

10. Bohlman HH, Kirkpatrick JS, Delamarter RB, et al: Anterior decompression for late pain and paralysis following fractures of the thoracolumbar spine. Clin Orthop 300:24–29, 1994.

11. Wynn-Parry CB: Pain in avulsion lesions of the brachial plexus. Pain 9:41–53, 1980.

12. Nashold BS: Paraplegia and pain. In Nashold BS, Ovelmen-Levitt J (eds): Advances in Pain Research and Therapy: vol. 19. Deafferentation Pain Syndromes Physiology and Treatment. New York, Raven Press, 1991, pp 302–319.

13. Esiri MM, Kennedy PGE: Virus diseases. In Adams JH, Duchen LW (eds): Greenfield's Neuropathology, ed 5. New York, Oxford University Press, 1992, p 353.

14. Rydevik BL: Etiology of sciatica. In Weinstein JN, Wiesel SW (eds): The Lumbar Spine. Philadelphia, WB Saunders, 1990, pp 132–159.

15. Howe JF, Loeser JD, Calvin WH: Mechanosensitivity of dorsal root ganglia and chronically injured axons: A physiological basis for the radicular pain of nerve root compression. Pain 3:25–41, 1977.

16. Macnab I: The mechanisms of spondylogenic pain. In Hirsch C, Zotterman Y (eds): Cervical Pain. New York, Pergamon Press, 1972, pp 89–95.

17. Smyth MJ, Wright V: Sciatica and the intervertebral disk: An experimental study. J Bone Joint Surg Am 40:1401–1418, 1958.

18. Tasker RR, de Carvalho G, Dostrovsky JO: The history of central pain syndromes, with observations concerning pathophysiology and treatment. In Casey KL (ed): Pain and Central Nervous System Disease: The Central Pain Syndromes. New York, Raven Press, 1991, pp 31–58.

19. Scadding JW: Neuropathic pain. In Asbury AK, McKhann GM, McDonald WI (eds): Diseases of the Nervous System, vol. II, ed 2. Philadelphia, WB Saunders, 1992, pp 858–872.

20. Maciewicz R, Bouckoms A, Martin JB: Drug therapy of neuropathic pain. Clin J Pain 1:39–49, 1985.

21. McQuay HJ: Pharmacologic treatment of neuralgic and neuropathic pain. Cancer Surv 7:141–159, 1988.

22. Dejerine J, Roussy G: Le syndrome thalamique. Rev Neurol 14:521–532, 1906.

23. Wilkins RH, Brody IA: The thalamic syndrome. Arch Neurol 20:559–562, 1969.

24. Holmes G: Pain of Central Origin: Contributions to Medical and Biological Research. New York, Paul B. Hober, 1919, pp 235–245.

25. Kendall D: Some observations on central pain. Brain 62:253–273, 1939.

26. Cassinari V, Pagini CA: Central Pain: A Neurosurgical Survey. Cambridge, Mass., Harvard University Press, 1969.

27. Willis WD: Central neurogenic pain: Possible mechanisms. In Nashold BS, Ovelmen-Levitt J (eds): Advances in Pain Research and Therapy: vol 19. Deafferentation Pain Syndromes: Pathophysiology and Treatment. New York, Raven Press, 1991, pp 81–101.

28. Lenz FA: The thalamus and central pain syndromes: Human and animal studies. In Casey KL (ed): Pain and Central Nervous System Disease: The Central Pain Syndromes. New York, Raven Press, 1991, pp 171–182.

29. Sjolund BH: Role of transcutaneous electrical nerve stimulation, central nervous system stimulation, and ablative procedures in central pain syndromes. In Casey KL (ed): Pain and Central Nervous System Disease: The Central Pain Syndromes. New York, Raven Press, 1991, pp 267–274.

30. Bainton T, Fox M, Bowsher D, et al: A double-blind trial of naloxone in central post-stroke pain. Pain 48:159–162, 1992.

31. Arner S, Meyerson BA: Lack of analgesic effect of opioids on neuropathic and idiopathic forms of pain. Pain 33:11–23, 1988.

32. Portenoy RK, Foley KM, Inturrisi CE: The nature of opioid responsiveness and its implications for neuropathic pain: New hypotheses derived from studies of opioid infusions. Pain 43:273–286, 1990.

33. Budd K: The use of the opiate antagonist, naloxone, in the treatment of intractable pain. Neuropeptides 5:419–422, 1985.

34. Leijon G, Boivie J: Central post-stroke pain: A controlled trial of amitriptyline and carbamazepine. Pain 36:27–36, 1989.

35. Davidoff G, Guarracini M, Roth E, et al: Trazodone hydrochloride in the treatment of dysesthetic pain in traumatic myelopathy: A randomized, double-blind, placebo-controlled study. Pain 29:151–161, 1987.

CHAPTER 22

Spastic Paresis

Robert R. Young, M.D.

DEFINITIONS

Theoretical

Spasticity was defined by Lance[37] as a motor disorder characterized by a velocity-dependent increase in tonic stretch reflexes (muscle tone) with exaggerated tendon jerks, resulting from hyperexcitability of the stretch reflex as one component of the upper motor neuron syndrome. To this rather narrow definition of spasticity, the following have been added, the sum of which is called *spastic paresis*[69]: other positive symptoms, such as exaggerated cutaneous reflexes (including nociceptive and flexor withdrawal reflexes); autonomic hyperreflexia; dystonia; contractures; and negative symptoms such as paresis, lack of dexterity, and fatigability. In toto, these constitute the upper motor neuron syndrome.

This definition, which is meant in part to differentiate spasticity from rigidity, is inadequate for several reasons. (1) In many patients, some muscles in a limb behave as though they are spastic and others in the same limb behave as though they are rigid. In a hemiparetic patient with a stroke, for example, some upper limb muscles may be spastic and others rigid, according to the definitions outlined in the following text. Hemiparetic dystonia often behaves as rigidity. In that circumstance, neurologists tend to classify the hypertonus (i.e., rigidity vs. spasticity) according to the overall clinical picture, which includes briskness of tendon jerks, presence of Babinski's response, and lability of flexor reflexes. That is, they call it *spastic*. (2) The definitions as listed invoke hypothetical physiologic mechanisms (exaggerated tonic stretch reflexes for both rigidity and spasticity). (3) Clearly different types of spasticity exist (e.g., the syndrome seen with cerebral lesions vs. that seen with spinal lesions) and rigidity (e.g., that seen with parkinsonism vs. that seen with an intrinsic tumor of the cervical cord). (4) Finally, all such definitions focus on discrete aspects of the overall clinical problem, much like the proverbial committee of blind men feeling an elephant. Inevitably, perception of the reality is altered to fit the theories in vogue at the time or to fit within the purview of contemporary understanding. As neurobiological details of the motor system are discovered, they will permit an accounting for clinical findings from first principles. It will then be possible to dispense with archaic terms such as *rigidity* and *spasticity*; clinical phenomena will finally be explicable in terms of objective dysfunction of fundamental subunits of the motor system.

Practical

Meanwhile, practical interim positions can be adopted that provide operational definitions of these phenomena with a minimum of speculation. *Rigidity* refers to increased muscle tone in patients with Parkinson's disease (PD). It is also found in other conditions without gross neuropathologic lesions (e.g., without encephalomalacia) in which the plantar reflex is normal and the tendon reflexes are usually normal, but because relaxation is difficult, muscle tone is increased even at rest. *Spasticity*, also an involuntary increase in muscle tone, occurs only during muscle stretch; is a result of structural lesions of the cerebrum, brain stem, or spinal cord; and is accompanied by Babinski's response and tendon reflexes that are usually increased.

When tonic stretch reflexes are increased, the limb adopts an abnormal posture as a consequence of the increased tone. In patients with rigidity accompanying extrapyramidal disorders such as PD, flexion of trunk

and limbs is present. With hemiplegia, the upper limb is flexed and adducted and the lower limb extended. With paraplegia or quadriplegia, lower limbs are flexed and adducted as are upper limbs if they are affected. These abnormalities of tone are referred to as *dystonia*; the hemiplegic and paraplegic varieties can be grouped under the term *spastic dystonia*. This term is useful in directing attention to chronic contraction of individual muscles, which may be treated by therapy that directly weakens muscle, such as neurectomy, phenol injection, and dantrolene or botulinum toxin administration (see following discussion).

SPASTICITY

The narrowest and most restrictive definitions of spasticity (items 1 and 2 in the following list) focus on a velocity-dependent increase in tonic stretch reflexes (compare Figs. 22–1 and 22–2) and ignore other positive symptoms, such as exaggerated nociceptive reflexes and autonomic hyperreflexia, which are also clinically important and are often more disturbing than abnormal stretch reflexes. Even more distressing and disabling are a variety of negative symptoms that are responsible for most of the functional deficits in patients with spastic paresis. A hierarchy of definitions, which are increasingly more comprehensive, follows:

1. Spasticity is a motor disorder characterized by a velocity-dependent increase in tonic stretch reflexes (muscle tone) with exaggerated tendon jerks, resulting from hyperexcitability of the stretch reflex, as one component of the upper motor neuron syndrome.[37]

2. Item 1 can be modified and updated to define spasticity as a motor disorder characterized by brisk tendon jerks, sometimes accompanied by clonus and a velocity-dependent elastic muscle hypertonia during stretch, which affects certain muscle groups preferentially. It results from a combination of hyperexcitability of the Ia pathway to motor neurons and disturbed processing at the

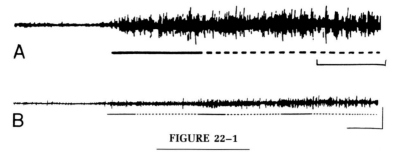

FIGURE 22–1

Electromyographic (EMG) recordings of stretch reflex activity in biceps brachii of a patient with Parkinson's disease and rigidity. Stretch is signified by the *solid line* and holding the muscle at the new length by the *dotted line*. Time line = 1 second. Note the length (not velocity) sensitivity of the EMG activity and the background EMG activity before stretching. (From Shimazu H, Hongo T, Kubota K, et al: Rigidity and spasticity in man. Arch Neurol 6:24–31, 1962.)

spinal cord level of other peripheral afferent messages (tonic stretch reflex).[17] To simplify, spasticity is a motor disorder characterized by a velocity-dependent increase in tonic stretch reflexes, which result from abnormal intraspinal processing of primary afferent input, as one component of the upper motor neuron syndrome.

3. Item 2 can be broadened to include other positive symptoms and signs such as flexor (or extensor) spasms, clasp-knife phenomenon, Babinski's sign, other exaggerated cutaneous (including nociceptive and flexor withdrawal) reflexes, autonomic hyperreflexia, dystonia, and contractures, which may restrain voluntary movement or cause discomfort.

4. Item 3 fails to address negative symptoms and should be expanded to include such abnormalities as paresis, lack of dexterity, synkinesias (inability to isolate individual finger movements, for example), and fatigability.

Altogether, the symptoms and signs that constitute item 4 define the upper motor neuron syndrome, an appropriate description of which is *spastic paresis*.[69]

Textbooks have long assumed that lesions of the corticospinal tract are responsible for all of these symptoms and signs, but in fact it is not known which descending motor tracts must be dysfunctional to cause them. Although lesions restricted to the corticospinal tract produce paresis (which improves) and Babinski's sign, they do not produce spastic dystonia or profound lasting weakness.[38] Pa-

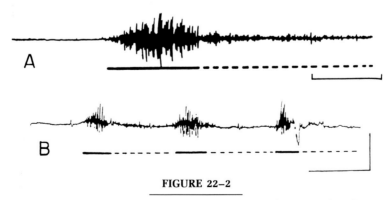

FIGURE 22–2

Electromyographic (EMG) recordings of stretch reflex activity in biceps brachii of a patient with hemiplegic spastic dystonia. Stretch is signified by the *solid line* and holding the muscle at the new length by the *dotted line*. Time line = 1 second. Note the velocity sensitivity of the EMG activity and the absence of EMG activity before stretching. (From Shimazu H, Hongo T, Kubota K, et al: Rigidity and spasticity in man. Arch Neurol 6:24–31, 1962.)

tients with pure motor hemiplegia due to a small lacunar infarction in the corticospinal system (usually in the internal capsule or basis pontis) are acutely hemiplegic but make remarkable recoveries. Such patients have little if any spastic dystonia. However, patients with hemiplegia or triplegia due to lesions of the parasagittal perirolandic area become acutely and severely dystonic.[52] This dystonia differs from the dystonia that commonly develops several weeks or more after most cerebral lesions in that it may gradually disappear if the patient's strength recovers. Lesions, usually traumatic but sometimes neoplastic, restricted to the parasagittal regions may produce spastic paresis and dystonia of both legs (the diplegic or paraplegic syndrome). A similar-appearing spastic diplegic syndrome is becoming more prevalent with increasing survival of tiny, preterm newborns.

Clearly different syndromes of spastic paresis appear with common cerebral lesions (e.g., the hemiplegic or hemiparetic syndrome, with more or less dystonia, but with the upper limb flexed and the lower limb extended in antigravity postures). These syndromes are easily distinguished from the spastic paresis seen with spinal cord lesions; the latter produces extremely labile flexor reflexes and tonically flexed and adducted lower limbs. Although all patients with spastic paresis are similar in some ways (i.e., they are spastic and paretic), many variations exist, which are a consequence of different lesion sites and amounts of central nervous system (CNS) damage. Neither one cause nor one type of spastic paresis exists, and one cure or therapy for it is unlikely.

Two alterations in single motor unit (SMU) behavior occur with spastic paresis; both probably reflect changes associated with paresis rather than with the positive symptoms. On the one hand, reduction takes place in the number of motor units that can be voluntarily recruited, which is difficult to quantify.[65, 68] On the other hand, changes take place in discharge properties of SMUs in spastic paretic muscles, which can be quantified.[14, 60, 65] In patients with spinal cord injuries, the average discharge rates of SMUs are reduced, the floating serial correlation coefficients are significantly more positive (i.e., short-term trends in interdischarge intervals occur, replacing the normal tendency for successive interdischarge intervals to alternate between being shorter and longer than the mean), and a measure that is similar to a coefficient of variation in these intervals becomes abnormal.[65] The last measure is best able to differentiate between normal and paretic SMU behavior; it is higher in paretic units in the biceps and the triceps brachii and either higher or lower than normal in the tibialis anterior.

Pathophysiology

Whereas positive symptoms result from the release of more or less intact motor subsystems from precise rostral control, most negative symptoms are a direct result of the disconnection of lower from higher motor centers. In either case, until techniques are devised that result in functional CNS regeneration, attention must be focused on therapeutic manipulations of the motor subsystems that remain operative caudal to the lesion. Increased knowledge of their neurobiology will permit rational pharmacologic and/or physiologic manipulations to reduce spasticity and, more important, to produce less automatic function of the motor system caudal to the lesion. For example, under special circumstances, such as noradrenergic receptor activation by the administration of clonidine plus electrical stimulation of perineal afferents, the isolated cat spinal cord can support such complex activity as locomotion.[4, 22, 25] Evidence is now being adduced that the isolated human cord also seems to contain a central pattern generator (CPG) for locomotion.[64] How can it be made to function more effectively? How can a more normal balance of excitatory and inhibitory synaptic activity be established? Most manipulations of the lower limbs in patients with spinal cord injuries produce gross, stereotyped flexor spasms that overwhelm any useful motor function. However, clonidine and electrical stimulation of rectal afferents are reported to reduce spasticity in patients with spinal cord injuries and thus may permit operation of the CPG for locomotion in the isolated human spinal cord.[28, 45, 57]

Although the spinal segmental stretch reflex arc contains monosynaptic connections on motor neurons by spindle primary endings that emerge from that muscle and synergistic muscles (via Ia fibers), most excitatory activity in the stretch reflex is mediated via oligosynaptic and polysynaptic pathways. That is, interneurons play a much larger role, even in the simplest of reflexes, than do direct connections between first-order sensory neurons and motor neurons. The stretch reflex arc also includes Renshaw cell recurrent inhibition, disynaptic (and more complex) reciprocal inhibition, nonreciprocal autogenic inhibition, presynaptic inhibition onto primary afferents, remote inhibition (and excitation) onto motor neurons, and a variety of other poorly understood or as yet unimagined circuitry. Fusimotor and skeletofusimotor systems are also involved.

Nociceptive reflexes are mediated by oligosynaptic and polysynaptic connections between "flexor reflex afferents" (FRA), interneurons, and motor neurons of extensor as well as flexor muscles. Many afferent fibers that mediate pain are identical with those responsible for nociceptive reflexes and share interneuronal pools in Rexed's spinal laminae II and III ("dorsal horn cells"). FRA, which are themselves multimodal, constitute only a fraction of the primary afferents entering through each dorsal root. These segmental afferent fibers and fibers of CNS origin, many of which descend from various levels of the neuraxis, converge on interneurons. Coordination and control of descending, segmental, and propriospinal activity are regulated by interneuronal systems and networks. These interneurons are more like pre–motor neuronal integrating centers than like simple relays that switch excitation to inhibition. Lundberg and colleagues have been particularly involved in the study of spinal interneuron behavior (for reviews of these essential networks see Baldissera et al[3] and Gordon[26]).

No experimental evidence exists to support the long-standing theory that exaggerated stretch reflexes are a result of increased sensitivity of muscle spindle primary endings, increased fusimotor activity, or other pathologic increase in peripheral input to the spinal cord.[27] Lesions of peripheral components of the stretch reflex arc obviously interfere with reflex function, including spasticity, but that fact does not support the contention that hyperactive reflexes are a result of increases in segmental afferent input. However, spindle secondary endings have not been ruled out as being important in the cause of spasticity.

Hyperexcitability of the alpha motor neurons themselves, due to either a primary change in their membrane properties (including reduction in area of dendritic membrane or hyperexcitable areas of deafferented dendrites) or a change in membrane potential secondary to alterations of synaptic input, may account for some aspects of spasticity. Normal excitatory/inhibitory balance at the motor neuron level is likely to be upset by changes in the continuous bombardment of these motor neurons that result from reduction in descending inhibition, for example. Such alterations may be accompanied by anatomically demonstrable changes in numbers and kinds of synaptic endings on motor neurons. Following certain injuries, death of some boutons and sprouting of surviving presynaptic terminals may take place, hence an abnormally large percentage of synapses might then be excitatory. Indirect evidence is accumulating, but no techniques exist to document or refute the presence of primary hyperexcitability of alpha motor neurons in human spasticity (see Delwaide[16]). Animal models of spasticity, although imperfect, are beginning to be studied with techniques that will be able to address this problem.

A principal current hypothesis states that spasticity is due to long-term reductions in inhibition rather than to permanent increases in excitation per se, but the differences between these alternatives are not always operationally clear and they need not be mutually exclusive. In their review, Pierrot-Deseilligny and Mazieres[49] assessed evidence for and against disorders of various types of inhibition as the underlying cause of spasticity. Among the types of inhibition recognized are: (1) recurrent Renshaw cell inhibition, (2) reciprocal Ia inhibition, (3) presynaptic inhibition of Ia terminals, (4) nonreciprocal Ib inhibition, and (5) inhibition from group II afferents. In brief, evidence exists against *decreased* Renshaw cell and group II inhibitions as a cause of spasticity, but some evidence is present for decreased presynaptic inhibition of Ia terminals, decreased reciprocal inhibition of antagonist motor neuron pools by Ia activity, and decreased nonreciprocal inhibition. All of this evidence is more or less indirect and none of it has settled the matter once and for all. Furthermore, with different types of spasticity, more than one of these mechanisms may be involved in any one patient. Further investigation of the neurobiology of spinal systems is needed to answer these questions more definitively.

Meanwhile, what about the three types of inhibition that may be reduced in certain types of spasticity? Presynaptic inhibition is mediated by axo-axonic gamma-aminobutyric acid (GABA)-ergic synapses on Ia terminals; these synapses, when activated, reduce the amount of transmitter released by the Ia terminals and thus decrease the efficacy of Ia input even before it gets to the first synapse. Interneurons involved in presynaptic inhibition are controlled by descending pathways; therefore, their activity will be altered (e.g., reduced) by rostral lesions. A tonic level of presynaptic inhibition is normally present and a reduction in it would increase any response generated by Ia input. Spasticity might therefore be due to reductions in presynaptic inhibition,[16] as a result of which normal Ia input following a tendon tap or muscle stretch produces an exaggerated tendon jerk or increased tonic stretch reflex.

Reciprocal Ia inhibition serves to reduce the likelihood that antagonistic muscle groups are co-activated primarily or that antagonists are activated by a stretch reflex when agonist muscles contract and shorten. For example, voluntary contraction of the tibialis anterior normally produces inhibition of the stretched soleus via the so-called Ia inhibitory interneurons, which mediate this important automatic inhibition of antagonist muscles during voluntary movement. In spastic patients who are seated, clonic reflex contraction of soleus is produced by voluntary or reflex-mediated contraction of the tibialis anterior. This inefficient spastic co-contraction of antagonistic muscle groups may also take place during walking, when increased muscle tone may be more impressive and important—as during other voluntary movements—than when it is tested with the patient at rest.[11] However, Dietz and colleagues[20] did not find increased reflex contraction of antagonist muscles at the ankle in walking spastic patients.

Ia inhibitory interneurons are also controlled by descending excitatory pathways, which may be damaged by rostral lesions of the CNS. The situation is more complex than was originally thought because evidence exists for both reduced excitability of the Ia inhibitory interneurons from flexor muscles to extensors and increased excitability from extensors to flexors.[2, 67] Abnormal reduced function of Ia inhibitory interneurons could thus give rise to some of the manifestations of spasticity, such as co-contraction of antagonistic muscle groups or weakness of the tibialis anterior as a result of increased activity in the gastrocnemius-soleus complex. Such weakness might then be diminished by use of botulinum toxin to weaken the overactive triceps surae and reduce their Ia input to the cord.

Delwaide and Gerard[17] found nonreciprocal Ib inhibition to be reduced or even replaced by facilitation in 27 patients with spastic paresis who had spastic dystonia (and tendon hyperreflexia), whereas no change was seen in this inhibition in 22 similar patients who had tendon hyperreflexia without spastic dystonia. This important observation both provides insights into the pathophysiologic features of spastic dystonia and demonstrates even more clearly that tendon hyperreflexia and increased tone in patients with spastic paresis are the result of two unrelated abnormalities. This insight, supported by other reports,[23, 62] resulted in the modification in the definition of spasticity listed as item 3 at the beginning of this chapter.

Recurrent inhibition via Renshaw cell activity is not decreased in patients with spastic paresis resulting from spinal cord lesions; it is *increased*,[54, 55] but can be reduced to normal levels with clonidine administration, which also diminishes the spastic dystonia.

In hemiplegic patients, recurrent inhibition is apparently also not reduced at rest, but is abnormally modulated during voluntary activation of the muscles.[35] Renshaw cells inhibit Ia interneurons as well as alpha motor neurons, so increased activity of the former in patients with spinal spasticity may account for some of the decreased reciprocal inhibition noted earlier.

Enhanced cutaneous (flexor or nociceptive) reflexes in spasticity also bear discussion. Inputs to neurons in Rexed's laminae II and III in the dorsal horn of the spinal cord come both from primary afferents (activity in many of which is generated by destructive, noxious, or potentially painful stimuli) and from descending fibers, which originate in the brain stem or further rostrally. Some dorsal horn neurons give rise to long axons, forming tracts that ascend to supraspinal areas. Other dorsal horn neurons have short, propriospinal axons that innervate motor areas of the cord. In rats, stimulation of the periaqueductal gray matter or the lateral reticular formation leads to suppression of both hindlimb flexion withdrawal reflexes and neural activity in spinothalamic tract neurons, caused by noxious skin stimuli. Rostral lesions within the CNS disrupt descending tracts such as these and alter normal gating functions within the spinal dorsal horn, so that a patient may experience pain as a result of afferent input to the cord that normally would be quite innocuous. This mishandling of segmental inputs, perhaps by failure of presynaptic inhibition (GABA-ergic synapses on primary afferents are found in the substantia gelatinosa), results in excessive activity in long-tract neurons, which, if it reaches consciousness, is felt as pain. Similar excessive activation of propriospinal neurons produces hyperactive nociceptive reflexes. The latter are ubiquitous in spasticity, ranging from a simple Babinski's response, through triple flexion of the leg, to gross flexor (and sometimes extensor) spasms. Furthermore, in spastic patients, these reflexes are produced by simple, non-noxious cutaneous stimuli. Procedures (such as surgical creation of lesions in the dorsal root entry zone) or administration of medications (i.e, opiates) that diminish excessive activation in these dorsal horn circuits reduces spastic nociceptive reflexes as well as pain. These circuits may share interneurons with other systems (such as the interneurons responsible for reciprocal Ia inhibition), so opiate pharmacotherapy may also reduce hyperactive stretch reflexes. Similarly, reductions in segmental input to the cord produced by a neurectomy in the leg result in generalized reductions in spasticity even in the arms.

Fleshman and colleagues[24] demonstrated short latency excitatory pathways from cutaneous afferents to hind-limb flexor motor neurons in the cat; these pathways are powerfully facilitated by the locomotor CPG and by fibers from the red nucleus and pyramidal tract. This system seems to funnel excitatory impulses from a variety of sources to flexor motor neurons. It is interesting that spasticity seems to be worse in patients with *incomplete* cord lesions. Could this be due to preservation of some of the descending pathways?

Seen clinicially, spasticity was always thought to be a manifestation of the superimposition of hyperactive reflexes on normal muscle. Whereas hyperactive reflexes account for most symptoms, Dietz and colleagues[20] and Hufschmidt and Mauritz[31] found that intrinsic mechanical properties of muscle changed in the presence of long-standing abnormalities of muscle tone. Increased passive stiffness of relaxed spastic (or rigid) muscle must be differentiated from underlying muscle contraction. The former may account for at least some clinical dysfunction, such as increased tone and contractures. Would increases in passive muscle stiffness be reduced following repeated stretching or paralysis by injections of botulinum toxin?

Clinical ratings (such as the Ashworth scale) are based on subjective assessment by an examiner of the resistance felt when muscles "at rest" are passively lengthened. Numerous attempts have been made to use mechanical techniques to objectify what the examiner feels, for example, by measuring torque-angle relationships at spastic joints during passive flexion and extension. These more objective techniques are an improvement over bedside clinical testing, but the results do not correlate well with signs and symptoms. Rather than using mechanical or electronic tools simply to do a more accurate version of the usual clinical examination, significant advances might result from study of other functional aspects of the various motor subsystems. For example, Powers and colleagues,[50] after measuring torque at a standard angle during constant velocity joint movements, suggest that stretch reflex threshold measurements correlate well with clinical severity of spasticity. It remains to be seen if this technique will be more useful than previous ones.

Classical reductionist tendencies have led many to hope that analyses, however indirect, of motor neuron pool excitability may be more meaningful than more finely grained studies of phenomenology, such as those just discussed. Delwaide,[16] Ashby and colleagues,[1] and Pierrot-Deseilligny and Mazieres[49] have all used clinically applicable neurophysiologic techniques to study H-reflex excitability curves, H/M ratios, H suppression by vibration, excitability of single motor neurons, and complex reflexology (see reviews by Delwaide and Pennisi[18] and Pierrot-Deseilligny and Mazieres[49]). These and similar techniques have proved valuable in dissecting the pathophysiologic characteristics of spasticity, but thus far, other investigators have not validated or compared these methods, nor have they been subjected to beta testing. It is time to undertake multicenter studies of spastic patients using such quantitative techniques.

Conrad and colleagues[10] and Benecke and co-workers[6] studied similar reflex functions of the human spinal cord during performance of everyday activities, a situation in which spastic paresis is apt to be most troublesome. Multichannel electromyographic (EMG) analyses, performed when patients bicycled on an ergometer or walked on a treadmill, yielded interesting data, which are more relevant to disabilities experienced by patients than data from studies that are done with patients at rest.

In patients with spastic paresis, suprasegmental lesions interfere with descending control of interneuronal systems in the cord. Interneuronal abnormalities may well account for increased stretch reflexes, hyperactive cutaneous reflexes, and even some of the weakness or loss of motor facility. Neurotransmitters and neuromodulators that are active in these interneuronal circuits are becoming known, and their pharmacologic manipulation should prove to be both instructive and therapeutically useful.

Therapy

The following concept has long been a favorite (albeit one for which there is little evidence) of those attempting to treat spasticity: Increased reflexes, particularly the tonic reflexes associated with abnormal tone, may somehow submerge remaining voluntary function of motor neurons. That is, if the spasticity/spastic dystonia could be alleviated, voluntary function of the limb would improve. Such has rarely proved to be the case clinically (see Duncan et al,[21] for example). Nevertheless, it is worth considering, and in its modern guise, this concept has been restated as follows: Lesions of the CNS that are rostral to the segment in question disrupt projections from higher centers, such as the brain stem, and adversely alter the function of interneuronal pools. Perhaps this dysregulation may increase reciprocal inhibitory input to motor neurons or to other inhibitory afferents, thus adding to the weakness seen clinically. The extent to which pharmacologic or other regulation of dystonia in spastic patients reduces negative symptoms, such as weakness, remains to be seen.

Before considering therapy for spasticity, it must be emphasized that spasticity, wherever and whenever diagnosed, should not automatically be treated. It is sometimes useful to the patient. For example, hemiplegic dystonia in extension of a leg may serve as a crutch or brace to support the patient's weight during stance or gait. Also, patients with spinal cord lesions sometimes induce flexor spasms to position their legs for putting on trousers and, as Babinski's nurse taught him, similar flexor spasms permit placement of a bedpan. Finally, when setting out to treat spasticity, both physician and patient must have realistic goals. The patient's disability is most likely the result of paresis, not spasticity, and relief of the latter may reduce discomfort and facilitate nursing care and/or hygiene, but it is unlikely to restore function.

Initial therapy for spasticity itself should involve the following, which must be considered before pharmacologic or invasive therapies are undertaken: First, an attempt should be made to discover factors that are increasing the severity of spasms or spastic dystonia in patients in whom CNS lesions are chronic and unchanging. For example, a urinary tract infection or another source of nociceptive input (e.g., pressure sore, unsuspected fracture, ingrown toenail) in a patient with spinal spasticity markedly worsens the symptoms and signs of spasticity. When the nonneurologic factors are alleviated, the patient's condition via-à-vis spasticity returns to its former state. Rarely, a new lesion, such as syringomyelia, is discovered. It should also be noted that non-tricyclic antidepressants (e.g., fluoxetine, trazodone, sertraline) have been reported to exacerbate spasticity,[61] perhaps by antagonizing the effects of baclofen. These antidepressants are serotonin reuptake inhibitors, and fluoxetine may also act on the $GABA_B$ receptor. If none of these accounts for the worsening of spasticity, pharmacologic treatment may be started, but before that (or in addition to it) the spastic muscles should be stretched several times a day. Even passive stretching is a remarkably effective therapy for spastic dystonia and is often overlooked.

Insofar as spasticity is the result of removal of supraspinal inputs to segmental interneurons, it is necessary to determine which neurotransmitters and neuromodulators are involved and to what extent they can be manipulated by agonists and antagonists. GABA has long been recognized as a mediator of presynaptic inhibition. Glycine is the strongest candidate for inhibitory postsynaptic potential production; a 50% reduction in glycine is seen in the segment of dog spinal cord caudal to a transection. Much activity has concerned the excitatory amino acids (EAAs), which include glutamate, aspartate, homocysteate, and cysteine sulphinate. Confusion still exists as to which substances, in addition to glutamate, are natural agonists and how many kinds of receptors are present.

Receptors have been named according to which agonist compound happens to have been used to study them. For example, glutamate activates at least the following five types of receptors: N-methyl-D-aspartate (NMDA), aminopropionic acid (AMPA), and kainate receptors, which are ionotropic (i.e., ligand-gated ion channels that open quickly), and amino-4-phosphonopropionic acid (L-AP4) and aminocyclopentyl dicarboxylic acid (ACPD) receptors (metabotropic), which are coupled to G proteins and operate on a slower time scale. This terminology continues to change, and clinically useful NMDA antagonists are being sought. Those available in the laboratory, such as MK-801, have untoward effects, including PCP (phencyclidine)-like actions, which limit their clinical use. PCP, itself an NMDA antagonist,[66] produces hallucinations, excitement, memory loss, depression, and hostile behavior. Evidence suggests that NMDA receptor activation releases nitric oxide (NO), which, acting as a neuromodulator like norepinephrine, diffuses to nearby synapses and alters their function.[43] This may play a role in plasticity as well as in neurotoxicity.

Flexor spasms and other cutaneous reflexes are thought to be released by lesions disrupting descending activity in the dorsal reticulospinal pathway. Axons in that system, which release norepinephrine (NE) and serotonin (5-HT), as well as non-monoaminergic transmitters, normally inhibit FRA input to the cord. Loss of this inhibition may account for increased flexor reflexes in spasticity. Endogenous opioids also reduce activity entering the cord via FRA and pain afferents. Substances, such as opiates, that reduce pain also alleviate spasticity, presumably by activating opioid receptors in the spinal dorsal horn. Neurotransmitters for each interneuronal circuit must be discovered and clinically useful agonists and antagonists developed so that a compilation similar to that seen in Table 22–1, but expanded and modified, can guide clinicians in the treatment of spastic paresis.

Useful pharmacotherapies for spasticity include baclofen, diazepam, and dantrolene[70] plus clonidine[45] and tizanidine (see *Neurology*, supplement 44 [in press]). Newer agents exist, such as tetrazepam, memantine,[5] and

TABLE 22–1

NEUROTRANSMITTERS AGONISTS AND ANTAGONISTS

SEGMENTAL ACTIVITY	NEUROTRANSMITTER
Alpha motor neuron collateral	Acetylcholine-N (nicotinic)
Ia EPSPs	EAAs (glutamate, aspartate)
Ia inhibitory interneuron	Glycine
Renshaw cell inhibition	Glycine
Presynaptic inhibition	GABA
Polysynaptic pathways	EAAs, 5-HT, substance P, TRH, etc.

DESCENDING ACTIVITY	NEUROTRANSMITTER
Reticulospinal (RST)	NE (inhibitory), Epi, DA, 5-HT (excitatory)
Dorsal RST	Non-monoaminergic
Ventral RST	Non-monoaminergic*
Rubrospinal	?EAAs
Vestibulospinal	?EAAs
Corticospinal	?EAAs, especially glutamate

NEUROTRANSMITTER	AGONIST
Acetylcholine-N	Nicotine, cytisine
EAAs	NMDA, AMPA, kainate
Glycine	Threonine
GABA with A-type receptors	Benzodiazepines, barbiturates
GABA with B-type receptors	Baclofen
5-HT	Sumatriptan, buspirone, LSD
Opioids	Morphine, other opiates

NEUROTRANSMITTER	ANTAGONIST
Acetylcholine-N	Trimethaphan
EAAs	2 APV, MK801
Glycine	Strychnine, tetanus toxin
GABA$_A$	Picrotoxin, bicuculline
GABA$_B$	Phaclofen, delta-aminovaleric acid
5-HT	Tricyclics, clozapine, clomipramine
Opioids	Naloxone, naltrexone
NE	Phenoxybenzamine
?Agmatine	
Adrenergic and imidazoline	Clonidine > tizanidine as alpha$_2$-agonists

*Does not inhibit flexor reflex afferents. EPSP = excitatory postsynaptic potentials; EAAs = excitatory amino acids; 5-HT = serotonin; NE = norepinephrine; TRH = thyroid-releasing hormone; Epi = epinephrine; DA = dopamine; NMDA = N-methyl-D-aspartate; AMPA = aminopropionic acid; LSD = lysergic acid diethylamide; 2 APV = 2-amino-S-phosphonovalerate.

mexiletine,[33] for which evidence is not yet convincing. (For a discussion of the mechanisms of action of the first three agents listed in this paragraph, see the 1981 review by Young and Delwaide[70]—little has changed regarding these substances.) Ivermectin, a GABA agonist used to treat onchocerciasis, has recently been reported to reduce spastic dystonia and spontaneous spasms in patients with spinal cord injury; it is presumed to act like baclofen.[12] Clonidine and tizanidine are alpha$_2$-adrenergic agonists, the effects of which on the spinal cord are generally inhibitory. Clonidine acts on structures within the spinal cord to restore noradrenergic inhibition, which may be deficient in spastic patients.[63] Clonidine also binds to the nonadrenergic imidazoline receptor, where agmatine may be the natural agonist.[39] It produces marked inhibition of short latency responses in alpha motor neurons to group II activity in the cat with spinal cord injury, presumably by increasing $alpha_2$-mediated presynaptic inhibition.[53] It also results in non-opiate analgesia by actions on $alpha_2$-receptors in the spinal dorsal horn, which inhibit release of substance P in that region.[46] This would diminish FRA-mediated actions and reduce flexor reflexes and spasms. Clinically, clonidine alleviates the stiffness of spastic dystonia in patients with spinal cord lesions, reduces the frequency and severity of spasms, and restores vibratory and Renshaw cell inhibitions to normal.[45, 54]

A uniquely direct and specific therapy diminishes the excessive muscle activity that accounts for spastic dystonia. Botulinum toxin injected into a muscle at its end-plate zone reduces or abolishes the release of acetylcholine from presynaptic motor axons and thereby weakens the muscle. The effect ("chemical denervation") develops over the course of a few days and lasts for several months, at which time, if the functional changes have been helpful, injections can be repeated. Although botulinum toxin is extremely potent, many thousands of patients have been treated with it worldwide without clinically significant systemic adverse reactions; it may diffuse locally to weaken muscles near to those being targeted, and occasionally short-lived tenderness is noted at the injection site. Overall, botulinum toxin is a remarkably safe and effective therapy. Clinical trials of botulinum toxin in the treatment of various types of spastic paresis are still under way, and details of its ultimate role in the therapy of these disorders remain to be worked out. In general terms, however, the following is already clear: Botulinum toxin is useful in treating spastic dystonia of cerebral palsy. In particular, injections into the triceps surae improve stance and gait (reduce toe walking) and forestall the need for surgical procedures to lengthen the Achilles tendon.[36] Injections into the same muscles in adults

with hemiplegic spasticity also improve stance and gait;[19] furthermore, they reduce "pistoning" of the lower limb out of an ankle-foot orthosis, thereby facilitating the use of this brace. Botulinum toxin injections reduce spastic dystonia seen in flexor muscles of hemiplegic upper limbs[30] and in adductor muscles of the lower limbs in patients with multiple sclerosis or other types of spinal cord impairment.[58] Even if these reductions in excessive muscle contraction are not associated with dramatic increases in function, they result in significant improvement in nursing care, hygiene, and patient comfort.[13, 42] Obviously botulinum toxin cannot be injected into all or even most of the spastic dystonic muscles of a patient with hemiparesis or paraparesis; the total amount of toxin needed would be too large and the task itself would be exhausting. The utility of botulinum toxin in this situation is restricted to treating a few particularly crucial muscles.[8]

Phenol or alcohol injections have also been used to damage nerves and weaken muscles. They damage both sensory and motor nerves, cause pain at the injection site, and are physically destructive, producing scarring and fibrosis. To minimize damage to surrounding structures, they must always be injected with EMG monitoring or as part of an open surgical procedure. Their effects last longer than those of botulinum toxin and are not fully reversible, but they can be considered for patients in whom therapy with botulinum toxin has failed.

Finally, several nonpharmacologic treatments are effective in reducing spastic dystonia. (1) Stretching spastic muscles, as noted earlier, is a very effective technique for reducing the dystonia, but it must be repeated daily (or several times a day), as the effects are relatively short-lived. (2) Microsurgical dorsal root entry zone lesions (DREZ-tomy) relieve both pain and spasticity by destroying the laterally placed small nociceptive fibers without producing loss of large fiber sensations.[57] Although they are invasive procedures, DREZ-tomy and selective dorsal rhizotomies[34] are replacing more destructive neurectomies and rhizotomies;[44] with the advent of more effective, less destructive therapies, fewer patients require procedures of this sort. (3) Nance and colleagues[45] demonstrated that electrostimulation with a rectal probe to activate perineal afferents reduces paraplegic dystonia and spasms for 3 to 24 hours. The principal side effect was autonomic dysreflexia, so patients were pretreated with nifedipine. Chronic dorsal column stimulation with an implanted device has also been reported to relieve spasticity,[41] but its efficacy is controversial. (4) Various orthoses are useful in compensating for paresis, and mechanical alterations of the lower limb (e.g., loading it to keep movement velocities below the threshold that must be reached before stretch reflex activity appears in antagonist muscles) may improve spastic gait.[40]

Intrathecal baclofen, a combined surgical/pharmacologic therapy using an implantable drug pump, is quite effective in relief of severe spastic paresis resulting from lesions of the spinal cord.[9, 47] It also relieves the spasms of tetanus and reduces the dystonia of spasticity due to cerebral lesions. Side effects, such as lethargy and respiratory depression, which are due to excessive concentrations of baclofen around the upper neuraxis, are infrequent when the lower limbs are the focus of therapeutic attention and the device is implanted in the thoracic region.

Finally, increasingly more effective therapies than those just discussed should emerge to minimize spastic dystonia and restore more normal reflex function to interneuronal circuits in the isolated cord; for example, spectacular improvements are expected in restoration of functions that have been lost because of disconnection of more cranial from more caudal motor centers within the CNS. The latter attempts to treat paralysis itself now include immunoactive therapies to permit regeneration and redirection of severed axons and grafting of fetal neural tissue into the damaged human nervous system. At least one pharmacotherapeutic agent is being used experimentally to overcome paralysis. 4-Aminopyridine, which blocks fast, voltage-gated potassium channels in neural membranes, has been shown to enhance motor unit recruitment in dogs[7] and humans[29] with spinal cord injuries and in patients with multiple sclerosis.[15, 59] 4-Aminopyridine is used to restore conduction in intact but demyelinated (and hence nonconducting) axons, thereby permitting function that otherwise appears to be irreversibly lost.

CONCLUSION

As it becomes better understood and as therapies for it improve, it is clear that spastic paresis is worthy of attention. It is a common and increasingly treatable disorder and is one of the focal points of neurorehabilitation.

REFERENCES

1. Ashby P, Mailis A, Hunter J: The evaluation of "spasticity." Can J Neurol Sci 14:497–500, 1987.
2. Ashby P, Wiens M: Reciprocal inhibition following lesions of the spinal cord in man. J Physiol 414:145–157, 1989.
3. Baldissera F, Hultborn H, Illert M: Integration in spinal neuronal systems. In Brooks VB (ed): Handbook of Physiology, sect 1: The Nervous System, vol. II. Motor Control, part 1. Bethesda, Md, American Physiological Society, 1981, pp 509–595.
4. Barbeau H, Julien C, Rossignol S: The effects of clonidine and yohimbine on locomotion and cutaneous reflexes in the adult chronic spinal cat. Brain Res 437:83–96, 1987.
5. Bauer HJ, Hanefeld FA: Multiple Sclerosis. Philadelphia, WB Saunders, 1993, pp 146–149.
6. Benecke R, Conrad B, Meinck HM, et al: Electromyographic analysis of bicycling on an ergometer for evaluation of spasticity of lower limbs in man. In Desmedt JE (ed): Motor Control Mechanisms in Health and Disease. New York, Raven Press, 1983, pp 1035–1046.
7. Blight AR, Toombs JP, Bauer MS, et al: The effects of 4-aminopyridine on neurological deficits in chronic cases of traumatic spinal cord injury in dogs: A phase I clinical trial. J Neurotrauma 8:103–119, 1991.
8. Borodic GE, Ferrante R, Wiegner AW, et al: Treatment of spasticity with botulinum toxin. Ann Neurol 31:113, 1992.
9. Coffey RJ, Cahill D, Steers W, et al: Intrathecal baclofen for intractable spasticity of spinal origin: Results of a long-term multicenter study. J Neurosurg 78:226–232, 1993.
10. Conrad B, Benecke R, Meinck HM: Gait disturbances in paraspastic patients. In Delwaide PJ, Young RR (eds): Clinical Neurophysiology in Spasticity. Amsterdam, Elsevier, 1985, pp 155–174.
11. Corcos DM, Gottlieb GL, Penn RD, et al: Movement deficits caused by hyperexcitable stretch reflexes in spastic humans. Brain 109:1043–1058, 1986.
12. Costa JL, Diazgranados JA: Ivermectin for spasticity in spinal-cord injury. Lancet 343:739, 1994.
13. Das TK, Park DM: Effect of treatment with botulinum toxin on spasticity. Postgrad Med J 19:208–210, 1989.
14. Davey NJ, Ellaway PH, Friedland CL, et al: Motor unit discharge characteristics and short term syn-

chrony in paraplegic humans. J Neurol Neurosurg Psychiatry 53:764–769, 1990.

15. Davis FA, Stefoski D, Rush J: Orally administered 4-aminopyridine improves clinical signs in multiple sclerosis. Ann Neurol 27:186–192, 1990.

16. Delwaide PJ: Spasticity, Motor Control Course No. 145. Minneapolis, American Academy of Neurology, 1993.

17. Delwaide PJ, Gerard P: Reduction of Non-reciprocal (Ib) Inhibition: A Key Factor for Interpreting Spastic Muscle Stiffness, International Congress on Stroke Rehabilitation. Berlin, November 1993.

18. Delwaide PJ, Pennisi G: Quantitative evaluation of the results of restorative neurology. In Young RR, Delwaide PJ (eds): Principles and Practice of Restorative Neurology. Oxford, Butterworth/Heinemann, 1992, pp 16–31.

19. Dengler R, Neyer U, Wohlfarth K, et al: Local botulinum toxin in the treatment of spastic drop foot. J Neurol 239:375–378, 1992.

20. Dietz V, Quintern J, Berger W: Electrophysiological studies of gait in spasticity and rigidity: Evidence that altered mechanical properties of muscle contribute to hypertonia. Brain 104:431–449, 1981.

21. Duncan GW, Shahani BT, Young RR: An evaluation of baclofen treatment for certain symptoms in patients with spinal cord lesions. Neurology 26:441–446, 1976.

22. Edgerton VR, de Guzman CP, Gregor RJ, et al: Trainability of the spinal cord to generate hindlimb stepping patterns in adult spinalized cats. In Shimamura M, Grillner S, Edgerton VR (eds): Neurobiological Basis of Human Locomotion. Tokyo, Japan Scientific Press, 1991, pp 411–423.

23. Fellows SJ, Ross HF, Thilmann AF: The limitations of the tendon jerk as a marker of pathological stretch reflex activity in human spasticity. J Neurol Neurosurg Psychiatry 56:531–537, 1993.

24. Fleshman JW, Rudomin P, Burke RE: Supraspinal control of a short-latency cutaneous pathway to hind limb motoneurons. Exp Brain Res 69:449–459, 1988.

25. Forssberg H, Grillner S: The locomotion of the acute spinal cat injected with clonidine i.v. Brain Res 50:184–186, 1973.

26. Gordon J: Spinal mechanisms of motor coordination. In Kandel ER, Schwartz JH, Jessell TM (eds): Principles of Neural Science, ed 3. Norwalk, Conn, Appleton & Lange, 1991, pp 581–595.

27. Hagbarth K-E, Wallin G, Lofstedt L: Muscle spindle response to stretch in normal and spastic subjects. Scand J Rehabil Med 5:156–159, 1973.

28. Halstead LS, Seager SWJ, Houston JM, et al: Relief of spasticity in SCI men and women using rectal probe electrostimulation. Paraplegia 31:715–721, 1993.

29. Hayes KC, Blight AR, Potter PJ, et al: Preclinical trial of 4-aminopyridine in patients with chronic spinal cord injury. Paraplegia 31:216–224, 1993.

30. Hesse S, Friedrich H, Domasch C, et al: Botulinum toxin therapy for upper limb flexor spasticity: Preliminary results. J Rehabil Sci 5:98–101, 1992.

31. Hufschmidt A, Mauritz KH: Chronic transformation of muscle in spasticity: A peripheral contribution to increased tone. J Neurol Neurosurg Psychiatry 48:676–685, 1985.

32. Jankowska E. Interneurons. In Adelman G (ed): Encyclopedia of Neuroscience. Boston, Birkhaeuser, 1987, pp 541–542.

33. Jimi T, Wakayama Y: Mexiletine for treatment of spasticity due to neurological disorders. Muscle Nerve 16:885, 1993.

34. Kasdon DL, Lathi ES: A prospective study of radio frequency rhizotomy in the treatment of posttraumatic spasticity. Neurosurgery 15:526–529, 1984.

35. Katz R, Pierrot-Deseilligny E: Recurrent inhibition of alpha-motoneurones in patients with upper motoneurone lesions. Brain 105:103–124, 1982.

36. Koman LA, Mooney JF, Smith B, et al: Management of cerebral palsy with botulinum-A toxin: Preliminary investigation. J Pediatr Orthop 13:489–495, 1993.

37. Lance JW: Symposium synopsis. In Feldman RG, Young RR, Koella WP (eds): Spasticity: Disordered Motor Control. Chicago, Year Book Medical Publishers, 1981, pp 485–494.

38. Lawrence DG, Kuypers HGJM: The functional organization of the motor system in the monkey: I. The effects of bilateral pyramidal lesions. Brain 91:1–14, 1968.

39. Li G, Regunathan S, Barrow CJ, et al: Agmatine: An endogenous clonidine-displacing substance in the brain. Science 263:966–969, 1994.

40. Maki BE, Rosen MJ, Simon SR: Modification of spastic gait through mechanical damping. J Biomechanics 18:504–511, 1985.

41. McBride GG: Dorsal column stimulation to control severe spasticity in spinal cord injury patients. J Am Paraplegia Soc 16:134, 1993.

42. Memin B, Pollak P, Hommel M, et al: Effects of botulinum toxin on spasticity. Rev Neurol 148:212–214, 1992.

43. Montague PR, Gancayco CD, Winn MJ, et al: Role of NO production in NMDA receptor-mediated neurotransmitter release in cerebral cortex. Science 263:973–977, 1994.

44. Munro D: Anterior-rootlet rhizotomy: A method of controlling spasm with retention of voluntary motion. N Engl J Med 246:161–166, 1952.

45. Nance PW, Shears AH, Nance DM: Reflex changes induced by clonidine in spinal cord injured patients. Paraplegia 27:296–301, 1989.

46. Ono H, Mishima A, Ono S, et al: Inhibitory effects of clonidine and tizanidine on release of substance P from slices of rat spinal cord and antagonism by alpha-adrenergic receptor antagonists. Neuropharmacology 30:585–589, 1991.

47. Penn RD, Savoy SM, Corcos D, et al: Intrathecal baclofen for severe spinal spasticity. N Engl J Med 320:1517–1521, 1989.

48. Petajan JH: Motor unit control in movement disorders. In Desmedt JE (ed): Motor Control Mechanisms in Health and Disease. New York, Raven, 1983, pp 897–905.

49. Pierrot-Deseilligny E, Mazieres L: Spinal mechanisms underlying spasticity. In Delwaide PJ, Young RR (eds): Clinical Neurophysiology in Spasticity. Amsterdam, Elsevier, 1985, pp 63–76.

50. Powers RK, Marder-Meyer J, Rymer WZ: Quantitative relations between hypertonia and stretch reflex threshold in spastic hemiparesis. Ann Neurol 23:115–124, 1988.

51. Roby-Brami A, Bussel B: Long-latency spinal reflex in man after flexor reflex afferent stimulation. Brain 110:707–725, 1987.

52. Russell WR, Young RR: Missile wounds of the parasagittal rolandic area. In Locke S (ed): Modern Neurology. Boston, Little, Brown, 1969, pp 289–302.

53. Schomburg ED, Steffens H: The effect of DOPA and clonidine on reflex pathways from group II afferents to alpha-motoneurons in the cat. Exp Brain Res 71:442–446, 1988.

54. Shefner JM, Berman SA, Sarkarati M, et al: Recurrent inhibition is increased in patients with spinal cord injury. Neurology 42:2162–2168, 1992.

55. Shefner JM, Berman SA, Young RR: The effect of nicotine on recurrent inhibition in the spinal cord. Neurology 43:2647–2651, 1993.

56. Shimazu H, Hongo T, Kubota K, et al: Rigidity and spasticity in man. Arch Neurol 6:24–31, 1962.

57. Sindou M: Microsurgical DREZ-tomy for the treatment of pain and spasticity. In Young RR, Delwaide PJ (eds): Principles and Practice of Restorative Neurology. Oxford, Butterworth/Heinemann, 1992, pp 144–151.

58. Snow BJ, Tsui JKC, Bhatt MH, et al: Treatment of spasticity with botulinum toxin: A double-blind study. Ann Neurol 28:512–515, 1990.

59. Stefoski D, Davis FA, Fitzsimmons WE, et al: 4-Aminopyridine in multiple sclerosis: Prolonged administration. Neurology 41:1344–1348, 1991.

60. Stein RB, Brucker BS, Ayyar DR: Motor units in incomplete spinal cord injury: Electrical activity, contractile properties and the effects of biofeedback. J Neurol Neurosurg Psychiatry 53:880–885, 1990.

61. Stolp-Smith KA, Wainberg M: Antidepressant exacerbation of spasticity. J Am Paraplegia Soc 16:140, 1993.

62. Thilmann AF, Fellows SJ: The time-course of bilateral changes in the reflex excitability of relaxed triceps surae muscle in human hemiparetic spasticity. J Neurol 238:293–298, 1991.

63. Unnerstall JR, Kopajtic TA, Kuhar MJ: Distribution of alpha-2 agonist binding sites in the rat and human central nervous system: Analysis of some functional, anatomic correlates of the pharmacologic effects of clonidine and related adrenergic agents. Brain Res 319:69–101, 1984.

64. Wernig A, Muller S: Laufband locomotion with body weight support improved walking in persons with severe spinal cord injuries. Paraplegia 30:229–238, 1992.

65. Wiegner AW, Wierzbicka MM, Davies L, et al: Discharge properties of single motor units in patients with spinal cord injuries. Muscle Nerve 16:661–671, 1993.

66. Wroblewski JT, Danysz W: Modulation of glutamate receptors: Molecular mechanisms and functional implications. Annu Rev Pharmacol Toxicol 29:441–474, 1989.

67. Yanagisawa N, Tanaka R, Ito Z: Reciprocal Ia inhibition in spastic hemiplegia of man. Brain 99:555–574, 1976.

68. Yang JF, Stein RB, Jhamandas J, et al: Motor unit numbers and contractile properties after spinal cord injury. Ann Neurol 28:496–502, 1990.

69. Young RR: Treatment of spastic paresis. N Engl J Med 320:1553–1555, 1989.

70. Young RR, Delwaide PJ: Drug therapy: Spasticity. N Engl J Med 304:28–33, 96–99, 1981.

71. Young RR, Wierzbicka MM: Behavior of single motor units in normal subjects and in patients with spastic paresis. In Delwaide PJ, Young RR (eds): Clinical Neurophysiology in Spasticity. Amsterdam, Elsevier, 1985, pp 27–40.

CHAPTER 23

Functional Electrical Stimulation and Its Application in the Management of Spinal Cord Injury

Timothy R. D. Scott, Ph.D.
P. Hunter Peckham, Ph.D.

Electrical stimulation of neural tissue provides a means of eliciting muscular activation of structures that are otherwise paralyzed when spinal cord pathways are interrupted. In the event that function does not return after the spinal injury, electrical stimulation may be used to restore functional capacity, for therapy to enhance the capabilities of the body, or to evoke a response of limited duration. Electrical stimulation has had an extensive history in its application to the human body.[46] However, the technology has now matured to the extent that it has become useful for persons with spinal cord injury.[93]

Electrical stimulation provides a nondestructive technique for selectively activating or silencing neural structures, despite the presence of the central nervous system (CNS) lesion. Furthermore, because neural structures remain electrically excitable, the technique can be applied in patients with recent or older injuries, unless secondary degeneration of axons due to the lesion has occurred. Thus, an opportunity exists to create an interface to a large number of organ systems to restore movement, sensation, waste control, respiration, reproductive function, and even certain types of homeostasis. Although the full achievement of potentially broad clinical impacts awaits future developments, several clinical systems that have an impact on the daily lives of individuals with spinal cord injuries are now in use or in clinical trials.

In this chapter, the basis for electrical stimulation of the peripheral nervous system and the present status of its clinical applications for spinal cord–injured individuals are reviewed.

OVERVIEW

Applied Motor Control

Electrical stimulation of a nerve via an extracellular current-carrying electrode results in a local depolarization of the axon membrane. This local depolarization results in an action potential that is propagated along the nerve. For nerves innervating muscle, the propagating action potential activates the muscle, causing it to contract. Functional electrical stimulation (FES) or functional neuromuscular stimulation (FNS) involves the coordination of muscles that are stimulated in this manner to produce purposeful movement.

By definition, FES must provide function for the person to whom it is administered. Equipment producing electrically stimulated muscle contractions therefore needs to meet certain criteria. It must produce coordinated movement, be safe, be user-controllable, be aesthetically acceptable, and provide significant benefit to the user.

Most persons who have undergone FES thus far have had complete traumatic spinal cord lesions. In its application to persons with incomplete lesions, considerations of whether neurologic function has stabilized, what functional benefits are expected, and toleration of stimulation should be addressed. Candidates with nontraumatic spinal cord lesions or impairments (if they are not associated with a progressive disease) can be assessed on the same basis as those with traumatic spinal cord lesions.[78]

To produce functional coordinated movement, the degree of activation of an individual muscle must be controlled and sets of muscles must be activated in synchrony (for review see Mortimer[85]). Requirements for each individual muscle that is to be utilized in the electrically activated movements are as follows: (1) generates little or no voluntary contraction, (2) has little or no denervation, and (3) is affected by negligible or pharmacologically controlled spasticity.

An important parameter with regard to safe electrical stimulation is the *stimulus waveform*. In addition to influencing the degree of recruitment of the target nerve and muscle being activated, the stimulus waveform influences the electrochemical reactions occurring at the electrode-tissue interface.[85] A constant-current source is generally used for stimulation because it produces a constant electrical field at the extracellular electrode site. This results in charge injection that is independent of local electrochemical reactions and is constant with repeated stimulation. A voltage-regulated source, the alternative to a current-regulated one, does not ensure this response.

The parameters of the stimulus waveform have a considerable influence on nerve recruitment. The stimulus consists of trains of pulses that are applied in sequence. As the width of the individual pulses is decreased, an increase in current amplitude is required to maintain the same degree of excitation. Modulation of these stimulus parameters thus regulates muscle activation and controls the strength of contraction of electrically stimulated muscles.[22]

When electrical stimulation is applied to a nerve, large-diameter axons are stimulated with less extracellular charge than smaller-diameter axons. Axons have a large membrane resistance and a small axoplasmic resistance. These resistances are inversely proportional to the axon radius, thus making larger-diameter axons (which innervate the larger motor units) more responsive to applied electrical current. Muscle activation can be controlled, even with stimulation of a single nerve, by modification of electrical stimulation, so as to differentiate between activating large and small axons. This is opposite to natural recruitment, in which smaller-diameter neurons are fired physiologically before larger-diameter neurons (Henneman's size principle). Small motor axons can be selectively activated electrically by modification of the stimulus waveform.[33] Proximity of the electrode to the nerve is also an important parameter in considering the degree of nerve stimulation (or recruitment) because the electrical field decreases radially from the electrode. With monopolar electrode stimulation, the field decreases as the inverse of the radius and with bipolar electrode stimulation, the field decreases as the inverse square of the radius.[89]

Along with electrode materials, size, and shape, the stimulus waveform has considerable influence on the electrochemical reactions that occur at the electrode-tissue interface. Some of the consequences of these reactions that can be avoided are electrode corrosion and tissue damage, both of which are detrimental to the function of the neuroprosthesis. Waveforms incorporating capacitative mechanisms and reversible faradic reactions for the delivery of a low overall charge density are considered to be safe, and they avoid the harmful irreversible reactions characteristic of high charge densities.[85] Biphasic stimulation is preferred over monophasic stimulation to reduce charge accumulation at the site of stimulation and resultant buildup of byproducts of the electrochemical reactions. The cathodic phase is applied for stimulation and the anodic phase is applied with the intention of reversing the electrochemical reactions.

Variation in the stimulus pulse frequency has been shown to alter muscle contraction by varying the rate of firing of active fibers. With gradual increase of stimulus frequency, the twitch contractions gradually fuse together to provide a tetanic increase in muscle force. Thus, muscle force is related strongly to the frequency of applied stimulation.[91] When modulating the frequency of applied stimulation, it is necessary to set limits to prevent muscle fatigue and damage. Nerve degeneration has been associated with stimulus frequencies of 50 Hz applied continuously for 2 hours.[1] Animal studies of diaphragm pacing using electrical stimulation of the phrenic nerve at 27 to 33 Hz for months reported ultrastructural damage to the muscle that did not occur with stimulation at 11 to 13 Hz.[21] For FES, the stimulation frequency must be high enough to produce a fused contraction with a usable force without compromising the safety of stimulation and causing undue muscle fatigue.

Techniques

Electrical stimulation for FES is undertaken using surface, percutaneous, implanted epimysial, or implanted neural electrodes.[108] These alternatives provide clinicians the opportunity to make the best choices for their patients, specific to the particular FES application.

Surface electrodes allow a quick and flexible means of noninvasive application of FES to subjects with spinal cord injury. However, the use of long-term surface stimulation in an FES system presents considerable disadvantages, which most likely limit its serious application to muscle exercise and conditioning. These disadvantages include a lack of specificity of which muscle is being stimulated, difficulty reaching deep muscles, and a greater likelihood of causing pain and discomfort through cutaneous stimulation. In addition, placement of surface electrodes on the skin is not likely to be entirely repeatable from day to day, electrode stimulation sites may vary with limb position, and the appearance of the electrodes is undesirable. Burns resulting from surface FES have also been reported.[7] Electrical stimulation has been shown in some cases to cause symptoms of autonomic dysreflexia,[4] which may be a result of the electrical activation of nociceptors that—via afferents to the spinal cord—cause a massive reflex sympathetic response. For these reasons, care should be taken when electrical stimulation—especially surface stimulation—is applied; surface stimulation is less specific and has an increased likelihood of activating nociceptors. When surface electrodes are used to apply rectangular pulses, threshold values are generally 30 mA or greater for a pulse width of 100 to 300 μsec,[92] although variations in the impedance at the skin-electrode interface are influential in determining these parameters.

Percutaneous intramuscular electrodes

used in the application of FES systems can easily be inserted via a hypodermic needle and placement can be relatively long term (months to years). This form of stimulation permits a single muscle to be individually stimulated. Some of the problems encountered with these electrodes include shearing stress and maintenance of the skin entry site. Shearing occurs when tissue layers, through which the electrode passes, move in opposing directions. The force on the wires is sufficient in some instances to fracture the electrode, making it useless. A lack of mobility is one of the problems with the percutaneous system, in which all components are external except the electrodes. Also, careful monitoring of the electrode skin entry site is necessary to check for the occurrence of problems such as infection and granuloma formation. Intramuscular electrodes generally elicit a maximal muscle contraction with stimulus parameters of 20 mA and 200 μsec pulse width.[92]

In a totally implantable system (telemetry controlled), stress on the electrodes and their leads is reduced and they are less subject to fracture or movement. Further benefits include the optimal location of electrodes on a particular muscle during surgery and elimination of the skin interface for the electrode. The most suitable choice for permanent FES applications is for the electrodes to be implanted surgically, either epimysially or neurally. An epimysial electrode is sutured to the muscle near the motor point. Stimulation parameters for epimysial electrodes are similar to those described for intramuscular electrodes. Recruitment following stimulation using an epimysial electrode is nonlinear and is also length-dependent, which means that the force output changes with muscle length as a result of changes in the electrode-nerve coupling.[92] This effect is added to the usual length-tension properties of the muscle. Neural electrodes are placed adjacent to, around (encircling), or within the nerve. Although these electrodes have the greatest potential for producing the best controllability for FES, they carry an increased risk of nerve damage. With an encircling nerve cuff electrode, maximal responses are elicited with stimuli of

approximately 2 mA and several hundred microseconds' duration.

RESPIRATORY FUNCTION

Electrical stimulation has been applied to treat some of the disorders of respiratory function that affect patients with spinal cord injury. The development of better interventional devices using electrical stimulation in the management of these problems is likely to result in reduced requirements for assistive care and in increased mobility for these patients.

Pacing

Considerable research has been undertaken in the application of FES to control breathing (for review see Nochomovitz et al.[90]). Candidates for this type of system are persons requiring respiratory support or assistance such as persons with high-level quadriplegia or those suffering from other syndromes that cause hypoventilation. Midcervical spinal cord injury results in paralysis of the diaphragm and intercostal muscles, which creates a requirement for interventional devices to maintain minimum respiration necessary for survival.

The primary muscle for inspiration is the diaphragm, which is innervated bilaterally by the phrenic nerves, the motor neuron pools of which are at C3, C4, and C5. Respiratory control is centered in the dorsal medulla at the base of the brain, where ventilatory rate is set to maintain normal values for arterial partial pressures of CO_2 and O_2 and where coordination of the muscles responsible for opening the upper airway and moving the rib cage takes place. An FES system activating the phrenic nerves aims to reestablish the control usually undertaken by the respiratory center in the brain and cervical spinal cord.

Remnant muscle function, generally available to individuals in this group with spinal cord injury, is in the upper airway and possibly in the sternocleidomastoid, although it may be compromised if the spinal accessory nerve is damaged. Paralyzed muscles with intact lower motor neuron innervation may be utilized for respiration through the application of electrical stimulation. In particular, electrical stimulation of the phrenic nerve causes contraction of the diaphragm. In clinical applications, stimulation is applied to as much of the phrenic nerve as possible to produce activation of both the costal and crural regions of the hemidiaphragm. Bilateral stimulation of the phrenic nerves provides a large benefit to respiration as it yields approximately twice the transdiaphragmatic pressure that is produced by unilateral phrenic nerve pacing.[90]

Scalene and intercostal muscles provide significant support to the rib cage when the diaphragm produces inspiration in normal breathing.[26, 27] Electrical stimulation of intercostal muscles in conjunction with that of the diaphragm has been suggested[90] and may provide a significant benefit. Together with increasing the inspiratory capability, intercostal stimulation might be used to eliminate upper rib cage paradoxical movements and to improve respiratory tidal volumes. Any benefit of using intercostal stimulation must be weighed against increased system complexity and risk of infection. Indeed, intercostal stimulation alone is likely to provide its most significant benefit to respiration when phrenic stimulation is unsuitable, such as when there has been damage to the diaphragm's innervation. In a study undertaken with dogs,[28] it was shown that electrical stimulation of the intercostal muscles alone provided up to 35% of normal inspiratory capacity.

Clinical application of electrical stimulation systems for respiratory pacing began with the development of an implantable device stimulating the phrenic nerve that was controlled externally by radiofrequency (RF) telemetered signals.[39, 40] Glenn's group is responsible for most of the clinical data derived from use of phrenic stimulators for over 20 years in approximately 600 people. This system, which was commercialized by Avery Laboratories, uses an external RF transmitter, the signal from which is decoded by the implant. The stimulus comes from the implant

via stainless steel monopolar or bipolar electrodes that are placed adjacent to or around the phrenic nerve. Application of the electrodes is generally undertaken in the chest via a thoracotomy, which avoids difficult neck surgery that would otherwise be required and which may also allow recruitment of extraphrenic nerve fibers that join the main phrenic trunk in the chest.

The main difficulties encountered in the application of this pacing system are fatigue and nerve damage resulting from electrical stimulation. Phrenic pacing requires the application of repetitive pulse trains and fatigue and possible nerve damage occur at stimulus frequencies between 27 and 33 Hz.[21] More recent investigations[55] have addressed low-frequency stimulation for phrenic pacing applications in quadriplegics. Damage was not observed with stimulation between 11 and 13 Hz. Two other phrenic pacing systems, one from Vienna, Austria (MedImplant GmbH) and one from Tampere, Finland (Atrotech OY), have addressed this question of fatigue and nerve damage by applying a migrating electrical field over the phrenic nerve cross section. These groups suggest that fatigue may be reduced by moving the electrical field throughout the nerve, although this hypothesis has not been proven.[90]

Researchers at Case Western Reserve University investigating phrenic pacing have used intramuscular electrodes in the diaphragm to stimulate the phrenic nerve.[89] With this method, similar maximal transdiaphragmatic pressures and tidal volumes were generated, as was the case with systems utilizing indwelling nerve cuffs in the neck. Peterson[100] showed that intramuscular phrenic nerve pacing provides 167% of ventilation necessary to support basal metabolism. Also, animal studies[100, 101] have shown that repeatable full-time bilateral stimulation can be achieved utilizing intramuscular electrodes without producing fatigue of the respiratory muscle. Other advantages of the intramuscular electrodes were that they showed no change in recruitment over time, caused no mechanical damage, and had sufficient anchoring properties to the muscle; in addition, a favorable tissue reaction to the electrodes and leads was noted. It was further shown that these intramuscular systems caused a nearly complete conversion of muscle fibers to the slow-twitch oxidative type.[100] This indicated that low-frequency stimulation is sufficient to produce a tetanic diaphragm contraction and supports the use of low-frequency bilateral stimulation from intramuscular electrodes to produce ventilation with reduced fatigue. A subsequent development of this technique involves the use of epimysial electrodes, which are placed laparoscopically for diaphragm activation.[113]

A significant problem with the current methods of electrically stimulated respiration is the requirement for tracheotomy, because the paced diaphragm is not synchronized with the spontaneous opening of the upper airways. The tracheotomy generally can be kept closed during the day, as volitional coordinated throat opening is possible; the tracheotomy must remain open during sleep to avoid airway obstruction. Research undertaken in addressing this problem of lack of coordination between the diaphragm and upper airway muscles concerns means of controlling the diaphragm pacing so that it is in synchrony with the opening of the airway. Airway opening has been assessed by recording from the sternocleidomastoid[111] or by measuring end-tidal CO_2 and changes in normal air temperature during breathing.[11, 109] More recent work monitors activity of the ala nasi muscle (nose flaring muscle, whose phasic activity usually aids respiration immediately prior to phrenic activity), which might provide a signal for triggering the onset of electrical stimulation of the phrenic nerve.[120]

In a multicenter study, Glenn and coworkers[39] found that of all of a group of phrenic pacers implanted, 47% were regarded as successful and patients did not require additional ventilatory support. The device was deemed to give significant benefit to another 36%, with a further 16% obtaining little or no support. In a subsequent study of 14 quadriplegic patients using bilateral diaphragm pacers,[31] 12 of 13 patients (1 of the 14 died of abdominal sepsis during hospitalization for the institution of diaphragm pacing) were able to receive full-time pacing. For these 12

patients, pacing continued for 2 to 15 years (mean, 7.6 years). At the time of this report, 7 patients were continuing to receive full-time pacing, with 2 using it part-time. Pacing provided normal tidal volumes and normal arterial blood gas values in all patients who received long-term pacing, and the nerve showed no loss of ability to be stimulated. The patients' quality of life was said to be improved when compared with that provided by positive-pressure ventilation. This improvement came in the form of increased independence, which contributed to a variety of educational, occupational, and social accomplishments. These results provide significant encouragement for the further clinical development and application of respiratory pacing systems using electrical stimulation.

Cough

Paralysis of abdominal muscles in individuals with spinal cord injury impairs their ability to cough and clear the airways of secretions. Traditional methods of management of this problem include positioning of the patient to passively drain secretions by gravity, applying active suction, or performing an assisted cough. In the assisted cough, an attendant applies pressure to the patient's abdomen while the patient, in coordination with this pressure, controls the opening or closing of the upper airways.

To produce a cough, investigators[58, 76] have stimulated the abdominal muscles electrically to increase pressure and flow in the airways. In a study of 24 tetraplegic individuals,[76] volitional, assisted, and electrical stimulation–induced methods of producing cough were compared. Normalized peak air flow rate was used as a quantitative measure of cough effectiveness. Electrical stimulation was applied via surface electrodes placed according to a skin surface map. Of the 24 patients studied, 5 could not tolerate electrical stimulation of the abdomen and 5 others had little or no response to electrical stimulation. For the remaining 14 subjects, assisted and electrically stimulated cough both had higher peak flow rates than the volitional cough.

Manually assisted cough was found to produce a higher peak air flow than the electrically stimulated cough. This study provides much encouragement for the use of electrical stimulation to produce cough, because although the performance of the stimulated cough was not as good as the assisted cough, an assisted cough requires an attendant, which decreases the patient's independence and may result in undertaking a cough less frequently than is desired. Also, the performance of the electrically activated cough may improve with optimization of electrode placement, a period of abdominal muscle conditioning, and the use of implantable electrodes with either a percutaneous interface or the development of an implantable stimulator. Current research into the dynamic events during cough[13] promises to increase understanding and improve application of electrical stimulation to produce an artificial cough.

BLADDER, BOWEL, AND SEXUAL FUNCTION

Persons with spinal cord injury lose the ability to control their sexual, bladder, and bowel function, which significantly affects their quality of life. Along with the social, hygiene, and psychological problems that this loss of function may cause, it also causes medical problems and reduces life expectancy.[125] In many cases, classical management of these problems has not provided an adequate solution, thus encouraging the application of FES in this area.

Micturition for Spinal Cord–Injured Patients Using FES

To produce micturition, FES has been applied directly to the bladder, to the conus medullaris, and to the sacral anterior roots or sacral nerves (for review see Creasey[24]). Electrical stimulation of the sacral anterior roots (the most successful of these techniques) or of the sacral nerves containing efferents to the lower urinary tract has been the most widely applied method of producing micturition. The following discussion of FES-controlled micturition deals predominantly with sacral root stimulation.

Two approaches to sacral root stimulation have been taken by Brindley and others[17, 19]: extradural and intradural. Intradural stimulation is used with separation of anterior and posterior roots so that posterior root stimulation, and therefore reflex urethral sphincter activation, may be minimized so as not to inhibit micturition. When arachnoiditis makes intradural placement of electrodes difficult, an extradural approach is taken. On stimulation of the mixed sacral roots, the detrusor and sphincter muscles both contract. The sphincter is striated muscle so it contracts and relaxes more rapidly than the smooth detrusor muscle. This property is exploited by the use of intermittent stimulation so that sphincter and bladder contractions are out of phase with one another. In this case, the sphincter relaxes rapidly at the end of each electrical burst, whereas the bladder pressure is maintained sufficiently long to produce micturition between the bursts. In the worldwide implementation of this device, at least 572 implants have been used so far.[126] Tanagho and colleagues[122] stimulated the sacral nerves or their motor components extradurally by placement of electrodes in the spinal canal. Surgical procedures, usually combined with implantation of the sacral root stimulator to reduce sphincter resistance, include peripheral neurectomy, myotomy (sphincterotomy), posterior rhizotomy, and selective pudendal neurectomy. In another approach, described by Talalla and Bloom,[121] extradural sacral nerve stimulation was undertaken without a sensory rhizotomy or pudendal neurectomy. This was initially successful and resulted in voiding using intermittent stimulation, but the reflex contraction of the bladder outlet that occurred concurrently was deemed to be unacceptable.

The two devices that predominate in the clinical implementation of sacral root stimulation are one distributed by Finetech, developed by Brindley, and one distributed by Medtronic, developed by Tanagho. Both are most suitable for persons with complete spinal cord lesions. In those with incomplete lesions, one should consider whether neurologic function has stabilized and whether the patient wishes to preserve sensory and reflex function (and not undertake posterior rhizotomy); also, the risk that the implant will cause pain should be taken into account (although tolerance can be evaluated prior to the implant).[78]

Co-activation of the urethral sphincter with stimulation of the sacral roots presents a major challenge. It can occur as a result of the electrical stimulation directly or reflexly and interferes with micturition by producing detrusor-sphincter dyssynergia. The latter is difficult to avoid because axons to the sphincter are intimately mixed in the sacral anterior roots and nerves with preganglionic parasympathetic efferent axons to the detrusor. Axons to the sphincter are easier to stimulate, which accounts for the difficulty encountered in activating motor fibers to the bladder without activating those to the sphincter as well. Reflex activation of the sphincter also occurs as a result of electrical stimulation of sensory fibers. The problem of reflex activation can be dealt with by surgically dividing sensory fibers from the sacral segments and applying electrodes to the motor fibers only. Posterior rhizotomy, which involves the division of all the posterior roots from S2–5, removes altogether the problem of reflex contractions of the sphincter. A further advantage of posterior rhizotomy in conjunction with sacral root stimulation is that it abolishes reflex bladder contractions, which increases bladder capacity and prevents reflex incontinence. Also, bladder compliance can be restored to normal, thus protecting the upper tracts, and autonomic dysreflexia arising from contraction of bladder or rectum is abolished. When a sacral root stimulator is implanted, posterior rhizotomy is generally recommended, although the clinician should consider each individual case on its own merits, especially in male patients. Some patients are able to activate reflex pathways to produce micturition, defecation, erection, and ejaculation. This might, for example, be done with vibratory stimulation. Posterior rhizotomy results in the loss of these reflex functions, although electrical stimulation, as has been reported,[24] in many cases restores these functions with increased peformance and re-

liability. Advantages and disadvantages of posterior rhizotomy should be examined by the clinician and potential patient with a view to its use with a sacral root stimulator.

To avoid the need for posterior rhizotomy, Sawan and colleagues[110] tried fatiguing the external sphincter in animals by electrical stimulation of the pudendal nerve. This fatigued state would result in reduction of the bladder outlet resistance, which could then be more easily overcome by bladder contraction controlled by sacral root stimulation. Hence, the effects of detrusor-sphincter dyssynergia would be reduced. Brindley and Craggs,[16] in addressing this problem, suggested blocking the propagating action potential in the large somatic axons while allowing signals to pass in the small parasympathetic fibers to the detrusor (as described by Fang and Mortimer[33]). Creasey[24] attempted this in a developmental study in dogs in whom it was possible to produce contraction of bladder and rectum without contraction of the external sphincters. Rijkhoff and others[107] also investigated the use of anodal block for this purpose in dogs; it shows a great deal of promise, although further investigations are necessary before it can be applied to humans.

Bowel Function

Stimulation of the lower sacral roots and spinal cord at the S3 level produces a response that should assist bowel function in spinal cord–injured persons (see Van Kerrebroeck et al.[126]; Banwell et al.[8]). Whereas lower sacral root stimulation causes contraction of the external anal sphincter and raises the pelvic floor, stimulation of S3 roots causes contraction of the lower bowel and increases the frequency of defecation (Mac-Donagh et al.[77]). This has been studied using the Finetech sacral implant, which was adjusted so that investigation of bowel function could be undertaken. Documentation of defecatory function using this stimulation indicates it produced moderate success (50% to 60%). Ongoing studies, including one described by Creasey,[24] are addressing the applicability of electrical stimulation for restoration of bowel function.

Electroejaculation

Electroejaculation (EE) has had a large degree of success in enabling men with spinal cord injuries to become biological fathers. Up to 95% of men with spinal cord injury are unable to ejaculate normally or by masturbation (Tarabulcy[123]), but current methods of semen collection, including vibratory stimulation, electrostimulation, and vas aspiration (see Bennett et al.[10] for review), followed by intrauterine insemination have resulted in successful conception in a large number of cases.

Over 3,600 EE procedures were evaluated in a study of 425 spinal cord–injured and other neurologically impaired men.[115, 116] Stimulation is applied using a rectal probe electrode with a higher voltage (10–15 V, 100–400 mA at 60 Hz) for patients injured below the T10 level than for those injured above this level (4–10 V, 100–400 mA at 60 Hz). If the patient has an incomplete lesion, spinal or general anesthesia may be required; for those with a complete injury, EE may be done as an outpatient procedure. Seager's study[116] suggests that this procedure may be promising. The average sperm count in 89 subjects was 505×10^6 per ejaculate, which far exceeds the count for men without spinal cord injury. In a study of 33 subjects who had been injured for 15 or more years (ages 17 to 41 years), EE produced semen adequate for insemination. In 14 of the subjects studied, spinal cord injury was sustained before age 11 years. The average age of the subjects at first EE was 27 years, and 10 of the 14 had semen of sufficient quality to be used for insemination. This suggests that spinal cord injury prior to puberty does not affect the potential fertility of males. Three subjects had semen evaluated preinjury and postinjury (preinjury: 9, 3, and 2 months; postinjury: 3, 4, and 6 months) with no significant change in motility or sperm count. These data suggest that spinal cord injury may not, as previously thought, have a negative effect on spermatogenesis. A single subject (40 years old) underwent EE 57 times in 68 months with no decline in the sperm quality or quantity. Thus, patients may not become refractory when EE is carried out over an extended period. With further increases in the frequency of EE in another subject (ten times over a 6-week period), the sperm count per ejaculate decreased from 476×10^6 to 160×10^6. These studies document significant improvements in EE in comparison with two previous studies by Brindley[14, 15] in which 154 men with spinal cord injury had EE; although semen was obtained from most men, good-quality semen was obtained from only a few, which led to only three pregnancies.

UPPER EXTREMITY FUNCTION

FES has been successfully used in the paralyzed upper extremity for restoration of hand function (see Gorman and Peckham[41] and Scott et al.[114] for reviews). Candidates benefiting from such a system are predominantly persons with traumatic cervical spinal cord injury. Minimum goals for FES systems in the upper limb are to provide grasp and release, which is controlled by the user. In addition to paralysis of hand grasp, a cervical spinal lesion may result in other deficits in motor control that increase the requirements for a functional upper extremity neuroprosthesis. These deficits may include wrist extension, pronation-supination, elbow extension or flexion, and shoulder control. As described in the following text, FES researchers are currently addressing these issues.

Keller and co-workers[65] demonstrated that normal subjects utilize predominantly two types of grasp: lateral prehension (or key grip) and palmar prehension (or three jaw chuck pinch). To provide users with considerable functional benefit from FES hand grasp systems, the Cleveland upper extremity neuroprosthesis (Fig. 23–1) has incorporated these two grasp patterns.[98] The current device consists of an implantable stimulator controlled and powered by external RF telemetry.[118] For lateral grasp, it was necessary to provide coordinated activation of thumb extensors, flexors, and adductors, together with finger flexors and extensors. Palmar grasp required the coordinated activation of thumb abductors, finger extensors, and finger flexors. As a minimum requirement for the system to be

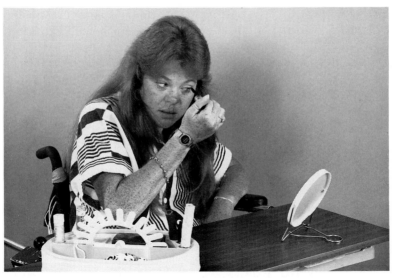

FIGURE 23–1

The implantable neuroprosthesis developed in Cleveland to provide functional electrical stimulation hand grasp has been shown to provide significant improvements in the ability of persons with C5 and C6 spinal cord injuries to perform activities of daily living, both in laboratory assessment and at home, thereby reducing their disability. A person with a C5 spinal cord injury is shown using the system for hand grasp to apply makeup.

applicable,[94] the candidate must produce at least a grade 3/5 muscle contraction (see Kendall and McCreary[66] for further description) with electrical stimulation of the following key muscles: extensor pollicis longus, extensor digitorum communis, and adductor pollicis brevis. In addition, at least a grade 4 contraction must be produced with electrical stimulation of adductor pollicis, flexor digitorum superficialis, and flexor digitorum profundus muscles. If one of these muscles is weak or denervated, accommodation may be possible using augmentative surgical procedures to modify hand biomechanics (see Keith et al.[64] for review).

Desired grasp, requiring coordinated muscle stimulation, was obtained by establishing a stimulus grasp map that translates the user-issued control signal into a stimulus level applied to each electrode.[67–70] The command signal is the sternoclavicular joint angle as measured by a skin-surface mounted joystick on the sternum, with an outwardly telescoping rod attached to the shoulder. This permits the user to have proportional and stable control of the hand system via shoulder movement.[60] Development of an implantable version of this sensor is currently under way.[61]

Wijman and others[128] reported that of 22 users of the Cleveland upper extremity neuroprosthesis who undertook a subset of 10 specified tasks, the median success rate across these tasks was 89% with the neuroprosthesis and 49% without the device. This demonstrated a significant benefit provided for users of the device. Further rigorous testing to quantify the users' independence, quality of performance, and preference, demonstrated that this system provides significant improvements in the ability of patients with C5 and C6 injuries to perform activities of daily living—both in the laboratory and at home—thereby reducing their disability.[129]

A multicenter study is presently under way to evaluate the utility of the implanted hand system across a population of patients when the procedure is performed by personnel at those centers (i.e., technology transfer). Candidate selection criteria to enhance the likelihood of a successful outcome for the hand grasp system, together with the minimum muscle-strength requirements with electrical stimulation as described previously, include additional medical, physical, and psychosocial requirements.[12] Medical requirements include freedom from infection, skin breakdown, uncontrolled spasticity, diabetes, chronic renal failure, and cardiac or pulmonary disease. Physical capabilities should include proximal control of hand positioning adequate to cover the user's functional work space, good trunk stability in the wheelchair, and a passive range of motion for the fingers and wrist that allows the formation of functional grasp and release. The arm should be tolerant of cutaneous stimulation. The candidate's neurologic function should have become stable (at least 1 year postinjury). This system has been implanted in 21 persons, with the longest implant period being more than 8 years; eight persons have been using the system for more than 1 year. The system enables users to perform activities at home (e.g., eating, self-care, entertainment), at work (e.g., writing, computer operation, telephoning), and during recreation (e.g., painting, chess, needlepoint, bingo), thus adding to both independence and quality of life.

In addition to the Cleveland device described here, implantable upper extremity neuroprostheses have been developed in Poland[71] and England,[99] although they have had limited application. Investigators at Sendai have developed an upper extremity neuroprosthesis for hand grasp that uses percutaneous electrodes[47] similar to those previously used in Cleveland.[96] Hand systems described thus far predominantly address the patient with C5 and weak C6 function. There have been limited studies of the application of FES systems for the reestablishment of functional hand grasp in patients with C4 level injuries. One system utilizes puff-sip commands to provide stimulation through percutaneous electrodes.[54] Another system effects voice-activated stimulation via surface electrodes.[87]

Investigators have attempted to control wrist extension to permit effective hand grasp by patients who have no volitional wrist extension, thereby removing the necessity of the wrist splint that is often worn during FES grasp for tenodesis resistance.[23, 87] Crago and co-workers[87] are also addressing the control of pronation and supination of the arm via FES. Research into the control of elbow extension is likely to result in its incorporation into forthcoming clinical FES systems[51, 54, 83]

that permit arm placement in the case of the user with C4 level injury and improved work space for the person with C5 or C6 level injury. It is likely that further improvement with arm placement for patients with C4 level injury will be possible with FES of the shoulder musculature,[48] thus enabling this user population to discard the awkward balanced forearm orthosis needed in FES systems described thus far.

LOWER EXTREMITY SYSTEMS

Applications of FES to the lower extremities of persons with spinal cord injury have predominantly addressed the restoration of standing, walking on flat surfaces, and climbing stairs (see Jaeger[56] for review). Potential candidates for such systems are those with complete or incomplete injuries in the thoracic region who have enough innervated muscles in the lower extremity to permit electrically stimulated functional movement. Many applications of FES for the lower extremity incorporate orthoses to limit the number of degrees of freedom and to produce stability and structural support which reduce fatigue and possible damage as a result of stress on the lower limbs and trunk. Devices using orthotics combined with electrical stimulation are known as *hybrid devices* (see Kantor et al.[63] and Marsolais et al.[80] for reviews).

The first FES-assisted standing devices[127] demanded that patients have electrically excitable quadriceps as a minimum criterion.[73] Since that time, a number of demonstrations of open-loop standing for transient periods have been made using balance aids.[59, 73] Attempts to achieve walking with FES devices have been made in the following different ways: direct stimulation of lower extremity muscles to provide the necessary movements,[79] stimulation of functional movement by reflex activation in concert with direct stimulation,[3, 6, 42, 105] or constant stimulation of the quadriceps to stabilize the knee and to allow crutch-assisted ambulation with a swing-to or swing-through gait.[52]

A review of 94 spinal cord–injured patients in Ljubljana, Slovenia, who received surface FES for standing, walking, and crutch-assisted gait[74] indicated that patients with T3- to 12-level injuries were the best candidates for this system. Standing was achieved by bilateral stimulation of quadriceps with the assistance of a standing frame. Four channels of stimulation were utilized for reciprocal gait assisted by a walker or crutches; two channels were used for quadriceps stimulation and two channels were used for bilateral activation of the flexion reflex. The flexion reflex was substituted for the swing phase of the gait cycle. Of the 94 patients, 62 achieved standing and walking with four-channel stimulation and 29 of the remaining 32 were able to utilize two-channel stimulation for standing. A major disadvantage of this system is that a flexion withdrawal reflex is not present bilaterally in all patients with spinal cord injury who might otherwise use the system. Also, when this reflex is present, it is often variable and can accommodate to the stimulation.[56] A device similar to the four-channel walking system, known as the Parastep, is commercially available in the United States (Sigmedics, Inc., Northfield, Ill.). Food and Drug Administration (FDA) approved clinical trials of the device have been undertaken at 20 sites with more than 100 patients since 1990.[63]

In Cleveland, Marsolais and Kobetic[63] have utilized implanted muscular stimulation that provides pivot transfers for persons with incomplete quadriplegia. Intramuscular electrodes are used to activate muscles[112] via their innervation. The pivot transfer incorporates quadriceps, hamstrings, posterior adductors, and erector spinae muscles bilaterally. Stimulation is derived from the eight-channel implanted stimulator described previously for upper extremity FES.

A 48-channel FES system using percutaneous electrodes was also developed in Cleveland to provide control of the spine, hip, knee, and ankle joints and to restore functional walking capabilities in persons with thoracic level paraplegia (see Kobetic et al.[72] for review). Some of the outcomes achieved in 20 patients with lesion levels between T4 and 12 include walking a maximum distance of 1200 m, achieving a maximum speed of

1.0 m/sec, side and back stepping, steady walking at 0.6 m/sec, and an intermittent capability of energy utilization at less than 50% of the maximum aerobic capacity.[63] The systems were used for walking in the laboratory, for seated exercise at home, and for limited, protocol-approved activities outside of the laboratory (Fig. 23–2).

With hybrid FES-orthotic devices, bracing has been used chiefly in combination with surface electrical stimulation to limit the degrees of freedom of the limb. Bracing reduces the need to continuously support total body weight, can provide an independent backup in the event of FES failure or fatigue, and can reduce stress on limbs and joints. Also, the number of degrees of freedom required for FES control is reduced. Modifications of the reciprocating gait orthosis (RGO), which provides standing balance and anti-gravity sup-

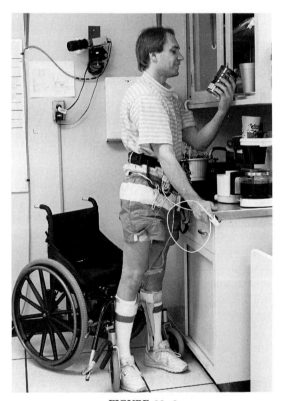

FIGURE 23–2

Functional electrical stimulation has been applied to the lower extremity of persons with spinal cord injury in the thoracic region for the purpose of restoring standing and gait. (Courtesy of Rudi Kobetic, Cleveland VA Medical Center.)

port, have been made by groups at Louisiana State University (LSU)[119] and Wright State University (WSU)[103] to incorporate electrical stimulation. The RGO features a mechanical reciprocating mechanism that forces the contralateral hip to flex when the ipsilateral hip extends. The WSU system also stimulates the gluteal and hamstring muscles with surface electrodes for ipsilateral hip extension, which causes the RGO to move the contralateral leg forward. Quadriceps are used for knee locking, which reduces the weight borne by the arm during crutch use and has been shown to double energy efficiency.[102] The LSU device uses surface electrodes on the quadriceps and hamstring muscles. In distinction to the WSU system, the knees are free to flex during walking. The LSU device was tested at speeds less than 0.3 m/sec and the energy cost of this device is 16% of that of the RGO without FES.[50] A hybrid device developed in the United Kingdom,[88] based on the ParaWalker orthotic from the Orthotic Research and Locomotor Assessment Unit (ORLAU), adds hip-extension capability, via stimulation of the gluteal muscles, to long-leg braces (LLB). A relatively high corset allows subjects to generate leg motions using upper body momentum, although it was found that ambulation was easier when no stimulation was used.[81, 88] Concerning the only hybrid device that does not rely on surface stimulation, teams from Cleveland and the University of Strathclyde, Glasgow, Scotland, have collaborated to develop a system making use of advanced orthotics and percutaneous electrodes.[9, 104] With this system it was possible to reduce significantly the amount of stimulation required to maintain stance (up to 80%), incorporate walking patterns, and develop strategies for incorporating standing rest periods during walking.

A successful FES system for standing and gait will need levels of function and convenience that at least approach those of a wheelchair while simultaneously falling within the boundaries of reasonable energy requirements. Research in this area suggests that these goals may be met, but successful clinical use of these FES systems has been limited.[56]

FUNCTIONAL ELECTRICAL STIMULATION AND THERAPEUTIC BENEFITS

Although users of neuroprostheses that incorporate FES obtain a significant functional benefit, evidence that therapeutic benefits result has also been seen. These benefits include improvements in muscle function, cardiovascular fitness, joint range of motion, and reduced spasticity.

Muscle

For FES to be effective, a prior course of chronic electrical stimulation is required to reestablish the functional metabolic capacity of weak and wasting paralyzed muscle. Muscles that have been paralyzed for a considerable time behave as type II muscle fibers (fast-twitch, anaerobic, glycolytic, white; Grimby et al.[44]), which are easily fatigued. These muscle fibers, following the chronic application of electrical stimulation for the purpose of exercise, gradually come to behave as type I fibers (slow-twitch, aerobic, oxidative red; Peckham et al.[91, 95]) which have increased fatigue resistance. Stimulation-induced exercise also results in increased muscle strength. Improved conditioning enables the muscle to participate effectively in coordinated movement via FES. Subsequent continued use of an FES system serves to maintain the muscle condition in this improved state.

Cardiovascular

Research has been undertaken to determine whether, with the application of FES over an extended period, increased cardiovascular fitness occurs (see Figoni[35] for review). This is based on the expectation that recruitment of the large lower extremity muscle mass and reactivation of the leg muscle pump will facilitate venous return and provide aerobic exercise. Studies undertaking electrically stimulated leg-cycle ergometry in quadriplegic subjects showed that these subjects have relatively high metabolic and cardiopulmonary stresses compared with those of nondisabled volunteers cycling at equivalent power outputs.[37, 38] Such an outcome may be beneficial with regard to stimulating aerobic metabolic and cardiovascular responses while minimizing orthopedic stresses. Leg-cycle ergometry training increased left ventricular chamber size and wall thickness, which indicated a reversal in myocardial disuse atrophy.[86] A further study,[32] which undertook submaximal electrically stimulated leg-cycle ergometry with quadriplegic subjects, showed that following a period of training, the subjects had decreased heart rate, increased blood pressure, increased stroke volume, and increased cardiac volume during exercise.

Combined volitional arm and electrically stimulated leg exercise in patients with spinal cord injury increased peak values of maximal oxygen uptake (VO_2), heart rate, stroke volume, and cardiac output,[36] although this type of exercise may be limited by circulatory factors particular to SCI individuals. For example, their legs may not be able to compete adequately with the arms for their portion of the limited cardiac output.[35] This may be especially evident when exercise hypotension, excessive venous pooling, and limited venous return occur in these patients. In subjects without spinal cord injury, adding arm exercise to leg exercise increased cardiac output but decreased leg blood flow, thereby indicating that the demands exceeded the heart's pumping capacity.[117] Subsequent exercise-induced hypotension might result in reduced perfusion of vital organs such as the brain[35] and cause extreme fatigue, vertigo, nausea, and syncope (to which individuals with spinal cord injury may have increased susceptibility). Thus, exercise that incorporates volitional arm and electrically activated leg motion may not be tolerated by all individuals, as their cardiac outputs might not be sufficient to satisfy requirements of both systems. Nonetheless, cardiovascular benefits have resulted from use of these hybrid systems, including increased VO_2 and cardiac output,[30, 53, 75] increased venous return,[106] and improved cardiovascular control during upper body exercise.[25] In FES exercise programs, lower limb contractions have aided venous return through the skeletal muscle venous pump. A result of this would be a greater end-diastolic volume and, thus, greater cardiac contractility (Frank-Starling relationship), with a resultant increase in stroke volume and cardiac output, which are known to have benefits for cardiac training.[35]

Range of Motion

Joint range of motion can be reduced as the result of immobilization or insult to the joint and surrounding tissue, damage and adhesions in the tendons, or muscle spasticity. It often follows nervous system trauma such as spinal cord injury. To prevent immobilization of the joint, it is important to preserve a functional range of motion. With FES, the joint is taken through the complete existing range of motion, which would not occur otherwise in individuals with spinal cord injury outside of therapy sessions. This movement, applied repeatedly, increasingly modifies interfering tissue that may immobilize the joint.[20]

Jaeger and Kralj[57] measured joint compliance of four patients with spinal cord injury before and after 20 to 30 minutes of repeated flexion reflex activity produced by stimulation of the peroneal nerve; they found that significant changes in joint compliance may be obtained using FES.

Spasticity

In the restoration of motor function to paralyzed muscles, spasticity can limit effectiveness. Spasticity following spinal cord injury[82] may be relieved following the application of electrical stimulation. If reduction of spasticity improves the function of a specific region of the body, this form of electrical stimulation might be termed FES. Transcutaneous electrical nerve stimulation (TENS) has also been applied to stimulate afferent nerves with the aim of decreasing spasticity. In three studies,[2, 5, 43] spasticity was reduced by TENS in 17 of 22 subjects with complete and incomplete spinal cord injury, although this effect did not last more than 2 hours. Perhaps the most effective relief of spasticity by electrical stimulation has been reported using rectal probe stimulation.[45] In a study of electroejaculation, clinical observation found spasticity to be reduced. In a subsequent single-blinded study of six men and three women with spinal cord injury, all subjects experienced a decrease in tone, frequency of spasms, and interference with activities of daily living, the mean duration of relief being 8.2 hours (range, 3 to 24 hours).

Seating Pressure

Due to immobility and absent sensation in areas of the bodies subjected to prolonged pressure, patients with spinal cord injury are very susceptible to pressure sores (decubitus ulcers). They are likely to occur in areas with bony prominences such as the trochanter and sacrum, in the ischial region, and on the heel. Pressure sores are often very resistant to healing and traditional prevention of pressure sores focuses on specialized seating surfaces and continual shifting of the person's weight (see Chapter 16). An alternative to these methods of prevention may be the use of FES to reduce ischial pressure. In a study of nine patients,[34] quadriceps were electrically stimulated with the lower legs restrained. Ischial pressures were measured during this stimulation and during periods of quiet sitting. FES resulted in a decrease in ischial pressure in most cases, which has encouraged the further development of such systems. However, the tissue tolerance threshold to pressure is likely to be only one in a series of interacting elements in the pathogenesis of pressure sores.

FES EQUIPMENT MARKET FOR SPINAL CORD INJURY USERS

The role for FES in rehabilitation is increasing as new applications demonstrate benefits to the patients' quality of life so the market for FES equipment has recently been reviewed.[124] Influences on whether a device reaches the market include technological limitations, government regulation, reimbursement status, and clinical training.

Technological limitations in bringing a device to market include manufacturability and reliability of intricate laboratory systems. Government regulation provides safeguards for the users and ensures that devices are of sufficient quality for human use. In the United States, the FDA regulates the availability of medical devices. Investigators wishing to introduce into the market a new device that is not similar to an existing device must submit an application for premarket approval (PMA). This PMA application provides a detailed description of the device and clinical data from controlled studies in humans. To obtain these data, approval must be made by an institutional review board (IRB), and for a device that might prove to be of significant risk to a user, an investigational device exemption (IDE) must be requested from the FDA.

A significant factor in the marketing, widespread distribution, and use of FES devices is clinician training. Without sufficient knowledge of the benefits and applications of a particular device, clinicians will not be confident in prescribing it for patients. For serious developers of FES systems, technology transfer forms an important component to ensure that the largest number of patients will have the opportunity to benefit from the neuroprosthesis (see, for example, Hart et al.[49]).

A number of FES devices are being marketed to persons with spinal cord injuries for the purpose of therapeutic muscle stimulation and cardiovascular exercise. Many of these devices incorporate surface stimulation. Market leaders in this area include Medtronic Inc. (Minneapolis, Minn.), Mettler Electronics (Anaheim, Calif.), Rich-Mar (Inola, Okla.), and Staodynamics (Longmont, Colo.). Portable and clinic-based systems are available to try to prevent some of the complications that result from immobility. Some FES devices incorporate surface stimulation into exercise equipment such as bicycle ergometers (Therapeutic Technologies, Inc., Tampa, Fla.; Sinties Scientific Corp., Tulsa, Okla.).

Currently, one fully FDA-approved device

is available in the United States to produce standing and stepping via lower extremity FES (Sigmedics, Inc., Northfield, Ill.) and one manufacturer (Petrofsky Center, Irvine, Calif.) is completing PMA applications to the FDA. The Sigmedics device uses pure FES, whereas that from the Petrofsky Center is a hybrid that combines orthotics and FES. In Japan, NEC San-ei Instruments, Ltd., have developed an FES system that uses percutaneous electrodes that can be applied to the upper or lower extremities. The implanted FES device for restoration of hand grasp developed in Cleveland is available to users for study under an IDE (NeuroControl Corp., Cleveland, Ohio), and clinical trials are currently being undertaken in the United States and Australia.

Phrenic nerve pacing FES devices are currently available in the United States and in Europe. The major manufacturer of implantable phrenic nerve pacers in the United States is Avery Laboratories (Glen Cove, N.Y.). In Europe, phrenic pacers are available from Atrotech Co. in Finland, Biotech in Austria, and Magstim Co., Ltd., in the United Kingdom. The device from Atrotech Co. is available is the United States under IDE status through Medlink Technical Corp. (Los Angeles).

Commercial systems have been developed for sacral root stimulation and are available in the United States (Avery Laboratories) and the United Kingdom (Finetech Ltd.). The Finetech device currently may be used in the United States under IDE status. Another such device is currently undergoing clinical trials in several patient populations under IDE status in the United States (Medtronic Inc., Neuro Division). A device providing electroejaculation developed at the National Rehabilitation Hospital (Washington, D.C.) has been applied successfully in clinical trials worldwide and is available under IDE status.

For FES systems to be exposed to and accepted by the international health care community, researchers and marketers should ensure that proper education and training of clinical professionals regarding the devices is available. The FES Information Center, established in Cleveland specifically for dissemination of information regarding the use of electrical stimulation in rehabilitation, is available to researchers, clinicians, and manufacturers (1–800–231–3257).

FUTURE PROSPECTS FOR FUNCTIONAL ELECTRICAL STIMULATION

FES will make greater contributions to clinical care as the technology continues to mature and evolve from controlled clinical studies and as clinicians become familiar with its appropriate utilization in clinical practice. Developers of these systems bear considerable responsibility to facilitate their transfer into clinical practice. Clinicians generally are unfamiliar with FES technology and, regardless of their desire to utilize it, training and guidance are necessary to ensure its safe and appropriate deployment. Building this interface is essential for broader accessibility of the technology, to make it available to both the clinician and the person with a disability.

Virtually every current clinical system has developments under way that should improve its performance for the patient, as described throughout this chapter. Not only will the systems continue to be smaller, lighter, and more efficient, but they also will be more powerful and provide finer, more natural control with fewer and "friendlier" external components that are easier to operate, both for the user and for the clinician.

All of these changes will result in more choices for both the person with spinal cord injury and the clinician. As the person with injury may benefit from several different FES devices, manufacturers must ensure that they operate compatibly, particularly with implanted technology. FES systems will improve with future developments, so the time when the individual chooses to participate should be thoughtfully considered. Particularly with implantable systems, the question of "upward compatibility" arises, as does the consideration of whether new advances can be provided for a person who elects to accept a system early in its evolution. Some measures of interchangeability and standardization by manufacturers would help to resolve this issue for clinicians, particularly as second-source manufacturers may be expected to introduce components of systems that may be more desirable than those from the original manufacturers.

Opportunity for the user to gain additional function through FES improves at an increasing rate. As more persons with spinal cord injury become users of FES systems and more clinicians are involved in their deployment, deficiencies will continue to be identified and resolved for the benefit of the user. Successful management of this clinical interaction will result in an increasing opportunity for better health, greater independence, and an improved quality of life for the person with spinal cord injury.

REFERENCES

1. Agnew WF, McCreery DB, Bullara LA, et al: Effects of prolonged electrical stimulation of peripheral nerve. In Agnew WF, McCreery DB (eds): Neural Prosthesis Fundamental Studies. Englewood Cliffs, NJ, Prentice Hall, 1990, pp 147–167.
2. Andrews BJ, Bajd T, Baxendale RH: Cutaneous electrical stimulation and reductions in spinal spasticity in man. J Physiol 367:86P, 1985.
3. Andrews BJ, Baxendale RH: A hybrid orthosis incorporating artificial reflexes for spinal-cord-damaged patients. J Physiol 380:19P, 1986.
4. Ashley EA, Laskin JJ, Olenik LM, et al: Evidence of autonomic dysreflexia during functional electrical stimulation in individuals with spinal cord injuries. Paraplegia 31:593–605, 1993.
5. Bajd T, Gregoric M, Vodovnik L, et al: Electrical stimulation in treating spasticity resulting from spinal cord injury. Arch Phys Med Rehabil 66:515–517, 1985.
6. Bajd T, Kralj A, Turk R, et al: The use of a four-channel electrical stimulator as an ambulatory aid for paraplegic patients. Phys Ther 63:1116–1120, 1983.
7. Balmaseda MT, Fatehi MT, Koozekanani SH, et al: Burns in functional electric stimulation: Two case reports. Arch Phys Med Rehabil 68:452–453, 1987.
8. Banwell JG, Creasey GH, Agarwal AM, et al: Management of the neurogenic bowel in patients with spinal cord injury. Urol Clin North Am 20(3): 517–526, 1993.
9. Barnicle K, Andrews BJ, Phillips GF, et al: A Hybrid Orthosis for Paraplegic Standing with Percutaneous Electrodes. Proceedings of the 10th Annual International Conference IEEE EMBS. New Orleans, 1988, pp 1645–1646.
10. Bennett CJ, Seager SW, Vasher EA, et al: Sexual dysfunction and electroejaculation in men with spinal cord injury: Review. J Urol 139:453–457, 1988.
11. Bilgutay AM, Bilgutay IM, Garanella JJ, et al: Augmented ventilation by synchronous phrenic nerve stimulation. Trans Am Soc Artif Intern Organs 16:213–217, 1970.
12. Billian C, Gorman PH: Upper extremity applica-

tions of functional electrical stimulation. Assist Tech 4:31–39, 1992.
13. Bobra S, Jaeger R: Dynamic Events During Cough. Proceedings of the Ljubljana FES Conference. Ljubljana, Slovenia, 1993, pp 171–173.
14. Brindley GS: Electroejaculation: Its technique, neurological implications and uses. J Neurol Neurosurg Psychiatry 44:9–18, 1981.
15. Brindley GS: The fertility of men with spinal injuries. Paraplegia 19:299, 1984.
16. Brindley GS, Craggs MD: A technique for anodally blocking large nerve fibres through chronically implanted electrodes. J Neurol Neurosurg Psychiatry 43:1083–1090, 1980.
17. Brindley GS, Polkey CE, Rushton DN: Sacral anterior root stimulators for bladder control in paraplegia. Paraplegia 20:365–381, 1982.
18. Brindley GS, Polkey CE, Rushton DN, et al: Sacral anterior root stimulators for bladder control in paraplegia: The first 50 cases. J Neurol Neurosurg Psychiatry 49:1104–1114, 1986.
19. Brindley GS, Rushton DN: Long-term follow-up of patients with sacral anterior root stimulator implants. Paraplegia 28:469–475, 1990.
20. Campbell JM, Meadows PM: Therapeutic FES: From rehabilitation to neural prosthetics. Assist Technol 4:4–18, 1992.
21. Ciesielski TE, Fukida Y, Glenn WWL, et al: Response of the diaphragm muscle to electrical stimulation of the phrenic nerve. J Neurosurg 58:92–100, 1983.
22. Crago PE, Peckham PH, Thrope GB: Modulation of muscle force by recruitment during intramuscular stimulation. IEEE Trans Biomed Eng 27(12):679–684, 1980.
23. Crago PE, Van Doren C, Keith MW, et al: Closed Loop Control of Functional Neuromuscular Stimulation. Quarterly Progress Report No. 2, 1993, NIH Neuroprosthesis Program Contract Number NO1–NS–2344.
24. Creasey GH: Electrical stimulation of sacral roots for micturition after spinal cord injury. Urol Clin North Am 20(3):505–515, 1993.
25. Davis GM, Servedio FJ, Glaser RM, et al: Cardiovascular responses to arm cranking and electrically induced leg exercise in paraplegics. J Appl Physiol 69:671–677, 1990.
26. De Troyer A, Estenne M: Coordination between rib-cage muscles and diaphragm during quiet breathing in humans. J Appl Physiol 57:899–906, 1984.
27. De Troyer A, Kelly S, Zin WA: Mechanical action of the intercostal muscles on the ribs. Science 220:87–88, 1983.
28. DiMarco AF, Altose MD, Cropp A, et al: Activation of inspiratory intercostal muscles by electrical stimulation of the spinal cord. Am Rev Respir Dis 136:1385–1390, 1987.
29. DiMarco AF, Budzinska K, Supinski GS: Artificial ventilation by means of electrical activation of the intercostal/accessory muscles alone in anesthetized dogs. Am Rev Respir Dis 139:961–967, 1989.
30. Edwards BG, Marsolais EB: Metabolic responses to arm ergometry and functional neuromuscular stimulation. J Rehabil Res Dev 27(2):107–114, 1990.
31. Elefteriades JA, Hogan JF, Handler A, et al: Long-term follow-up of bilateral pacing of the diaphragm in quadriplegia. N Engl J Med 326:1433–1434, 1992.

32. Faghri PD, Glaser RM, Figoni SF, et al: Feasibility of using two FNS exercise modes for spinal cord injured patients. Clin Kinesiol 43:62–68, 1989.

33. Fang Z-P, Mortimer JT: Selective activation of small motor axons by quasitrapezoidal pulses. IEEE Trans Biomed Eng 38:168–174, 1991.

34. Ferguson ACB, Keating JF, Delargy MA, et al: Reduction of seating pressure using FES in patients with spinal cord injury: A preliminary report. Paraplegia 30:474–478, 1992.

35. Figoni SF: Exercise responses and quadriplegia. Med Sci Sport Exer 25(4):433–441, 1993.

36. Figoni SF, Glaser RM, Rodgers MM, et al: Haemodynamic responses of quadriplegics to arm, ES-leg, and combined arm + ES-leg ergometry. Med Sci Sport Exerc 21(2):S96, 1989.

37. Glaser RM, Figoni SF, Collins SR, et al: Physiologic responses of SCI Subjects to electrically Induced Leg Cycle Ergometry. Proceedings of the 10th Annual International Conference of IEEE EMBS. 1988, vol 10, pp 1638–1640.

38. Glaser RM, Figoni SF, Hooker SP, et al: Efficiency of Leg Cycle Ergometry. Proceedings of the 10th Annual International Conference of IEEE EMBS. 1989, vol 11, pp 961–963.

39. Glenn WWL, Brouillette RT, Dentz B, et al: Fundamental considerations in pacing of the diaphragm for chronic ventilatory insufficiency: A multicenter study. PACE 11:2121–2127, 1988.

40. Glenn WWL, Hageman JH, Mauro A, et al: Electrical stimulation of excitable tissue by radio-frequency transmission. Ann Surg 160:338–350, 1964.

41. Gorman PH, Peckham PH: Upper extremity functional neuromuscular stimulation. J Neuro Rehabil 5:3–11, 1991.

42. Graupe D: EMG pattern analysis for patient-responsive control of FES in paraplegics for walker-supported walking. IEEE Trans Biomed Eng 36(7):711–719, 1989.

43. Gregoric M, Peterlin-Potisk K: Transcutaneous Electrical Stimulation in the Treatment of Spasticity: I. Effects on Muscle Hypertonia. Proceedings of the Ljubljana FES Conference, 1993, Ljubljana, Slovenia, pp 140–143.

44. Grimby G, Broberg C, Krotkiewska I, et al: Muscle fiber composition in patients with traumatic spinal cord lesions. Scand J Rehabil Med 8:37–42, 1976.

45. Halstead LS, Seager SWJ, Houston JM, et al: Relief of spasticity in SCI men and women using rectal probe stimulation. Paraplegia 31:715–721, 1993.

46. Hambrecht FT: A brief history of neural prostheses for motor control of paralyzed extremities. In Stein RB, Peckham PH, Popovic DP (eds): Neural Prostheses: Replacing Motor Function After Disease or Disability. New York, Oxford University Press, 1992.

47. Handa Y, Hoshimiya N: Functional electrical stimulation for the control of the upper extremities. Med Prog Technol 12:51–63, 1987.

48. Handa Y, Kameyama J, Hoshimiya N: FES-Control of Shoulder Motion in Hemiplegic and Quadriplegic Patients. Proceedings of the Vienna International Workshop for Functional Electrostimulation. Vienna, Austria, September 1992, pp 127–129.

49. Hart RL, Thrope GB, Stroh KC, et al: Technology Transfer of an Upper Extremity Functional Neuromuscular Stimulation Program. RESNA 12th Annual Conference. New Orleans, 1989.

50. Hirokawa S, Grimm M, Thanh Le MS, et al: Energy consumption in paraplegic ambulation using the reciprocating gait orthosis and electrical stimulation of the thigh muscles. Arch Phys Med Rehabil 71:687–694, 1990.

51. Hollander JB: Integration of functional neuromuscular stimulation control of elbow extension and hand grasp, Master's Thesis. Cleveland, Case Western Reserve University, 1993.

52. Holle J, Frey M, Gruber H, et al: Functional electrostimulation of paraplegics: Experimental investigations and first clinical experience with an implantable stimulation device. Orthopedics 17:1145–1156, 1984.

53. Hooker SP, Figoni SF, Rodgers MM, et al: Metabolic and hemodynamic responses to concurrent voluntary arm crank and electrical stimulation exercise in quadriplegics. J Rehabil Res Dev 29(3):1–11, 1992.

54. Hoshimiya N, Naito A, Yajima M, et al: A multichannel FES system for the restoration of motor functions in high spinal cord injury patients: A respiration-controlled system for multijoint upper extremity. IEEE Trans Biomed Eng 36(7):754–760, 1989.

55. Ilbawi MN, Idriss FS, Hunt CE, et al: Diaphragmatic pacing in infants: Techniques and results. Ann Thorac Surg 40:323–329, 1985.

56. Jaeger RJ: Lower extremity applications of functional neuromuscular stimulation. Assist Technol 4:19–30, 1992.

57. Jaeger RJ, Kralj A: Functional electrical stimulation changes joint compliance. Proceedings of the 5th Annual Conference on Rehabilitation Engineering. Houston, 1982.

58. Jaeger RJ, Turba RM, Yarkony GM, et al: Cough in spinal cord injured patients: Comparison of three methods to produce cough. Arch Phys Med Rehabil 74:1358–1361, 1993.

59. Jaeger RJ, Yarkony GM, Smith RM: Standing the spinal cord injured patient by electrical stimulation: Refinement of a clinical protocol for clinical use. IEEE Trans Biomed Eng 36:720–728, 1989.

60. Johnson MW, Peckham PH: Evaluation of shoulder movement as a command control source. IEEE Trans Biomed Eng 37:876–885, 1990.

61. Johnson MW, Peckham PH: An Implantable Two-Degree-of-Freedom Joint Angle Sensor. Proceedings of the 12th Annual International Conference on IEEE EMBS. 1990, vol 12(2), pp 510–511.

62. Judson JP, Glenn WWL: Radio-frequency electrophrenic respiration: Long-term application to a patient with primary hypoventilation. JAMA 203:1033–1037, 1968.

63. Kantor C, Andrews BJ, Marsolais EB, et al: Report on a conference on motor prostheses for workplace mobility of paraplegic patients in North America. Paraplegia 31:439–456, 1993.

64. Keith MW, Kilgore KL, Peckham PH, et al: Tendon transfers and functional electrical stimulation for reconstruction of hand function in spinal cord injury. J Hand Surg (submitted).

65. Keller AD, Taylor CL, Zahm V: Studies to Determine the Functional Requirements for Hand and Arm Prostheses, final report, National Academy of Science contract No. VAm–21:223, 1947.

66. Kendall FP, McCreary EK: Muscles: Testing and Function. Baltimore, Williams & Wilkins, 1983, p 12.

67. Kilgore KL, Peckham PH: Grasp synthesis for upper extremity FNS: 1. Automated method for synthesising the stimulus map. Med Biol Eng Comput 31:607–614, 1993.

68. Kilgore KL, Peckham PH: Grasp synthesis for upper extremity FNS: 2. Evaluation of the influence of electrode recruitment properties. Med Biol Eng Comput 31:615–622, 1993.

69. Kilgore KL, Peckham PH, Keith MW, et al: Electrode characterization for functional application to upper extremity FNS. IEEE Trans Biomed Eng 37(1):12–21, 1990.

70. Kilgore KL, Peckham PH, Thrope GB, et al: Synthesis of hand grasp using functional neuromuscular stimulation. IEEE Trans Biomed Eng 36(7):761–769, 1989.

71. Kiwerski J, Pasniczek R: An apparatus making possible restoration of simple functions of the tetraplegic hand. Paraplegia 22:316–319, 1984.

72. Kobetic R, Marsolais EB, Samame P, et al: The next step: Artificial walking. In Rose J (ed): Inman's Human Walking, ed 2. Baltimore, Williams & Wilkins, 1993, chap 10.

73. Kralj A, Bajd T: Functional Electrical Stimulation: Standing and Walking after Spinal Cord Injury. Boca Raton, Fla, CRC Press, 1989.

74. Kralj A, Turk R, Bajd T, et al: FES utilisation statistics for 94 patients. Proceedings of the Ljubljana FES Conference. Ljubljana, Slovenia, 1993, pp 79–81.

75. Laskin JJ, Ashley EA, Olenik LM, et al: Electrical stimulation-assisted rowing exercise in spinal cord injured people: A pilot study. Paraplegia 31:534–541, 1993.

76. Linder SH: Functional electrical stimulation to enhance cough in quadriplegia. Chest 103:166–169, 1993.

77. MacDonagh RP, Sun WM, Smallwood R, et al: Control of defecation in patients with spinal injuries by stimulation of sacral anterior roots. Br Med J 300:1494–1497, 1990.

78. Madersbacher H, Fischer J: Sacral anterior root stimulation: Prerequisites and indications. Neurourol Urodyn 12(5):489–494, 1993.

79. Marsolais EB, Kobetic R: Functional walking in paralyzed patients by means of electrical stimulation. Clin Orthop 175:30–36, 1983.

80. Marsolais EB, Kobetic R, Chizeck HJ, et al: Orthoses and electrical stimulation for walking in complete paraplegia. J Neurol Rehabil 5:13–22, 1991.

81. McClelland M, Andrews BJ, Patrick JH, et al: Augmentation of the Owestry ParaWalker orthosis by means of surface electrical stimulation: Gait analysis of three patients. Paraplegia 25(1):32–38, 1987.

82. Merritt JL: Management of spasticity in spinal cord injury. Mayo Clin Proc 56:614–622, 1981.

83. Miller LJ, Peckham PH, Keith MW: Elbow extension in the C5 quadriplegic using functional neuromuscular stimulation. IEEE Trans Biomed Eng 36:771–780, 1989.

84. Mizrahi J, Braun Z, Najenson T, et al: Quantitative weightbearing and gait evaluation of paraplegics using functional electrical stimulation. Med Biol Eng Comput 23:101–107, 1985.

85. Mortimer JT: Motor prostheses. In Brooks VB (ed): Handbook of Physiology: The Nervous System II. Bethesda, Md, American Physiological Society, 1981, pp 155–187.

86. Nash MS, Bilsker S, Marcillo AE, et al: Reversal of left ventricular atrophy following electrically stimulated exercise training in human quadriplegics. Paraplegia 29:590–599, 1992.

87. Nathan RH, Ohry A: Upper limb functions regained in quadriplegia: A hybrid computerized neuromuscular system. Arch Phys Med Rehabil 71:415–421, 1990.

88. Nene AV, Jennings SJ: Hybrid paraplegic locomotion with the ParaWalker using intramuscular stimulation: A single subject study. Paraplegia 27:125–132, 1989.

89. Nochomovitz ML, Peterson DK, DiMarco AF, et al: The effect on tidal volume of rib cage paradox during diaphragm activation. Am Rev Respir Dis 127:325–329, 1983.

90. Nochomovitz ML, Schmit BD, Mortimer JT: Electrical activation of the diaphragm. Prob Respir Care 3(3):507–533, 1990.

91. Peckham PH: Control of Contraction Strength of Electrically Stimulated Muscle by Pulse Width and Frequency Modulation. Proceedings of the 29th ACEMB. Boston, 1976, 116.

92. Peckham PH: Functional electrical stimulation. In Webster JG (ed): Encyclopedia of Medical Devices and Instrumentation. New York, John Wiley & Sons, 1988, vol 2, pp 1331–1352.

93. Peckham PH, Creasey GH: Neural prostheses: Clinical applications of functional electrical stimulation in spinal cord injury. Paraplegia 30:96–101, 1992.

94. Peckham PH, Kilgore KL, Keith MW, et al: An Implanted Neuroprosthesis for Restoration of Grasp and Release. Proceedings of the Ljubljana FES Conference. Ljubljana, Slovenia, 1993, pp 199–202.

95. Peckham PH, Mortimer JT, Marsolais EB: Alteration in the force and fatigueability of skeletal muscle in quadriplegic humans following exercise induced by chronic electrical stimulation. Clin Orthop Rel Res 114:326–334, 1976.

96. Peckham PH, Mortimer JT, Marsolais EB: Controlled prehension and release in the C5 quadriplegic elicited by functional electrical stimulation of the paralyzed forearm musculature. Ann Biomed Eng 8:369–388, 1980.

97. Peckham PH, Mortimer JT, Van Der Meulen JP: Physiologic and metabolic changes in white muscle of cat following induced exercise. Brain Res 50:424–429, 1973.

98. Peckham PH, Thrope GB, Buckett JR, et al: Coordinated two-mode grasp in the quadriplegic initiated by functional neuromuscular stimulation. In Campbell RM (ed): Control Aspects of Prosthetics and Orthotics. Elmsford, NY, Pergamon, 1983, pp 29–32.

99. Perkins TA, Brindley GS, Donaldson ND, et al: Implant provision of key, pinch and power grips in a C6 tetraplegic. Med Biol Eng Comp (in press).

100. Peterson DK: Chronic Intramuscular Activation of the Phrenic Nerve, doctoral thesis. Case Western Reserve University, Cleveland, 1988.

101. Peterson DK, Nochomovitz MN, DiMarco AF: Intramuscular electrical activation of the phrenic nerve. IEEE Trans Biomed Eng 33:342–351, 1986.

102. Petrofsky JS, Phillips CA, Douglas R, et al: A computer-controlled walking system: The combination of an orthosis with functional electrical stimulation. J Clin Eng 11(2):121–133, 1986.

103. Phillips CA: Electrical stimulation for ambulation of selected paraplegics and quadriplegics. J Neurol Orthop Med Surg 10(2):145–146, 1989.

104. Phillips GF, Andrews BJ, Chizeck HJ, et al: Finite State Control of Paraplegic Gait using a Hybrid FNS Orthosis. Proceedings of the 10th Annual International Conference of IEEE EMBS. New Orleans, 1988, p 1671.

105. Popovic D, Tomovic R, Schwirtlich L: Hybrid assistive system—the motor prosthesis. IEEE Trans Biomed Eng 36:729–737, 1989.

106. Ragnarsson KT, Pollack S, O'Daniel W, et al: Clinical evaluation of computerized functional electrical stimulation after spinal cord injury: A multicenter pilot study. Arch Phys Med Rehabil 69:672–677, 1988.

107. Rijkhoff NJM, Koldewijn EL, Van Kerrebroeck PEV, et al: Sacral Root Stimulation in the Dog: Reduction of Urethral Resistance. Proceedings of the 15th Annual International Conference of IEEE EMBS. San Diego, 1993, pp 1257–1258.

108. Rushton DN: Surface versus implanted electrodes in the daily application of FES. In Pedotti A (ed): Restoration of Walking for Paraplegics. Milan, Edizione Pro Juventute, 1992, pp 363–364.

109. Sato I, Hogan JF, Glenn WWL, et al: A demand diaphragm pacemaker. Trans Am Soc Artif Intern Organs 23:456–463, 1977.

110. Sawan M, Hassouna M, Li JS, et al: A Multichannel Implant for Total Bladder Evacuation. Proceedings of the Ljubljana FES Conference. Ljubljana, Slovenia, 1993, pp 53–55.

111. Scharf SM, Feldman NT, Goldman MD, et al: Vocal cord closure: A cause of upper airway obstruction during controlled ventilation. Am Rev Respir Dis 117:391–397, 1978.

112. Scheiner A, Polando G, Marsolais EB: Design and clinical application of a double helix electrode for functional electrical stimulation. IEEE Trans Biomed Eng 41(5):425–431, 1994.

113. Schmit BD, Mortimer JT: Electrical Activation of the Diaphragm using Epimysial Electrodes. Proceedings of the 15th Annual International Conference of IEEE EMBS. San Diego, 1993, vol 12, pp 1251–1252.

114. Scott TRD, Peckham PH, Keith MW: Upper extremity neuroprostheses utilising functional electrical stimulation. In Brindley GS, Rushton DN (eds): Bailliere's Clinical Neurology: 3.3. Neuroprostheses. London, Bailliere Tindall (in press).

115. Seager SWJ, Halstead LS: Fertility options and success after spinal cord injury. Urol Clin North Am 20(3):543–548, 1993.

116. Seager SWJ, Halstead LS, Houson JM: Electroejaculation and Fertility Evaluation in 425 Spinal Cord Injured (SCI) and Other Neurologically Impaired Men. Proceedings of the Ljubljana FES Conference. Ljubljana, Slovenia, 1993, pp 185–189.

117. Secher NH, Clausen JP, Klausen K, et al: Central and regional circulatory effects of adding arm exercise to leg exercise. Acta Physiol Scand 100: 288–297, 1977.

118. Smith B, Peckham PH, Keith MW, et al: An externally powered, multichannel, implantable stimulator for versatile control of paralyzed muscle. IEEE Trans Biomed Eng 34(7):499–508, 1987.

119. Solomonow M: Biomechanics and physiology of a practical FES powered walking orthosis for paraplegics. In Stein RB, Peckham PH, Popovic DP (eds): Neural Prostheses: Replacing Motor Function After Disease or Disability. Oxford Press, London, 1992.

120. Strohl KP, Hensley MJ, Hallett M, et al: Activation of upper airway muscles before the onset of inspiration in normal man. J Appl Physiol 49:638–642, 1980.

121. Talalla A, Bloom J: Sacral electrical stimulation for bladder control. In Illis L (ed): Functional Stimulation (Spinal Cord Dysfunction III). Oxford, England, Oxford University Press, 1992, pp 206–218.

122. Tanagho EA, Schmidt RA, Orvis BR: Neural stimulation for control of voiding dysfunction: A preliminary report in 22 patients with serious neuropathic voiding disorders. J Urol 142:340–345, 1989.

123. Tarabulcy E: Sexual function in the normal and in paraplegia. Paraplegia 10:201, 1979.

124. Teeter JO: A review of the functional electrical stimulation equipment market. Assist Technol 4:40–45, 1992.

125. Van Kerrebroeck PEV, Debruyne FMJ: Electrical stimulation in the management of neurogenic bladder dysfunction. Urology (in press).

126. Van Kerrebroeck PEV, Koldewijn EL, Debruyne FMJ: Worldwide experience with the Finetech-Brindley sacral anterior root stimulator. Neurourol Urodyn 12(5):497–503, 1993.

127. Vodovnik L, Bajd T, Trncoczy A, et al: Functional electrical stimulation for control of locomotor systems. CRC Crit Rev Bioeng 6(2):63–131, 1983.

128. Wijman CAC, Stroh KC, Van Doran CL, et al: Functional evaluation of quadriplegic patients using a hand neuroprosthesis. Arch Phys Med Rehabil 71:1053–1057, 1990.

129. Wuolle KS, Van Doren CL, Thrope GB, et al: Development of a quantitative hand grasp and release test for patients with tetraplegia using a hand neuroprosthesis. J Hand Surg 19A(2):209–218, 1994.

CHAPTER 24

Psychiatric Aspects of Spinal Cord Injury

Michael Mufson, M.D.
Manish Fozdar, M.D.

THE INITIAL PSYCHIATRIC EVALUATION

"Of the many forms of disability which can beset mankind, a severe injury or disease of the spinal cord undoubtedly constitutes one of the most devastating calamities in human life."[1] So opens Guttman's classic text on spinal cord injuries. He goes on to point out that "A disaster in human life of such magnitude as a sudden transection or severe injury to the spinal cord, which throws the body completely out of gear, inevitably disrupts the psychophysical entity of the organism resulting in profound effects on the paralyzed patient's mind."[2]

Following a spinal cord injury, the patient suddenly finds himself in a dramatically transformed state. Depending on the site of the injury, alterations may occur in all or some voluntary movements, in bowel and bladder control, in sexual function, and even in respiration and cardiac regulation. The individual finds that he is dependent on others for basic daily care, his habitual style of relating to the world radically transformed.

This chapter examines the psychiatric aspects of spinal cord injury. The first part of this chapter describes the effect of the spinal cord injury on an individual's sense of self and how it relates to loss and suffering. An understanding of the sense of loss allows discussion of issues of adaptation and coping in the adjustment period following spinal cord injury.

Second, the variety of causes of altered mental status in the patient with spinal cord injury is discussed, and the major psychiatric disorders associated with spinal cord injury, with an emphasis on psychiatric management in the hospital setting, are examined.

Loss, Suffering, Adaptation, and Coping

The individual who suffers a spinal cord injury experiences a massive insult to the sense of self. From the physiologic standpoint, a sudden loss of basic daily function takes place, ranging from voluntary movement to loss of such personal functions as bowel and bladder control. In addition to these losses, the individual undergoes a change in the psychological sense of self. This most fundamental change is a loss of independence. A major change occurs in how the individual functions in basic roles, particularly in the family and at work. Just as significant is the change of the internal sense of self including self-esteem, capacity to love and be loved, and capacity to relate to the world as an injured self, rather than as the former "whole" self.

Cassell's book on the nature of suffering contains an extensive examination of the impact of chronic illness on the sense of self. Suffering is seen as a feeling state that occurs when an individual perceives an impending destruction of self. It can continue until the integrity of the person is restored and most often occurs in relation to pain and bodily symptoms. In the most general terms, suffering may be defined as severe distress associated with events that threaten a person's "intactness."[3] The spinal cord–injured patient is thrust into this state of suffering and distress; suffering often continues throughout the adjustment period, if not beyond.

Cassell describes the complexity of suffering in chronic illness and its related feelings of isolation, pain, and loss of self-integrity. He emphasizes that suffering is ultimately a personal matter, known primarily to the sufferer but existing in the context of others including wife, children, parents, employer, and physicians. He describes how life experi-

ences, previous illness, and experiences with doctors and hospitals form a psychological background for adjustment to traumatic illness. Cassell also points out that "suffering arises in chronic illness because of the conflicts within the person that are generated by the simultaneous need to respond to the demands and limitations of the body and to the forces of society in group life."[4] This is a central area of psychological conflict for the spinal cord–injured patient.

An individual with spinal cord injury also undergoes a change in how he or she experiences the emotional world inside himself or herself. An initial general and medical psychiatric assessment of the patient with spinal cord injury not only requires an evaluation of the patient's suffering but also requires listening to the patient's personal experience of the injury. Suffering associated with this change may be expressed in anger, grief, sadness, or rage. The physician must begin by acknowledging the individual's losses, fears, and, ultimately, the suffering arising from the injury. In the initial phase of adjustment, the patient begins to reassess his sense of self and identity. The patient may feel humiliated by new dependency needs and may experience feelings of shame, which can lead to social withdrawal indifference, or denial. This picture contrasts with the angry, anxious state, in which the patient feels enraged at the loss and responds with anger and hostility toward caretakers.

It is imperative that physicians understand that while the patient is being stabilized medically, he or she is already experiencing an altered sense of self and is attempting to cope with loss and suffering. This process may initially interfere with an individual's ability to respond and adapt to the demands of spinal cord injury treatment, which can be quite rigorous. This should not be interpreted as defiant or oppositional behavior.

The spinal cord physician needs also to understand that an individual patient's response to injury is in great part determined by his or her premorbid personality structure, which, more than anything, influences his coping style. As Leigh and Reiser point out, identifying the personality type of a patient allows the physician to understand the meaning of illness for that patient and, in turn, the influence of personality style on "sick role" performance.[5] Understanding the patient's premorbid personality style and the ways in which he or she is attempting to cope in the early phase of adjustment during hospitalization can lead to psychological approaches that maximize the individual's emotional strengths. This subject is reviewed exhaustively in the discussion of Kahana and Bibring[6] on personality types in medical management, which elucidates the psychological characteristics of different personality styles and the meaning of illness to each type. In addition to premorbid personality style, the maturity of the patient's ego functioning and the stage of his or her life cycle also helps determine how the patient adjusts to the acute injury.[7]

Psychological defense mechanisms brought to bear by each individual must also be evaluated when assessing responses to a traumatic experience such as spinal cord injury. Patients attempt to minimize anxiety and distress through the use of psychological defense mechanisms. These mechanisms can either be helpful in adaptation (mature defenses) or lead to difficulties in adaptation (immature defenses). Understanding this aspect of the patient's adjustment can be useful in setting forth treatment plans and in treating a patient's behavior on the ward. It is important to note that defense mechanisms, even if they distort reality, may provide an adaptive function early in adjustment. Only if they continue to interfere with the patient's functioning or adjustment should concern be raised about particular coping strategies. The psychiatric consultant can help the staff understand the precise defense mechanisms and personality style of the patient and can point out appropriate strategies for management of the patient based on that assessment.

Finally, an evaluation of whether the patient suffers from a major psychiatric disorder, such as affective disorder, and/or psychosis must be performed in the initial evaluation, with specific focus on whether the patient poses a risk for suicide.

In summary, the patient with spinal cord injury is transported into a frightening world of modern medical treatment, and is descended on by numerous specialists attempting to stabilize the acute medical condition. Although in need of rapid medical and/or neurosurgical care, the patient is simultaneously entering a period of acute emotional turmoil and stress. This period of stress necessitates a period of adaptation and coping that brings into play a variety of psychological defense mechanisms and coping strategies. The individual must begin to cope with changes in self-image and the associated psychological suffering. The initial evaluation must be alert to and address all of these aspects of patient care[8], which includes an assessment of the meaning of the injury to the patient, an understanding of the role of suffering in the patient's illness, an evaluation of psychological defenses and premorbid personality structure, an analysis of social support, an assessment of vulnerability toward major psychiatric disorders, and an evaluation of suicide risk (Table 24–1).

ALTERED MENTAL STATUS IN THE SPINAL CORD–INJURED PATIENT

It is not uncommon for patients with spinal cord injury to display an altered mental status. Psychiatric consultation is often sought during periods in which the patient appears

TABLE 24–1

INITIAL PSYCHIATRIC EVALUATION OF SPINAL CORD–INJURED PATIENTS

1. Evaluation of the meaning of the injury to the patient
2. Understanding of the nature of the patient's suffering
3. Assessment of defense mechanisms and premorbid personality style
4. Assessment of social support
5. Evaluation for major psychiatric disorders (depression, psychosis, substance abuse) and risk of suicide
6. Assessment of mental status
7. Assessment of adjustment reaction to injury and associated emotional features (demoralization, depression, anger)
8. Assessment for acute pain syndrome

either out of touch with reality or in a confusional state. It is imperative for the psychiatrist and medical and neurologic staff to be alert to the common causes of altered mental status in the spinal cord–injured patient. Mental status changes most often fall into one of the following categories: (1) delirium, (2) dementia (and dementia with superimposed confusional state), (3) sleep disorders, (4) major psychiatric disorders, and (5) psychological reactions to the spinal cord injury (Table 24–2).

The acute confusional state and its underlying causes are exhaustively reviewed by Lishman,[9] Lipowski,[10] and Taylor and Lewis.[11] Taylor and Lewis[11] point out that delirium is common in the hospital setting and often goes undiagnosed in the early stages. In a patient with spinal cord injury, the most common causes of delirium are sepsis, central nervous system (CNS) injury, toxic metabolic states, alcohol and drug withdrawal or intoxication, and adverse effects of medications. Sepsis is often due to urinary tract infection, pressure sores, or pneumonia. Spinal cord–injured patients are vulnerable to such infections, and a change in mental status characteristic of delirium is often the first symptom of infection that is manifested. The pharmacologic treatment of delirium is outlined in Table 24–3. Pharmacotherapy is aimed primarily at gaining control of agitation and psychotic symptoms. Often, the symptoms do not cease until the underlying cause of the delirium is removed. Haloperidol or lorazepam can be effective in reducing agitation; haloperidol will be more useful when psychotic symptoms are present. Both can have adverse effects, which must be monitored closely, especially if confusion worsens or any symptoms of neuroleptic malignant syndrome emerge.

It is also not uncommon for patients in the spinal cord injury unit to have suffered a head injury during the trauma that caused the spinal cord injury, and post-traumatic head injury syndromes can present with altered mental status. Clinicians treating patients with spinal cord injury must familiarize themselves with the classic syndromes associated with traumatic brain injury, especially in patients with a history of alcoholism. Patients can display syndromes associated with minor head injury; the most common of these is postconcussion syndrome, in which symptoms of headaches, dizziness, impaired concentration, a faulty memory, irritability, and lack of energy occur.[12] Patients may also appear depressed, and a postconcussion syndrome must be distinguished from a major depressive disorder. Patients with more severe head injury who have lost consciousness may manifest a syndrome that includes memory loss, denial of illness, confabulation, perseveration, sleep/wake disturbance, and confusion.[13] Recovery from head injury with a stage of mute responsiveness must always be evaluated in patients who are being assessed for withdrawal and mutism before those disorders are attributed to a psychological origin. Other post-traumatic states that must be considered include post-traumatic aphasia

TABLE 24–2

ALTERED MENTAL STATUS IN THE SPINAL CORD–INJURED PATIENT

DELIRIUM
    Sepsis secondary to infection (urinary tract infection, pressure sore, pneumonia, subcutaneous abscess, peritonitis)
    CNS injury: head trauma with postconcussive states, seizure disorder
    Toxic-metabolic encephalopathy
    Medication: steroids, baclofen, minor tranquilizers, antidepressants, cimetidine, morphine
    Anoxia: pneumonia, congestive heart failure, respiratory failure, silent myocardial infarction, arrhythmia
    Endocrine dysfunction
DEMENTIA
    Alzheimer's disease, multi-infarct dementia, Parkinsonism
    Confusion (delirium) superimposed on dementing illness
SLEEP DISORDERS
    Sleep apnea
    Sleep deprivation
    Sleep cycle reversal
MAJOR PSYCHIATRIC DISORDERS
    Psychotic disorders
    Major depressive disorder, unipolar and bipolar
    Anxiety disorders
    Substance abuse with intoxication or withdrawal
    Paranoid disorders
PSYCHOLOGICAL REACTION TO INJURY
    Adjustment reactions
    Dissociative reactions
    Mutism
    Personality disorder with impulsivity and outbursts

TABLE 24–3

PHARMACOTHERAPEUTIC MANAGEMENT OF DELIRIUM

CLINICAL SYNDROME	DRUG	DOSAGE RANGE*	ADVERSE EFFECTS
Delirium: confusion, acute agitation; paranoia and hallucinations may be present	Haldol (haloperidol)	0.5–2 mg, PO mild agitation, 5–10 mg, moderate agitation, 10–15 mg, severe agitation, IM or IV (may repeat in 1 hour if agitation is not controlled; monitor the level of sedation)	Acute dystonias, akathisia, tremor, rigidity, bradykinesia, hypotension, neuroleptic malignant syndrome (characterized by rigidity, fever, autonomic instability, delirium, increased creatine kinase levels)
	or		
	Ativan (lorazepam)	1–2 mg (IM/IV for acute agitation); 0.5–1 mg PO or IM b.i.d.–q.i.d. until agitation is controlled	Short-term memory impairment, paradoxical agitation, confusion, oversedation with lethargy

* IV = intravenous; IM = intramuscular; PO = by mouth; b.i.d. = twice daily; q.i.d. = four times daily.

and post-traumatic epilepsy, for which altered mental status can be the presenting symptom.

In the acute phase of spinal cord injury, patients are vulnerable to metabolic disorders that can cause confusion, so evaluation of renal function, liver function, acid-base status, and electrolytes is imperative, as is the case with confusional states in all patients.

Given the association of spinal cord injury with drug and alcohol abuse, confusional states may be associated with alcohol-related syndromes including Wernicke's encephalopathy, Korsakoff's psychosis, and alcohol withdrawal, including delirium tremens. Confusional states due to sedative hypnotic intoxication and withdrawal and toxic ingestion of opiates, antidepressants, and minor tranquilizers need to be assessed as well. In patients prone to drug abuse, intoxication with medications prescribed for the spinal cord injury, including diazepam, baclofen, and narcotic analgesics, can lead to altered mental states. Finally, given the use of steroids in the acute phase of treatment, affective changes and/or paranoid states and paranoid psychosis secondary to steroid administration can be observed.[14]

Dementia in the patient with spinal cord injury may present as nocturnal confusion and intermittent acute confusional states (i.e., beclouded dementia). Dementia syndromes can be exacerbated by medications, sleep deprivation, and many of the other toxic-metabolic insults described earlier.

Mental status changes in the context of sleep disorders, including sleep apnea, sleep deprivation, and sleep cycle reversal, occur in this patient population. Patients with sleep deprivation complain of daytime fatigue and may display mental status changes, including psychotic features. A study of patients with spinal cord injury showed some degree of obstructive sleep apnea in 45% of 22 patients, which illustrates the need for close evaluation of sleep disorders.[15] Sleep apnea may be an exacerbation of a prior sleep apnea syndrome or may be due to impaired ventilatory function resulting from the spinal cord injury. Medications used to treat spasticity, such as diazepam, baclofen, and dantrolene, may also contribute to the higher incidence of sleep apnea in this group. Sleep apnea is well known to produce daytime symptoms, including depression, decreased cognitive alertness with memory impairment, confusion, irritability, and daytime fatigue.[16]

Alterations in sensation produced by spinal cord lesions, including potential alterations in function of the reticular activating system, may also contribute to disorders of sleep that can produce sleep deprivation and sleep cycle reversal. This syndrome can be made worse, obviously, by the hospital environment, in which patients often have difficulty sleeping at night, and in the early stages of spinal cord injury, sleep deprivation due to pain and emotional distress is not uncommon. A full workup, including polysomnography, may be necessary to document the level of sleep impairment in such individuals.

Given the increased incidence of spinal cord injury associated with major psychiatric disorders, including major depression, psychosis, alcoholism, and antisocial personality disorder,[17] these syndromes must be considered in patients with mental status changes. Schizophrenic individuals are more prone to psychotic and paranoid symptoms on the spinal cord unit. Patients with substance abuse can appear in states of intoxication or withdrawal. Patients with mania can appear in hypomanic or manic states, characterized by euphoria, irritability, paranoia, increased motor activity, and pressured speech. Patients with major depression can present in withdrawn, apathetic states, and patients with delusional depression can appear acutely paranoid, delusional, and preoccupied with morbid depressive themes.

Finally, patients with spinal cord injury must adapt to enormous psychological stress. Patients can present with withdrawal and mutism and/or dissociative reactions. Such states can be quite disturbing to medical and nursing staff who are caring for the patient. It may take days for patients to begin to talk after an initial episode of mutism. A patient with a dissociative reaction can feel detached and outside his or her body, or he or she may not recall important information relating to the acute experience. These dissociative states must be distinguished, of course, from true postconcussive states or states secondary to memory disorders based on CNS injury.

In summary, multiple etiologies account for changes in mental status in the patient with spinal cord injury. The neuropsychiatric assessment must be thorough and not simply rely on a diagnosis of "psychological causes" to explain behavioral changes. Considering the complexity of mental status changes in the patient with spinal cord injury, the physician should be open to early involvement of the psychiatrist. This consultation can help both in the evaluation of mental status changes and in the formulation of treatment plans to manage behavioral problems and acute psychiatric states, such as psychosis and depressive disorders.

MANAGEMENT OF PSYCHIATRIC SYNDROMES IN THE SPINAL CORD–INJURED PATIENT

Spinal cord injury may occur in a patient who has a premorbid psychiatric disorder (e.g., mood disorder, psychotic disorder, substance abuse disorder) or it may occur de novo in an individual who has no prior psychiatric history.

In patients with no prior history of psychiatric disorder, treatment most often revolves around an adjustment disorder. If a patient has an active psychiatric disorder, treatment of that problem must be undertaken conjointly with the medical treatment and the treatment of the acute psychological adjustment.

A team approach remains most useful in the psychiatric management of patients with spinal cord injuries. The team includes psychiatrists, nurses, social workers, and rehabilitation therapists who work with the medical and spinal cord injury staff. This interdisciplinary team can create effective psychiatric treatment that enhances the basic medical treatment.

Adjustment Reactions and Dissociative States

The patient who has suffered a spinal cord injury is subjected to an acute period of psychological disruption. This period is accompanied by a wide range of emotional responses including anxiety, depression, overt expressions of anger and hostility, denial of the severity of the injury, increased dependency, withdrawal, and, in the extreme, mutism and noncompliance.

Hammell reviewed theoretical approaches to understanding the nature of adjustment in the patient with spinal cord injury. In the acute stage, patients experience a variety of psychiatric and somatosensory alterations including a sense of unreality, anesthesia and/or acute pain, sleep cycle disruption, indigestion and appetite disturbance, muscle tension and aches, rashes, anxiety, dysphoria, and demoralization.[18] The severity of the loss and changes resulting from a spinal cord injury can impair an individual's ability to reason clearly and to concentrate, which can contribute to the state of "denial" that is seen in the acute adjustment phase. This type of denial needs to be distinguished from the denial in which patients psychologically do not accept the severity of their injuries.

Initial treatment of the adjustment reaction includes emotional support from nursing and medical staff to help diminish fear and anxiety. Acknowledgment of the reality of how frightening and anxiety provoking the situation is to the patient can be very reassuring. The psychiatrist can often be of help in reassuring the patient that he or she is not "losing [his or her] mind." The emotional turmoil in the early period of adjustment can make a patient feel quite out of control and cause either a feeling of unreality or a feeling that he or she is "going crazy."

In the face of life-threatening danger, patients can also experience a variety of depersonalization phenomenona including feelings of unreality, slowing of time, lack of emotion, feelings of detachment, heightening of certain perceptions, dream-like states, and mystical experiences.[19] Sensory disruption caused by a spinal cord injury can exacerbate the state of depersonalization and lead to distortion of bodily sensations, such as feelings of reduplication of limbs, of telescoping of limbs, and of floating above one's own body.

Following the acute phase of adjustment, patients begin to cope with the resulting disability and dependency caused by the spinal cord injury. This period necessitates a close working relationship among caregivers, especially the rehabilitation specialists, nurses, and psychiatrists. In this phase of treatment, the patient needs to begin learning how to live with and adapt to disability and chronic illness and how to address the psychological issues of suffering and loss. The psychiatrist can help the patient deal with feelings of depression, anger, and frustration, which often impede rehabilitation. In this period, intense feelings of loss, shame, and guilt can surface. In the individual meetings between the psychiatrist and the patient, these feelings often are the focus of psychotherapy.

The final phase of treatment incorporates the patient's acceptance of the injury and addresses the transition from the hospital ward to the home or rehabilitation setting. This can be a period of acute stress for the patient and may reactivate anxieties and psychological issues from earlier in the course of treatment. Family support needs to be mobilized, if available, to help the transition occur effectively.

Adjustment to spinal cord injury does not always go smoothly. Demoralization and dysphoria can become protracted and evolve into a major depressive disorder, for which antidepressant medication is indicated (see following discussion on mood disorders). Anxiety can be extremely intense and can approach or include panic attacks; anxiolytic drugs and/or behavioral therapy are indicated in these situations.

Couples need to address the many issues regarding daily care, sexual functioning, and ongoing rehabilitation. These can be addressed in ward groups or in meetings with the couple and a trained social worker or psychologist.

There is also considerable variation in the time at which different phases of adjustment take place. Some patients pass from acute adjustment to acceptance within months; others are still in the acute phase after 6 months, and enter the acceptance phase later. The key for the clinician is to identify the psychological state of the patient, to have an interdisciplinary team available for support and treatment, and not to expect the patient to fit any preconceived picture of adjustment. This flexible approach reduces conflict with the patient and allows for more successful treatment on all fronts.

Certain patients who are injured in life-threatening situations, such as a car accident, airplane crash, or military combat, may experience development of what is termed *posttraumatic stress disorder*. In this disorder, patients report reexperiencing the trauma in recurrent recollections, dreams, nightmares, or intrusive sudden feelings of reliving the event (in the extreme, a dissociative flashback), and they experience severe distress when exposed to events that remind them of the traumatic event. Patients report the need to avoid thoughts or activities associated with the trauma, feel distant from important persons in their lives, and have a lessened ability to feel close to loved ones. Associated symptoms include insomnia, angry outbursts, and difficulty in concentrating. Patients may appear depressed and anxious.[20, 21]

In such cases, psychiatric consultation is indicated both to evaluate for pharmacotherapy (anxiolytics and antidepressants) and ongoing psychotherapy and to assess suicide risk. The latter can complicate the adjustment to injury and may present as a psychiatric emergency.

Personality Disorders

Personality disorder is another psychiatric problem that can complicate adjustment to spinal cord injury. Personality disorders, behaviors that are characteristic of a person's long-term style, impair social and occupational functioning and cause, in some cases, subjective distress, such as chronic depression. These individuals display emotional lability and cause disruption on hospital wards.

Patients with unstable personality disorders (also called borderline personality) often exhibit substance abuse and impulsive behavior, which lead to accidents that give rise to spinal cord injury. These patients may cause management problems on the ward. Their behavior reflects intense expressions of affect characterized by anger and hostility, rapid shifts in mood in relation to how they perceive their treatment by the staff, and inappropriate anger at staff. Such patients feel the staff may not be meeting their needs, are sensitive to feeling abandoned, and tend to distort reality, place blame on others, and split staff into the "good" vs. the "bad."

These patients are best treated by an organized team approach. The team must agree on the limits to be set and present them to the patient in an open fashion; this often involves written contracts. The patient must take responsibility for his or her behavior on the ward and is expected to participate in recommended treatment without dictating the terms of treatment.

Patients with personality disorders can be very demanding and drain the staff's emotional energy. In certain instances, having a primary nurse and primary doctor relating to the patient helps avoid "splitting" and begins formation of the much-needed therapeutic alliance. A psychiatrist can help provide additional and consistent support to the patient and should be involved to help evaluate the patient for co-morbid substance abuse, affective disorder, and suicide risk.

At the other end of the spectrum is the patient with dependent personality disorder, who regresses and becomes totally dependent on staff for self-care. Such patients can cause frustration for nursing and rehabilitation staff, and need a structured treatment plan to help mobilize them out of a state of dependency into a more active role in self-care.

Again, psychiatric consultation can be invaluable for assessment of the severity of character pathology in the patient, planning with staff how best to treat such patients, and addressing problems that arise on the ward and during the transition from the ward to the outside world.

The key to managing personality disorders on the spinal cord injury unit revolves around having an organized team approach that promotes dialogue among doctors, nurses, and auxiliary caretakers and presents a treatment plan to the patient that the spinal cord injury team supports and can work on with the patient. At times, patients with personality disorders try to defeat such treatment, and caretakers must accept the limits of what can be accomplished with such patients.

Alcoholism and Substance Abuse

A substance abuser on the spinal cord injury ward presents difficult management problems. A new patient who is suffering from alcoholism or substance abuse (narcotics, minor tranquilizers, cocaine, or mixed substance abuse) must receive psychiatric evaluation to address issues of acute toxicity or risk of withdrawal. Issues of drug-seeking behavior in the hospital or after discharge must also be addressed.

The most important part of the psychiatric evaluation involves documenting the pattern of abuse. Often, the substance abuser distorts the history or mimics withdrawal symptoms to influence the amount of drugs he will receive. Obtaining a history from family or friends, if possible, can help define the severity of the abuse and the recent history. The drug history must include types of drugs used, duration of abuse, frequency of use, amounts used, route of ingestion, and time and date of last doses. The initial medical evaluation must address evidence of withdrawal or toxicity. Special attention should be paid to medical problems associated with drug use including hepatitis, tuberculosis, acquired immunodeficiency syndrome (AIDS), and other infections. Patients with mixed substance abuse (e.g., barbiturates or alcohol plus narcotics) must receive evaluation to assess the possibility of mixed withdrawal states, especially given the morbidity associated with sedative withdrawal.

It is important to note that drug and alcohol use are factors associated with increased risk of suicide. Patients with spinal cord injury who are substance abusers should always be assessed for suicidal ideation. In some cases, these patients present with accidental overdoses or impulsive suicide attempts. In these contexts, psychiatric evaluation is imperative to help with placement and treatment decisions, especially regarding the need for detoxification.

Specific types of drug dependency necessitate appropriate intervention. The opiate abuser may show signs of withdrawal (e.g., craving, nervousness, yawning, perspiration, achiness, cramps, insomnia, fever) and advanced withdrawal (e.g., vomiting, diarrhea, tachycardia, and hypertension). Acutely injured patients can receive maintenance doses of opiates and drug detoxification can be addressed later in the treatment. In such cases, a patient may be started on methadone, 20 to 30 mg/day (10 to 20 mg is usually sufficient),

with a tapering of 5 mg every 48 hours in the patient whose condition is stabilized.

Patients with narcotic dependency may demand analgesics to treat pain syndromes. Drug-seeking behavior such as drug hoarding, seeking analgesics from more than one physician, dose escalation, or requests for renewals of analgesics before they are due should alert the physician that there is a problem. Psychiatric consultation helps define the nature of the substance abuse, determine the presence of a co-morbid psychiatric disorder (such as depression or character disorder), and manage drug-seeking behavior. Narcotic-dependent individuals present difficult management problems in both hospital and outpatient settings. The narcotic dependence must be addressed as a primary problem and treated as such. Referral for drug treatment, inpatient or outpatient, is often a necessity.

Similarly, the alcoholic spinal cord injury patient should be treated as if the alcohol problem were an independent problem. The spinal cord injury should not allow the patient to bargain for special treatment or to deny the severity of the alcohol problem. Referral to an alcohol treatment program or Alcoholics Anonymous may be necessary.

Alcoholic patients need early assessment for withdrawal when admitted to the spinal cord injury unit. This is true on initial admission and on subsequent admissions for spinal cord injury care. Chronic alcoholics should not be allowed to use their drinking problems to gain admission to spinal cord injury units; they should receive referral to inpatient detoxification facilities that can accommodate patients with spinal cord injury. If no such facilities are available, psychiatric consultation can be of use in facilitating detoxification and in evaluating any mental status changes secondary to chronic alcohol abuse, which include alcoholic hallucinosis, amnestic syndrome, Wernicke's encephalopathy, and alcoholic paranoia.

Mood Disorders

The catastrophic nature of spinal cord injury evokes varied responses in patients, which range from adjustment reactions to major depressive disorders. Mood disorders include major depressive disorder, bipolar disorder (manic depressive illness), and dysthmyia. Alterations in mood are also seen in adjustment reactions.

The incidence of depressive illness in the population with spinal cord injury is higher than in the general population. Certain authors have stated that depression should be considered normal in all spinal cord injury patients and that if a patient is not depressed, he or she should be considered to be in denial. Studies have not supported such statements. Unfortunately, few studies exist that systematically assess the incidence of depressive illness in this population.[22] Trieschmann[23] has concluded that spinal injury does not lead to severe depressive reactions in all patients, and the absence of depression does not seem to imply either denial of illness or poor adjustment to disability.

The differential diagnosis of depressed mood in patients with spinal cord injury includes adjustment reaction with depressed mood, demoralization, "conservation-withdrawal," and major depressive disorder.

Adjustment reaction with depressed mood is a common reaction to serious illness, but it is usually brief, nonpervasive, and not accompanied by ongoing vegetative, cognitive, and behavioral symptoms of depression. Adjustment reactions are not treated with antidepressant medications. Psychotherapy is the treatment of choice in addition to activation of the patient's support system, including friends and family. Certain patients also benefit from the support of a clergyman as they struggle with the meaning of injury within the context of their religious beliefs, especially if feelings of guilt or punishment are associated with the injury.

Conservation-withdrawal has been described as the ordinary self-limited biological reaction pattern of withdrawal and inactivity that protects the organism against overstimulation or excessive deprivation. Physical and psychological concomitants of conservation-withdrawal, such as weakness, fatigue, diminished energy, diminished muscle tone, and loss of interest in the environment, may readily be confused with symptoms of depression.[24]

Major depressive disorder refers to both unipolar depression and the depressed phase of bipolar illness. It is characterized by a pervasive feeling of depression with diminished interest and pleasure in all or almost all activities (anhedonia). Other symptoms include psychomotor agitation or retardation, loss of energy or fatigue, feelings of worthlessness and hopelessness, poor concentration, inappropriate or excessive guilt, slowed thinking, and suicidal ideation. Patients with major depression are at high risk for suicide.

Some of the neurovegetative symptoms of depression, such as sleep and appetite disturbances, can also be secondary to the medical complications of spinal cord injury. In these cases, cognitive symptoms of depression, such as guilt, hopelessness, anhedonia, and suicidal ideation, are of more importance in signaling a major depressive disorder. Risk factors for depressive disorder include previous history of major depressive illness, family history of depression, past suicide attempt, and history of alcohol and drug abuse.

Failure to recognize major depression or the incorrect assumption that depression is a "normal response" to injury may adversely influence both the short- and long-term rehabilitation of the patient. After major depression is diagnosed, several steps should be taken to treat it rapidly. Careful selection of an antidepressant is imperative (Table 24–4). After selection of an antidepressant medication, the patient should be started on the lowest efficacious dose, which is increased gradually to achieve a full response or until side effects become intolerable. In the latter case, administration of a second antidepressant medication can be initiated. In general, tricyclics have more troublesome side effects, such as dry mouth, constipation, urinary retention, blurred vision, and orthostatic hypotension. Given the vulnerability of spinal cord–injured patients to autonomic dysreflexia, the tricyclics are no longer the drugs of choice for major depression in this group of patients and the serotonin reuptake inhibitors constitute the first-line drugs of choice. Serotonin reuptake inhibitors, such as fluoxetine, sertraline, and paroxetine, have a different side effect profile, including stimulation, daytime sleepiness, sexual dysfunction,

TABLE 24-4

PHARMACOLOGIC MANAGEMENT OF MAJOR DEPRESSIVE DISORDER

CLINICAL SYNDROME	DRUG	DOSAGE RANGE	ADVERSE EFFECTS
Major depressive disorder	Tricyclics Imipramine Desipramine } Amitriptyline } Nortriptyline	150–300 mg/day PO; elderly may need lower dosages, in 25–100 mg range (blood level monitoring of plasma levels guide dosage) 50–150 mg/day	Anticholinergic side effects such as dry mouth, constipation, urinary retention, blurred vision; orthostatic hypotension, sedation, intracardiac conduction abnormalities, weight gain, sexual dysfunction
	Monoamine oxidase (MAO) inhibitors Phenelzine Tranylcypromine	45–90 mg/day 30–50 mg/day	Orthostatic hypotension, sexual dysfunction, sedation, insomnia, stimulation, weight gain, headache; **patient must follow MAO diet to avoid hypertensive crisis**
	Serotonin reuptake inhibitors Fluoxetine Sertraline Paroxetine	20–80 mg/day 50–200 mg/day 20–40 mg/day	Nausea, diarrhea, drowsiness, dizziness, confusion, asthenia, insomnia, somnolence, headache, restlessness, anxiety, sexual dysfunction
	Aminoketone Bupropion	200–450 mg/day (single dose should not exceed 150 mg)	Nausea, stimulation, higher incidence of seizures in doses >450 mg/day; relatively contraindicated in patients with seizures, head injury, eating disorders

407

and headaches, but cause much less anticholinergic activity; as such, they are more useful as the first choice in treatment. Nonetheless, patients with spinal cord injury must also be closely monitored for these side effects, which can be quite troublesome and may necessitate a switch to bupropion.

Suicidal ideation must be taken seriously in all cases and represents a psychiatric emergency. Patients who have experienced the losses associated with spinal cord injury can become quite depressed and demoralized and are at risk for suicide even if no evidence of a major depressive disorder is seen.

Some patients with major depression may present with depressive delusions. Administration of neuroleptics in addition to antidepressants is indicated in the treatment of these patients. Electroconvulsive therapy (ECT) may be more effective in the treatment of delusional depression. Patients with depression refractory to medication or severe suicidal ideation also may require ECT. Response to ECT is often more rapid than response to medications, and ECT is safer in the treatment of elderly patients with heart disease. ECT is not contraindicated in patients with spinal cord injury and can be used safely when clinically indicated.

A patient with mania presents with euphoria or irritable mood, pressured speech that is hard to interrupt, grandiosity, inflated self-worth, history of spending sprees, and increased sexual activity. These patients can show serious impairment in judgment, which can lead to dangerous and impulsive activities. Sometimes delusions and hallucinations are present. Patients with bipolar disorder can "cycle" from mania to depression or present in a "mixed state," with features of both depressive disorder and mania.

A previous history of mania and family history of affective disorder or alcoholism may assist in making the diagnosis of bipolar disorder. An extremely manic patient can be very difficult to manage and may require physical or chemical restraints. Mood stabilizers such as lithium, carbamazepine, and valproic acid are the drugs of choice to treat a manic episode, but they may take two to four weeks to exert their full effect. In the interim, neuroleptic agents or benzodiazepines may be used to control agitation (Table 24–5).

It should be noted that neurologic and medical causes of mood disorders (e.g., CNS lesions, infectious or metabolic causes, or any endocrine disorder) must be ruled out as etiological factors for mood changes. A complete laboratory workup includes thyroid function tests, rapid plasma reagin test, and vitamin B_{12} and folate assays. In appropriate cases, CT and/or MRI should be ordered to rule out CNS lesions that present with mood disorder (e.g., subdural hematoma or tumor).

Between the extremes of adjustment reactions and major depessions exists a relatively milder, chronic form of depression, termed *dysthymia*. Sometimes patients with dysthymia develop major depression; the term *double depression* is used to describe this disorder. Antidepressants may help in the treatment of dysthymia.

In summary, a patient who experiences spinal cord injury is vulnerable to depression and demoralization. The physician must be able to distinguish features of an adjustment disorder from a more severe depressive disorder that can present as a psychiatric emergency and, if untreated, can hamper short- and long-term rehabilitation. Psychiatric consultation is most useful in establishing the diagnostic and treatment guidelines for patients, especially as regards administration of antidepressants, supportive therapy, ongoing psychotherapy, and family therapy, all of which play a role in the treatment of depression.

Anxiety Disorders

Patients with spinal cord injury are vulnerable to a variety of anxiety states. These include an adjustment reaction with anxious mood and anxiety related to such specific issues as bowel training or rehabilitation demands. Individuals with preexisting generalized anxiety disorder or panic disorder may present with exacerbations of these disorders.

Adjustment to spinal cord injury can produce an anxiety state. It is often related to feelings of loss of control, fear of what the

TABLE 24–5

PHARMACOTHERAPEUTIC MANAGEMENT OF BIPOLAR DISORDER

CLINICAL SYNDROME	DRUG	DOSAGE RANGE	ADVERSE EFFECTS
Manic-depressive illness	Lithium	600–1800 mg/day; elderly people and patients with impaired renal function need lower dosages; levels must be monitored closely and kept between 0.6–1.0 ml/L to avoid lithium toxicity	Nausea, vomiting, diarrhea, polyuria, cognitive side effects (such as memory disturbances), neurologic side effects (such as tremors, lethargy), hypothyroidism, ECG changes (such as T-wave flattening), acne, psoriasis, benign leukocytosis, weight gain, acute lithium toxicity (blood level >2–3 mmol/L) is a medical emergency that may necessitate saline infusion or hemodialysis
	Carbamazepine	200–1800 mg/day (blood levels guide dosage)	Sedation, dizziness, ataxia, diplopia, gastrointestinal upset, reversible mild leukopenia and reversible mild elevation in liver function tests; tremor, memory disturbances, and confusional states are less common; hepatitis and blood dyscrasias are rare but serious side effects
	Valproic acid	1800–3000 mg/day (blood levels guide dosage)	Sedation; gastrointestinal upset; mild cognitive impairment; elevation in liver function tests tremor; platelet dysfunction

future holds, and fear of being abandoned by loved ones. In addition, patients who have been respirator-dependent can become exquisitely anxious when being weaned from the respirator and during changes in respiratory state (in which the patient fears the loss of independent breathing). In cases of severe situational anxiety, benzodiazepines are quite useful in conjunction with supportive psychotherapy.

Patients with premorbid generalized anxiety or panic disorder may present difficult management problems. Such patients may experience intensification of generalized anxiety characterized by minor tension, restlessness, shortness of breath, sweating, nausea, insomnia, and intense worry about all aspects of spinal cord care. In these individuals, vigorous treatment with minor tranquilizers and/or buspirone is indicated, along with supportive therapy to address the acute issues of adjustment (Table 24–6).

Panic disorder differs from generalized anxiety by the appearance of discrete episodes of panic accompanied by autonomic dysfunction, including dyspnea, dizziness, tachycardia, diaphoresis, nausea, chest pain, and a fear of dying. These episodes occur daily or episodically and make the patient extraordinarily frightened. In some instances, the patient suffers from both generalized anxiety and panic.

Panic disorder necessitates pharmacotherapy including antidepressants and/or anxiolytics, often in conjunction with behavior therapy.

Symptoms of anxiety in patients with spinal cord injury may also be associated with substance abuse, especially of stimulants, and nicotine or drug withdrawal. Caffeine ingestion can exacerbate anxiety as well. Common medical conditions such as hyperthyroidism, anoxia, congestive heart failure, pneumonia, and migraine headaches can exacerbate anxiety. Medications including antidepressants, steroids, sympathomimetics, and baclofen have increased or produced anxiety.

Finally, patients taking neuroleptics can experience akasthisia, a syndrome of restlessness that must be distinguished from anxiety.

The Spinal Cord–Injured Patient with Chronic Pain: Psychiatric Aspects

Patients with spinal cord injury are vulnerable to chronic pain syndromes. Chapter 21 describes the variety of pain syndromes seen in patients with spinal cord injury, including local pain, radiating pain, and diffuse pain.

In some patients, however, the pain syndrome becomes associated with a psychiatric

TABLE 24–6

PHARMACOTHERAPY OF ANXIETY

CLINICAL SYNDROME	DRUG	DOSAGE RANGE	ADVERSE EFFECTS
Anxiety disorders			
Generalized anxiety	Benzodiazepines		
	Lorazepam	1–6 mg/day	Sedation, dizziness, ataxia, anterograde amnesia,
	Diazepam	5–40 mg/day	nausea, slight hypotension
	Oxazepam	30–60 mg/day	
	Alprazolam	1–4 mg/day	
Adjustment reactions with anxious mood	Antihistamines		
	Atarax	200–400 mg/day	Drowsiness, dry mouth
	Vistaril	50–100 mg/day	
	Buspirone	15–40 mg/day	Headache, nausea, dizziness, tension
	Benzodiazepines		Sedation, dizziness, ataxia, anterograde amnesia, nausea, slight hypotension
Panic disorder	Antidepressants		
	Desipramine	50–300 mg/day	As in Table 24–4
	Fluoxetine	20–60 mg/day	

disorder or an underlying psychological disorder. In these cases, psychiatric consultation can help be helpful in diagnosis, treatment, and management.

Mufson described the integration of medical and psychiatric evaluation and treatment in patients with chronic pain.[25] The important diagnostic issue is that patients can suffer primary chronic pain syndromes associated with the spinal cord injury, which eventually become part of a pain syndrome exacerbated by psychological factors or a psychiatric disorder.

Psychological factors associated with exacerbation of chronic pain include unresolved grief, marital discord, family discord, sexual conflict in the couple, anger at doctors, and unaddressed suffering. Patients with psychosocial histories of physical or sexual abuse are also at risk for complex chronic pain syndromes.

Chronic pain syndromes are associated with a variety of psychiatric disorders including major depression, psychosis, somatoform pain disorder, drug abuse, paranoid disorders, and hypochondriasis.

The psychiatrist can be of great assistance in helping the physician ascertain whether a primary pain syndrome has become part of a broader psychological or psychiatric problem. In these instances, treatment of the psychiatric issues are imperative if therapy of the pain syndrome is to be effective. This may include administration of antidepressants, individual psychotherapy, or couples therapy. Psychological testing, including a Minnesota Multiphasic Personality Inventory, can be useful in diagnosis of somatoform disorders.

Psychotic Disorders

Psychotic disorders constitute a heterogeneous group of states characterized by the presence of symptoms that interfere with an individual's reality testing. Impaired reality testing leads to impairment of the person's ability to think, function, or organize goal-directed behavior.

Psychotic symptoms include delusions, hallucinations, and thought disorder often characterized by loose associations or personalized and illogical thinking. The patient may present in a very guarded state with paranoia, and it may be difficult to interview such a patient. The acutely psychotic patient is in a disorganized emotional state, and the hospital setting can be quite frightening and stressful, leading to a worsening of the psychotic symptoms. Psychosis occurs with a wide variety of medical, neurologic, and toxic states as well as with formal psychiatric disorders, such as schizophrenia or bipolar illness. It is important for the clinician to determine whether the psychosis is due to an underlying medical or neurologic condition, because treatment of such a condition as substance abuse, metabolic imbalance, infection, vitamin deficiency, or a CNS lesion would lead to resolution of the psychosis in almost all cases. In these cases, the psychosis is secondary to a confusional state or reflects what is termed an *organic delusional state*. Careful history-taking, including a thorough cognitive evaluation, is the most important step in establishing the organic etiology. Confusional states may continue days beyond the resolution of the primary problem.

The patient with spinal cord injury may already carry a diagnosis of a chronic psychotic condition such as schizophrenia and may develop an acute exacerbation of the chronic condition on the spinal cord injury unit. Psychotic patients are prone to act in response to their delusional beliefs and hallucinations and may incur a spinal cord injury while engaging in dangerous activities, e.g., jumping from the roof due to command hallucinations.

Elderly patients with dementia may develop psychotic symptoms secondary to the dementing process. This may include delusions, paranoia and hallucinations.

Management of psychotic conditions involves understanding the correct etiology. Neuroleptic therapy constitutes the mainstay of treatment of psychosis (Table 24–7). The various groups of neuroleptics are, generally speaking, equipotent in equitherapeutic dosages. They should be started in the lowest possible doses and the dose should be increased gradually. It is important to note that certain psychotic symptoms, such as delu-

TABLE 24–7

PHARMACOTHERAPY OF PSYCHOTIC DISORDERS

CLINICAL SYNDROME	DRUG	DOSAGE RANGE	ADVERSE EFFECTS
Psychotic disorders (e.g., schizophrenia, manic psychosis)	Haloperidol Fluphenazine Perphenazine Chlorpromazine	5–30 mg 5–30 mg 8–64 mg 50–400 mg	Orthostatic hypotension, anticholinergic side effects (such as dry mouth, constipation, urinary retention), extrapyramidal side effects, acute dystonias, neuroleptic malignant syndrome (characterized by rigidity, fever, dysautonomia, delirium, increased creatine kinase levels)
	Clozapine	200–500 mg/day; start with 25 mg/day and gradually increase to 200 mg/day	Sedation, orthostatic hypotension, tachycardia, seizures, agranulocytosis, salivation, fever. Extrapyramidal signs and neuroleptic malignant syndrome very rare. Weekly blood monitoring makes use difficult in outpatients.
	Risperidone	2–10 mg	Anxiety, somnolence, dizziness, constipation, nausea, tachycardia.

sions, may persist despite treatment with neuroleptics, and that increasing the dose in such situations only exposes the patient to a higher incidence of side effects, but does little to diminish symptoms.

While on the spinal cord injury ward, supportive therapy from a consistent figure (psychiatrist, psychiatric nurse, psychologist, social worker) can be extremely helpful in stabilizing the psychotic patient's condition and creating a milieu in which the patient feels less threatened.

SUMMARY

Psychiatric assessment and treatment of the patient with spinal cord injury is complex and should accompany ongoing medical treatment. Psychiatric assessment includes an initial evaluation of adjustment to the injury that focuses on issues of loss, diminished self-esteem, suffering, and coping and adaptation. An initial evaluation of premorbid personality style and defense mechanisms guides the psychological treatment throughout the phases of adjustment.

Spinal cord injury patients may show mental status changes in the acute or chronic phases of treatment. These changes necessitate a thorough evaluation for potential causes, including delirium, dementia, and

psychiatric disorders. Finally, spinal cord injury is associated with a variety of major psychiatric disorders, including psychosis, drug and alcohol abuse, and major depression. The physician should be familiar with the guidelines set out in this chapter for management of such patients in the spinal cord injury setting.

The psychiatrist can be called on to help provide both diagnostic evaluation and ongoing treatment of the many psychiatric and neuropsychiatric problems encountered in this patient population.

REFERENCES

1. Guttman L: Spinal Cord Injuries: Comprehensive Management and Research. Oxford, Blackwell Scientific Publications, 1976, pp 1–5.
2. Guttmann L: Spinal Cord Injuries: Comprehensive Management and Research. Oxford, Blackwell Scientific Publications, 1976, pp 506–511.
3. Cassel E: The Nature of Suffering and the Goals of Medicine. New York, Oxford University Press, 1991, pp 60–65.
4. Cassel E: The Nature of Suffering and the Goals of Medicine. New York, Oxford University Press, 1991, pp 60–65.
5. Leigh H, Reiser M: The Patient: Biological, Psychological and Social Dimensions of Medical Practice. New York, Plenum, 1985.
6. Kahana R, Bibring G: Personality types in medical management. In Zinberg N (ed): Psychiatry and Medical Practice in a General Hospital. New York, International Universities Press, 1964, pp 108–123.
7. Green SA: Principles of medical psychotherapy. In Stoudemire A, Fogel B (eds): Psychiatric Care of the

Medical Patient. New York, Oxford University Press, 1993, pp 3–18.

8. Stewart T: Spinal cord injury: A role for the psychiatrist. Am J Psychiatry 134:538–541, 1977.

9. Lishman WA: Organic Psychiatry. Oxford, Blackwell Scientific Publications, 1987, pp 137–186.

10. Lipowski Z: Delirium: Acute Confusional States. New York, Oxford University Press, 1990.

11. Taylor D, Lewis S: Delirium. Neurol Neurosurg Psychiatry 56:742–751, 1993.

12. Rutherford W: Post concussive symptoms: Relationship to acute neurologic indices, individual differences, and circumstances of injury. In Levin H, Eisenberg H, Benton A (eds): Mild Head Injury. New York, Oxford University Press, 1989, pp 218–228.

13. Alexander MP: Traumatic brain injury. In Benson DF, Blumer D (eds): Psychiatric Aspects of Neurologic Disease, vol II. New York, Grune & Stratton, 1982, pp 219–221.

14. Ling M, Perry P, Tsuang M: Side effects of corticosteroid therapy: Psychiatric aspects. Arch Gen Psychiatry 38:471–476, 1981.

15. Short DJ, Stradling JR, Williams SJ: Prevalence of sleep apnea in patients over 40 years of age with spinal cord lesions. Neurol Neurosurg Psychiatry 55:1032–1036, 1992.

16. Guilleminault C: Clinical features and evaluation of obstructive sleep apnea. In Kryger M, Roth T, Dement W (eds): Principles and Practice of Sleep Medicine. Philadelphia, WB Saunders, 1989, pp 552–558.

17. Fullerton D, Harvey R, Klein M, et al: Psychiatric disorders in patients with spinal cord injury. Arch Gen Psychiatry 38:1369–1371, 1981.

18. Hammell KR: Psychological and sociological theories concerning adjustment to traumatic spinal cord injury: The implications for rehabilitation. Paraplegia 30:317–326, 1992.

19. Noyes R, Kletti N: Depersonalization in the face of life threatening danger: A description. In Garfield C (ed): Stress and Survival: The Emotional Realities of the Life Threatening Illness. St Louis, CV Mosby, 1979, pp 367–375.

20. Brett E, Spitzer R, Williams D: DSM III-R criteria for post-traumatic stress disorder. Am J Psychiatry 145:1232–1235, 1988.

21. Gersons B, Carlier I: Post-traumatic stress disorder: The history of a recent concept. Br J Psychiatry 161:742–748, 1992.

22. Judd FK, Burrows GD, Brown DJ: Depression following acute spinal cord injury. Paraplegia 24:358–363, 1986.

23. Trieschmann RB: Spinal Cord Injuries: Psychological, Social and Vocational Adjustment. New York, Pergamon Press, 1980, pp 35–85.

24. Weiner MF, Lovitt R: Conservation-withdrawal versus depression. Gen Hosp Psychiatry 4:347–349, 1979.

25. Mufson M: Chronic pain syndrome: Integrating the medical and psychiatric treatment. In Branch WT Jr (ed): Office Practice of Medicine, ed 3. Philadelphia, WB Saunders, 1994, pp 1019–1027.

CHAPTER 25

Clinical Pharmacology of Spinal Cord Injury

Jack L. Segal, M.D.

Longevity and the quality of life in humans who have sustained a spinal cord injury have increased significantly since World War I when survival was measured in terms of weeks or months. Most survivors now go on to live full lives, and the average life span of even the most gravely disabled person now approaches that enjoyed by able-bodied populations.[1] The extended longevity and improved quality of life in patients who have sustained traumatic spinal myelopathy are not mere happenstance, but represent the result of an increasingly more comprehensive body of knowledge of the pathobiology of spinal cord injury and the applied expertise of knowledgeable health care professionals.

Patients with spinal cord injury receive many medications during the acute and chronic phase of injury, and the number of conditions afflicting patients with spinal cord injury that are responsive to ameliorative or curative drug therapy has expanded. Consequently, the risk of therapeutic misadventure or toxicity has been magnified. Although the relevance of applying pharmacokinetic and pharmacodynamic analyses to development of rational drug prescribing has been recognized for populations distinguished by altered drug metabolism, e.g., the elderly or neonates, relatively few studies of drug disposition kinetics or drug effects have been carried out in patients with spinal cord injury, and criteria or effective strategies for optimizing pharmacotherapy based on pharmacokinetic principles have yet to evolve.

Treatment strategies available to the physician who is managing patients with spinal cord injury have been extrapolated, often uncritically, from anecdotal experience or experimental data obtained in able-bodied populations.[2, 3]

Drug therapies in spinal cord injury have been almost exclusively directed toward the treatment of diseases common to both the able-bodied and the spinal cord–injured patient. Few drug therapies have been developed specifically as pharamacologic interventions in patients with pathophysiologic and altered metabolic processes that are uniquely the sequelae of a spinal cord injury, and the medications discussed in this chapter represent the small number of therapeutic agents for which any effort to characterize population-specific pharmacokinetic/pharmacodynamic profiles for patients with spinal cord injury have been attempted. Only recently have population-specific drug therapies for patients with spinal cord injury been developed that include medications to enhance the survival of acutely traumatized neurons and to contribute to the restoration of voluntary motor function in long-standing injury.

Myriad changes in human physiology caused by acute trauma to the spinal cord or associated with a chronic spinal cord injury involve nearly every organ system,[4] and demodulation or disruption of the autonomic nervous system is a ubiquitous phenomenon.[5, 6] Hemodynamic abnormalities and cardiac dysrhythmias that may influence drug disposition are common, particularly with acute cervical and high-level thoracic lesions.[7–10] Segal, Shizgal, Nuhlicek, Greenway and their colleagues described variations in gross body composition, shifts in body fluid compartments, changes in drug distribution, and alterations in electrolyte concentrations.[11–14] During the acute and chronic phase of injury, ventilatory compromise and respiratory failure are frequent complications of spinal cord injury.[15–17] Both restrictive and obstructive changes in pulmonary function occur simultaneously with acute spinal cord trauma and reflect sudden alterations in anatomy of the thorax and demodulation of the autonomic nervous system. These and other alterations in physiology caused by spinal cord injury have been observed in association with clinically significant changes in pharmacokinetics and pharmacodynamics.[18, 19] Their magnitude reflects the extent of disruption in homeostasis that contributes to many problems confronting the clinician and confounding the clinical decision-making process.[20, 21]

Safe, effective use of medication in the spinal cord–injured patient is often biased by critiera or therapeutic strategies derived from sparse, fragmentary data or limited clinical experience. Thus the patient with spinal cord injury and a pharmacologically modifiable disease process, iatrogenic or otherwise, poses a formidable therapeutic challenge that has neither been adequately delineated nor systematically addressed. Even prescribing over-the-counter medications, commonly acknowledged as posing little or no risk in the able-bodied, can be associated with an increased frequency of adverse reactions in spinal cord–injured patients, who, for example, share with cardiac transplant recipients the altered responses of a denervated heart.[22]

Because of our lack of knowledge of the clinical pharmacology of spinal cord injury, increased incidence of population-specific therapeutic misadventures should be anticipated, and equivocal outcomes associated with drug therapies, particularly pharmacologic interventions designed to limit the acute injury or restore function, may be mistakenly attributed. Problems of this nature, often unrecognized, are ubiquitous and reflect the magnitude of the therapeutic dilemma in patients with spinal cord injury.

THERAPEUTIC CONSIDERATIONS

Analgesics

In general, effects of a drug, beneficial or toxic, depend on the concentration of drug at sites of action. Blood and tissue drug concentrations reflect the rate and completeness of drug absorption (bioavailability). Intravenously administered drugs are considered to be 100% bioavailable, as no absorptive or metabolic processes impede their entry into the systemic circulation.

Spinal cord injury population-specific research into the pharmacokinetic/pharmacodynamic behavior of commonly prescribed analgesic medications such as the nonsteroidal anti-inflammatory drugs (NSAIDs) (e.g., acetaminophen, ibuprofen, naproxen, aspirin) and the opiates or narcotic analogs is virtually nonexistent. The only guidelines available to assist in therapeutic decision-making concerning the administration of acetaminophen or similar analgesics must be inferred from research in a relatively small population of spinal cord–injured humans or extrapolated to such patients from studies in the able-bodied (neurologically intact).

Acetaminophen (Tylenol) is widely prescribed to patients with spinal cord injury as an analgesic/antipyretic. Following oral administration to able-bodied subjects, acetaminophen is passively absorbed from the gastrointestinal (GI) tract. Gastric emptying and GI motility appear to influence the absorption of acetaminophen and other drugs in the able-bodied. Halstead and co-workers[23] recognized the need to study effects of pathophysiology in spinal cord injury on variables that influence the efficiency of GI absorption. Riboflavin and acetaminophen were chosen because they are absorbed by distinctly different mechanisms. Riboflavin absorption is dependent on active transport in the upper small intestine and is influenced by changes in gastric emptying. Acetaminophen absorption is also influenced by GI motility, but acetaminophen appears to be absorbed passively. These authors assessed the GI uptake of riboflavin and acetaminophen under fasting and nonfasting conditions. They found no significant difference in the peak excretion rate, the time required to achieve peak serum riboflavin levels, and the cumulative percent of riboflavin recovered from urine (Fig. 25–1) between nonfasting able-bodied controls and patients. A fasting state for both controls and patients with spinal cord injury was, however, associated with a statistically significant change in riboflavin absorption parameters.

GI uptake of acetaminophen was significantly impaired in spinal cord–injured pa-

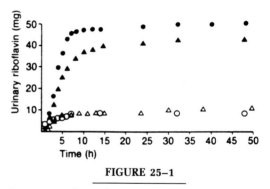

FIGURE 25–1

Comparison of cumulative urinary excretion of oral riboflavin, 150 mg, vs. time during fasting and nonfasting conditions for an able-bodied subject and a patient with spinal cord injury. *Solid dot* indicates nonfasting patient; *open dot*, fasting patient; *solid triangle*, able-bodied nonfasting subject; *open triangle*, able-bodied fasting subject. (From Halstead LS, Feldman S, Claus-Walker J, et al: Drug absorption in spinal cord injury. Arch Phys Med Rehabil 66:298–301, 1985.)

tients, and pathophysiology of spinal cord injury was implicated as a presumptive etiology for the change in intestinal absorption parameters for orally administered acetaminophen (Table 25–1). A similar reduction in the rate of absorption of acetaminophen was achieved in able-bodied subjects by Nimmo and colleagues[24] using an anticholinergic drug to delay gastric evacuation. These observations are highly suggestive of a causal association between the impairment in postprandial gastric emptying characteristic of spinal cord injury and changes of potential clinical significance in the efficacy of orally administered drugs when absorption efficiency is dependent on gastric motility or emptying rate.[25–28] Rajendran and co-workers,[29] in a study of gastric emptying in a small number of patients with spinal cord injury, were unable to demonstrate impaired evacuation of gastric contents. Their study was uncontrolled and differed significantly in methodology from previous studies. Nevertheless, the weight of experimental evidence implicates a spinal cord injury population-specific impairment in gastric emptying,[25, 27] supports recommendations to modify oral dosing regimens of selected drugs in recognition of altered physiology in spinal cord injury, and emphasizes the need to implement dosing algorithms derived from population-specific pharmacokinetic/pharmacodynamic profiles.

TABLE 25–1

COMPARISON OF ABSORPTION AND DISPOSITION PARAMETERS (MEAN ± SD) OF PARACETAMOL (ACETAMINOPHEN) IN SERUM ASSAYS IN SPINAL CORD–INJURED PATIENTS AND ABLE-BODIED SUBJECTS

SUBJECTS (NO.)	t_{max}* (hr)	C_{max}* (mg/L)	t_{lag}* (min)	AUC[†] (mg/L·h)	$t_{1/2}$[†] (hr)	k_e[†] (hr^{-1})
Control (3)[‡]	0.51 ± 0.06	14.50 ± 6.85	8.90 ± 7.80	27.36 ± 7.30	2.60 ± 0.10	0.26 ± 0.01
Control (18)[§]	0.76 ± 0.12	11.99 ± 1.02	4.20 ± 0.25	26.82 ± 6.11	2.55 ± 0.14	Not reported
SCI (5)	1.35 ± 0.60	6.80 ± 2.68	18.18 ± 1.83	21.75 ± 6.72	2.89 ± 1.81	0.30 ± 0.13

From Halstead LS, Feldman S, Claus-Walker J, et al: Drug absorption in spinal cord injury. Arch Phys Med Rehabil 66:298–301, 1985.

C_{max} = peak serum drug concentration; t_{max} = time to C_{max}; t_{lag} = lag time; AUC = area under the concentration-time curve; $t_{1/2}$ = serum half-life; k_e = elimination rate constant; SCI = spinal cord injury; hr^{-1} = reciprocal hours.

* Differences between controls and patients statistically significant (P < 0.05).

[†] Differences between controls and patients not statistically significant.

[‡] Lee WH, Kramer WG, Granville GE: Effect of obesity on acetaminophen pharmacokinetics in man. J Clin Pharmacol 21:284–287, 1981.

[§] Ameer B, Divoll M, Abernathy DR, et al: Absolute and relative bioavailability of oral acetaminophen preparations. J Pharm Sci 72:955–958, 1983.

It would appear that the amounts of analgesic administered need only be increased to compensate for diminished absorption and to titrate to an acceptable state of pain relief. This, in fact, may be all that is required. Still, for drugs such as acetaminophen, which exhibit dose-dependent kinetics and nonlinear elimination, or whose biotransformation is dependent on hepatic oxidative metabolism, simply increasing the dose until a desired level of analgesia or antipyresis is achieved may result in untoward effects and toxicity. Unlike the able-bodied who, when ill, do not necessarily experience liver dysfunction, it appears that many "healthy" patients with spinal cord injury have altered hepatic metabolism of unknown clinical significance,[30] thereby rendering conventional dosing regimens and titration-to-effect of highly biotransformed drugs unreliable and risky. Less conventional drug therapies directed toward achieving pain relief (e.g., anticonvulsants and tricyclic antidepressants) are prescribed empirically and in the absence of population data.[31] The efficacy of these interventions in the treatment of patients with spinal cord injury will remain unreliable, unpredictable, and equivocal until their pharmacokinetic/pharmacodynamic profiles are characterized and used to augment clinical judgment.

We may ask why, if spinal cord injury population-specific pharmacokinetic/pharmacodynamic knowledge is so critical, is the absence of this knowledge not more conspicuous and why are not more clinical manifestations of untoward reactions or side effects documented in patients with spinal cord injury who are being medicated. The answers lie in understanding that such patients *are* experiencing clinically significant untoward reactions and therapeutic misadventures, many of which are often not recognized. It is important to realize that clinical manifestations of side effects and untoward reactions to drugs have been characterized almost exclusively in patients with intact spinal cords. Logically, drug reactions or side effects in patients with spinal cord injury and altered physiology should not be expected to appear as the recognizable, familiar patterns observed in persons with an intact spinal cord (intact neuraxis) and normally functioning autonomic nervous system. In fact, the extensive, mosaic pathophysiology of spinal cord injury (acute or chronic) often precludes the use of pattern recognition or set-piece algorithmic approaches to identifying drug side effects or defining cause-and-effect relationships.

Some comments on the parenteral administration of analgesics to spinal cord–injured patients are of clinical significance: (1) Neither pharmacokinetic nor drug concentration-effect relationships following the intravenous administration of analgesics has been delineated in spinal cord–injured persons and (2) the bioavailability (rate and completeness of absorption) of narcotic analgesics or the newer NSAIDs following subcutaneous or intramuscular administration is, however, more than likely to be impaired. Following spinal cord injury, blood flow through the muscle and overlying tissue of paralyzed limbs is markedly diminished.[32] Hence, it should be anticipated that flow-dependent drug uptake from injected depots will be impaired.[33] For the narcotic analgesics and parenterally administered NSAIDs, titration-to-effect, monitored with occasional serum levels, may be the most effective way to optimize therapy.

Antibiotics

Relatively few classes of antibiotics have been studied in spinal cord–injured persons even though antibiotics are among the most commonly prescribed medications. Spinal cord injury population-specific pharmacokinetic/pharmacodynamic behavior for the aminoglycoside antibiotics (gentamicin and amikacin) has been the most extensively profiled. Sparse, fragmentary data on cefotiam (a cephalosporin antibiotic) and doxycycline are available, but are not sufficient to predict serum levels, to monitor therapy, or to develop optimal dosing strategies. Essentially nothing is known about the penicillins, third-generation cephalosporins, carbapenems, or antibiotic/beta-lactamase inhibitor combinations such as Unisyn and Augmentin in patients with spinal cord injury.

Following intramuscular administration, the bioavailability of gentamicin is impaired in patients with spinal cord injury and is characterized by lower peak serum levels and a slower rate of absorption than that seen following an intramuscular injection into normally innervated muscle (Fig. 25–2). Although intramuscular injection of gentamicin is routinely done below the neurologic level of injury and is justified as a humane, efficacious, cost-effective method of administration, the impairment in bioavailability that has been demonstrated must invariably result

in diminished therapeutic efficacy.[34] This pharmacokinetically defined impediment to effective therapy is not generally recognized, and the intramuscular administration of aminoglycosides continues to provide caregivers with a false sense of efficacy and security. Hence, in patients with spinal cord injury, the intramuscular administration of drugs should be discouraged.

While the pharmacokinetic profile of the aminoglycosides gentamicin and amikacin is altered following a spinal cord injury, the clinical utility of these observations is somewhat less relevant today than when these findings were first reviewed in 1989.[19] Research supports the efficacy of simplified dosing regimens that are less dependent on the complexity, extent, and magnitude of pharmacokinetic changes.[35] Nevertheless, recognition of an increase in volume of distribution and total body clearance of aminoglycosides attributable to spinal cord injury continues to be a prerequisite to individualizing and optimizing therapy.[36, 37]

Interstitial fluid serves as a medium for propagation of infection and is also the primary path by which antibiotics are transported to a site of sepsis. Segal and colleagues[38] measured amikacin concentrations in the interstitial fluid of viable tissue surrounding pressure sores that developed following spinal cord injury. The elimination half-life of amikacin in interstitial fluid (time required for a given amikacin concentration in interstitial fluid to decrease by 50%) was far longer than the serum half-life of amikacin calculated for these patients. This could not have been predicted from conventional pharmacokinetic models which usually do not incorporate antibiotic levels measured directly in infected tissue fluids. In demonstrating the prolonged half-life and persistence of amikacin in tissues (Fig. 25–3), these authors found evidence to support a currently recommended therapeutic rationale for the once-a-day administration of aminoglycoside antibiotics and to explain the clinical observation of residual postantibiotic effect.[39]

Once-daily dosing in both able-bodied and spinal cord–injured persons could supplant the currently accepted approach for administering aminoglycosides and other antibiotics

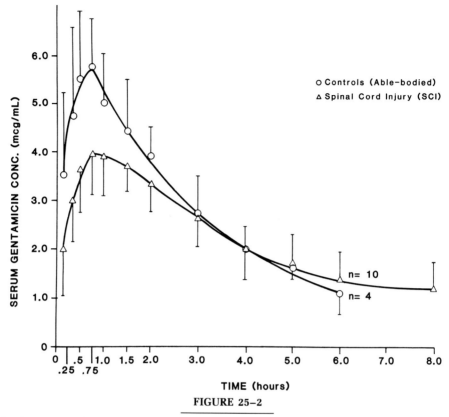

o Controls (Able-bodied)
Δ Spinal Cord Injury (SCI)

n= 10
n= 4

FIGURE 25-2

The time-course of serum gentamicin concentration is compared in all tetraplegic plus paraplegic subjects and in able-bodied control subjects. Serum gentamicin concentrations are significantly lower and are achieved more slowly in subjects with spinal cord injury than in control subjects, which suggests an impairment in the absorption of intramuscularly administered gentamicin. Both time-course profiles are consistent with a first-order elimination process. (From Segal JL, Brunnemann SR, Gray DR, et al: Impaired absorption of intramuscularly administered gentamicin in spinal cord injury. Curr Ther Res 36:961–969, 1986.)

that exhibit minimal serum protein binding.[40] Calculation of the correct initial loading doses, individualization of therapy, and therapeutic monitoring of serum levels in patients with spinal cord injury, however, remain dependent on strategies incorporating population-specific pharmacokinetic parameters.[18, 41, 42]

For the penicillins, cephalosporins, and other antibiotics that are extensively protein bound (greater than 70% to 80%) in serum, development of population pharmacokinetic/pharmacodynamic parameter profiles and models of pharmacokinetic behavior in spinal cord injury, as yet unaccomplished, remain clinically significant prerequisites to rational prescribing. The limited research on cefotiam[43] and doxycycline[44] has not been reproduced and available data are inadequate

to delineate the disposition kinetics of these antibiotics in patients with spinal cord injury. Failed or only marginally successful antibiotic therapy continues to be reflected in unexplained morbidity, mortality, and cost-ineffective treatment strategies.

Anticoagulants

The increased risk of thromboembolic disease in patients with spinal cord injury, particularly during the immediate postinjury period,[45] has resulted in diverse therapeutic strategies.[46] Prophylactic anticoagulant therapy has been recommended empirically even though the use of preventive anticoagulation is controversial and its efficacy has not been unequivocally established.[47] In addition to

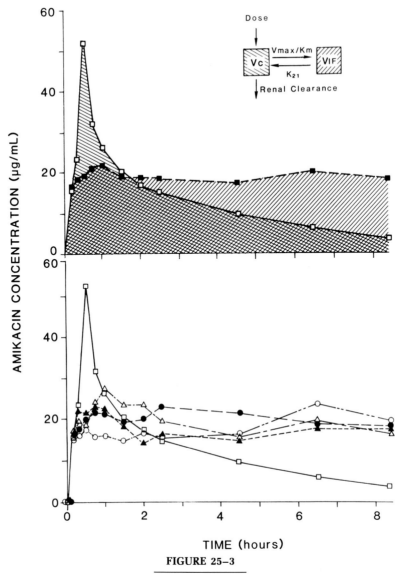

FIGURE 25–3

Amikacin time-concentration data (*top*) for the serum (*open squares*) and interstitial fluid (IF) (*solid squares*) of a representative patient with spinal cord injury. No statistically significant difference exists between amikacin concentrations measured in IF at a pressure sore margin and those in the IF of uninvolved healthy adjacent tissue (*bottom*). *Open triangles* and *solid triangles* indicate amikacin concentrations measured in paired tapes implanted in the pressure sore margin; *open circles* and *solid circles*, measurements of amikacin concentrations in paired tapes in healthy tissue at a distance of not less than 10 cm from the wound margin. V_C = volume of central compartment; V_{IF} = volume of interstitial fluid; Vmax/Km = transfer rate constant, central to interstitial fluid compartment; K_{21} = transfer rate constant, interstitial fluid compartment to central compartment. (From Segal JL, Brunnemann SR, Eltorai IM: Pharmacokinetics of amikacin in serum and in tissue contiguous with pressure sores in humans with spinal cord injury. Antimicrob Agents Chemother 34:1422–1428, 1990; with permission.)

suggestions that the increase in deep vein thrombosis (DVT) is due to immobilization, hematologic and metabolic sequelae of spinal cord injury have been implicated in the pathogenesis of vascular thrombosis and em-bolic phenomena.[48, 49] While the clinical pharmacology of the anticoagulants heparin and warfarin has not been adequately charac-terized in the spinal cord–injured patient, the efficacy of intravenously administered heparin as a treatment for DVT remains unquestioned, regardless of whether the recipient's neuraxis is intact. Overall, these observations suggest that spinal cord injury–altered pharmacokinetic/pharmacodynamic behavior exists and probably contributes to the diminished efficacy of heparin observed after subcutaneous administration.[32]

Green and co-workers[50] and Merli and colleagues[51] discussed the seemingly equivocal therapeutic efficacy of subcutaneously administered heparin in patients with spinal cord injury as a function of the heparin molecule's physical properties or absorption profile from a subcutaneous depot. Merli and colleagues showed the pharmacokinetic behavior of conventional heparin following subcutaneous administration is altered and spinal cord–injured patients absorb less heparin than do neurologically intact patients. Green and co-workers, in comparing low molecular weight heparin to a standard heparin mixture for prevention of DVT, demonstrated enhanced efficacy for the low molecular weight, more readily absorbed heparin and recommended its use in patients with spinal cord injury. These findings are reflective of, and consistent with, well-described changes in postinjury physiology, such as the impaired musculocutaneous blood flow seen in paralyzed limbs.[32] They may disclose a shared mechanism that also contributes to the impairment in bioavailability of the aminoglycoside antibiotics observed following intramuscular administration.[33]

Benefits derived from research into the prevention and treatment of DVT and thromboembolic disease in spinal cord–injured patients clearly demonstrate the utility of applying population-specific pharmacokinetic/pharmacodynamic principles to the development of rational, objective approaches to drug therapy and clinical decision-making. While most authorities acknowledge that all patients with spinal cord injury and motor paralysis should receive thromboprophylaxis, modes of therapy, indications for prophylactic administration of heparin, dosing, and duration of treatment are often based on anecdotal evidence, and drug treatment strategies incorporating population-specific criteria need to be developed to assist in eliminating uncertainty.

Anticonvulsants/Anxiolytics/Sedative-Hypnotics

Data experimentally derived from studies of spinal cord injury describing the population-specific pharmacokinetic/pharmacodynamic behavior of phenytoin (Dilantin), carbamazepine (Tegretol), or other anticonvulsants is inadequate to develop sound therapeutic strategies. For example, Menard and Hahn[52] observed the occurrence of toxic serum phenytoin levels in association with drug- and environment-induced hypothermia in a quadriplegic patient. From this single observation they deduced, probably correctly, that hypothermia appears to affect the metabolism of phenytoin in the presence of spinal cord injury. Implications of this and similar findings scattered throughout the literature pertaining to spinal cord injury, however, remain as yet unintegrated into efforts to develop rational drug-prescribing patterns. Published case studies and clinical experience in patients with spinal cord injury tend to corroborate the efficacy of phenytoin and carbamazepine as anticonvulsants,[53] but treatment strategies that recognize the potential influence of the injury on drug disposition or that incorporate this information into treatment regimens designed to maximize drug efficacy do not exist.

Benzodiazepines are multipurpose drugs commonly prescribed to the spinal cord–injured patient. In addition to their muscle relaxant properties, benzodiazepines exhibit seemingly disparate activities such as seizure suppression, sedation, antiemesis, and lysis of anxiety; members of this class of drugs have a very high abuse potential. Extensive literature exists on the pharmacokinetics and pharmacodynamics of benzodiazepines in neurologically intact populations, but the only population-specific pharmacokinetic data available on this important class of drugs in patients with spinal cord injury have been obtained from a single study of lorazepam (Ativan).[54]

Lorazepam is an intermediate-acting benzodiazepine whose unique metabolic profile in the able-bodied confers on it highly desirable properties and a distinct clinical advantage over many members of its class. The biotransformation of lorazepam is thought to proceed by hepatic conjugation. Presumably, this metabolic pathway makes the metabolism of lorazepam, unlike that of diazepam, independent of hepatic microsomal oxidation and the formation of highly bioactive metabolites characterized by long elimination half-lives. Hence, in the neurologically intact patient, biotransformation of lorazepam should proceed uninfluenced by concurrent administration of drugs that are capable of inhibiting or inducing hepatic oxidation. From a practical standpoint, certain adverse effects, such as excessive sedation and respiratory depression, should be avoidable when lorazepam is administered in conjunction with commonly prescribed medications (e.g., the H_2-antagonist cimetidine) that interfere with hepatic oxidation. It remains to be established, however, whether the adverse reaction and therapeutic profile of lorazepam is unchanged following spinal cord injury. Extrapolating knowledge and clinical experience from studies in neurologically intact populations to patients with spinal cord injury, as is commonly done, cannot be relied on to ensure the safety and therapeutic effectiveness of lorazepam in spinal cord–injured patients because the pharmacokinetic behavior of lorazepam is demonstrably different from that observed in individuals with an intact neuraxis (Table 25–2). Whether these observations hold true for other benzodiazepines, or, for that matter, other psychotropic drugs, also remains to be determined.

In persons with spinal cord injury, the rate of elimination of lorazepam is slowed. If lorazepam disposition kinetics in spinal cord injury are impaired because of altered hepatic metabolism (Fig. 25–4) or because of exaggerated and erratic enterohepatic recirculation,[54, 55] the prescribing of benzodiazepines as anticonvulsants, anxiolytics, or sedative-hypnotics will need to take into account population-specific pharmacokinetic behavior to be safe and optimally effective.

Regulation of Blood Pressure/Dysreflexia

Hemodynamic sequelae of spinal cord trauma reflect the neurologic level and completeness of injury. Acute injuries at or above T6 are often associated with profound hypotension[56] whereas hemodynamic lability is more characteristic of a chronic injury.[57] Cardiovascular consequences of spinal cord injury are attributable to disruption of autonomic nervous system control that invariably accompanies a high-level spinal cord injury. The most dramatic of these sequelae, dysreflexia or autonomic hyperreflexia, often constitutes a medical emergency requiring sophisticated pharmacologic intervention to control sympathetic hyperactivity and paroxysmal hypertension.[58, 59]

Clinical syndromes associated with arterial hypertension in the able-bodied are also seen in the spinal cord–injured, and cardiovascular diseases may have a higher incidence in the population with spinal cord injury than that observed in age-matched neurologically intact humans.[60–62] In either population, disposition kinetics of drugs used to alter arterial blood pressure are of lesser importance than the pharmacodynamics (drug effects) in developing effective treatment strategies. Titration of dose to an acceptable end point (i.e., normalization of blood pressure) before emergence or recognition of adverse effects is the sought-after outcome. This approach to blood pressure control is routinely employed irrespective of whether hypertension or hypotension is the clinical presentation.

In patients with spinal cord injury, antihypertensive drug therapies, most commonly administered for dysreflexia, are most effective when directed toward modifying sympathetic efferent tone. Vasoactive drugs or adrenolytic agents, such as nifedipine or prazosin, are more likely to be effective than centrally acting sympatholytic drugs, such as clonidine.[59, 63]

Orthostatic hypotension frequently complicates the management of spinal cord in-

TABLE 25–2

LORAZEPAM PHARMACOKINETIC PARAMETERS AND SERUM PROTEIN BINDING

SUBJECT	CL (mL/min/m² BSA)	AUC_∞ (ng/mL·hr)	AUC_{10} (ng/mL·hr)	V_{ss} L/kg	$V_{D(area)}$ (L/kg)	$t_{1/2\beta}$ hr	LRZ Protein Binding (% Bound)
A Tetraplegic (95% CI) n = 9	26.49 ± 5.70 (21.84–31.14)	716.50 ± 142.67 (600.18–832.82)	233.99 ± 72.89 (174.57–293.43)	1.58 ± 0.41 (1.27–1.90)	1.64 ± 0.37 (1.36–1.92)	31.06 ± 12.82 (20.01–41.51)	87.36 ± 13.22 (76.59–98.14)
B Paraplegic (95% CI) n = 6	37.07 ± 10.55 (24.94–49.20)	505.27 ± 120.55 (366.69–643.85)	167.57 ± 35.04 (127.29–207.85)	1.64 ± 0.41 (1.21–2.07)	1.63 ± 0.45 (1.16–2.09)	24.75 ± 9.25 (14.12–35.38)	88.64 ± 8.71 (76.54–100.73) n = 5
C Control (95% CI) n = 9	41.98 ± 19.12 (26.39–57.57)	480.31 ± 261.66 (266.98–693.64)	169.00 ± 54.34 (124.70–213.30)	1.38 ± 0.40 (1.08–1.68)	1.50 ± 0.48 (1.13–1.87)	20.19 ± 11.76 (10.60–29.78)	88.24 ± 12.70 (73.64–102.83) n = 6
P Value Cohort	NS .03 A vs. B A vs. C	.01 .02 A vs. B A vs. C	.047 .045 A vs. B A vs. C	NS NS A vs. B A vs. C	NS NS A vs. B A vs. C	NS .07 A vs. B A vs. C	NS NS A vs. B A vs. C

From Segal JL, Brunnemann SR, Eltorai IM, et al: Decreased systemic clearance of lorazepam in humans with spinal cord injury. J Clin Pharmacol 31:651–656, 1991.
CL = total body clearance; BSA = body surface area (m²); AUC = area under the concentration-time curve; AUC_∞ = to infinity; AUC_{10} = to 10 hours; V_{ss} = volume of distribution at steady-state; LRZ = lorazepam; $t_{1/2\beta}$ = beta-phase elimination half-life; 95% CI = 95% confidence interval; control = able-bodied subjects (intact neuraxis); $V_{D(area)}$ = volume of distribution (area).

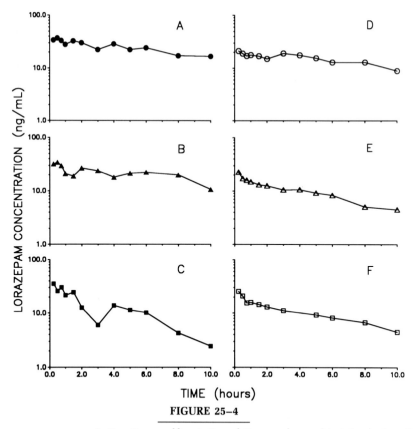

TIME (hours)

FIGURE 25–4

Lorazepam serum concentration-time profiles A, B, and C were observed in tetraplegic patients. The widely fluctuating sinusoidal pattern is characteristic of this population after the intravenous administration of a single 2.0 mg dose of lorazepam and probably reflects impaired and/or exaggerated enterohepatic circulation. D, E, and F are representative profiles of the time-course of intravenous lorazepam in able-bodied (intact CNS) subjects. The mean of the natural log transformed, weighted sum of squared residuals obtained from a linear, least-squares regression fit of individual lorazepam serum concentration vs. time data over the 10-hour interval after administration was significantly larger in the paraplegic and tetraplegic patients than in the able-bodied subjects (mean$_{tetraplegic}$ = 5.553 ± 0.893, P = 0.04; 95% CI for able-bodied subjects, 3.33–5.213). No significant difference was observed, however, between paraplegic and tetraplegic patients. Area under the concentration-time curve (AUC) over the 10-hour interval after lorazepam administration was significantly increased only in patients with tetraplegia. (From Segal JL, Brunnemann SR, Eltorai IM, et al: Decreased systemic clearance of lorazepam in humans with spinal cord injury. J Clin Pharmacol 31:651–656, 1991.)

jury, and the acquired dysautonomia that characterizes spinal cord damage, particularly with high thoracic and cervical injuries, frequently results in precipitous and paradoxical changes in arterial blood pressure. As in the drug treatment of hypertension, treatment of this condition requires titration of medication to achieve some consistent level of arterial blood pressure that maintains an asymptomatic state. Adrenoreceptor agonists, mineralocorticoids, or vasopressors are commonly employed with varying degrees of success, usually in the absence of population-specific pharmacokinetic/pharmacodynamic

guidelines.[64–66] Development of spinal cord injury population-specific pharmacokinetic profiles should promote better understanding of the pathogenesis of the conditions being treated and will be of value in establishing safe and effective drug treatment regimens.

Spasticity

The sustained muscle tone and increased resistance to passive movement that develop after spinal cord injury as a result of upper motor neuron lesions represent only part of the clinical syndrome of spasticity. In addition to hypertonia, weakness or paralysis, loss of dexterity, hyperreflexia, and flexor spasms contribute to postinjury morbidity and are formidable obstacles to rehabilitation. Drug therapy represents only one aspect of the multimodal approach to the treatment of spasticity.[67, 68] Often, treatment is begun with physical therapy. Pharmacologic interventions are usually an adjunct to exercise programs, and baclofen, dantrolene, or diazepam are the drugs most commonly prescribed (see also Chapter 22).

In terms of efficacy and risk-benefit ratio, baclofen (Lioresal), a centrally acting, gamma-aminobutyric acid (GABA)-ergic agent structurally similar to carbamazepine, is arguably the least toxic and most effective medication. While the absolute bioavailability of peroral baclofen in disease processes associated with or causing spasticity is generally thought to be unimpaired, most studies of baclofen pharmacokinetic/pharmacodynamic behavior have been carried out in mixed populations of patients, only some of whom suffered from spinal cord injury. Although knowledge of baclofen pharmacokinetic parameters (e.g., elimination half-life and bioavailability) derived from these studies is relevant and useful, extrapolation of these data and validation of their usefulness or applicability in patients with spinal cord injury has not been accomplished.

Capobianco and colleagues,[69] in a controlled study of simultaneous pharmacokinetic/pharmacodynamic behavior, demonstrated a clinically significant impairment in oral baclofen absorption in patients with chronic spinal cord injury (greater than 1 year's duration). In a study of spinal cord–injured patients receiving baclofen in higher doses, Aisen and others[70] observed prolongation in the time required to attain peak plasma levels and a decrease in the rate of elimination of baclofen from the systemic circulation following oral administration. Although these investigators attributed the delay in attaining steady-state blood levels to impaired renal clearance, it is more likely that nonlinear, dose-dependent baclofen pharmacokinetics or altered metabolism may cause this phenomenon in spinal cord–

injured patients. Data of this type are of particular importance in spinal cord injury and have special utility in the development of population-specific pharmacotherapy.[18] Numerous "trial-and-error" clinical studies carried out in mixed patient cohorts have failed to provide information needed to explain the equivocal outcomes and therapeutic failures often observed when baclofen is administered orally to spinal cord–injured patients.

The pharmacokinetic behavior of any drug, however, is of most concern in the development of safe and effective therapies when drug administration is at a distance from the putative site of drug action. Thus, intrathecal administration of baclofen, which bypasses the blood-brain barrier, minimizes these concerns. This mode of drug delivery avoids systemic influences of spinal injury on drug disposition by placing the drug in direct contact with the damaged spinal cord. For patients who are refractory to or intolerant of oral baclofen, intrathecal administration represents an efficacious alternative to standard drug therapy.[71, 72]

Benzodiazepines, such as diazepam and lorazepam, are centrally acting skeletal muscle relaxants, which are often prescribed alone or in conjunction with other drugs to relieve spasticity.[73] Their primary mode of action is through inhibition of reflex activity in the central nervous system, but direct effects on skeletal muscle contractility also have been postulated. The clinical pharmacokinetic behavior of this class of drug, to the extent that it has been studied in patients with spinal cord injury, is briefly summarized in the previous section of this chapter on anticonvulsants. While benzodiazepines have addictive potential, their adverse reaction profile is relatively benign in comparison to that of dantrolene. Spinal cord injury population-specific pharmacokinetic behavior of diazepam (Valium) has not been characterized, and the disposition kinetics of lorazepam in spinal cord–injured patients[54] are not necessarily representative of, nor can they be uncritically substituted for, those of diazepam in developing dosing regimens. Nevertheless, the exaggerated, enhanced hepatobiliary recirculation and prolonged elimination half-life exhibited by lorazepam in patients with spinal cord injury should alert a prescribing physician to the possibility of enhanced side effects or impaired efficacy in patients receiving benzodiazepines.[54]

Dantrolene (Dantrium) is highly lipid soluble and is sterically similar to hydantoins such as phenytoin (Dilantin). Its direct effect on skeletal muscle is mediated through modulation of calcium efflux from the sacroplasmic reticulum. The adverse reaction profile of dantrolene includes significant hepatotoxicity. As with nearly all drugs prescribed to patients with spinal cord injury, the pharmacokinetics and pharmacodynamics of dantrolene have been studied most thoroughly in able-bodied, neurologically intact recipients.[74] Population-specific disposition parameters estimated from analysis of changes in dantrolene serum concentrations over time can be used to calculate an absolute bioavailability ranging from 50% to 70% of an oral dose in patients with spinal cord injury and 30% to 70% in able-bodied subjects.[74–77] Although this suggests there is little or no impairment in peroral dantrolene bioavailability associated with spinal cord injury, a study of dantrolene bioavailability in otherwise healthy spinal cord–injured patients demonstrated a significant decrease in the rate and completeness of absorption of peroral dantrolene that could be reversed by the intravenous administration of a GI prokinetic drug, metoclopramide (Reglan).[78] Segal and Brunnemann[78] were also able to show that the systemic clearance of dantrolene can become dose-dependent and nonlinear following intravenous metoclopramide administration. Hence, the safety and effectiveness of dantrolene in patients with spinal cord injury may be altered by the co-administration of metoclopramide (Reglan). These findings need to be reproduced and corroborated in larger study populations so that their clinical significance can be better understood.

A new antispasticity drug has become available. Tizanidine, an alpha$_2$-adrenergic agonist with properties similar to those of clonidine, has been compared to tetrazepam, a benzodiazepine, and baclofen in a double-blind study of efficacy. Although subjective improvement was reported by multiple sclerosis patients within each treatment group, statistically significant differences between quantitative outcome variables were not demonstrated.[79] Mathias and co-workers,[80] in a study of tizanidine pharmacokinetic/pharmacodynamic behavior in patients with spinal cord injury, estimated an elimination half-life of 2.7 hours. Plasma levels following oral administration rose rapidly, and peak levels at 1 hour coincided with a significant reduction in spasticity lasting for up to 4 hours. Rapid attainment of peak serum levels following oral administration suggests that population-specific tizanidine bioavailability (absorption) is unimpaired in patients with spinal cord injury. Studies of temporal relationships between emergence of drug effect and associated blood levels[81, 82] provide insights into metabolic pathways and enantioselective drug disposition kinetics.[83] Such information is in short supply in patients with spinal cord injury and is precisely what is needed for incorporation into models of population-specific drug behavior that are needed to develop effective, safe strategies for the therapeutic use of antispasticity drugs.[69, 70, 81]

Bronchodilators

Theophylline is a bronchodilator of proven efficacy that has been shown to enhance the strength and prolong the duration of contraction of muscles of respiration.[84] Therapeutic benefits of this drug are potentially greater in patients with high thoracic and cervical spinal cord injury who are prone to diaphragmatic and intercostal muscle dysfunction.

Segal and colleagues[85, 86] profiled the pharmacokinetics of theophylline in patients with spinal cord injury. "Healthy" paraplegic and tetraplegic patients were compared with an able-bodied control group. These investigators observed an increase in systemic theophylline clearance and a decreased elimination half-life in both patients and neurologically intact control subjects who smoked tobacco. They were unable, however, to demonstrate differences in these parameters between patients who denied smoking (nonsmokers) and their able-bodied counterparts. Among the nonsmoking patients and control subjects, theophylline volume of distribution, half-life of elimination, and rate of clearance did not differ significantly, and these parameters were identical in magnitude to parameters published in the literature as being characteristic in neurologically intact adult recipients of this drug.

Bioavailability, the rate and completeness of absorption of a drug when administered by any non-intravenous pathway, is an important parameter in determining drug safety and effectiveness. The bioavailability of theophylline is impaired following oral administration to patients with spinal cord injury, and this impairment is most consistent with high thoracic and cervical cord injuries (Fig. 25–5).[26, 87] Time required to reach peak serum theophylline concentration was prolonged to 2.2 hours and the peak serum concentration decreased to 7.35 mg/L in comparison with values of 1.5 hours and 10.09 mg/L for these variables in an able-bodied control group. The absolute bioavailability of peroral theophylline (i.e., the ratio of the amount of an oral dose reaching the systemic circulation to the amount administered intravenously)

was less than 0.70 (less than 70% of the oral dose) in most patients with cervical injuries in contrast to an oral bioavailability approximating 100% in able-bodied persons.[26]

As the biotransformation (metabolism) of theophylline is not altered in patients with spinal cord injury, an alternative explanation for the impaired bioavailability was sought. Segal and others[25, 26] demonstrated impairment of gastric emptying in association with the diminished theophylline bioavailability observed in patients with spinal cord injury, and they corroborated previous population-specific findings of impaired bioavailability. A significant correlation between the magnitude of impairment in drug absorption and the neurologic level of injury was shown to exist (Fig. 25–6), and these authors concluded that spinal cord injury population-specific pharmacokinetic profiles can be employed to describe more accurately the extent and neurologic level of an injury. Fealey and others,[27] in a small sample of patients, demonstrated the existence of a delay in gastric emptying in spinal cord–injured patients. These authors did not observe, as did Segal

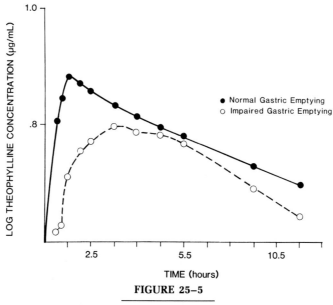

FIGURE 25–5

Representative profiles of the time-course of serum theophylline concentrations following the oral administration of 4.8 mg/kg to a tetraplegic subject with impaired gastric emptying (*open circle*) and an able-bodied control (*solid circle*) are compared. In the tetraplegic subject, maximum serum concentration and area under the curve are decreased while time to maximum serum concentration is prolonged. (From Segal JL, Brunnemann SR, Gordon SK, et al: Decreased theophylline bioavailability and impaired gastric emptying in spinal cord injury. Curr Ther Res 38:831–846, 1985; with permission.)

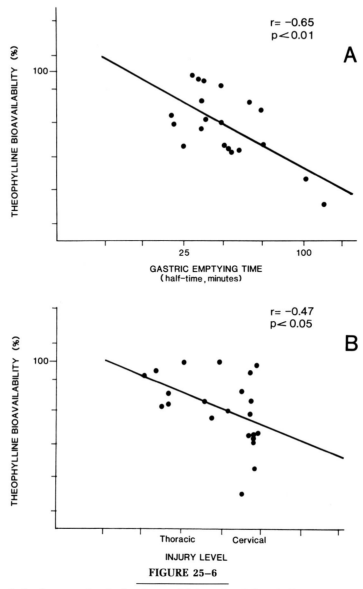

FIGURE 25–6

Linear correlation between the absolute bioavailability of oral theophylline and gastric emptying half-time (A) or level of cord injury (B). (From Segal JL, Brunnemann SR, Gordon SK, et al: Decreased theophylline bioavailability and impaired gastric emptying in spinal cord injury. Curr Ther Res 38:831–846, 1985.)

and colleagues,[26] a subset of patients with cervical cord injury in whom postprandial gastric emptying appears to be accelerated and is associated with a "normal" or increased rate of peroral theophylline absorption.

Approximately 20% of patients with cervical cord injury exhibit "normal" or accelerated absorption of orally administered theophylline.[26] This phenomenon is found in association with rapid gastric emptying simi-

lar to that seen in the classic "dumping syndrome" and is clinically significant. For example, in changing from intravenous to oral theophylline therapy a potentially dangerous situation involving an increased risk of theophylline toxicity exists. In these patients, oral administration of theophylline based on the assumption that delayed gastric emptying characterizes all high-level spinal myelopathy might easily result in toxicity caused by a rapid displacement of the total dose of theophylline into the proximal small intestine as a single bolus. In spinal cord–injured patients with enhanced gastric emptying or "dumping," theophylline absorption can be astonishingly fast, and significantly higher-than-anticipated serum levels, similar to those obtainable with an intravenous infusion, can be readily attained. Had patients been receiving theophylline, albeit with serum levels in the subtherapeutic range, toxic levels could still result. Unfortunately, though no simple method exists for predicting patterns of gastric emptying or anticipating bioavailability in patients with spinal cord injury, reliable restoration to normal of impaired gastric emptying can be achieved in the vast majority of patients with the gastrointestinal prokinetic drug metoclopramide (Reglan).[25] Studies of gastric emptying in tetraplegic and paraplegic patients have demonstrated the efficacy of metoclopramide in correcting postprandial gastric emptying time to normal (Fig. 25–7) and in restoring a normal pattern of gastric emptying to injured patients with impaired postprandrial gastric evacuation. The positive, reproducible response of gastric emptying to metoclopramide suggests that the target organ (stomach) is intact in these patients. It was concluded from these studies that altered gastric motility in spinal cord injury is causally associated with clinically significant changes in the bioavailability of oral theophylline. The application of a multicompartmental, nonlinear model (modified to estimate an early prolonged, adynamic phase of gastric evacuation) to the analysis of gastric emptying data in spinal cord injury was recommended.[25]

Although altered drug disposition does not invariably follow the oral administration of medication to the spinal cord–injured patient,[88] it is probably safest to anticipate that an impairment of gastric emptying exists and that, subsequently, a decrease in oral bioavailability characterizes the vast majority of patients with spinal cord injury, particularly those with high-level thoracic or cervical cord dysfunction. While alternative GI sites of drug absorption (e.g., the colon or rectum) exist, it remains unclear at this time if they offer any advantages or have clinical utility in patients with spinal cord injury.

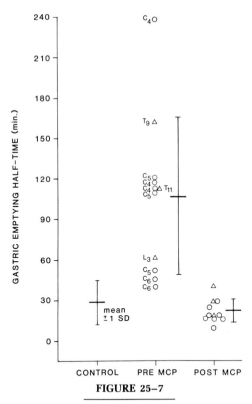

FIGURE 25–7

Pretreatment and posttreatment results compared in eight quadriplegic subjects (*open circles*) and three paraplegic subjects (*open triangles*) who received an intravenous dose of metoclopramide, 10 mg. Gastric emptying half-time ($t_{1/2 \, GE}$) decreased markedly ("normalized") in all treated subjects and was indistinguishable from that observed in the control population (n = 8). Spinal cord injury patients treated with metoclopramide had a pretreatment $t_{1/2GE}$ of more than 30 minutes. Mean posttreatment $t_{1/2GE}$ differs significantly from the pretreatment mean (P < 0.01). In each subject $t_{1/2GE}$ declined by not less than 50%. Spinal injury levels are displayed adjacent to corresponding data points (premedication), and the mean (±SD) for premedication or postmedication data appears to the right of the respective column. (From Segal JL, Milne N, Brunnemann SR, et al: Metoclopramide-induced normalization of impaired gastric emptying in spinal cord injury. Am J Gastroenterol 82:1143–1148, 1987; with permission.)

Modulation of Cytokine Bioactivity

Cytokines are ubiquitous, soluble cell products that act as hormone-like intercellular signals. They function as immunomodulators and influence activities of many tissues. In health, these molecules are essential to maintain physiologic and metabolic equilibrium (i.e., homeostasis).[89] The bioactivity of cytokines is modulated by an intact central nervous system (CNS), and cytokines are humoral components of bi-directional control loops that mediate the maintenance and function of virtually every organ system.[90, 91] As with many naturally occurring bioregulatory mechanisms, the expression of bioactivity may become exaggerated or perverted when homeostasis is challenged by the imposition of trauma or illness. Cytokines have been implicated both as mediators of disease and indicators of pathogenesis in neurologically intact humans.[92] As a corollary, questions have arisen about spinal cord–injured patients that address the role of cytokines in the etiopathogenesis of acute axonal damage and subsequent pathophysiologic sequelae.[21, 93, 94] The therapeutic implications of a role for cytokines in preventing or mediating axonal dysfunction and cell death have yet to be systematically explored.[95] Evidence exists, however, that these bioactive molecules exert a regulatory action on synaptic transmission and may contribute both to axonal regeneration and to pathogenesis of neuronal dysfunction following CNS injury.[96–98]

Regulation of in vivo cytokine activity is partly mediated by endogenously secreted cell products that block or antagonize cytokine receptors.[95] These regulatory processes occur both in the CNS and peripherally. In systemic illness or following CNS injury, disruption of these otherwise homeostatic mechanisms can initiate or sustain pathologic changes in cellular function.[99] To the extent that these changes are deleterious, it is possible, to a limited extent, to beneficially alter the effects of cytokines by manipulating or blocking specific receptors on the membranes of cells targeted by these molecules.[95]

A major impediment to the development of therapeutic strategies incorporating the manipulation of cytokines is our ignorance of their spinal cord injury population-specific pharmacokinetic behavior in blood or CSF. Although limited data exist on the pharmacokinetics of cytokines in neurologically intact study populations,[100] drug disposition differs significantly between humans and animals and among neurologically intact and spinal cord–injured humans. It follows, then, that the uncritical translation of pharmacokinetic data between populations characterized by major differences in physiology or metabolism (e.g., neurologically intact vs. spinal cord–injured humans) is inherently unreliable and likely to be inaccurate. Although methods have been developed for extrapolating data from one physiologically or metabolically different population to another,[101] these techniques have yet to be applied in translating drug disposition parameters estimated in able-bodied persons to those with spinal cord injury. Perhaps these techniques have been overlooked in spinal cord injury research. More likely, however, the need to conceptualize patients with spinal cord injury as a physiologically distinct "population within a population" has engendered a conscious or subconscious resistance to developing the objectivity needed to deal effectively with differences between neurologically intact and spinal cord–injured humans.

In summary, the manipulation or blockade of cytokines presents a novel and potentially productive approach to developing therapeutic interventions in acute spinal cord damage and the pathobiologic sequelae of chronic injury. This will not be readily accomplished until population-specific cytokine pharmacokinetic and pharmacodynamic behavior is characterized in patients with spinal cord injury.

Bioavailability of Micronutrients/Nutrition

Undernutrition is commonly observed in patients with spinal cord injury.[102] A catabolic state characterized by negative nitrogen balance and resistance to enhanced caloric intake persists for many weeks following the acute injury,[103] and a general impairment in nutritional status of unknown etiology is commonly observed during the chronic phase. Body composition is altered and body fat increases both absolutely and as a proportion of total body weight.[12, 13] Anemia and hypoalbuminemia of unknown etiology are endemic,[4, 104, 105] and, although readily attributable to a state of chronic disease, their cause has been addressed neither in terms of spinal cord injury induced changes in caloric requirements nor as a result of injury-associated changes in the absorption and metabolism of calories and micronutrients.

Although spinal cord injury frequently results in disorders of GI motility,[25-27, 55, 106] frank malabsorption has not been observed. And although an association between altered drug efficacy and diminished bioavailability of medication administered orally has been suspected,[26] little consideration has been accorded to assessing the impact of spinal cord injury on the mechanisms of GI uptake or the pharmacokinetics of micronutrients such as vitamins, minerals, and trace elements.

The bioavailability of certain drugs and micronutrients appears to be altered in patients with spinal cord injury.[26, 33, 104, 107, 108] The clinical pharmacologist studies these changes by following the time-course of serum drug or micronutrient concentrations, estimating pharmacokinetic parameters, and modeling concentration-effect relationships. Often, the physiologic mechanisms mediating changes in drug/nutrient disposition kinetics can be identified or inferred from pharmacokinetic/pharmacodynamic studies. Information of this type is, however, usually acquired from studies of physiology or metabolism that are not necessarily carried out in concert with studies of clinical pharmacology. The intestinal transport of drugs or micronutrients has traditionally been of intense interest to researchers studying neurologically intact populations; only limited effort has been directed toward documenting clinically significant changes in the intestinal transport or GI absorption of vitamins as sequelae of spinal cord injury.[104, 108]

Halstead and co-workers[23] and McDeavitt and others,[107] in what are probably the first studies of their kind in spinal cord injury, sought to assess the adequacy of intestinal absorption of the vital micronutrients riboflavin (vitamin B$_2$) and folic acid. These investigators did not observe significant impairment in GI uptake of either vitamin and concluded that the active transport-dependent uptake of riboflavin and folic acid in the small intestine is not significantly altered in persons with spinal cord injury. In contrast, the peroral bioavailability of the NSAID acetaminophen, which is dependent on both gastric emptying and passive diffusion in able-bodied subjects, was significantly impaired.[23] It is therefore possible to infer for micronutrients whose intestinal uptake depends on passive diffusion and/or the efficiency of gastric emptying that clinically significant deficiencies of these factors might occur.

Data gathered in a study of vitamin D levels in spinal cord–injured patients suffering from pressure sores showed significant reductions in serum 25(OH)-vitamin D. Nutritional deficiencies associated with altered intestinal transport of micronutrients were among the etiologies considered.[104] Brunnemann and others,[108] seeking hypovitaminosis or avitaminosis C (ascorbic acid) as a contributing factor to delayed wound healing, documented a statistically significant deficiency state in patients with spinal cord injury who were fed a standard hospital diet. Furthermore, spinal cord–injured patients receiving supplemental vitamin C were unable to attain serum levels significantly higher than levels observed in neurologically intact controls fed an unenhanced standard diet. These authors concluded that factors other than mere dietary inadequacy (e.g., altered bioavailability of ascorbic acid) contribute to the lowering of serum ascorbate levels following spinal cord injury.

Population pharmacokinetic studies of metabolism, turnover, or bioavailability of nutrients, minerals, and trace elements in patients with spinal cord injury are rare. Nutrient/caloric requirements and physiologic or metabolic factors that may confound the restoration and maintenance of nutritional equilibrium are clearly less well understood in spinal cord–injured persons than in neurologically intact persons. Studies of pharmacokinetics and pharmacodynamics in the former population, however, have a high likelihood of providing the information needed to identify population-specific impediments to nutritional homeostasis and of contributing to the development of effective therapeutic strategies.

Drug Therapy of Acute and Chronic Injury

The numerous, diverse pharmacologic interventions under investigation and the extensive array of putative mechanisms implicated in the etiopathogenesis of acute spinal cord damage or its pathobiologic effects suggest that neither a single drug therapy nor a unique mechanism of pathogenesis will be found that is both necessary and sufficient to effect cure or explain the sequelae of spinal cord injury. Certainly, pessimism is inappropriate; yet optimism expressed in the literature[109, 110] is not supported when a critical analysis of the data and clinical significance of outcomes (i.e., restoration of useful motor and sensory function as opposed to theoretically significant improvements in voluntary motor activity or electrophysiological correlates) is made. Bracken[111] nicely summarizes the status of pharmacologic treatments of acute spinal cord injury, but he and other researchers do not adequately address the paucity of, or the need to delineate and apply, population-specific pharmacokinetic/pharmacodynamic profiles for development of effective pharmacotherapy.[109–115] In fact, this information is unavailable, and the influence of pathophysiologic sequelae of spinal cord injury on population-specific pharmacokinetic/pharmacodynamic behavior remains virtually unknown. It is thus reasonable to speculate that equivocal clinical outcomes and often contradictory conclusions found in the current literature will probably continue as long as population-specific alterations in pharmacokinetic/pharmacodynamic behavior are not sought as probable contributing factors.

Drug therapies under investigation can be classified in terms of either (1) their putative efficacy in reversing or limiting anatomic, cellular, and functional defects associated with the acute injury, or (2) their efficacy in enhancing or restoring functional integrity to the spinal cord during the chronic phase of injury.

Methylprednisolone and the 21-aminosteroids (Tirilazad), naloxone, N-methyl-D-aspartate receptor antagonists, thyrotropin-releasing hormone and its analogs, GM$_1$ ganglioside, and 4-aminopyridine (an axonal voltage-sensitive potassium channel blocker) are among the many pharmacologic interventions reported to be beneficial in reducing tissue damage and enhancing recovery following spinal cord injury.[110, 112–118] And although it is beyond the scope of this chapter

to review the clinical pharmacology of all these drugs, two interventions are particularly noteworthy in terms of their efficacy and as representatives of specific categories of drug therapy.

In humans, recovery of neurologic function following acute spinal cord injury has been observed after the administration of high-dosage methylprednisolone. Significance of the magnitude and duration of return of motor function was inferred using rigorous statistical analyses. Actual clinical improvement was insubstantial, and recovery of useful motor function was not demonstrated.[109, 110, 117] On the basis of similar analyses, the comparative efficacy of naloxone was deemed insignificant. In fact, conclusions of the principal investigators of the Second National Acute Spinal Cord Injury Study[109] and a 1-year follow-up study concerning the efficacy of methylprednisolone or the lack of efficacy associated with the use of naloxone[119] are equally tenuous. While the use of methylprednisolone appears still to hold promise, the reason for methylprednisolone's efficacy or, for that matter, the reason for naloxone's apparent failure in patients with spinal cord injury has not been adequately analyzed in terms of population-specific pharmacokinetic behavior in humans.[120, 121] Nockels and Young[118] acknowledge this impediment to developing effective pharmacotherapy and conclude that "pharmacokinetics of the drug must be known so that the experimenter can be reasonably assured that the drug reaches the target in sufficient concentration."[118]

Pharmacokinetics of 4-aminopyridine have been investigated in neurologically intact subjects and patients with spinal cord injury; the kinetics vary with the mode of administration.[122, 123] 4-Aminopyridine is considered a nonregenerative therapy that enhances axonal conduction and functional recovery in animal models of spinal cord injury by inhibiting potassium ion flux across demyelinated axons.[124, 125] Hansebout and co-workers[126] and Hayes and colleagues[127, 128] demonstrated significant electrophysiologic changes in association with restoration of useful motor and sensory function in spinal cord–injured patients receiving a single intravenous dose of 4-aminopyridine. Human studies of 4-aminopyridine serum concentration-response relationships and pharmacokinetics following administration in capsule form are currently under way. These studies anticipate the existence of spinal cord injury population-specific drug behavior and will provide the population models, the pharmacokinetic/pharmacodynamic profiles, and the criteria needed to develop an oral sustained-release formulation.

Results of experimental trials with Tirilazad, GM_1 ganglioside, thyrotropin releasing hormone, N-methyl-D-aspartate receptor antagonists, and flunarizine, although interesting, are inconclusive and will probably remain debatable until well-designed pharmacokinetic/pharmacodynamic studies in humans with spinal cord injury are implemented.[110, 112, 116, 129, 130]

CLINICAL IMPLICATIONS: THE RELEVANCE OF POPULATION-SPECIFIC PHARMACOKINETIC/ PHARMACODYNAMIC MODELING

Characterizing the typical pharmacokinetic behavior and effects (pharmacodynamics) of a drug in a population of patients has the greatest potential for improving individual patient care.[3, 42, 131] It provides the best opportunity for studying physiologic and metabolic characteristics of the population that influence drug disposition. Methods are available simultaneously to model drug disposition and effects in patients with spinal cord injury and to estimate the population pharmacokinetic profiles needed to predict the parameters that govern pharmacokinetic decision-making in an individual patient. These methods have significant limitations but are clearly superior to previous approaches that ignore interindividual kinetic differences and that have been shown to be inaccurate and imprecise.[42, 132]

The adaptation of Bayes' theorem and the application of bayesian analysis to pharmacokinetic decision-making is a significant advance in clinical therapeutics and has allowed quantification of the decision-making process. Assigning levels of probability to the likelihood of accuracy of each of several decision-making factors enables us to arrive at an aggregate estimate of decision quality.[132] Mean population pharmacokinetic parameters generated by research into the clinical pharmacology of spinal cord injury,[19, 54, 69, 80, 88] serum drug concentrations measured in individual patients, and descriptive/demographic data can be used in a bayesian analysis. A priori information derived from the spinal cord injury population can be incorporated into the bayesian algorithm along with individual serum levels to improve the accuracy of predicting serum concentrations and of estimating individual pharmacokinetic parameters. By iteratively minimizing a bayesian least-squares fitting function, a feedback loop can be created for control of serum drug concentrations and estimation of pharmacokinetic parameters.[133]

Alternative approaches to determining population-specific drug disposition have been assigned the acronyms NONMEM (nonlinear mixed effects model) and NPEM (nonparametric expectation maximization). Both NONMEM and NPEM are sophisticated computational software programs for carrying out statistical analyses and calculations required to study, predict, and quantitatively characterize population-specific pharmacokinetics.[134, 135] Population statistics that are independent of subject-specific kinetic parameter estimates can be generated from sparse, fragmentary data. NPEM, however, employs nonparametric (relatively assumption-free) approaches to statistical analysis.[18, 135] NPEM, NONMEM, and the bayesian method are able to analyze data (drug levels, renal function, weight changes) obtained during routine clinical patient care. Use of data generated during routine patient care allows extraordinary flexibility and cost-effectiveness to be achieved by all three methods.

A population model for the aminoglycoside antibiotic gentamicin that incorporates population-specific pharmacokinetic parameters and individual patient characteristics has been developed for patients with spinal cord injury (Fig. 25–8).[18] Comprehensive, sophisticated software that uses these data in developing rational approaches to the administration and monitoring of aminoglycoside

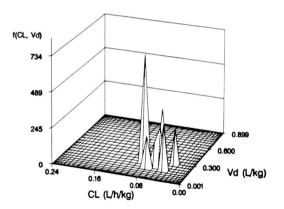

Gentamicin Joint Density: Surface Plot
Able – Bodied Subjects (11)

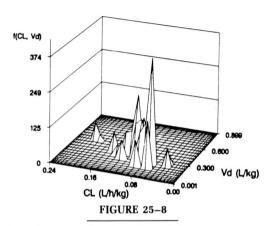

Spinal Cord Injured Patients (29)

FIGURE 25–8

Three-dimensional surface plots of the nonparametric expectation maximization (NPEM) joint density functions over the clearance (CL) vs. volume of distribution (Vd) grid. It is clear that the joint density for CL and Vd is considerably more dispersed in the spinal cord–injured population (bottom) than it is in the able-bodied population (top). NPEM analyses support serendipity and the NPEM algorithm can be used as a hypothesis-generating engine. f(CL, Vd) = joint density function. (From Gilman TM, Brunnemann SR, Segal JL: Comparison of population pharmacokinetic models for gentamicin in spinal cord-injured and able-bodied patients. Antimicrob Agents Chemother 37:93–99, 1993; with permission.)

therapy is available (e.g., CAPCIL and SIMKIN).[136–138]

Recognition of the need for more critical approaches to prescribing practices in spinal cord–injured patients is evidenced by the quantity and quality of recent pharmacokinetic/pharmacodynamic studies.[38, 47, 50, 54, 70, 80, 127] For the time being, however, lack of population-specific dosing guidelines dictates that we continue to implement phar-

macologic interventions developed and standardized in able-bodied patients.[2] More sophisticated studies of serum drug concentration-effect/response relationships (simultaneous pharmacokinetic/pharmacodynamic modeling) are the logical next step in delineating the clinical pharmacology of spinal cord injury.[81] Relatively simple mathematical expressions that simultaneously relate changes in the concentration of drugs in biologic fluids and tissues to drug effects are accessible as tools to optimize clinical therapeutics in patients with spinal cord injury.[139] When fully characterized and tested for predictive performance, descriptor/demographically sensitive approaches to population modeling that incorporate experimentally derived population-specific pharmacokinetic/pharmacodynamic data can be used to define more completely the pathophysiology of spinal cord injury and to develop optimal strategies for determining dosing regimens of clinically important, commonly prescribed medications.[136]

Systematic study of the clinical pharmacology of spinal cord injury has revealed characteristic patterns of drug metabolism and disposition. These metabolic, pharmacodynamic, and pharmacokinetic profiles reflect the changed physiology that accompanies spinal cord injury; they correlate well with the neurologic level, magnitude, or completeness of the injury. Their greatest value is realized when they are used to develop criteria and strategies for optimal prescribing of drugs and therapeutic drug monitoring. Rational, efficacious, and cost-effective approaches to pharmacotherapy in spinal cord–injured patients can only come about when population-specific pharmacokinetic/pharmacodynamic behavior is used to develop therapeutic guidelines.

REFERENCES

1. Stover SL, Fine PR, Go BK, et al (eds): Spinal Cord Injury: The Facts and Figures. ed 1. Birmingham, The University of Alabama at Birmingham, 1986.
2. Halstead LS, Claus-Walker J: Neuroactive Drugs of Choice in Spinal Cord Injury: A Guide for Using Neurologically Active Medications in Spinal Injured Patients, ed 1. New York, Raven Press, 1980.
3. Scharf S, Christophidis N: Relevance of pharmacokinetics and pharmacodynamics. Med J Aust 158:395–402, 1993.

4. Vaziri ND, Eltorai IM, Segal J, et al: Erythropoietin profile in spinal cord injured patients. Arch Phys Med Rehabil 74:65–67, 1993.

5. Mathias CJ, Frankel HL: Clinical manifestations of malfunctioning sympathetic mechanisms in tetraplegia. J Autonom Nerv Sys 7:303–312, 1983.

6. Bannister R. Autonomic Failure: A Textbook of Clinical Disorders of the Autonomic Nervous System, ed 2. New York, Oxford University Press, 1988.

7. Greenhoot JH, Mauck HP: The effect of cervical cord injury on cardiac rhythm and conduction. Am Heart J 83:659–662, 1972.

8. Mathias CJ, Christensen NJ, Frankel HL, et al: Cardiovascular control in recently injured tetraplegics in spinal shock. Quart J Med 48:273–287, 1979.

9. Welply NC, Mathias CJ, Frankel HL: Circulatory reflexes in tetraplegics during artificial ventilation and general anaesthesia. Paraplegia 13:172–182, 1975.

10. Lehmann KG, Lane JG, Piepmeier JM, et al: Cardiovascular abnormalities accompanying acute spinal cord injury in humans: Incidence, time course, and severity. J Am Coll Cardiol 10:46–52, 1987.

11. Segal JL, Brunnemann SR, Gray DR: Gentamicin bioavailability and single-dose pharmacokinetics in patients with spinal cord injury. Drug Intell Clin Pharm 22:461–465, 1988.

12. Shizgal HM, Roza A, Ludec B, et al: Body composition in quadriplegic patients. J Parenteral Enteral Nutr 10(4):364–368, 1986.

13. Nuhlicek DN, Spurr GB, Barboriak JJ, et al: Body composition of patients with spinal cord injury. Eur J Clin Nutr 42:765–773, 1988.

14. Greenway RM, Houser HB, Lindan O, et al: Long-term changes in gross body composition of paraplegic and quadriplegic patients. Paraplegia 7:302–308, 1970.

15. Sassoon CSH, Laurente-Tjoa F, Rheeman C, et al: Neuromuscular compensation with changes in posture during hypercapnic ventilatory and occlusion pressure responses in quadriplegia. Chest 103:165S, 1993.

16. Saltzstein R, Melvin J: Ventilatory compromise in spinal cord injury—A review. J Am Paraplegia Soc 9(1–2):6–9, 1986.

17. Spungen AM, Dicpinigaitis PV, Almenoff PL, et al: Pulmonary obstruction in individuals with cervical spinal cord lesions unmasked by bronchodilator administration. Paraplegia 31(6):404–407, 1993.

18. Gilman TM, Brunnemann SR, Segal JL: Comparison of population pharmacokinetic models for gentamicin in spinal cord-injured and able-bodied patients. Antimicrob Agents Chemother 37(1):93–99, 1993.

19. Segal JL, Brunnemann SR: Clinical pharmacokinetics in patients with spinal cord injuries. Clin Pharmacokinet 17(2):109–129, 1989.

20. Desmond J: Paraplegia: Problems confronting the anaesthesiologist. Can Anaesth Soc J 17:435–451, 1970.

21. Segal JL: Spinal cord injury: Are interleukins a molecular link between neuronal damage and ensuing pathobiology? Perspect Biol Med 36(2):222–240, 1993.

22. Lake KD, Nolen JG, Slaker RA, et al: Over-the-counter medications in cardiac transplant recipients: Guidelines for use. Ann Pharmacother 26:1566–1577, 1992.

23. Halstead LS, Feldman S, Claus-Walker J, et al: Drug absorption in spinal cord injury. Arch Phys Med Rehabil 66:298–301, 1985.

24. Nimmo J, Heading RC, Tothill P, et al: Pharmacological modification of gastric emptying: Effects of propantheline and metoclopramide on paracetamol absorption. Br Med J 1(853):587–589, 1973.

25. Segal JL, Milne N, Brunnemann SR, et al: Metoclopramide-induced normalization of impaired gastric emptying in spinal cord injury. Am J Gastroenterol 82(11):1143–1148, 1987.

26. Segal JL, Brunnemann SR, Gordon SK, et al: Decreased theophylline bioavailability and impaired gastric emptying in spinal cord injury. Curr Ther Res 38(6):831–846, 1985.

27. Fealey RD, Szurszewski JH, Merritt JL, et al: Effect of traumatic spinal cord transection on human upper gastrointestinal motility and gastric emptying. Gastroenterology 87:69–75, 1984.

28. Ibarra A, Kretschmer R, Guizar-Sahagun G, et al: Acute spinal cord injury alters the bioavailability of oral and intraperitoneal cyclosporine-A in contused rats. J Neural Transplant Plast 3(4):317–318, 1992.

29. Rajendran SK, Reiser JR, Bauman W, et al: Gastrointestinal transit after spinal cord injury: Effect of cisapride. Am J Gastroenterol 87(11):1614–1617, 1992.

30. Segal JL, Brunnemann SR: Altered catecholamine levels are associated with changes in hepatic oxidative metabolism in humans with spinal cord injury (abstract). J Clin Pharmacol 31(9):844, 1991.

31. Sanford PR, Lindblom LB, Haddox JD: Amitriptyline and carbamazepine in the treatment of dysesthetic pain in spinal cord injury. Arch Phys Med Rehabil 73(3):300–301, 1992.

32. Seifert J, Lob G, Stoephasius E, et al: Blood flow in muscles of paraplegic patients under various conditions measured by a double isotope technique. Paraplegia 10:185–191, 1972.

33. Segal JL, Brunnemann SR, Gray DR, et al: Impaired absorption of intramuscularly administered gentamicin in spinal cord injury. Curr Ther Res 39(6):961–969, 1986.

34. Segal JL, Brunnemann SR, Gray DR: Gentamicin bioavailability and single-dose pharmacokinetics in spinal cord injury. Drug Intell Clin Pharm 22:461–465, 1988.

35. International Antimicrobial Therapy Cooperative Group of the European Organization for Research and Treatment of Cancer: Efficacy and toxicity of single daily doses of amikacin and ceftriaxone versus multiple daily doses of amikacin and ceftazidine for infection in patients with cancer granulocytopenia. Ann Intern Med 119:584–593, 1993.

36. Segal JL, Gray DR, Gordon SK, et al: Gentamicin disposition kinetics in humans with spinal cord injury. Paraplegia 23:47–55, 1985.

37. Segal JL, Brunnemann SR, Gordon SK, et al: Amikacin pharmacokinetics in patients with spinal cord injury. Pharmacotherapy 8(2):79–81, 1988.

38. Segal JL, Brunnemann SR, Eltorai IM: Pharmacokinetics of amikacin in serum and in tissue contiguous with pressure sores in humans with spinal cord injury. Antimicrob Agents Chemother 34(7):1422–1428, 1990.

39. Zhanel GG, Hoban DJ, Harding GKM: The postantibiotic effect: A review of in vitro and in vivo data. Ann Pharmacother 25:153–163, 1991.

40. Brunnemann SR, Segal JL: Amikacin serum pro-

tein binding in spinal cord injury. Life Sci 49(2):PL1–PL5, 1991.

41. Evans WE, Schentag JJ, Jusko WJ (eds.): Applied Pharmacokinetics: Principles of Therapeutic Drug Monitoring, ed 2. Spokane, Wash., Applied Therapeutics, 1986, pp 465.

42. Grasela TH: Population pharmacokinetics: Application to clinical trials. In Smith RB (ed): Pharmacokinetics and Pharmacodynamics: Research Design and Analysis. Cincinnati, Harvey Whitney Books, 1986.

43. Ishikawa M, Watanabe M, Mashimo K: An evaluation of antibiotic dosage regimen for urinary tract infection in spinal cord injury patients. Chemotherapy 31(6):628–633, 1983.

44. Livshits AV, Yakovlev VP: Dynamics of doxycycline levels in cases with trauma of the spinal marrow. Antibiotkhimioter 17(9):844–847, 1972.

45. Myllynen P, Kammonen M, Rokkanen P, et al: Deep venous thrombosis and pulmonary embolism in patients with acute spinal cord injury: A comparison with non-paralyzed patients immobilized due to spinal fractures. J Trauma 25:541–543, 1985.

46. Hull RD: Venous thromboembolism in spinal cord injury. Chest 102(6):568S–663S, 1992.

47. Merli GJ, Herbison GJ, Ditunno JF, et al: Deep vein thrombosis: Prophylaxis in acute spinal cord injured patients. Arch Phys Med Rehabil 69:661–664, 1988.

48. Vaziri ND, Patel B, Alikhami A, et al: Protein C abnormalities in spinal cord injured patients with end-stage renal disease. Arch Phys Med Rehabil 68(11):791–793, 1987.

49. Hachen HJ, Rossier AB, Bouvier CA, et al: Deficiency within intrinsic prothrombin activator system in patients with acute spinal cord injury. Paraplegia 12:132–138, 1974.

50. Green D, Lee MY, Lim AC, et al: Prevention of thromboembolism after spinal cord injury using low-molecular-weight heparin. Ann Intern Med 113:571–574, 1990.

51. Merli GJ, Crabbe SJ, Doyle L, et al: An evaluation of the effect of subcutaneous low dose heparin in patients with and without spinal cord injury (abstract). Paraplegia 14(2):70, 1991.

52. Menard MR, Hahn G: Acute and chronic hypothermia in a man with spinal cord injury: Environmental and pharmacologic causes. Arch Phys Med Rehabil 72(6):421–424, 1991.

53. Meythaler JM, Tuel SM, Cross LL: Spinal cord seizures: A possible cause of isolated myoclonic activity in traumatic spinal cord injury: Case report. Paraplegia 29(8):557–560, 1991.

54. Segal JL, Brunnemann SR, Eltorai IM, et al: Decreased systemic clearance of lorazepam in humans with spinal cord injury. J Clin Pharmacol 31:651–656, 1991.

55. Milne N, Segal JL, Rypins EB, et al: Biliary kinetics in spinal cord injury (abstract). J Nucl Med 28:688, 1987.

56. Meyer GA, Berman IR, Doty DB, et al: Hemodynamic responses to acute quadriplegia with or without chest trauma. J Neurosurg 34:168–177, 1971.

57. Krum H, Howes LG, Brown DJ, et al: Blood pressure variability in tetraplegia patients with autonomic hyperreflexia. Paraplegia 27:284–285, 1989.

58. Amzallag M: Autonomic hyperreflexia. Int Anesthesiol Clin 31(1):87–102, 1993.

59. Mathias CJ: Role of sympathetic efferent nerves in blood pressure regulation and in hypertension. Hypertension 18(5 suppl III):22–30, 1991.

60. Krum H, Howes LG, Brown DJ, et al: Risk factors for cardiovascular disease in chronic spinal cord injury patients. Paraplegia 30:381–388, 1992.

61. Bauman WA, Spungen AM, Raza M, et al: Coronary artery disease: Metabolic risk factors and latent disease in individuals with paraplegia. Mt Sinai J Med 59(2):163–168, 1992.

62. Yekutiel M, Brooks ME, Ohry A, et al: The prevalence of hypertension, ischaemic heart disease and diabetes in traumatic spinal cord injured patients and amputees. Paraplegia 27:58–62, 1989.

63. Kooner JS, Edge W, Frankel HL, et al: Haemodynamic actions of clonidine in tetraplegia—Effects at rest and during urinary bladder stimulation. Paraplegia 26:200–203, 1988.

64. Hollister AS: Orthostatic hypotension: Causes, evaluation, and management. West J Med 157(6):652–657, 1992.

65. Hoeldtke RD, Streeten DH: Treatment of orthostatic hypotension with erythropoietin. N Engl J Med 329(9):611–615, 1993.

66. Robertson RM, Biaggioni I, Mosqueda-Garcia R, et al: Autonomic dysfunction: Diagnosis guided by therapy. Transact Am Clin Climatol Assoc 103:228–237, 1992.

67. Katz RT: Management of spasticity. Am J Phys Med Rehabil 67(3):108–116, 1988.

68. Young RR: Physiologic and pharmacologic approaches to spasticity. Neurology Clin 5(4):529–539, 1987.

69. Capobianco M, Brunnemann SR, Segal JL: Baclofen pharmacokinetics (PK) and pharmacodynamics (PD) in spinal cord injury (abstract). Clin Autonom Res 3:212, 1993.

70. Aisen ML, Dietz MA, Rossi P, et al: Clinical and pharmacokinetic aspects of high dose oral baclofen therapy. J Am Paraplegia Soc 15(4):211–216, 1992.

71. Penn RD: Intrathecal baclofen for spasticity of spinal origin: Seven years of experience. J Neurosurg 77:236–240, 1992.

72. Lewis KS, Mueller WM: Intrathecal baclofen for severe spasticity secondary to spinal cord injury. Ann Pharmacother 27:767–774, 1993.

73. Madorsky JG: The role of benzodiazepines in the management of neurological and muscular disorders. J Psychoact Drugs 15(1–2):45–48, 1983.

74. Ward A, Chaffman MO, Sorkin EM: Dantrolene: A review of its pharmacodynamic and pharmacokinetic properties and therapeutic use in malignant hyperthermia, the neuroleptic malignant syndrome, and an update on its use in muscle spasticity. Drugs 32:130–168, 1986.

75. Katogi Y, Tamaki N, Adachi M, et al: Simultaneous determination of dantrolene and its metabolite, 5-hydroxydantrolene, in human plasma by high-performance liquid chromatography. J Chromatogr 228:404–408, 1982.

76. Flewellen EH, Nelson TE, Jones WP, et al: Dantrolene dose response in awake man: Implications for management of malignant hyperthermia. Anesthesiology 59(4):275–280, 1983.

77. Pinder RM, Brogden RN, Speight TM, et al: Dantrolene sodium: A review of its pharmacological properties and therapeutic efficacy. Drugs 13(1):22–23, 1977.

78. Segal JL, Brunnemann SR: Pharmacological modi-

fication of dantrolene bioavailability in humans with spinal cord injury (abstract). J Clin Pharmacol 29:835, 1989.

79. Pellkofer M, Paulig M: Comparative double-blind study of the effectiveness and tolerance of baclofen, tetrazepam and tizanidine in spastic movement disorders of the lower extremities. Med Klin 84(1):5–8, 1989.

80. Mathias CJ, Luckitt J, Desai P, et al: Pharmacodynamics and pharmacokinetics of the oral antispastic agent tizanidine in patients with spinal cord injury. J Rehabil Res Dev 26(4):9–16, 1989.

81. Holford NHB, Sheiner LB: Understanding the dose-effect relationship: Clinical application of pharmacokinetic-pharmacodynamic models. Clin Pharmacokinet 6:429–453, 1981.

82. Girard P, Boissel J: Clockwise hysteresis or proteresis (letter to the editor). J Pharmacokinet Biopharm 17(3):401–402, 1989.

83. Mehvar R: Pitfalls in pharmacodynamic modeling of racemic drugs. In From Controversy to Resolution: Bioequivalence of Racemic Drugs. A Symposium on Dynamics, Kinetics, Bioequivalence and Analytical Aspects of Stereochemistry. Atlanta, American College of Clinical Pharmacology 20th Annual Meeting, 1991, pp 9–10.

84. Aubier B, De Troyer A, Sampson M, et al: Aminophylline improves diaphragmatic contractility. N Engl J Med 305(5):249–252, 1981.

85. Segal JL, Smith CM, Gordon SK, et al: Theophylline pharmacokinetics in paraplegic subjects. Clin Pharm 4:448–451, 1985.

86. Segal JL, Gordon SK, Eltorai IM: Theophylline disposition in tetraplegic man. South Med J 80(6):720–724, 1987.

87. Segal JL, Brunnemann SR, Gordon SK, et al: The absolute bioavailability of oral theophylline in patients with spinal cord injury. Pharmacother 6(1):26–29, 1986.

88. More DG, Watson CJ, Boutagy JS, et al: Pharmacokinetics of ranitidine in quadriplegics. Br J Clin Pharmacol 20:166–169, 1985.

89. Dinarello CA: Interleukin-1 and its biologically related cytokines. Adv Immunol 44:153–205, 1989.

90. Banks WA, Kastin AJ: Blood to brain transport of interleukin links the immune and central nervous systems. Life Sci 48(25):PL117–PL121, 1991.

91. Berkenbosch F, De Goeij DE, Rey AD, et al: Neuroendocrine, sympathetic and metabolic responses induced by interleukin-1. Neuroendocrinol 50(5):570–576, 1989.

92. Fridman WH, Michon J: Pathophysiology of cytokines. Leukemia Res 14(8):675–677, 1990.

93. Segal JL, Brunnemann SR: Circulating levels of soluble interleukin-2 receptors are elevated in the sera of humans with spinal cord injury. J Am Paraplegia Soc 16(1):30–33, 1993.

94. Giulian D, Robertson C: Inhibition of mononuclear phagocytes reduces ischemic injury in the spinal cord. Ann Neurol 27:33–42, 1990.

95. Dinarello CA, Thompson RC: Blocking IL-1: Interleukin-1 receptor antagonist in vivo and in vitro. Immunol Today 12(1):404–410, 1991.

96. Sawada M, Hara N, Maeno T: Reduction of the acetylcholine-induced K^+ current in identified Aplysia neurons by human interleukin-1 and interleukin-2. Cell Molec Neurobiol 12:439–445, 1992.

97. Giulian D, Chen J, Ingeman JE, et al: The role of mononuclear phagocytes in wound healing after traumatic injury to adult mammalian brain. J Neurosci 9(12):4416–4429, 1989.

98. Carman-Krzan M, Vige X, Wise BC: Regulation by interleukin-1 of nerve growth factor secretion and nerve growth factor mRNA expression in rat primary astroglial cultures. J Neurochem 56:636–643, 1991.

99. Guénard V, Dinarello CA, Weston PJ, et al: Peripheral nerve regeneration is impeded by interleukin-1 receptor antagonist released from a polymeric guidance channel. J Neurosci Res 29:396–400, 1991.

100. Bocci V: Interleukins: Clinical pharmacokinetics and practical implications. Clin Pharmacokinet 21(4):274–284, 1991.

101. Ritschel WA, Vachharajani NN, Johnson RD, et al: The allometric approach for interspecies scaling of pharmacokinetic parameters. Comp Biochem Physiol 103C(2):249–253, 1992.

102. Lee BY, Agarwal N, Corcoran L: Assessment of nutritional and metabolic status of paraplegics. J Rehabil Res Dev 22:11–15, 1985.

103. Rodriguez DJ, Clevenger FW, Osler TM, et al: Obligatory negative nitrogen balance following spinal cord injury. J Parenteral Enteral Nutr 15(3):319–322, 1991.

104. Zhou XJ, Vaziri ND, Segal JL, et al: Effects of chronic spinal cord injury and pressure ulcer on 25(OH)-vitamin D levels. J Am Paraplegia Soc 16:9–13, 1992.

105. Hirsch GH, Menard MR, Anton HA: Anemia after traumatic spinal cord injury. Arch Phys Med Rehabil 72(3):195–201, 1991.

106. Glick ME, Meshkinpour H, Haldeman S, et al: Colonic dysfunction in patients with thoracic spinal cord injury. Gastroenterology 86:287–294, 1984.

107. McDeavitt JT, Emery EA, Harton S, et al: Folate deficiency in the spinal cord injured with decubiti (abstract). J Am Paraplegia Soc 15(2):146, 1992.

108. Brunnemann SR, Eltorai IM, Segal JL, et al: Vitamin C: Depressed serum levels in humans with spinal cord injury. J Am Paraplegia Soc (in review).

109. Young W, Bracken MB: The Second National Acute Spinal Cord Injury Study. J Neurotrauma 9(suppl 1):S397–S405, 1992.

110. Geisler FH, Dorsey FC, Coleman WP: Recovery of motor function after spinal-cord injury—A randomized, placebo-controlled trial with GM-1 ganglioside. N Engl J Med 324:1829–1838, 1991.

111. Bracken MB: Pharmacological treatment of acute spinal cord injury: Current status and future prospects. Paraplegia 30:102–107, 1992.

112. Faden AI: Effects of TRH-analog treatment on tissue cations, phospholipids and energy metabolism after spinal cord injury. J Pharmacol Exp Ther 255:608–614, 1990.

113. Holtz A, Gerdin B: MK 801, an OBS N-methyl-D-aspartate channel blocker, does not improve the functional recovery nor spinal cord blood flow after spinal cord compression in rats. Acta Neurol Scand 84:334–338, 1991.

114. Fowl RJ, Patterson RB, Gewirtz RJ, et al: Protection against postischemic spinal cord injury using a new 21-aminosteroid. J Surg Res 48:597–600, 1990.

115. Young W: Strategies for the development of new and better pharamcological treatment for acute spinal cord injury. Adv Neurol 59:249–256, 1993.

116. Gentile NT, McIntosh TK: Antagonists of excitatory

amino acids and endogenous opioid peptides in the treatment of experimental central nervous system injury. Ann Emerg Med 22:1028–1034, 1993.

117. Simpson RK, Hsu CY, Dimitrijevic MR: The experimental basis for early pharmacological intervention in spinal cord injury. Paraplegia 29:364–372, 1991.

118. Nockels R, Young W: Pharmacologic strategies in the treatment of experimental spinal cord injury. J Neurotrauma 9(suppl 1):S211–S217, 1992.

119. Bracken MB, Shepard MJ, Collins WF, et al: Methylprednisolone or naloxone treatment after acute spinal cord injury: 1-year follow-up data. J Neurosurg 76:23–31, 1992.

120. Hall ED: Importance of pharmacologic considerations in the evaluation of new treatments for acute spinal cord injury. J Neurotrauma 9(2):173–176, 1992.

121. Iwai A, Monafo WW, Eliasson SG: Methylprednisolone treatment of experimental spinal cord injury. Paraplegia 31:417–429, 1993.

122. Uges DRA, Sohn YJ, Greijdanus B, et al: 4-Aminopyridine kinetics. Clin Pharmacol Ther 31(5):587–593, 1982.

123. Evenhuis J, Agoston S, Salt PJ, et al: Pharmacokinetics of 4-aminopyridine in human volunteers: A preliminary study using a new GLC method for its estimation. Br J Anaesthesiol 53:567, 1981.

124. Blight AR, Gruner JA: Augmentation by 4-aminopyridine of vestibulospinal free fall responses in chronic spinal-injured cats. J Neurol Sci 87:145–159, 1987.

125. Hayes KC: 4-Aminopyridine and spinal cord injury: A review. Restor Neurol Neuro Science 6:259–270, 1994.

126. Hansebout RR, Blight AR, Fawcett S, et al: 4-Aminopyridine in chronic spinal cord injury: A controlled, double-blind, crossover study in eight patients. J Neurotrauma 10(1):19–24, 1993.

127. Hayes KC, Blight AR, Potter PJ, et al: Preclinical trial of 4-aminopyridine in patients with chronic spinal cord injury. Paraplegia 31(4):216–224, 1993.

128. Hayes KC, Potter PJ, Wolfe DL, et al: 4-Aminopyridine sensitive neurological deficits in patients with spinal cord injury. J Neurotrauma 11:433–446, 1994.

129. Hall ED, Braughler JM, McCall JM: Antioxidant effects in brain and spinal cord injury. J Neurotrauma 9(suppl 1):S165–S172, 1992.

130. Rich KM, Hollowell JP: Flunarizine protects neurons from death after axotomy or NGF deprivation. Science 248:1419–1421, 1990.

131. Ratain MJ: Therapeutic relevance of pharmacokinetics and pharmacodynamics. Semin Oncol 19(4 suppl 11):8–13, 1992.

132. Schumacher GE, Barr JT: Bayesian approaches in pharmacokinetic decision making. Clin Pharm 3:525–530, 1984.

133. Jelliffe RW, Schumitzky A, Van Guilder M, et al: Individualizing drug dosage regimens: Roles of population pharmacokinetic and dynamic models, Bayesian fitting, and adaptive control. Therap Drug Monitoring 15:380–393, 1993.

134. Sheiner LB, Beal SL: NONMEM Users Guide. part 1: Users Basic Guide. San Francisco, Regents of the University of California, 1988.

135. Schumitzky A: Nonparametric EM Algorithms for Estimating prior Distributions, Laboratory of Applied Pharmacokinetics. Technical report 90-2, Los Angeles, University of Southern California School of Medicine.

136. D'Argenio DZ, Schumitzky A: ADAPT II, Interactive Mathematical Software for Pharmacokinetic/Pharmacodynamic Systems Analysis, User's Guide. Los Angeles: Biomedical Simulations Resource, University of Southern California, 1988.

137. Robinson JD: CAPCIL (Continuous Assessment of Pharmaceutical Care to Improve Life) System with Kinetics 5.0. Gainesville, Fl., Simkin, 1994.

138. Segal JL, Robinson JD: Population-specific pharmacokinetic profile for the use of aminoglycoside antibiotics in patients with spinal cord injury. The SIMKIN Pharmacokinetics System Version 4.2. Gainesville, Fla., Simkin, 1991.

139. Schwinghammer TL, Kroboth PD: Basic concepts in pharmacodynamic modeling. J Clin Pharmacol 28:388–394, 1988.

CHAPTER 26

Functional Restoration of the Upper Extremity in Tetraplegia

Vincent R. Hentz, M.D.
Amy L. Ladd, M.D.

With continued improvements in the emergency resuscitation of patients with cervical spinal cord injuries, greater numbers of patients with higher-level injuries are surviving. These patients reach rehabilitation facilities with heightened expectations regarding recovery and with significant rehabilitative demands.

In addition, because of the increasing acceptance of the important role played by surgery in restoring function to the paralyzed upper extremity, greater numbers of tetraplegic patients are knowledgeable about upper extremity surgery and inquire about the appropriateness of surgery for their hands and arms. Tetraplegic patients express a greater desire to have function restored to their hands than to have, for example, sexual function restored.

HISTORY

In the minds of both physiatrists and surgeons, the appropriateness of surgical reconstruction of the upper extremity in tetraplegic patients has waxed and waned in acceptance since the initial reports of Bunnell[1] in the 1940s. The many factors that are responsible for the varying attitudes toward surgery are discussed here.

In 1949, Bunnell[1] described his results with procedures designed to provide an automatic finger grasp and release and a tip-to-tip, or so-called *opposition pinch*, for tetraplegic patients possessing active wrist extension. This was accomplished by multiple tenodeses (implanting a tendon into bone) so that the fingers would automatically flex with wrist extension and would automatically open with wrist flexion. Additionally, with wrist extension, the thumb and the index and middle fingertips were brought together in so-called opposition, or three-jawed chuck pinch. Muscle transfers were used occasionally rather than tenodeses, but Bunnell's goal for the thumb remained focused on achieving tip-to-tip pinch, since this was felt to represent refined function. In general, Bunnell's patients would be classified at C6 and 7 functional levels according to current standards.

Some years later, at Rancho Los Amigos Hospital, Nickel and colleagues[2] attempted to extend hand surgery to tetraplegic patients with less residual upper extremity function. They devised a complex operation that involved multiple joint fusions to pre-position the fingers and thumb and multiple tenodeses to achieve an automatic opposition-type or tip-to-tip pinch between thumb and index and middle fingers. In actuality, it was difficult to achieve the precise digital posture needed for accurate thumb opposition. Some patients were unhappy with the stiffness of the fingers, which was a consequence of the joint fusions. Although this surgical procedure fell into disfavor, its external corollary, which is a mechanical device or orthosis that holds the fingers and thumbs in the necessary position, became the standard orthosis. The design of the wrist-driven flexor hand splint, with subsequent modifications, remains the standard functional hand orthosis for the tetraplegic patient (Fig. 26–1).

During the 1960s and early 1970s several pioneer reconstructive extremity surgeons, including Lamb and Landry[3] in Scotland and Zancolli[4] in Argentina, were reporting good results using active muscle-tendon transfers to substitute for lack of function. However during the decades of the 1950s and 1960s, surgery had not been held in high regard because of more than occasionally poor results. The results of muscle-tendon transfers were sometimes unpredictable because the trans-

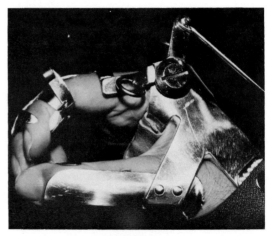

FIGURE 26–1

The wrist-driven flexor hinge splint remains the most commonly prescribed orthosis for the tetraplegic patient. A series of metal supports acts to stabilize all but the metacarpophalangeal joints of the index and middle fingers. The mechanical assembly serves to translate wrist flexion and extension into digital extension and flexion at these two joints. The thumb becomes a rigid post against which the other digits act.

ferred muscle was frequently spastic. Patients did not appreciate the stiff, contracted fingers that might result from transfer of such spastic muscles. In his textbook on spinal cord management, Guttmann[5] stated that fewer than 5% of tetraplegic patients were candidates for hand surgery.

In 1975 a Swedish hand surgeon, Erik Moberg,[6] published his philosophy regarding the role of hand surgery in tetraplegia and described his results in reconstructing two important functions that were lacking in the majority of tetraplegic patients. The four main constituents of Moberg's philosophy are:

1. Aside from the brain, the hand of the tetraplegic patient represents his or her most important residual resource. However, the tetraplegic uses the hands differently from any other patient in that he or she must "walk on [the] hands." Failure to recognize the functional demands of the tetraplegic's hands led to poorly designed fusions and tenodeses, which broke down in response to these demands.

2. As the most important residual resource, the hand has three primary

roles: gripping, feeling, and establishing human contact. Moberg believed that supple hands are preferred for human contact and that stiff, clawed hands are unacceptable.

3. When limited functional resources remain after injury, surgery should pose essentially no risk to these residual resources. Therefore, especially for patients in whom cervical cord injuries are more cranial, surgery should be reversible.

4. The key grip, or lateral pinch, between the broad pulp of the thumb and the side of the index finger is far more useful for the tetraplegic patient than the opposition-type pinch favored earlier. For the patient with C5–6 injury (this constitutes the largest single group of tetraplegic patients), the goal of surgery should be reconstruction of active elbow extension and provision of key grip for at least one extremity.

Moberg remained a champion of the role of surgery for tetraplegic patients until his death in 1993. His philosophy has personally guided the development of our program in surgical reconstruction for tetraplegic patients at the Palo Alto Veterans Administration Medical Center Spinal Cord Injury Center over the past 18 years. We and others[7–9] have enlarged on Moberg's philosophy as we have gained experience. Tetraplegic patients with greater numbers of residual motor resources are candidates for the reconstruction of more functional hands than can be achieved by the creation of only a key or lateral pinch. A minimal risk for these patients is acceptable. After 20 years' experience we still follow Moberg's dictums, especially for the patients who have little remaining function in the upper limb.

CLASSIFICATION OF THE TETRAPLEGIC UPPER EXTREMITY

An injury to the cervical spinal cord has been classified in many ways, including by the skeletal level of injury or according to the most distal remaining functional cervical root. No two patients, however, even with injuries at the same skeletal level, are exactly alike; the same is frequently true of the function of the right and left extremities in the same patient. Discrepancies may occur in the motor and sensory distribution of an individual patient's injury. To develop useful recommendations for treatment, it was necessary to develop a more precise method of classification for upper limb function in the tetraplegic patient (Table 26–1). From these needs the international classification was developed, which is based not on the spinal level of injury but rather on the limb's remaining useful motor and sensory resources. Muscle strength is assessed using the standard 0 to 5 scale, and the limb is classified according to the number of grade 4 or 5 muscles that remain functional distal to the elbow. The grade 4 level was chosen because a grade 4 muscle can be transferred and still perform useful work. A grade 3 muscle loses so much of its power in transfer that it cannot be reliably expected to do useful work after transfer.

Moberg[10, 11] encouraged us to also consider remaining sensory resources. If sufficient proprioception remains in any part of the hand (typically the thumb and index fingers), the patient can control the hand without having to keep it in view. If the hand lacks proprioception, the patient must instead use the eyes for afferent control. However, lack of proprioception still limits performance of bimanual activities. We now equate static two-point discrimination of less than 12 to 15 mm as being indicative of the presence of proprioception. The classification has been extended somewhat to include a determination of the presence or absence of active elbow extension. This system has been adopted by the International Federation of Hand Surgery Societies and is used by essentially all surgeons involved in the care of the upper extremities of tetraplegic patients.

FORMING A TEAM

Moberg also stressed the need to develop a "critical mass" of like-minded professionals into a team, which should include physia-

TABLE 26-1

INTERNATIONAL CLASSIFICATION FOR SURGERY OF THE HAND IN TETRAPLEGIA, EDINBURGH (1978)

SENSIBILITY*			
O OR Cu GROUP		MOTOR CHARACTERISTICS*	DESCRIPTION OF REGIONAL FUNCTION
	0	No muscle below elbow suitable for transfer	Flexion of elbow, supination of forearm
	1	BR	Flexion of elbow, supination of forearm
	2	ECRL	Extension of wrist (weak or strong)
	3†	ECRB	Extension of wrist (strong)
	4	PT	Wrist extension, pronation of forearm
	5	FCR	Flexion of wrist
	6	Finger extensors	Extrinsic extension of fingers (partial or complete)
	7	Thumb extensors	Extrinsic extension of thumb
	8	Partial digital flexors	Extrinsic flexion of fingers (weak)
	9	Lacks only intrinsic muscle function	Extrinsic flexion of fingers

Modified from McDowell CL, Moberg EA, House JA: Second International Conference on Surgical Rehabilitation of the Upper Hand in Tetraplegia. J Hand Surg 11A:604–608, 1986

* O = ocular afferents; Cu = sufficient remaining digital sensibility; BR = brachioradialis; ECRL = extensor carpi radialis longus; ECRB = extensor carpi radialis brevis; PT = pronator teres; FCR = flexor carpi radialis.

† It may not be possible to determine the strength of the ECRB without surgical exposure.

trists and spinal cord medicine specialists involved in the rehabilitation and long-term care of tetraplegic patients. Critical to the concept of a team are well-trained therapists, either physical therapists or occupational therapists (preferably both). The hand and upper extremity surgeon, whose primary background may be in either orthopedics or plastic and reconstructive surgery, constitutes the remaining professional resource. Others, including social workers and psychologists, may play unique roles. However, the most important part of the team is the patient; equally important is the patient's support group, including family, spouse, and attendant. The role of the professionals in this team seems relatively clear-cut. The physiatrist or spinal cord medicine specialist should assist in determining the appropriateness of surgery as well as the appropriate timing of surgery relative to overall rehabilitation goals and schedules. The therapist frequently serves as the patient's advocate. He or she knows the patient better than anyone else, understands the patient's motivation and intellectual capabilities, and, most important, is aware of the patient's voiced and unvoiced expectations.

For the tetraplegic patient, upper extremity surgery has perhaps greater emotional impact than it does for most other patients. The tetraplegic patient is aware of the somewhat precarious nature of his or her life. While the goal of surgical reconstruction for the upper extremity is greater independence, this can only be achieved at the expense of an occasionally prolonged period of greater dependence. For family and attendants, this greater period of dependence translates into more inconvenience and effort. All of the team members must play a role in the decision-making process and must share in the frustrations as well as the rewards.

PATIENT EVALUATION AND SELECTION

It is our strong belief that the hand and upper extremity team should participate in the routine evaluation of even newly injured patients. The patient with cervical cord injury usually arrives at a rehabilitation facility or spinal cord injury unit with fairly supple upper limbs, though volitional movement is absent or minimal. Most therapists involved with patients in the early days or weeks following injury are aware of the need for protective splinting to avoid insidious development of pathologic contractures of the shoulders, elbows, wrists, and digits.

Once the vertebral injury has stabilized and the patient can be placed in a wheelchair, an assessment by the upper extremity team takes on new meaning. By the third or fourth month following injury, the eventual functional level is clearly established in the majority of patients. At this time, and based on the patient's ability to use adaptive devices for feeding and hygiene, an early determination can be made regarding the applicability of more complex functional orthoses. For some patients, early measurement, fabrication, and fitting of a functional orthosis, such as a wrist-driven flexor hinge splint, advances the rate of rehabilitation. For patients with early but weak recovery of wrist extension, the wrist-driven flexor hinge splint represents an excellent exercise therapy directed toward strengthening wrist extensors so that they may eventually actuate a surgically reconstructed pinch or grip.

Hand or upper extremity surgery is rarely indicated during the initial months of rehabilitation following injury. The patient needs time to experience neurologic and psychological stability. From a practical standpoint, too many more important rehabilitation activities are taking place. However, a dogmatic philosophy embracing tired dicta such as "never operate on a patient before 12 months" has no basis in science. Some patients are clearly candidates for surgery before this calendar interval. For example, early surgical intervention to relieve the pathologic effects of a fixed elbow flexion contracture may allow a patient to participate more vigorously in necessary rehabilitation activities. There exists a good rationale for surgically paralyzing a spastic and shortened biceps muscle for a period of some months by performing an open crush of the musculocutaneous nerve. A good argument can be made for early release of a fixed elbow flexion contracture with simultaneous transfer of the contracted biceps muscle to the triceps. This removes a pathologic or deforming force and reinforces or restores some power to the antagonist muscle.

Once the patient seems to have achieved neurologic and psychological stability, a formal evaluation to establish the appropriateness of upper extremity surgery can be accomplished by the team. The evaluation should focus on not only tangible evidence of recovery, ascertained by assessment of remaining motor and sensory resources, but also important intangible contributors to recovery, such as motivation and intelligence. In addition, the assessment should include an evaluation of the means by which the patient accomplishes tasks of daily living, with particular attention paid to how he or she performs transfers and pushes the wheelchair (Fig. 26–2).

The motor examination includes an assay of residual motor groups as well as identification of pathologic conditions such as contracted, painful, or unstable joints. The sensory evaluation includes measurement of two-point discrimination in the digits to assess proprioception and identification of pathologic conditions such as painful hypersensitivity. Any residual grip or pinch power

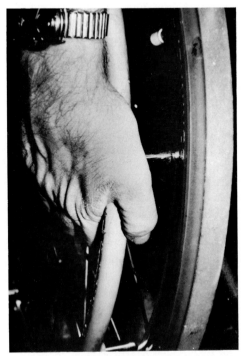

FIGURE 26–2

A careful analysis of the patient's hand and thumb posture during wheelchair mobility is critical to ensure that the benefits of surgery are not compromised by persistent overstress of tenodeses or fusions.

is measured using standard dynamometers or pinch gauges. It may be necessary to construct a more useful measuring tool for these patients, such as a squeeze ball attached to a mercury manometer.

The patient's current functional status is assessed. Does he or she perform bed mobility tasks dependently or independently? How are transfers performed? Is a manual or electric wheelchair employed? What adaptive devices are used for dressing, grooming, and feeding? If surgery is to be performed, is there sufficient support for the patient during a period of greater functional dependence, or will the extra burden of care result in the patient's attendant quitting? For many patients, upper extremity surgery means restriction to an electric-powered wheelchair. Can this be made available? Does the home situation permit use of an electric wheelchair? Are the controls on the chair mounted on the correct side? We have come to rely on therapists for the attention to detail necessary in resolving these issues.

Often some aspect of the examination identifies features that indicate that surgery is inadvisable at the moment. Perhaps a motor group can be made significantly stronger by a period of directed exercise, which may mean the difference between a mediocre and a truly beneficial surgical result. Occasionally we can assess the level of patient motivation by the response to a course of functional therapy. Does the patient respond favorably? Does he or she demonstrate the commitment to achieve a goal? The input and ideas of all team members are sought in the decision-making process. While the surgeon must accept the ultimate responsibility for the decision, the decision is a team effort. The fact that decisions are a team effort is made abundantly clear to the patients, which permits all participants to share in the rewards of a good result and to help bear the frustrations of a disappointing result.

GENERAL GUIDELINES FOR RECONSTRUCTION

The surgical procedures for improving upper limb function in tetraplegia include surgically immobilizing a joint (fusion); anchoring tendons to bone (tenodesis), so that another movement will result in the passive tightening of the anchored tendon; and with this tightening, movement of a more distally located joint and transfer of the power of an expendable muscle-tendon unit that is under good volitional control to compensate for the absence or ineffectiveness of function of another (tendon transfer). These are all well-established surgical techniques, many of which date from the era of polio reconstructive surgery. A fourth reconstructive technique has been introduced. Termed *functional electrical stimulation* (FES), this technique utilizes the residual contractile properties of upper motor neuron–paralyzed muscles when stimulated by an extraneural source (see Chapter 23).

The remainder of this chapter is devoted to a discussion of the role of surgery for improving function at the elbow, wrist, and fingers. The objective is not to teach surgical techniques. References are provided if more information is required. Our goal is to discuss the procedures that are available to patients with injuries at the various international classification levels and the expected outcomes of surgical reconstruction. Admittedly, it is difficult to present this in a fashion that does not bring to mind a cookbook; however, each patient, and indeed each upper extremity, must be evaluated and each treatment plan must be individualized. This cannot be stressed enough.

For cervical spinal cord injuries at the most cranial anatomic level, no expendable, and thus transferable, muscles exist. For patients injured at the more caudal anatomic extreme, many potentially transferable muscles of grade 4 or 5 power exist. Thus, reconstructive possibilities range from straightforward procedures to merely simplify the mechanics of the hand (e.g., fusing a wrist joint so that it no longer requires external stabilization by an orthosis) to complex multi-staged procedures involving many muscle-tendon transfers. The choice of procedure depends primarily on the residual resources and, secondly, on the intangible factors such as motivation and support. While the surgical techniques are exactly those used to overcome functional loss in patients with peripheral nerve injuries, matching the patient and procedure requires an understanding of the real difference between the tetraplegic patient and someone with, for example, a brachial plexus injury or a combined high median and ulnar nerve palsy. A cautious approach while the surgeon gains experience pays great dividends in terms of obtaining the acceptance of team members and patients and promoting greater independence for the patients. A poor outcome early in the team's experience creates a tremendous hurdle.

ORTHOSES

For the patient with no muscles functioning at a grade 4 or 5 level distal to the elbow, few reconstructive possibilities exist. For the majority of these patients, some type of functional orthosis must suffice. For the O or OCu–0 patient, fusion of the wrist might rarely permit the use of a less cumbersome functional orthosis (e.g., a self-donned universal cuff rather than a long opponens splint, for which the patient needs assistance in donning and doffing).

Surgery may also be useful in repositioning a badly positioned part. For example, osteotomy of the radius may be useful in placing the hand in a more favorable pronated position, which might permit easier manipulation of the joystick control for an electric wheelchair than can be accomplished by a perpetually supinated hand.

SURGICAL RECONSTRUCTION

Elbow Extension

Moberg brought to our attention the importance of active elbow extension for the spinal cord–injured patient. The wheelchair-bound individual depends on good shoulder and elbow power and stabilization to push a wheelchair, transfer from bed to chair, and perform pressure releases to prevent pressure sores. For the tetraplegic patient, lack of functional elbow extension results in a much reduced functional environment. The world of the tetraplegic patient is determined by the range of motion of his or her upper extremity. Without the ability to extend the elbow, the patient's

"sphere of influence" is much reduced. The ability to extend the hand in space by an additional 12 in. results in an additional 800% of space that the hand can reach.

There are other reasons that reconstruction of active elbow extension is tremendously useful. Without active elbow extension, the tetraplegic patient's hands frequently fall into the face when he or she is lying supine. A manual wheelchair cannot be pushed up an incline without triceps function. Even as simple a task as turning on a room lightswitch may be impossible without active elbow extension.

DELTOID TO TRICEPS TRANSFER

Two surgical procedures are advocated for restoring active elbow extension. In the United States, transfer of the power of the posterior half of the deltoid to the triceps tendon, as described by Moberg,[10] is preferred. We prefer this procedure when the posterior deltoid is strong and the elbow has near-normal passive extension. The procedure, performed with the patient under general anesthesia, involves detaching the insertion of about half of the deltoid (usually the posterior half) from the humerus and connecting this portion of the muscle via the triceps tendon insertion into the olecranon process of the ulna (Fig. 26–3). Several technical modifications have been described but the goals are similar. After surgery the elbow is immobilized in full or nearly full extension for several weeks, and then the elbow is exercised for several additional weeks by allowing progressively greater elbow flexion. Some months of cautious use are necessary to prevent overstretching of the transfer, and many months pass before maximal strength is obtained.

The results have been reasonably consistent in our experience. The great majority of patients can achieve full or nearly full extension against gravity (Fig. 26–4). This allows more accurate positioning of the arm in space and control of its movements. A patient occasionally achieves sufficient power to permit independent transfer in all circumstances, but this is not a realistic goal for most patients. The majority find that they achieve more efficient transfers and pressure

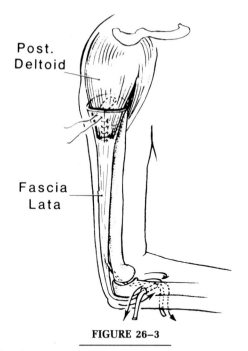

Post.
Deltoid

Fascia
Lata

FIGURE 26–3

The elements of the deltoid to triceps transfer to regain active elbow extension are depicted. A wide strip of fascia lata, harvested from the lateral thigh, is tubularized around the fibrous insertion of the deltoid muscle after the deltoid is elevated off the humerus. The fascia lata is woven into the olecranon distally to provide for the transfer of power from the posterior deltoid to the ulna when the elbow is extended.

releases, and have more efficient wheelchair mobility.

Complications are rare, provided the patient follows the exercise protocol and does not overstretch the transfer by performing full elbow flexion too rapidly. In two patients we have transferred the entire deltoid muscle without measurably changing shoulder function. This makes sense as surgery has merely moved the point of attachment of the muscle more distally on the limb.

BICEPS TO TRICEPS TRANSFER

A second procedure has been advocated to improve elbow extension. The biceps tendon can be detached from its insertion on the greater tuberosity of the radius, the muscle-tendon unit routed either medially or laterally, and the tendon attached to the triceps aponeurosis. We have performed this transfer when a preexisting flexion contracture of the

elbow of greater than 30 degrees is present. In this case, the biceps is usually a deforming force, which must be treated either by tendon lengthening or tenotomy. Rather than lengthen the biceps tendon, we prefer to transfer it. One might anticipate that the transfer of an antagonist would cause problems during rehabilitation of the transfer. However, we have learned that by teaching the patient to conjointly supinate the forearm and extend the elbow, the supinator function of the biceps can be used in reeducation. The results of biceps-to-triceps transfer are not as impressive as those of deltoid-to-triceps transfer. Typically the patient cannot actively extend through a large range against the force of gravity. However, the patient does appreciate a gain in the ability to position the arm more accurately in space, and the removal of a deforming force with strengthening of the antagonist decreases the chances for recurrence of elbow contracture.

Reconstruction of elbow extension has been the single most satisfying reconstruction for our patients. Even though the overall time for rehabilitation can be relatively lengthy, the functional gain is substantial, predictable, and easily appreciated by the patient. Furthermore, the risks to residual preoperative function are practically nil. It represents an important addition to our reconstructive surgical armamentarium.

IMPROVING WRIST EXTENSION THE O OR OCu–1 PATIENT

In the class O or OCu–1 patient, the brachioradialis is typically the only muscle with grade 4 function distal to the elbow. However, grade 2+ to 3+ radial wrist extensor function is typically present as well. The patient may be able to extend the wrist against gravity but cannot exert any force between digits and thumb through any existing natural tenodesis effect of the paralyzed finger and thumb flexors, or cannot utilize a wrist-driven flexor hand splint unless it is equipped with a ratchet mechanism lock and release. For this patient, wrist extensor strength can be augmented by transferring the power of the brachioradialis into the more central of the radial wrist extensors, the ex-

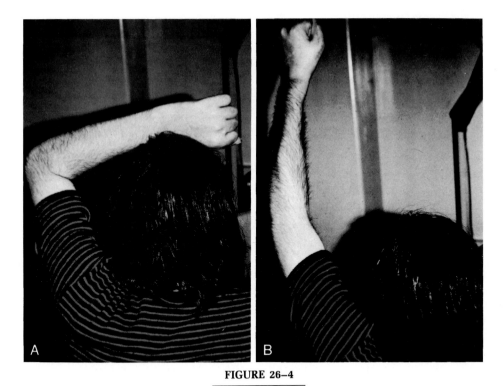

FIGURE 26–4

A and *B*, Approximately 6 months after deltoid to triceps transfer surgery, the patient can fully extend the elbow even with the shoulder fully abducted.

tensor carpi radialis brevis (ECRB) tendon, which attaches to the base of the third metacarpal. From several biomechanical studies it has been determined that the brachioradialis becomes a more effective wrist extensor following transfer if the patient can stabilize the elbow in space. If no active elbow extension is present, the brachioradialis, because it crosses the elbow joint, may waste some of its excursion and power in flexing the elbow rather than in extending the wrist. For this reason, we prefer to first reconstruct active elbow extension; we occasionally combine deltoid to triceps and brachioradialis to ECRB transfers. Following surgery and over time, we have observed impressive gains in wrist extensor strength. The patient is able to better utilize a wrist-driven flexor hand splint; in the best cases, the patient may become a candidate for surgical reconstruction of key pinch. The brachioradialis is truly a useful "spare part."

KEY PINCH PROCEDURE

Patients functioning at the O or OCu–2 level can actively extend the wrist against gravity and against some resistance. This is a presenting feature in a large number of our patients, and it correlates to the C5–6 functional classification. Wrist extension may be relatively weak or very strong, as grade 4 is a subjective parameter.

Patients in the O or OCu–2 category are potential candidates for creation of a lateral or key pinch as described by Moberg.[6] Conceptually, this is a very simple operative procedure; what is more important, it is essentially totally reversible should the patient decide he or she had better function before surgery. This is a consideration for a patient with weak wrist extension many years after injury. The key pinch procedure may be combined with brachioradialis to ECRB transfer if greater wrist extensor power is deemed advantageous. Key pinch procedure represents an automatic pinch in that the tendon of the thumb flexor, the flexor pollicis longus (FPL), is anchored to the palmar surface of the radius under such tension that with wrist extension, the thumb tip is pulled against the side of the index finger (Fig. 26–5). The other fingers are usually left in a supple state, and the patient frequently must learn to roll these digits into some degree of flexion to provide a platform against which the thumb can act (Fig. 26–6). Gravity is needed to flex the wrist, which releases tension on the tenodesed FPL and allows opening of the grip. This implies that the wrist must have a good passive range of motion preoperatively and that the patient can be sitting much of the time so that gravity can affect the opening of the grip.

Several technical modifications have been described to accommodate individual anatomic variations.[12, 13] Typically, the hand and wrist are immobilized for 4 to 5 weeks and cautious use is required for an additional 1 to 2 months to allow firm adherence of the tenodesis. We have performed this procedure on more than 50 hands and the results have been very satisfying. We can measure the gain in pinch strength, and it is typically proportional to the strength of the wrist extensor power but somewhat depends on the stability of the thumb and finger joints. Pinch strengths between 1 and 5 kg have been uniformly achieved. No patient has asked to have the operative procedure reversed.

ACTIVE KEY PINCH

After gaining experience with the key pinch procedure described by Moberg, we chose to modify the key pinch operation for the patient with very strong wrist extension meaning a patient in class O, OCu–2, or OCu–3. These patients do not require augmentation of wrist extension by, for example, brachioradialis transfer. Instead of performing tenodesis of the FPL to the radius in a single-stage procedure, as described earlier, the following steps are accomplished:

1. The carpometacarpal (CMC) joint is fused to pre-position the thumb tip to contact the index and middle fingers.

2. The extensor pollicis longus (EPL) tendon is anchored to the extensor retinaculum on the dorsum of the wrist.

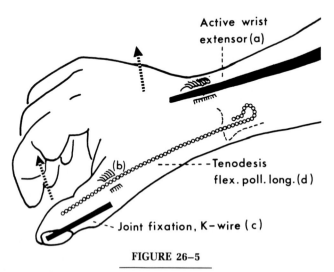

FIGURE 26–5

The elements of the key pinch operation described by Moberg are depicted. The flexor pollicis longus tendon is detached from the muscle tendon juncture and is anchored to the radius. The interphalangeal joint of the thumb is immobilized in nearly full extension by a large Steinmann pin. If indicated, the annular ligament at the metacarpophalangeal joint is released and the tendons of the extensor pollicis longus and brevis are anchored to the dorsum of the thumb just proximal to the metacarpophalangeal joint.

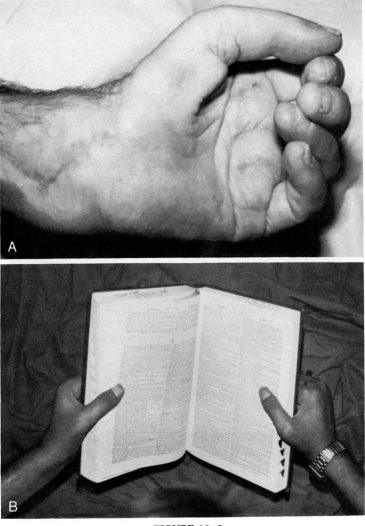

FIGURE 26–6

A, With wrist extension, the broad pulp surface of the thumb comes into contact with the radial side of the index finger. The slight bowstringing of the flexor pollicis longus tendon can be appreciated. *B*, After bilateral key pinch procedure, the patient is able to support even relatively heavy objects.

3. The brachioradialis muscle-tendon unit is transferred to the tendon of the flexor pollicis longus.

With this procedure, the patient depends on gravity to flex the wrist and tighten the extensor pollicis longus tenodesis, thus opening the grip. Then by actively contracting the brachioradialis, the thumb flexes against the side of the index finger regardless of wrist position (Fig. 26–7). Further wrist extension augments the power of the brachioradialis transfer. Although we have had less experience with this transfer, other colleagues have enjoyed good results and patients have been very satisfied. In several instances we have performed bilateral hand surgery in class OCu–2 or OCu–3 patients and have chosen to provide a traditional key pinch via FPL tenodesis on one side, and active key pinch via brachioradialis muscle transfer to the FPL tendon on the opposite side. The patients have enjoyed the different functional attributes of each method and find that certain functions are easier with one extremity, whereas others are more efficiently performed with the opposite hand.

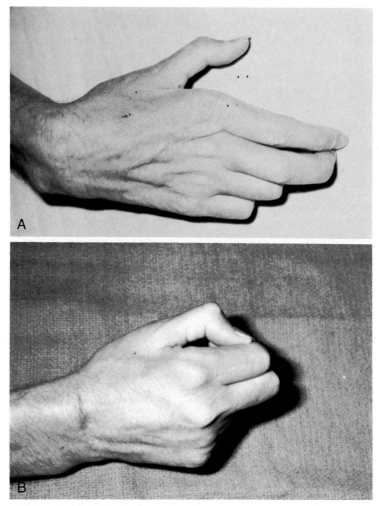

FIGURE 26–7

When sufficient wrist extension strength exists, the brachioradialis muscle may be used to power the tendon of the flexor pollicis longus to create an active key pinch that is somewhat independent of wrist position. *A*, The wrist is shown in flexion secondary to gravity. Tenodesis of the extensor pollicis longus to the radius acts to fully extend the thumb. *B*, Forceful pinch is demonstrated. Note that relatively excessive flexion occurs at the thumb interphalangeal joint (Froment's sign) as a consequence of absent thumb intrinsic muscle power and balance.

GRASP AND RELEASE PROCEDURES

For tetraplegic patients who possess additional motor resources distal to the elbow, more complicated reconstructions are possible but not always indicated. These patients are, of course, also candidates for either procedure described earlier if reversibility seems an important consideration. In the early years of our experience, we frequently offered only key pinch reconstruction for OCu–4 and even OCu–5 patients. As we have gained experience, so have we gained confidence in the team's decisions. With the achievement of reliable outcomes, we have extended the risk-benefit equation to include more complex procedures.

The OCu–4 patient has four strong muscles functioning distal to the elbow, usually the brachioradialis, the two radial wrist extensors, the extensor carpi radialis longus (ECRL), and ECRP; frequently, the pronator teres muscle is also functional. In addition, the majority of class OCu–4 patients have some function, albeit minimal, in the flexor carpi radialis. They can flex the wrist with some force when the forearm is pronated with gravity, thereby assisting the weak flexor carpi radialis. For these patients, we have devised a two-stage procedure that takes advantage of the presence of two expendable muscles for transfer, the ECRL and the brachioradialis. Prerequisites for surgery include near-normal passive wrist movement and reasonably flexible fingers. At the initial procedure, the power of the ECRB is tested under local anesthesia to be certain that this muscle is sufficiently strong to extend the wrist. If this is the case, we proceed to fuse the CMC joint of the thumb to pre-position the thumb ray for pinch and, at the same time, attach the tendons of the extensor digitorum communis and EPL to the dorsum of the radius. This is referred to as the *release phase*. After a period of healing with wrist flexion, the fingers and thumb extend. This is a very natural and synergistic motion and is easily learned.

Some weeks to months later, the *flexor phase* is performed. Two active muscle-tendon transfers are performed, including transfer of the extensor carpi radialis to the combined tendons of the flexor digitorum profundus, so that this muscle smoothly flexes all of the fingers, and transfer of the brachioradialis to the tendon of the FPL. The transfers permit the patient to actively close the fingers around an object and to flex the fingers to provide a platform against which the thumb can actively pinch through the power of the brachioradialis transfer. The hand and wrist are immobilized for about 4 weeks and then exercises are performed under the supervision of a therapist. Because the transfers are synergistic, reeducation is relatively easy and quick. Many months are necessary before full strength is achieved. Also, as the patient lacks active finger extension, daily digital extension exercises are necessary to avoid the development of finger flexion contractures. A static night splint that maintains the proximal interphalangeal joints in nearly full extension should be worn indefinitely.

We have seen so few patients of this functional category that we cannot determine outcome in a meaningful manner. Nonetheless, outcome of the procedure is predictable.

STRONG GRASP AND RELEASE

Patients in the international classification of OCu–5 category usually have a functioning triceps. They also function at a reasonable level of efficiency because they frequently have some residual effective natural flexor tenodesis in the paralyzed fingers and thumb. Decisions regarding the appropriateness of surgery for patients in this category need careful consideration.[14, 15] However, these patients have the most to gain from carefully planned and executed surgery.

We have performed several variations of the two-stage grasp-and-release procedure just described for the OCu–4 group except that an additional muscle is available for transfer. Typically, we have tried to avoid fusion of any joints. Extension of the fingers or the release phase is obtained either via extensor tenodesis, as described earlier, or, occasionally, by active muscle transfer to the combined tendons of the thumb and finger extensors. The flexor phase includes several procedures to maximize the versatility of thumb pinch and to provide powerful finger flexion. This includes provision for some ability to abduct the thumb away from the palm. The goal of pinch is still directed toward a more lateral, side, or key pinch, but frequently the patient can also pinch closer to the index fingertip and can manipulate smaller objects, such as coins into a pay telephone, with some efficiency.

These patients have truly gained the most from surgery, particularly in terms of efficiency of movement and function. Instead of requiring an hour to dress themselves in the morning, they accomplish the same tasks in 10 to 15 minutes. Few do many more tasks postoperatively, but all perform these tasks with much greater efficiency and less expenditure of energy (Fig. 26–8).

OCu–6, OCu–7, AND OCu–8 LEVEL PATIENTS

Patients classified at the OCu–6 level possess active digital extension but lack thumb extension. These patients, as is true of those in the OCu–5 category, already have very functional hands, and surgery should be ap-

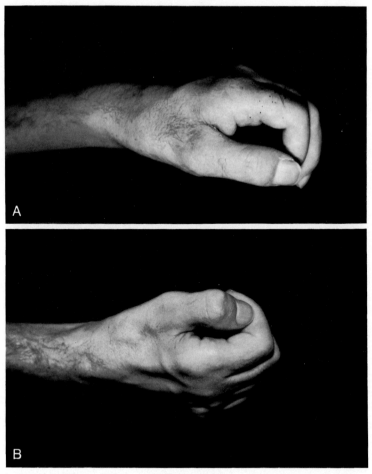

FIGURE 26–8

This patient has undergone bilateral grasp-release procedures. A, For the right hand, the thumb carpometacarpal joint has been fused to pre-position the thumb ray for pinch against the index finger. B, For the left hand, an opposition-like transfer was performed. The thumb demonstrates great adaptation in the pinch position. This case illustrates the principle of creating a somewhat different grasp and pinch pattern for each hand when bilateral hand surgery is contemplated.

proached cautiously. Again, however, they can achieve truly spectacular results by all parameters, including pinch strengths equal to 5 kg and grasp strengths between 10 and 15 kg. The results of surgery can be nearly normal hands except for lack of ulnar intrinsic function. They require only addition of an extensor force for the thumb and, at the same operation, multiple tendon transfer to achieve balanced thumb pinch and strong finger grasp. Therefore, only one procedure is necessary, and the period of dependence is minimal (Fig. 26–9).

Patients with an even greater number of remaining resources can be approached somewhat like a patient with a lower periph-

eral nerve injury. The surgical procedures are more directed at reconstructing some aspect of hand intrinsic muscle function and balance (Fig. 26–10). Relatively few tetraplegic patients are included in this category compared with numbers in the OCu–2 or OCu–5 categories, and we have operated on insufficient numbers of such patients to draw useful conclusions.

Other Presentations

Some injury patterns do not fit easily into the international classification. Patients with so-called central cord injuries have hands

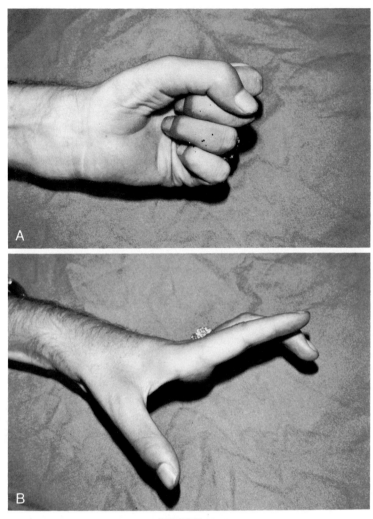

FIGURE 26–9

This patient was able to actively extend his fingers preoperatively, but lacked thumb extension (group 6). He had no digital or thumb flexion. Surgery involved both tenodesis and active transfers to permit active thumb extension (A) and multiple muscle tendon transfers to provide strong finger flexion and an adaptable and strong thumb pinch (B).

that defy classification. These patients require prolonged studies and frequent reexamination before a surgical plan can be formulated. Temporary nerve blocks have been particularly helpful in determining the procedure of choice.

Functional Electrical Stimulation

We have had experience implanting a system of electronics, including a programmable stimulator that controls an array of eight epimysial electrochannels. This system, developed by surgeons and engineers from the Case Western Reserve University and the Cleveland Veterans Administration Medical Center (see Chapter 23), has the capability of allowing a patient with a very high spinal injury to activate and control a preprogrammed sequence of muscle contractions and thus achieve a useful grasp for one hand. The control mechanism is mounted externally about the opposite shoulder allowing active and volitional shoulder movement to open and close the grip and modulate the force. Some additional movements can lock the grip in a closed position at the desired

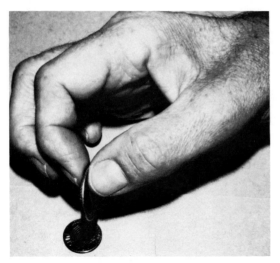

FIGURE 26–10

This patient (group 8) had muscle tendon transfers to provide a refined pinch position.

force of closure. This system of electrodes placed on predetermined upper motor neuron–paralyzed muscles has the potential to restore useful function in limbs heretofore deemed useless and unreconstructable by standard surgical techniques.

Postoperative Care

The operative procedure is only the prelude to a series of important, if not critical, steps in the rehabilitation of upper limb function. All of our patients have benefited from the skills of the therapy team members. Much of the therapy takes place at home; some takes place in the unit on an outpatient basis. Frequently the patient is discharged from the hospital 2 to 3 days following surgery, once therapists have determined it is safe to do so. Safety means having a suitable electric wheelchair with an overhead support to assist in elevation of the hand that has been operated on and an adequately instructed attendant or family member. The patient is readmitted at the proper time for removal of the cast or splint, and several days are spent in instructing the patient in the exercise protocols and, more important, in activities that must be avoided or modified, particularly

transfers and activities related to wheelchair mobility. Removable protective splints are fashioned at this time. Depending on circumstances, the patient may be discharged to continue the exercise regimen at home. Frequent follow-up is not particularly necessary for the majority of patients once transfers or tenodeses have achieved stability through healing. However, long-term follow-up is absolutely essential, because the tetraplegic hand is a dynamic structure and changes occur over time. Surgical revisions may be necessary if tenodeses stretch out or joints become malpositioned secondary to contractures.

CONCLUSIONS

With continued experience, we have found it necessary to modify surgical indications and procedures more or less continually. We recommend videotaping the patient's hand performing several standard functions, such as opening a package or holding a pen, both preoperatively and postoperatively. We recommend formalizing the record-keeping process, the team dynamics, and decision-making processes.

As mentioned earlier, few of our patients perform many new activities. Typically, a good or excellent result means that the patient performs many of the same functions with much greater efficiency. The rewards for surgeons, rehabilitation medicine specialists, and therapists are best expressed by one of our patients who, when asked about the outcome of his surgery, said, "It's not as much as I hoped for, but it's much more than I ever had."

REFERENCES

1. Bunnell S: Tendon transfer in the hand and forearm, vol VI. American Academy of Orthopedic Surgeons Instructional Course Lectures. St Louis, CV Mosby, 1949, pp 106–112.
2. Nickel VL, Perry J, Garrett AL: Development of useful function in the severely paralyzed hand. J Bone Joint Surg (Am) 45:933, 1963.
3. Lamb DW, Landry R: The hand in quadriplegia. Hand 3:31–7, 1971.
4. Zancolli E: Surgery for the quadriplegic hand with active, strong wrist extension preserved. Clin Orthop Rel Res 112:101, 1975.
5. Guttman L: Spinal Cord Injuries: Comprehensive

Management and Research, ed 2. Oxford, Blackwell Scientific Publications, 1976, p 588.

6. Moberg E: Surgical treatment for absent single-hand grip and elbow extension in quadriplegia. J Bone Joint Surg Am 57:196, 1975.

7. Hentz VR, Keoshian LA: Reconstruction of the hand in quadriplegia. Plast Reconstruct Surg 64:509, 1979.

8. Hentz VR, Keoshian LA, Brown M: A functional assessment of hand surgery in quadriplegia. J Hand Surg 8:19, 1983.

9. Hentz VR: Historical background and changing perspectives in surgical reconstruction of the upper limb in quadriplegia. J Am Paraplegia Soc 7:36, 1984.

10. Moberg E: Reconstructive hand surgery in tetraplegia, stroke and cerebral palsy: Some basic concepts in physiology and neurology. J Hand Surg 1:29, 1975.

11. Moberg E: The Upper Limb in Tetraplegia: A New Approach to Surgical Rehabilitation. Stuttgart, Thieme, 1978.

12. Bryan RS: The Moberg deltoid-triceps replacement and key pinch operations in quadriplegia: Preliminary experiences. Hand 9:209, 1977.

13. Newman JH: The use of the key grip procedure for improving hand function in quadriplegia. Hand 9:215, 1977.

14. House JH, Gwathmey FW, Lundsgaard DK: Restoration of strong grasp and lateral pinch in tetraplegia due to cervical spinal cord injury. J Hand Surg 1:152–159, 1976.

15. Zancolli E: Structural and Dynamic Bases of Hand Surgery, ed 2. Philadelphia, JB Lippincott, 1979.

Index

Note: Page numbers in *italics* indicate illustrations; those followed by t indicate tables.

Chain muscle spindle fibers, 31
Chance fracture, Luque rod fixation of, *128*
Charcot's disease. See *Amyotrophic lateral sclerosis (ALS)*.
Chemical neuroanatomy, 9
Chemonucleolysis, chymopapain, acute transverse myelopathy and, 71
Chemotherapy, cerebrospinal fluid infusion in, 90
  myelopathy and, 71
Chest pain, in coronary artery disease, 311
Chiari malformation, in syringomyelia, 93
  magnetic resonance imaging of, 194, *195*
Childbirth, 263
Chlorpromazine, for psychotic disorders, 412t
Cholecystokinin, in gray matter, 10, 11t, 13, 14
Cholesterol, high-density lipoprotein, coronary artery disease and, 311, *311*
  serum levels of, reduction of, 313
Cholinergic drugs, for detrusor arreflexia, 228
Chondrosarcoma, magnetic resonance imaging of, 186
Chordoma, *61*
  magnetic resonance imaging of, 185
Chromatolysis, central, 58, 60
Chronic bacterial prostatitis, urinary tract infection and, 204–205
Chronic cerebral paraplegia, 142–143
Chronic meningomyelopathy, 100–101
Chronic myelopathy, 84–101
  incidence of, 84–85
Chronic pain. See also *Pain*.
  causes of, 136
  psychiatric aspects of, 410–411
Chronic pyelonephritis, 306, *307*
Chronic spastic paraplegia/quadriplegia, with gait ataxia, 141
Chymopapain chemonucleolysis, acute transverse myelopathy and, 71
Cigarette smoking, coronary artery disease and, 310–311, 313
  theophylline and, 426–427
Circ-O-Lectric turning frame, 292–293
Cisapride, for constipation, 337
Clarke's column, 7
Claudication, spinal cord, atherosclerotic, 73
Clean intermittent self-catheterization, 226–227, 240–241
  drug therapy with, 228
Cleveland upper extremity neuroprosthesis, 385–387, *386*
Clonidine, for spasticity, 372–373
Clotting disorders. See *Coagulopathy*.
Clozapine, for psychotic disorders, 412t
Coagulopathy, ischemic myelopathy and, 77
  venous thrombosis and, 302
Coarctation of aorta, repair of, ischemic complications in, 74–75
Cobalamin, malabsorption of, in subacute combined degeneration of spinal cord, 96
Coccidioidomycosis, 57
Coccygeal nerve, *122*
Cock robin position, 104
Cockcroft-Gault equation, 308
Colon. See also under *Anal; Bowel; Colorectal; Rectal; Rectum*.
  acute inflammatory conditions of, 339–340
  cancer of, 341
  innervation of, 332
  obstruction of, 341
    fecal impaction and, 335–339, 341
  structure and function of, 332, 333

Colonic motility, alterations in, 334
  stimulation of, Brindley stimulator for, 337
  prokinetic agents for, 337
Colonoscopy, in cancer diagnosis, 341
  in fecal impaction, 335
Color Doppler ultrasonography, in venous thrombosis diagnosis, 302
Colorectal cancer, 341
Colorectal compliance, alterations in, 334
Colorectal emergencies, 339–340
Colorectal physiology, in spinal cord disorders, 333–342
  normal, 332–333
Colostomy, for neurogenic bowel, 338–339
Commissural myelotomy, for pain, 22
Complete cord syndrome, 140–141, *141*
Compound muscle action potentials (CMAPs), in cervical myelopathy/spondylosis, 155–156
Compression neuropathies, in spinal cord injury, 148
Compressive myelopathy, 317–329
  AIDS-related, 97
  causes of, 91, 318t
  clinical presentation of, 318–319
  differential diagnosis of, 317
  disk protrusion and, 62
  epidural abscess and, 328–329
  in cervical spondylosis, 64, 86–88, 319–322
  in spondylosis deformans, 62, 64, 88
  ligamentum flavum compression and, 320
  motor disturbances in, 318
  neck hyperextension and, 320
  pain in, 318
  schistosomiasis and, 50, 70–71, 91
  sensory disturbances in, 319
  traumatic. See *Spinal cord injury*.
  tumors and, 61, *61*, 62, 90–91. See also *Metastatic epidural spinal cord compression*.
    magnetic resonance imaging in, 180–186, *180–186*
  vs. paraneoplastic myelopathy, 90
Computed tomography (CT), in cervical radiculopathy, 190
  in cervical spondylosis, 321
  in degenerative disk disease, 188–189
  in ischemic myelopathy, 78
  in multiple sclerosis, *190*, 190–191
  in spinal cord injury, in initial evaluation, 117
  limitations of, 178, *179*
  renal, 217
Conal lesions, bladder management in, 140, 242
Conditioning, for disabled patients, 278
Condom catheter, 227
  urinary tract infection and, 238
Confusional states, 411
Congenital malformations, magnetic resonance imaging of, 193–195, *194–196*
  pathologic findings in, 48–51
Conservation-withdrawal, 406
Constipation, 335–339
  assessment in, 338–339
  bowel regimen for, 338–339
  colostomy for, 338–339
  evaluation of, 335–336
  fecal impaction and, 335–339, 341
  in acute inflammatory gastrointestinal conditions, 339
  prokinetic agents for, 338–339
Continent augmentation, 236–238, *237*
Continent urinary diversion, *235*, 235–236
Contraction. See *Muscle contraction*.

ISBN 0-7216-5447-9